Anesthesiology

MW01154588

Linda S. Aglio · Richard D. Urman
Editors

Anesthesiology

Clinical Case Reviews

Springer

Editors
Linda S. Aglio, MD, MS
Associate Professor of Anesthesia
Harvard Medical School
Director of Neuroanesthesia
Clinical Director of Operating Room Suites
Brigham and Women's Hospital
Boston, MA
USA

Richard D. Urman, MD, MBA
Associate Professor of Anesthesia
Harvard Medical School
Director, Center for Perioperative Research
Brigham and Women's Hospital
Boston, MA
USA

ISBN 978-3-319-50139-0 ISBN 978-3-319-50141-3 (eBook)
DOI 10.1007/978-3-319-50141-3

Library of Congress Control Number: 2016959180

© Springer International Publishing AG 2017
This work is subject to copyright. All rights are reserved by the Publisher, whether the whole or part of the material is concerned, specifically the rights of translation, reprinting, reuse of illustrations, recitation, broadcasting, reproduction on microfilms or in any other physical way, and transmission or information storage and retrieval, electronic adaptation, computer software, or by similar or dissimilar methodology now known or hereafter developed.
The use of general descriptive names, registered names, trademarks, service marks, etc. in this publication does not imply, even in the absence of a specific statement, that such names are exempt from the relevant protective laws and regulations and therefore free for general use.
The publisher, the authors and the editors are safe to assume that the advice and information in this book are believed to be true and accurate at the date of publication. Neither the publisher nor the authors or the editors give a warranty, express or implied, with respect to the material contained herein or for any errors or omissions that may have been made.

Printed on acid-free paper

This Springer imprint is published by Springer Nature
The registered company is Springer International Publishing AG
The registered company address is: Gewerbestrasse 11, 6330 Cham, Switzerland

Preface

For several years, we have felt the necessity for a concise, readable but comprehensive clinical review book. Such a book should be easy to read and provide sound practical advice for both trainees and practitioners.

Our intention was to develop updated, concise, and easy-to-read content that is designed to be read by trainees preparing for anesthesiology examinations and to serve as a succinct and practical reference for more experienced practitioners.

We are grateful to all who have helped in this important endeavor. There is an advantage in having a multi-authored text, as our contributors have significant expertise in the topics they discuss in our book. Also, they have been generous in permitting the section and book editors to undertake revision of the manuscript in an attempt to achieve conformity and accuracy. Many authors are from the Boston area teaching hospitals, but overall are drawn from institutions nationwide. We believe this provides a broad perspective in the field of anesthesiology. The book contains 12 parts and 60 chapters. Each part is specialty-specific, with chapters devoted to the most important clinical scenarios found in the practice of anesthesia.

The editors wish to express their gratitude to Ms. Marcia Rosen for providing valuable editorial assistance. Likewise, the editors appreciate the support of Springer Publishers in the preparation of this book, and our families for encouragement. We hope this book will prove to be a valuable resource that will enrich the libraries of our readers and help promote clinical excellence for our patients.

Boston, MA, USA

Linda S. Aglio, MD, MS
Richard D. Urman, MD, MBA

Contents

Part I Cardiovascular System
Section Editors: Jill Lanahan and Martin Zammert

1 **Coronary Artery Disease** 3
Suzana M. Zorca and K. Annette Mizuguchi

2 **Myocardial Infarction** 13
Hanjo Ko

3 **Heart Failure** 19
Dirk J. Varelmann

4 **Hypothermia** 29
Dirk J. Varelmann

5 **Anesthetic Considerations in Patients with Valvular Heart Disease** 33
Heather L. Lander and Martin Zammert

6 **Mitral Stenosis** 37
Agnieszka Trzcinka

7 **Eisenmenger Syndrome** 41
Marilyn Diane Michelow

8 **Subacute Bacterial Endocarditis Prophylaxis** 47
Marilyn Diane Michelow

9 **Hypertrophic Cardiomyopathy (HCM)** 49
Pingping Song

10 **Pacemakers and Implantable Cardioverter Defibrillators** 55
Ciorsti J. MacIntyre

11 **Pericardial Tamponade** 61
Kate Mitchell Liberman

12 **Non-cardiac Surgery After Heart Transplantation** 67
Elliott Woodward

13 **Anesthesia for Coronary Artery Bypass Graft (CABG)** 73
Jamahal Luxford and Levi Bassin

Part II The Respiratory System
Section Editor: Ju-Mei Ng

14 **One-Lung Ventilation** 89
Thomas Hickey

Part III The Central Nervous System
Section Editor: Leslie C. Jameson

15 Anesthesia Management for Posterior Fossa Craniotomy 97
Mihaela Podovei and Lisa Crossley

16 Intracranial Aneurysm 103
Penny P. Liu

17 Carotid Endarterectomy 113
Reza Gorji and Lu'ay Nubani

18 Spine Surgery and Intraoperative Monitoring 121
Fenghua Li and Reza Gorji

19 Transsphenoidal Hypophysectomy 133
Saraswathy Shekar

Part IV The Neuromuscular System
Section Editor: Zhiling Xiong

20 Depolarizing Neuromuscular Blocking Agents 143
Caroline S. Gross and Zhiling Xiong

21 Nondepolarizing Neuromuscular Blocking Agents 149
Erin Bettendorf and Zhiling Xiong

22 Myasthenia Gravis 155
Huan Wang and Zhiling Xiong

23 Malignant Hyperthermia 161
Milad Sharifpour and Raheel Bengali

Part V The Endocrine System
Section Editor: Sibinka Bajic

24 Diabetes Mellitus 167
Amit Prabhakar, Jonathan G. Ma, Anthony Woodall, and Alan D. Kaye

25 Thyrotoxicosis 175
Mark R. Jones, Rachel J. Kaye, and Alan D. Kaye

26 Pheochromocytoma 183
Julie A. Gayle, Ryan Rubin, and Alan D. Kaye

Part VI The Abdomen
Section Editor: Michael T. Bailin

27 The Full Stomach 193
Scott Switzer and Derek Rosner

28 Anesthesia for Liver Transplantation 199
John Stenglein

29 Anesthesia for Open Repair of Abdominal Aortic Aneurysm 215
Stefan Alexandrov Ianchulev

30 Anesthesia for Endovascular Aortic Aneurysm Repair (EVAR) 227
Stefan Anexandrov Ianchulev

31 **Morbid Obesity** 237
John Stenglein

32 **Laparoscopy** 247
Carmelita W. Pisano

33 **Carcinoid Disease** 255
Tara C. Carey

34 **Kidney Transplantation** 263
Jonathan Ross

Part VII Eye, Ear, and Throat Surgery
Section Editor: Dennis J. McNicholl

35 **Open Eye Injury** 273
Alvaro Andres Macias

36 **Anesthesia for Tympanomastoidectomy** 281
Martha R. Cordoba Amorocho

37 **The Difficult Airway** 287
Dennis J. McNicholl

38 **Pediatric Tonsillectomy and Adenoidectomy** 297
Makara E. Cayer

39 **Laser Surgery of the Airway** 305
Dongdong Yao

Part VIII Blood/Hematologic System
Section Editor: Charles P. Plant

40 **Transfusion Reactions** 315
Charles P. Plant and Jonathan H. Kroll

41 **Intraoperative Coagulopathies** 319
Alimorad G. Djalali and Anil K. Panigrahi

42 **Hemophilia** 327
Shamsuddin Akhtar

43 **Sickle Cell Disease: Anesthetic Management** 333
Gustavo A. Lozada

Part IX Orthopedic Surgery
Section Editor: Kamen Vlassakov

44 **Total Hip Replacement** 341
Vijay Patel, Kamen Vlassakov, and David R. Janfaza

45 **Local Anesthetics** 347
Cyrus A. Yazdi

46 **Spinal Anesthesia** 357
Benjamin Kloesel and Galina Davidyuk

47 **Brachial Plexus Block** 367
Nantthasorn Zinboonyahgoon and Kamen Vlassakov

Part X Obstetrics
Section Editor: Jie Zhou

48 Labor and Delivery 379
Vesela Kovacheva

49 Preeclampsia 385
Dan Drzymalski

50 Abruptio Placenta and Placenta Previa 389
Annemaria De Tina and Jie Zhou

51 Nonobstetric Surgery During Pregnancy 395
Jeffrey Huang

Part XI Pediatrics
Section Editors: Craig D. McClain and and Kai Matthes

52 Neonatal Resuscitation 407
Jonathan R. Meserve and Monica E. Kleinman

53 Gastroschisis and Omphalocele 415
Laura Downey

54 Congenital Diaphragmatic Hernia 421
Bridget L. Muldowney and Elizabeth C. Eastburn

55 Pyloric Stenosis 427
Hyun Kee Chung

56 Tracheoesophageal Fistula 435
Herodotos Ellinas

57 Congenital Heart Disease: Atrioventricular Septal Defects 441
Viviane G. Nasr and Annette Y. Schure

58 Premature Infant 449
Lisa M. Hammond

Part XII Critical Care
Section Editor: Suzanne Klainer

59 Trauma Anesthesia 459
Kevin Handy

60 Burns 465
Sara E. Neves

Index 475

Contributors

Shamsuddin Akhtar, MD Department of Anesthesiology and Pharmacology, Yale University School of Medicine, New Haven, CT, USA

K. Annette Mizuguchi, MD, PhD, MMSc Department of Anesthesiology, Perioperative and Pain Medicine, Harvard Medical School, Brigham and Women's Hospital, Boston, MA, USA

Michael T. Bailin, MD Department of Anesthesiology, Baystate Health, Springfield, MA, USA

Sibinka Bajic, MD, PhD Department of Anesthesiology, Perioperative and Pain Medicine, Brigham and Women's Hospital, Boston, MA, USA

Levi Bassin, MBBS, PhD, FRACS Cardiac Surgery, Brigham and Women's Hospital, Boston, MA, USA

Raheel Bengali, MD Department of Anesthesiology, Perioperative and Pain Medicine, Brigham and Women's Hospital, Boston, MA, USA

Erin Bettendorf MD Department of Anesthesiology, Perioperative and Pain Medicine, Brigham and Women's Hospital, Boston, MA, USA

Tara C. Carey, MD Department of Anesthesiology, Perioperative, and Pain Medicine, Harvard Medical School, Brigham and Women's Hospital, Boston, MA, USA

Makara E. Cayer, MD Department of Anesthesiology, Massachusetts Eye and Ear Infirmary, Boston, MA, USA

Hyun Kee Chung, MD Division of Pediatric Anesthesia, Department of Anesthesiology and Perioperative Medicine, University of Massachusetts Medical School, Worcester, MA, USA

Martha R. Cordoba Amorocho, MD Department of Anesthesiology, Perioperative and Pain Medicine, Brigham and Women's Hospital, Boston, MA, USA

Lisa Crossley, MD Department of Anesthesiology, Perioperative and Pain Medicine, Harvard Medical School, Brigham and Women's Hospital, Boston, MA, USA

Galina Davidyuk, MD, PhD Department of Anesthesiology and Perioperative Pain Medicine, Brigham and Women's Hospital, Boston, MA, USA

Annemaria De Tina, MD, FRCPC Department of Anesthesiology, Perioperative and Pain Medicine, Harvard Medical School, Brigham and Women's Hospital, Boston, MA, USA

Alimorad G. Djalali, MD, PhD Department of Anesthesiology, Perioperative, and Pain Medicine, Stanford University Medical Center, Stanford, CA, USA

Laura Downey, MD Pediatric Cardiac Anesthesiology, Emory University, Atlanta, GA, USA

Dan Drzymalski, MD Department of Anesthesiology, Perioperative and Pain Medicine, Brigham and Women's Hospital, Boston, MA, USA

Elizabeth C. Eastburn, DO Department of Anesthesiology, Perioperative and Pain Medicine, Boston Children's Hospital, Boston, MA, USA

Herodotos Ellinas, MD Department of Anesthesiology, Children's Hospital of Wisconsin, Medical College of Wisconsin, Milwaukee, WI, USA

Julie A. Gayle, MD Department of Anesthesiology, Louisiana State University School of Medicine, New Orleans, LA, USA

Reza Gorji, MD Department of Anesthesiology, SUNY Upstate Medical University, Syracuse, NY, USA

Caroline S. Gross, MD Department of Anesthesiology, Perioperative and Pain Medicine, Brigham and Women's Hospital, Boston, MA, USA

Lisa M. Hammond, MD Department of Anesthesia, Harvard Medical School, Clinical Instructor, Boston Children's Hospital, Boston, MA, USA

Kevin Handy, MD, MS Department of Anesthesia, Critical Care and Pain Medicine, Massachusetts General Hospital, Boston, MA, USA

Thomas Hickey, MD, MS Department of Anesthesiology, VA Connecticut Healthcare System, Yale University School of Medicine, West Haven, CT, USA

Jeffrey Huang, MD Department of Anesthesiology, Anesthesiologists of Greater Orlando & University of Central Florida, Maitland, FL, USA

Jill Lanahan, MD Department of Anesthesiology, Perioperative and Pain Medicine, Harvard Medical School, Brigham and Women's Hospital, Boston, MA, USA

Stefan Alexandrov Ianchulev, MD Department of Anesthesiology, Tufts Medical Center, Boston, MA, USA

Leslie C. Jameson, MD Department of Anesthesiology, University of Colorado, Aurora, CO, USA

David R. Janfaza, MD Department of Anesthesiology, Perioperative and Pain Medicine, Brigham and Women's Hospital, Boston, MA, USA

Mark R. Jones, BA Beth Israel Deaconess Medical Center, Harvard Medical School, Resident in Anesthesiology, Boston, MA, USA

Alan D. Kaye, MD, PhD, DABA, DABPM, DABIPP Department of Anesthesiology, Louisiana State University School of Medicine, New Orleans, LA, USA

Rachel J. Kaye, MD Bowdoin College, Brunswick, ME, USA

Suzanne Klainer, MD Department of Anesthesiology, Perioperative and Pain Medicine, Brigham and Women's Hospital, Boston, MA, USA

Monica E. Kleinman, MD Department of Anesthesiology, Perioperative and Pain Medicine, Boston Children's Hospital, Boston, MA, USA

Benjamin Kloesel, MD, MSBS Department of Anesthesiology, Perioperative and Pain Medicine, Boston Children's Hospital, Boston, MA, USA

Hanjo Ko, MD Department of Anesthesiology, Perioperative and Pain Medicine, Brigham and Women's Hospital, Philadelphia, PA, USA

Vesela Kovacheva, MD, PhD Department of Anesthesiology, Perioperative and Pain Medicine, Harvard Medical School, Brigham and Women's Hospital, Boston, MA, USA

Jonathan H. Kroll, MD Department of Medicine, MedStar Union Memorial Hospital 201 E University Parkway, Baltimore, MD, USA

Heather L. Lander, MD Department of Anesthesiology, Perioperative and Pain Medicine, Brigham and Women's Hospital, Boston, MA, USA

Fenghua Li, MD Department of Anesthesiology, SUNY Upstate Medical University, Syracuse, NY, USA

Kate Mitchell Liberman, MD Department of Anesthesiology, Perioperative and Pain Medicine, Brigham and Women's Hospital, Boston, MA, USA

Penny P. Liu, MD Department of Anesthesiology, Tufts Medical Center, Boston, MA, USA

Gustavo A. Lozada, MD Department of Anesthesiology, Tufts Medical Center, Boston, MA, USA

Jamahal Luxford, MBBS, FANZCA Department of Anesthesiology, Perioperative and Pain Medicine, Brigham and Women's Hospital, Boston, MA, USA

Jonathan G. Ma, BS, MD Louisiana State University Health and Sciences Center, New Orleans, LA, USA

Alvaro Andres Macias, MD Department of Anesthesiology, Perioperative and Pain Medicine, Brigham and Women's Hospital/Massachusetts Eye and Ear, Boston, MA, USA

Ciorsti J. MacIntyre, MD Arrhythmia Service, Harvard School of Medicine, Brigham and Women's Hospital, Boston, MA, USA

Kai Matthes, MD, PhD Division of Gastroenterology, Department of Anesthesiology, Perioperative and Pain Medicine, Boston Children's Hospital, Harvard Medical School, Boston, MA, USA

Craig D. McClain, MD, MPH Department of Anesthesiology, Perioperative and Pain Medicine, Boston Children's Hospital, Boston, MA, USA; Harvard Medical School, Boston, MA, USA

Dennis J. McNicholl, DO Department of Anesthesiology, Perioperative and Pain Medicine, Brigham and Women's Hospital, Boston, MA, USA

Jonathan R. Meserve, MD Department of Anesthesiology, Perioperative and Pain Medicine, Boston Children's Hospital, Boston, MA, USA

Marilyn Diane Michelow, MD Department of Anesthesiology, Perioperative and Pain Medicine, Brigham and Women's Hospital, Boston, MA, USA

Bridget L. Muldowney, MD Department of Anesthesiology, University of Wisconsin School of Medicine and Public Health, Madison, WI, USA

Viviane G. Nasr, MD Division of Cardiac Anesthesia, Department of Anesthesiology, Perioperative and Pain Medicine, Harvard Medical School, Boston Children's Hospital, Boston, MA, USA

Sara E. Neves, MD Department of Anesthesia, Critical Care and Pain Medicine, Beth Israel Deaconess Medical Center, Cambridge, MA, USA

Ju-Mei Ng, FANZCA Department of Anesthesia, Perioperative and Pain Medicine, Brigham and Women's Hospital, Boston, MA, USA

Lu'ay Nubani, MD Department of Anesthesiology, University Hospital, Syracuse, NY, USA

Anil K. Panigrahi, MD, PhD Department of Anesthesiology, Perioperative, and Pain Medicine, Stanford University Medical Center, Stanford, CA, USA

Vijay Patel, MD Department of Anesthesiology, Lenox Hill Hospital, New York, NY, USA

Carmelita W. Pisano, MD Department of Anesthesiology, Perioperative and Pain Medicine, Brigham and Women's Hospital, Boston, MA, USA

Charles P. Plant, MD, PhD Department of Anesthesia, Tufts Medical Center, Boston, MA, USA

Mihaela Podovei, MD Department of Anesthesiology, Perioperative and Pain Medicine, Harvard Medical School, Brigham and Women's Hospital, Boston, MA, USA

Amit Prabhakar, MD, MS Department of Anesthesiology, University Medical Center, New Orleans, LA, USA

Derek Rosner, DO Department of Anesthesiology, Baystate Medical Center, Springfield, MA, USA

Jonathan Ross, MD, PhD Department of Anesthesia, Baystate Medical Center, Springfield, MA, USA

Ryan Rubin, MD, MPH Department of Anesthesiology, Louisiana State University School of Medicine, New Orleans, LA, USA

Annette Y. Schure, MD Division of Cardiac Anesthesia, Department of Anesthesiology, Perioperative and Pain Medicine, Harvard Medical School, Boston Children's Hospital, Boston, MA, USA

Milad Sharifpour, MD, MS Department of Anesthesia, Critical Care, and Pain Medicine, Massachusetts General Hospital, Boston, MA, USA

Saraswathy Shekar, MB, BS, FFARCS(I) UMass Medical Center, University of Massachusetts Medical School, Worcester, MA, USA

Pingping Song, MD Department of Anesthesiology, Perioperative and Pain Medicine, Brigham and Women's Hospital, Boston, MA, USA

John Stenglein, MD Department of Anesthesiology, Baystate Medical Center, Tufts University School of Medicine, Springfield, MA, USA

Scott Switzer, DO Department of Anesthesiology, Baystate Medical Center, Springfield, MA, USA

Agnieszka Trzcinka, MD Department of Anesthesiology, Perioperative and Pain Medicine, Harvard Medical School, Brigham and Women's Hospital, Boston, MA, USA

Dirk J. Varelmann, MD, DESA, EDIC Department of Anesthesiology, Perioperative and Pain Medicine, Harvard Medical School, Brigham and Women's Hospital, Boston, MA, USA

Kamen Vlassakov, MD Department of Anesthesiology, Perioperative and Pain Medicine, Brigham and Women's Hospital, Boston, MA, USA

Huan Wang, MD Department of Anesthesiology, Perioperative and Pain Medicine, Brigham and Women's Hospital, Boston, MA, USA

Anthony Woodall, MD Department of Anesthesiology, Louisiana State Hospital, New Orleans, LA, USA

Elliott Woodward, MB, Bch BAO, MSc Department of Anesthesiology, Perioperative and Pain Medicine, Brigham and Women's Hospital, Boston, MA, USA

Zhiling Xiong, MD, PhD Department of Anesthesiology, Perioperative and Pain Medicine, Brigham and Women's Hospital, Boston, MA, USA

Dongdong Yao, MD, PhD Department of Anesthesiology, Perioperative and Pain Medicine, Brigham and Women's Hospital, Boston, MA, USA

Cyrus A. Yazdi, MD Department of Anesthesiology/Pain Medicine, UMass Memorial Medical Center, Worcester, MA, USA

Martin Zammert, MD Department of Anesthesia, Perioperative and Pain Medicine, Brigham and Women's Hospital, Boston, MA, USA

Jie Zhou, MD, MS, MBA Department of Anesthesiology, Perioperative and Pain Medicine, Harvard Medical School, Brigham and Women's Hospital, Boston, MA, USA

Nantthasorn Zinboonyahgoon, MD Department of Anesthesiology, Siriraj Hospital, Bangkok, Thailand

Suzana M. Zorca, MD Department of Anesthesiology, Perioperative and Pain Medicine, VABHS, Massachusetts General Hospital, West Roxbury, MA, USA

Part I

Cardiovascular System

Section Editors: Jill Lanahan and Martin Zammert

Jill Lanahan
Department of Anesthesiology, Perioperative and Pain Medicine, Harvard Medical School, Brigham and Women's Hospital, Boston, MA, USA

Martin Zammert
Department of Anesthesia, Perioperative and Pain Medicine, Brigham and Women's Hospital, Boston, MA, USA

1 Coronary Artery Disease

Suzana M. Zorca and K. Annette Mizuguchi

Clinical Vignette

A 64-year-old man with a past medical history relevant for hypertension, dyslipidemia, 3-vessel coronary artery disease (70% right coronary artery, 50% left main, 75% left circumflex artery stenosis), nicotine dependence, and pancytopenia secondary to myelodysplastic syndrome presents with acute abdominal pain, vomiting, and obstipation. Imaging studies reveal an incarcerated hernia. He is brought to the operating room for emergent laparoscopy.

During abdominal insufflation, ST depressions are seen in leads II, III, and aVF and the patient becomes acutely bradycardic and hypotensive. The ST depressions improve after transient exsufflation, initiation of norepinephrine infusion, as well as red blood cell (RBC) transfusion for a hematocrit of 20. However, postoperatively, the patient experiences angina accompanied by recurrence of inferior lead depressions and 2nd degree AV block. A high-sensitivity troponin is positive for myocardial injury.

Past Medical History
Hypertension
Hyperlipidemia
Chronic stable CAD, with a positive stress test 2 years ago (mild inferolateral perfusion defect on stress MIBI) and a coronary angiogram revealing 3-vessel coronary artery disease as above.
EF 65% with moderate LVH, mild MR/TR
Myelodysplastic syndrome without excess blasts, complicated by pancytopenia requiring RBC transfusions every other month
Gastroesophageal reflux disease
Depression/PTSD
Benign prostatic hypertrophy
Nicotine dependence, 45-pack-year smoking history, transitioned to the nicotine patch 3 weeks ago.

Outpatient medications	
Aspirin	81 mg EC daily
Atenolol	50 mg daily
Hydrochlorothiazide/Triamterene	25/37.5 mg daily
Lisinopril	20 mg daily
Simvastatin	20 mg daily
Sertraline	50 mg daily
Tamsulosin	0.4 mg daily
Famotidine	20 mg daily
Folic acid	1 mg daily
Ferrous Sulfate	325 mg three times daily
Nicotine	21 mg/24 h patch
Allergies	Penicillin (rash)
Physical Exam (ED)	Vitals: HR 78, BP 184/91, RR 18-22, SpO2 98% on RA
Airway exam	Mallampati II, thyromental distance >3 finger breadths, good mouth opening, slight limitation to neck extension, edentulous with removable upper and lower dental plates

S.M. Zorca (✉)
Department of Anesthesiology, Perioperative and Pain Medicine, VABHS, Massachusetts General Hospital, 1400 VFW Parkway, West Roxbury, MA 02132, USA
e-mail: szorca@gmail.com

K. Annette Mizuguchi
Department of Anesthesiology, Perioperative and Pain Medicine, Harvard Medical School, Brigham and Women's Hospital, 75 Francis Street, Boston, MA 02115, USA
e-mail: amizuguchi@gmail.com

© Springer International Publishing AG 2017
L.S. Aglio and R.D. Urman (eds.), *Anesthesiology*,
DOI 10.1007/978-3-319-50141-3_1

General	Cooperative, alert, but uncomfortable and slightly dyspneic
Cardiopulmonary	RRR, no murmurs, rubs or gallops, CTAB
Abdominal	Soft but tender and tense to palpation, with guarding and tap tenderness in left lower quadrant
EKG	Sinus rhythm at 78 bpm, normal axis, QTc 418 ms, meeting LVH criteria, small Q-wave in lead III, J-point elevation V2–V3 with inverted T-waves in V1–V2

Discussion Questions

1. **What is Coronary Artery Disease (CAD)?**

Coronary artery disease (CAD) is defined as the progressive, pathological development of atherosclerotic plaque within the lumen and walls of the coronary vasculature. CAD results in compromised supply of blood to the myocardium, and can gradually or suddenly result in regional myocardial ischemia and infarction. Although previously understood as a slowly progressive lipid storage disorder, CAD is now viewed as a complex interplay between advancing atherogenesis, inflammation, endothelial cell dysfunction, collagen synthesis defects, fibrous plaque thinning, plaque rupture, and immune cell dysfunction [1–4]. Globally, the high prevalence of CAD is associated with extensive morbidity and high health care costs. Chronic CAD can manifest acutely with exacerbations known as acute coronary syndromes (ACS), and it remains the leading cause of death in the developed world.

2. **Define the anatomy of the coronary vasculature.**

The **left main coronary artery** and right coronary artery (RCA) arise from the aortic root, just above the left and right aortic coronary cusps (Fig. 1.1). The left main coronary artery (L main) branches early to form the **left anterior descending artery** (LAD), which courses anteriorly over the left ventricle and interventricular septum, and the **left circumflex artery** (LCx), which travels laterally and posteriorly in the atrioventricular groove.

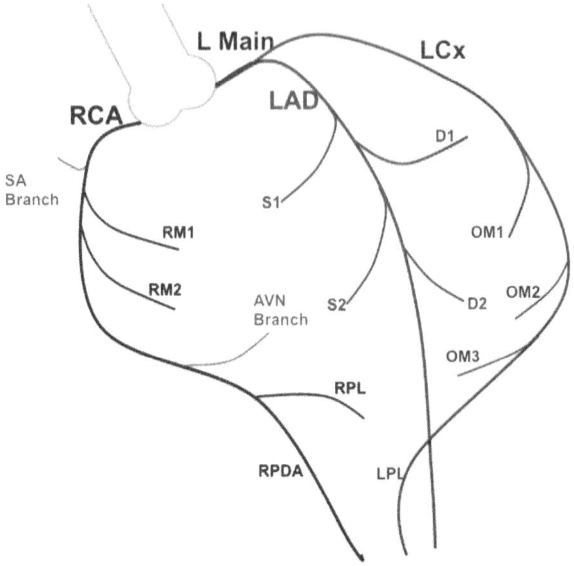

Fig. 1.1 Schematic of normal (right-dominant) coronary artery anatomy. Abbreviations: Left main coronary artery (L Main), right coronary artery (RCA), left anterior descending artery (LAD), left circumflex artery (LCx), septal (S) and diagonal (D) branches of the LAD, obtuse marginal branches (OM) of the LCx, marginal branches of RCA (RM), branch to SA node (SA branch), branch supplying AV node (AVN branch), right posterior descending artery (RPDA), right posterolateral artery (RPL), and left posterolateral branch (LPL)

Primary branches of the LAD include septal perforators (S1, S2, etc.), which supply the interventricular septum, and the diagonal branches (D1, D2, etc.) that supply the anterior LV wall. The primary branches of the LCx are called obtuse marginals (OM1, OM2) and distal posterolateral branches (LPL).

The **right coronary artery** (RCA) travels laterally in the right atrioventricular groove, giving off marginal branches to supply the more anterior portion of the RV free wall (RM1, RM2, etc.) and lateral branches, such as the right posterior lateral (RPL) artery to supply the lateral free wall.

The RCA generally also supplies the **SA node and AV node**, and thus plays a key role in perfusing the conduction system of the heart. In the majority of patients (85%), the distal RCA turns into the **posterior descending artery** (RPDA), which supplies the inferior free wall and posterior interventricular septum. The RCA also gives off AV nodal arteries, resulting in a pattern of coronary anatomy termed "right **coronary dominance**."

The left circumflex artery supplies the PDA (left PDA or LPDA) as well as the AV node in only 7% of patients (termed "left dominant" circulation), whereas 8% of patients receive dual blood supply and are termed "co-dominant" or "non-dominant" [5, 6]. Although the clinical significance of coronary dominance is not established, several studies have demonstrated that patients with left dominant or co-dominant circulation have worse outcomes after an acute coronary event [7, 8].

3. **Describe the perfusion of the cardiac conduction system**.

The **SA node** is nearly always supplied (exclusively or primarily) by the RCA. In 70% of patients, the RCA alone perfuses the SA node. In approximately 25% of persons, the LCx contributes blood flow to the SA node, but only in a small minority of patients is the primary blood supply to the SA node from the LCx artery alone. Ischemia to the SA node, therefore, is generally caused by very proximal RCA lesions that result in loss of sinus automaticity. Typically this results in a junctional escape rhythm characterized by bradycardia and the absence of anterograde p-waves [9, 10].

The **AV node** is supplied primarily by the RCA in 85% of the population. In patients with left or co-dominant coronary anatomy, the AV node may be supplied by both the RCA and the left circumflex (8% of persons) or entirely by the left circumflex artery (7%). Ischemia to the AV node leads to atrioventricular block. This can manifest as a prolongation of the PR interval (1st degree AV block), progressive prolongation of PR interval (Type I 1st degree AV block), or complete loss of conduction via the AV node (complete heart block). It is more common for type II 1st degree AV block, high-grade AV block, and complete heart block to result from loss of perfusion to the proximal bundle of His, which is generally supplied by the same vasculature as the AV node itself [6, 9].

The **distal bundle of His and proximal Purkinje network** are contained within the interventricular septum, which is supplied anteriorly by the LAD and posteriorly by the PDA. Loss of the PDA rarely causes significant cardiac conduction disease, however. Lesions in the LAD or its septal perforators can result in new left bundle branch block through ischemia to these conduction elements.

4. **Describe the expected patterns of injury due to ischemia or infarction in each coronary territory**.

Ischemia to a vascular territory resulting from a non-occlusive lesion can lead to subendocardial injury or infarction. Mild ischemia often results in impaired relaxation (i.e., ventricular stiffening), followed by impaired contraction (**hypokinesis**). Infarction, generally resulting from complete occlusion of the blood supply to a territory, can manifest as loss of contraction (**akinesis**), or even systolic bulging (**dyskinesis**) of the affected segment.

The **left anterior descending artery** (LAD) supplies the anterior 2/3 of the interventricular septum and the LV anterior wall in its entirety (Fig. 1.2). Severe ischemia in this territory often results in marked reduction in ejection fraction and septal dyskinesis. Infarction of this territory can also result in significant left bundle branch block. ECG changes generally occur in the anterior precordial leads (V2–V4) [9].

The **left circumflex artery** (LCx) supplies the lateral wall of the left ventricle. Ischemia or infarction in this territory results in ischemic changes in the lateral ECG leads, including I, aVL, V5, and V6, with evidence of reduced contraction of the lateral wall on echocardiography. In patients with a left dominant circulation, LCx infarction will also result in inferior ischemia due to loss of the left PDA perfusion supply.

The **right coronary artery** (RCA) gives rise to the PDA in right-dominant circulations, so distal RCA ischemia results in loss of blood supply to the LV inferior wall. Severe ischemia can cause dysfunction or infarction of the posterior papillary muscle, which can lead to acute severe mitral regurgitation.

In contrast, the anterior papillary muscle typically benefits from a dual blood supply and is less likely to become dysfunctional. The more proximal RCA also supplies the RV and usually supplies the proximal conduction system of the heart. Acute ischemia to these territories can lead to arrhythmias (see Question 3) and also to acute shock due to sudden hypokinesis of the RV. If supported through the first few hours after ischemic injury, persons with isolated RV infarcts generally recover RV function because of collateral

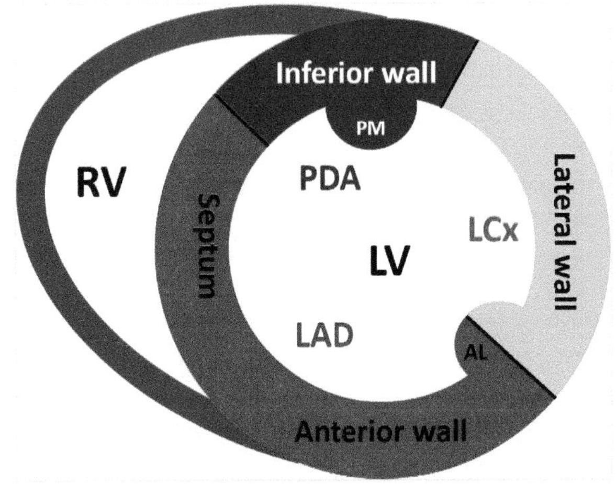

Fig. 1.2 Schematic of normal coronary perfusion. Abbreviations: Left ventricle (LV), right ventricle (RV), left anterior descending artery (LAD, red), right coronary artery (RCA, blue), left circumflex artery (LCx, green), anterolateral papillary muscle (AL), posteromedial papillary muscle (PM)

blood flow and decreased oxygen requirements of the RV compared to LV myocardium.

5. **What are the major established risk factors for coronary artery disease?**

The literature supports the following major risk factors for CAD: hypertension, dyslipidemia, advanced age, gender (with male gender conferring higher risk), a positive family history of premature atherosclerosis manifesting with acute coronary events and early CAD, diabetes mellitus (DM), and smoking. In addition, chronic inflammatory comorbidities also pose a risk for early CAD. A lipid-rich/pro-inflammatory diet and a sedentary lifestyle and lack of exercise also predispose to CAD, constituting modifiable risk predictors. In women, unique additional predictors for cardiovascular disease also include hypertensive disorders of pregnancy as well as migraines and polycystic ovarian syndrome [11]. A high HDL cholesterol level (>60 mg/dL) has been shown to be associated with decreased CAD risk [12].

In both men and women, poor glycemic control has been tightly linked to the development of cardiometabolic syndrome, with macrovascular and microvascular complications rising precipitously and in parallel to worsened glucose control. In a multicenter, prospective observational study of 3642 UK patients with type 2 DM, the hazard ratio for MI and heart failure rose linearly in relation to mean hemoglobin A1c concentration. The rates of fatal and non-fatal MI decreased by approximately 14% per 1% A1c reduction, and the rate of clinically manifest heart failure decreased by 16% per 1% reduction in mean HbA1c [13]. Exposure to excess glycemia over time increased the risk of both macro- and microvascular complications.

Furthermore, exercise attenuates the progression of macrovascular CAD by promoting collateralization, increasing myocardial blood flow, and stabilizing and possibly retarding the progression of atherosclerotic lesions [14].

6. **What are the clinical manifestations of chronic coronary artery disease?**

Chronic CAD is typically heralded by a history of angina pectoris, or chest pain worsened by exertion and alleviated by rest. However, coronary artery disease can progress silently for decades prior to manifesting with acute thrombotic exacerbations such as ST segment elevation myocardial infarction (STEMI) or non-ST elevation MI (NSTEMI), arrhythmias, congestive heart failure, and/or death. The global burden of morbidity and mortality due to CAD is enormous and it is estimated that in the United States alone, a myocardial infarction or cardiac death occurs and is reported every 34 s [14].

New understandings into the mechanism of chronic stable CAD, and its acute manifestations, have emerged in recent years. In particular, the old paradigm of progressive coronary artery luminal narrowing predisposing to sudden flow strangulation at the site of critical stenosis has been challenged. Rather, coronary artery plaque formation does not simply narrow the vessel lumen early on in the disease process; outward vessel wall expansion compensates instead for diffuse plaque deposition and results in a continued and ongoing inflammatory process. This process remodels the coronary arterial walls and involves the coronary tree diffusely. Supporting evidence includes the observation that plaque rupture and the resulting inflammatory cascade often occur at sites of non-critical stenoses. The subsequent infarction occurs in segments of the coronary arterial tree that would not have been easily predicted by angiography [4]. Please see Question 9 for a more detailed description of these new mechanistic insights into CAD progression and triggering of ACS [15, 16].

7. **What are associated extracardiac manifestations of atherosclerotic disease?**

Although chronic CAD progression is typically silent until acute exacerbations manifest as acute coronary syndromes (unstable angina, STEMI, NSTEMI), extracardiac manifestations of chronic atherosclerosis can strongly suggest the presence of CAD. Concomitant comorbidities in at-risk patients often include peripheral arterial disease, such as carotid artery disease predisposing to cerebrovascular events, chronic kidney disease resulting in renal insufficiency, peripheral vascular disease manifesting as claudication, hypertension, and the formation of aortic aneurysms.

8. **What are common perioperative adverse outcomes in patients with atherosclerotic disease? Define MACE.**

Perioperative outcomes seen with disproportionately larger frequency in CAD patients include MI (STEMI/NSTEMI), congestive heart failure, hemodynamically significant arrhythmias, and death. The cardiovascular outcomes literature references **Major Adverse Cardiac Events (MACE)** as primary endpoints of medical and surgical interventions. However, no consensus or standard definition of MACE exists. Rather, MACE consist of composite clinical events that reflect safety and effectiveness of medical or surgical interventions.

In aggregate, most studies include safety endpoints (MI, death, and need for repeat revascularization), as well as effectiveness endpoints as part of MACE. However, individual outcomes comprising MACE vary significantly by study. In a recent study of the heterogeneity and validity of

MACE, the authors highlight the substantial heterogeneity in study-specific individual outcomes used to define MACE. They conclude that this heterogeneity makes inconsistency among study results inevitable. They recommend a focus on safety outcomes, separate from effectiveness outcomes, and avoidance of the combined term MACE [17].

Nevertheless, it is worth noting that the most recent (2014) ACC/AHA guidelines on perioperative cardiovascular evaluation and management of patients undergoing noncardiac surgery utilizes the terminology **MACE, defined as myocardial infarction and death**, to categorize procedures into low-risk profiles (MACE risk <1%, such as for cataract surgery, superficial plastic surgery) and elevated risk profiles (MACE risk >1%) [18]. An intermediate category of 1–5% risk for MACE is no longer part of the current guidelines' dialog [18].

9. **Define the mechanism of chronic stable CAD and its acute thrombotic complications, including STEMI and NSTEMI**.

Chronic stable CAD has long been viewed as a disorder of lipid storage, with modifiable and non-modifiable risk factors predisposing to progressive coronary luminal narrowing to the point of critical occlusion. The resulting high-grade lesions, visible on coronary angiography, were presumed to be the primary site of plaque rupture causing **acute coronary syndromes (ACS)**. Plaque rupture at these sites was known to trigger an inflammatory response that activates platelets, endothelial cells, and immune cells, resulting in acute thrombosis (STEMI, NSTEMI).

The traditional concepts of flow limitation due to critical luminal narrowing have been revolutionized by the understanding that coronary arterial walls dilate to accommodate growing plaques. As a result, coronary vessel wall remodeling occurs early and continuously at sites of obstructive and non-obstructive plaque. An ongoing cycle of inflammation, endothelial injury, platelet activation, collagen cap thinning, with potential for plaque rupture ensues. Thus it is currently thought that the inflammatory cascade associated with coronary arterial remodeling produces diffuse plaque vulnerability in all parts of the coronary arterial tree, not only at sites of critical stenoses [2, 19].

10. **How do the new insights into the pathophysiology of CAD inform modern approaches to treating CAD and its acute thrombotic complications?**

Disruption of atherosclerotic plaques at sites of high-grade stenoses, visible by angiography, may manifest clinically as unstable angina and/or ischemia, and result in perfusion defects. Acute thrombotic complications (STEMI, NSTEMI) following plaque rupture at critical stenoses can be treated with percutaneous transluminal coronary angioplasty (PTCA) and stenting, or surgically with coronary artery bypass grafting (CABG).

Given the extensive and prevalent nature of coronary arterial remodeling, plaque rupture can also occur at sites of non-obstructive CAD. These non-obstructive or non-critical lesions cannot be easily spotted by angiography, stress testing, or other coronary imaging. Non-obstructive plaques vastly outnumber the critical stenoses, and may have larger lipid cores and thinner fibrous caps, making them particularly susceptible to rupture.

Non-stenotic plaques may be clinically silent for many years, but can manifest suddenly with unstable angina or MI when plaque rupture or thrombosis occurs. As a result, lifestyle modification with a balanced healthy diet, exercise, and pharmacotherapy (statin use, beta-blockade) can impact the clinical management of non-obstructive CAD. Lifestyle modifications and pharmacotherapy help stabilize diffuse, vulnerable plaques and increase collateral coronary perfusion. By limiting the expansion of lipid cores, strengthening the collage cap, decreasing the exposure to products of glycoxidation associated with hyperglycemia and pro-inflammatory cytokines generated by excess adipose tissue, lifestyle modifications, and pharmacotherapy help contain the cycle of vessel wall inflammation and arterial remodeling.

11. **Review conventional therapies for stable angina and its acute thrombotic complications**.

Medical therapy with beta-blockers, statins, antiplatelet, and anti-hypertensive agents titrated to optimal blood pressure control remain the mainstay of chronic CAD management. They are used to optimize perfusion and myocardial oxygen demand balance, and to prevent acute thrombotic complications. When acute complications occur, revascularization by means of fibrinolysis, coronary stenting (with bare metal or drug-eluting stents) or surgical revascularization is necessary. Revascularization is attempted emergently in order to minimize the inflammatory thromboembolic cascade associated with myocardial injury.

12. **What are the unique characteristics, etiologies, and mechanisms of perioperative coronary events?**

Cardiac complications represent the most common cause of perioperative morbidity and mortality. Perioperative myocardial infarction differs from typical, non-operative acute coronary syndromes in that demand ischemia (classified as Type 2 MI in the most recent convention) is much more prevalent than Type 1 MI (MI due to plaque rupture or erosion). The expert consensus published in 2012 by the ESC/ACCF/AHA/WHF Task Force for Redefinition of Myocardial Infarction stratified and redefined MI in light of the evolving literature on new biomarkers and interventions [20, 21].

Type 1	Spontaneous MI associated with ischemia due to plaque rupture, erosion, fissuring, or coronary dissection
Type 2	MI secondary to ischemia due to increased oxygen demand or decreased supply, such as results from coronary artery spasm, coronary embolism, anemia, arrhythmias, hypertension, or hypotension

13. **Describe the mechanism of demand ischemia by reviewing the key determinants of myocardial oxygen consumption.**

Demand ischemia occurs when myocardial oxygen demand exceeds myocardial oxygen supply. If uncorrected, it will progress to infarction and subsequent myocardial necrosis. In patients with chronic progressive atherosclerotic narrowing of the coronaries, demand ischemia can manifest with ST changes such as ST depressions, arrhythmias, and AV block.

Key determinants of myocardial oxygen consumption include oxygen supply (dependent on coronary blood flow, hemoglobin concentration, oxygen saturation, oxygen extraction ratio), and the determinants of myocardial oxygen demand (including heart rate, contractility, and wall stress determinants such as preload and afterload).

14. **What are the overarching goals of perioperative cardiac risk stratification?**

The goals of perioperative risk stratification, as outlined in the most recent ACC/AHA guidelines on perioperative cardiovascular evaluation and management of patients undergoing noncardiac surgery, include the following:

1. Identification of patients at risk for perioperative MACE.
2. Adjusting the timing of surgery in order to minimize the risk of MACE.
3. Optimization of long-term medical therapy regardless of the ultimate timing of surgery.

15. **What do the most recent (2014) ACC/AHA guidelines for perioperative risk stratification specify regarding patients preparing for noncardiac surgery?**

The 2014 ACC/AHA guidelines (Table 1.1) for perioperative risk stratification for noncardiac surgery stress that most patients do not require an extensive cardiac work-up prior to elective noncardiac procedures. The guidelines recommend evaluating patients based on patient- and surgery-specific risk factors using the national surgical quality improvement program (NSQIP) risk calculator or the revised cardiac risk index (RCRI) assessment tools. Patients with a low risk of perioperative MACE (<1%) should proceed to surgery without further work-up or risk stratification.

For patients with moderate-to-high risk of MACE (>1%), clinical evaluation for functional capacity is recommended.

Table 1.1 2014 AHA/ACC guidelines: a brief summary

Level of evidence	Guideline recommendations
	Valvular Heart Disease
I-C	Patients with moderate or severe valvular disease should undergo echocardiography within 1 year or if there has been a clinical change
I-C	Valvular intervention before noncardiac surgery is effective in reducing perioperative risk
IIa-B	It is acceptable to perform surgery in patients with asymptomatic severe AS
IIa-C	It is acceptable to perform surgery on patients with asymptomatic severe MR or AR w/preserved EF
IIb-C	It is acceptable to proceed with noncardiac surgery in asymptomatic severe MS patients if the valve anatomy is not favorable to balloon commissurotomy
	ICDs/Pacemakers/Systemic Prostanoid Therapy
I-C	The perioperative team should communicate with the patient's cardiologist, electrophysiologist, or pulmonary hypertension specialist regarding perioperative planning
I-C	Chronic pulmonary vascular-targeted therapy should be continued unless contraindicated
I-C	Cardiac monitoring should be continuous when an ICD has been deactivated, and external defibrillation equipment available. ICD reactivation prior to hospital discharge is recommended
IIa-C	Preoperative evaluation by a pulmonary hypertension expert can be valuable for perioperative patient management of patients with significant pulmonary hypertension

(continued)

Table 1.1 (continued)

Level of evidence	Guideline recommendations
	ECGs and Echocardiography
IIa-B	ECGs are reasonable for patients with known CAD or CHF undergoing non-low risk surgery
IIa-C	It is reasonable for patients with dyspnea of unknown origin or worsening dyspnea and CHF to undergo LV function assessment with echocardiography
IIb-B	It may be helpful for asymptomatic patients undergoing non-low risk surgery to receive preoperative ECGs
IIb-C	Re-evaluation of LV function in stable patients w/CHF may be reasonable if there has been no evaluation in the past year
III-B	Routine preoperative echocardiography evaluation is not recommended
	Perioperative Risk Stratification
IIa-B	Use of a perioperative risk stratification tool to assess MACE risk is recommended
III-B	Patients with a low risk of MACE should not undergo further testing preoperatively
	Exercise and Stress Testing
IIa-B	In patients with elevated MACE risk but excellent functional capacity (>10 METS), no further cardiac testing is recommended prior to surgery
IIa-B	It is reasonable for patients who are at elevated MACE risk and have poor functional capacity (<4 METS) to undergo noninvasive pharmacological stress testing if it will change management
IIb-B	For patients with elevated MACE risk and moderate-to-good functional capacity (> or equal to 4 METS), it may be reasonable to forego further testing and proceed to surgery
IIb-B	Cardiopulmonary exercise testing may be done for patients with elevated risk & unknown functional capacity
IIb-C	For patients with elevated risk and poor or unknown functional capacity, exercise testing with cardiac imaging for ischemia may be reasonable if it will change perioperative management
III-B	Routine noninvasive exercise or stress testing is not useful for perioperative evaluation
	Perioperative angiography and coronary intervention
I-C	Revascularization before noncardiac surgery is recommended if revascularization would normally be indicated by current guidelines
III-B	It is not recommended that coronary revascularization be performed before noncardiac surgery exclusively to reduce perioperative cardiac events
III-C	Routine perioperative coronary angiography is not recommended
	Timing of Surgery after Percutaneous Coronary Intervention (PCI)
I-B	If possible, surgery should be delayed for 14 days after PTCA & 365 days after DES placement
IIa-C	Consensus decisions regarding antiplatelet therapy are helpful
IIb-B	Consider noncardiac surgery 180 days after DES placement if the risk of further delay outweighs the risks of ischemia and stent thrombosis
III-B	Elective surgery should not be performed within 30 days of BMS implantation or within 12 months of DES implantation if dual antiplatelet therapy must be discontinued perioperatively
III-C	Elective surgery should not be performed within 14 days of PTCA if dual antiplatelet therapy must be discontinued perioperatively
	Perioperative Beta-Blockade
I-B	Continue beta-blocker therapy in patients on beta-blockers preoperatively
IIa-B	Post-operative beta-blockade should be guided by clinical circumstances
IIb-B	In patients with 3 or more RCRI risk factors, it may be reasonable to begin beta-blockade
IIb-B	In patients with a compelling long-term indication for beta-blockade but without RCRI risk factors, initiating beta-blockers is of unclear benefit
IIb-B	It is preferred that perioperative beta-blockade be initiated long enough in advance of surgery to assess safety and tolerability, preferably more than one day prior to surgery/intervention
IIb-C	In patients with intermediate or high-risk ischemia on preoperative testing, it may be reasonable to begin beta-blockade
III-B	Beta-blocker therapy should not be started on the day of surgery

(continued)

Table 1.1 (continued)

Level of evidence	Guideline recommendations
	Perioperative Statin Therapy
I-B	Continue statin therapy in patients taking statins preoperatively
IIa-B	It is reasonable to initiate statins in patients undergoing vascular surgery
IIb-C	Consider initiating statins in patients with clinical indications who are preparing to undergo elevated risk procedures
	Alpha-2 Agonists
III-B	Alpha-2 agonists are not recommended for noncardiac surgery
	ACE Inhibitors (ACEIs) and Angiotensin Receptor Blockers (ARBs)
IIa-B	It is reasonable to continue ACE inhibitors and/or ARBs perioperatively
IIa-C	If ACEIs or ARBs are held perioperatively, they should be resumed once clinically feasible
	Antiplatelet Therapy
I-C	Consensus building among the perioperative team and outpatient specialists is helpful
I-C	Continuation of dual antiplatelet therapy (DAPT) is recommended for 4–6 weeks after BMS or DES implantation unless the risk of bleeding outweighs the risk of stent thrombosis
I-C	If one must discontinue a P2Y12 inhibitor, it is recommended to continue aspirin and resume the P2Y12 inhibitor as quickly as possible
IIb-B	It may be reasonable to continue aspirin after PCI if the potential increased risk for cardiac events outweighs the risks of bleeding
IIIb-B	Initiation or continuation of aspirin is not beneficial in patients who have not had previous coronary stenting (except in carotid surgery)
IIIb-C	Initiation or continuation of aspirin is not beneficial in patients who have not had previous coronary stenting (except in carotid surgery) unless the risk of ischemic events outweighs the risks of surgical bleeding

The guidelines recommend proceeding with surgery without further cardiac assessment in patients with moderate (>4 METS) or excellent functional capacity (>10 METS).

For patients with low or unknown functional capacity, exercise testing or pharmacologic stress testing with perfusion imaging is reasonable prior to surgery. This is recommended only when the diagnosis of ischemic disease would make a therapeutic impact. Exercise and stress testing results should lead to coronary interventions only if established evidence-based criteria for intervention are met, regardless of the need for surgery. Interventions for the sole purpose of mitigating cardiac risk perioperatively *are not recommended* and possibly harmful. Interventions that optimize therapeutic management for the long term—regardless of the specific timing of surgery—are encouraged. Conversely, if the patient has evidence of ACS during the perioperative evaluation, then standard evidence-based therapies including immediate invasive intervention should be considered.

References

1. Nabel EG, Braunwald E. A tale of coronary artery disease and myocardial infarction. N Engl J Med. 2012;366(1):54–63.
2. Libby P, Theroux P. Pathophysiology of coronary artery disease. Circulation. 2005;111:3481–8.
3. Libby P. Mechanisms of acute coronary syndromes. N Engl J Med. 2013;369(9):883–4.
4. Libby P. Mechanisms of acute coronary syndromes and their implications for therapy. N Engl J Med. 2013;368(21):2004–13.
5. Barash PG, Cullen BF, Stoelting RK, Cahalan MK, Stock MC, Ortega R. Clinical Anesthesia. 7th ed. Philadelphia: Lippincott Williams & Wilkins. In: Pagel PS, Kampine JP, Stowe DF, editors. Chapter 10: Cardiac anatomy and physiology. 2013. p. 239–262.
6. Futami C, Tanuma K, Tanuma Y, Saito T. The arterial supply of the conducting system in normal human hearts. Surg Radiol Anat. 2003;25(1):42–9.
7. Veltman CE, van der Hoeven BL, Hoogslag GE, Kharbanda RK, de Graaf MA, Delgado V, van Zwet EW, Schalij MJ, Bax JJ, Scholte AJ. Influence of coronary vessel dominance on short- and long-term outcome in patients after ST-segment elevation myocardial infarction. Eur Heart J. 2015;36(17):1023–30.
8. Goldberg A, Southern DA, Galbraith PD, Traboulsi M, Knudtson ML, Ghali WA. Alberta provincial project for outcome assessment in coronary heart disease (APPROACH) investigators. Coronary dominance and prognosis of patients with acute coronary syndrome. Am Heart J. 2007;154(6):1116–22.
9. Lilly LS, Pathophysiology of Heart Disease. 5th ed. Philadelphia: Lippincott Williams & Wilkins. In: Lin KY, Edelman ER, Strichartz G, Lilly LS, editors. Chapter 1: basic cardiac structure and function. 2011. p. 1–28.
10. Abuin G, Nieponice A, Barcelo A, Rojas-Granados A, Herrera-Saint Leu P, Arteaga-Martinez M. Anatomical reasons for the discrepancies in atrioventricular block after inferior myocardial infarction with and without right ventricular involvement. Tex Heart Inst J. 2009;36(1):8–11.
11. Gill SK. Cardiovascular risk factors and disease in women. Med Clin N Am. 2015;99:535–52.

12. Awtry EH, Jeon C, Ware MG. Blueprints in Cardiology. 2nd ed. Hoboken: Blackwell Publishing. In: Chapter 9: coronary artery disease—pathophysiology. 2006. p. 42–46.
13. Stratton IM, Adler AI, Neil HA, Matthews DR, Manley SE, Cull CA, Hadden D, Turner RC, Holman RR. Association of glycaemia with macrovascular and microvascular complications of type 2 diabetes (UKPDS 35): prospective observational study. BMJ. 2000;321(7258):405–12.
14. Bruning RS, Sturek M. Benefits of exercise training on coronary blood flow in coronary artery disease patients. Prog Cardiovasc Dis. 2015;57(5):443–53.
15. Braunwald E. Coronary plaque erosion: recognition and management. JACC Cardiovasc Imaging. 2013;6:288–9.
16. Renker M, Baumann S, Rier J, Ebersberger U, Fuller SR, Batalis NI, Schoepf UJ, Chiaramida SA. Imaging coronary artery disease and the myocardial ischemic cascade: clinical principles and scope. Radiol Clin North Am. 2015;53(2):261–9.
17. Kip KE, Hollabaugh K, Marroquin OC, Williams DO. The problem with composite end points in cardiovascular studies: the story of major adverse cardiac events and percutaneous coronary intervention. J Am Coll Cardiol. 2008;51(7):701–7.
18. Fleisher LA, Fleischmann KE, Auerbach AD, Barnason SA, Beckman JA, Bozkurt B, Davila-Roman VG, Gerhard-Herman MD, Holly TA, Kane GC, Marine JE, Nelson MT, Spencer CC, Thompson A, Ting HH, Uretsky BF, Wijeysundera DN. ACC/AHA Guideline on perioperative cardiovascular evaluation and management of patients undergoing noncardiac surgery: executive summary. J Am Coll Cardiol. 2014;64(22):e77–137.
19. Duncker DJ, Koller A, Merkus D, Canty JM. Regulation of coronary blood flow in health and ischemic heart disease. Prog Cardiovasc Dis. 2015;57(5):409–22.
20. Landesberg G, Beattie WS, Mosseri M, Jaffe AS, Alpert JS. Perioperative myocardial infarction. Circulation. 2009;119: 2936–44.
21. Thygesen K, Alpert JS, Jaffe AS, Simoons ML, Chaitman BR, White HD. Third universal definition of myocardial infarction. J Am Coll Cardiol. 2012;60:1581–98.

Suggested Reading

22. Keely EC, Hills LD. Primary PCI for myocardial infarction with ST-segment elevation. N Eng J Med. 2007;356:47–54.
23. Alfonso F, Byrne RA, Rivero F, Kastrati A. Current treatment of in-stent restenosis. J Am Coll Cardiol. 2014;63:2659–73.
24. Antman EM, Anbe DT, Armstrong PW, Bates ER, Green LA, Hand M, et al. ACC/AHA guidelines for the management of patients with ST-elevation myocardial infarction—executive summary: a report of the American College of Cardiology/American Heart Association Task Force on practice guidelines. Circulation. 2004;100:588–636.
25. Fibrinolytic Therapy Trialists (FFT) Collaborative Group. Indications for fibrinolytic therapy in suspected acute myocardial infarction: collaborative overview of early mortality and major morbidity results from all randomized trials of more than 1000 patients. Lancet. 1994: 343:311022.
26. Grines CL, Cox DA, Stone GW, Garcia E, Mattos LA, Giambartolomei A, et al. Coronary angioplasty with or without stent implantation for acute myocardial infarction. Stent primary angioplasty in myocardial infarction study group. N Eng J Med. 1999;341:1949–56.
27. Hochman JS, Sleeper LA, Webb JG, Sanborn TA, White HD, Talley JD, et al. Early revascularization in acute myocardial infarction complicated by cardiogenic shock. SHOCK investigators. Should we emergently revascularize occluded coronaries for cardiogenic shock? N Eng J Med. 1999;341:625–34.
28. Indermuehle A, Bahl R, Lansky AJ, Froehlich GM, Knapp G, Timmis A, et al. Drug-eluting balloon angioplasty for in-stent restenosis: a systematic review and meta-analysis of randomized control trials. Heart. 2013;99:327–33.
29. Ozaki K, Tanaka T. Molecular genetics of coronary artery disease. J Hum Genet. 2015;2(10):1038.
30. Podgoreanu MV, Schwinn DA. New paradigms in cardiovascular medicine: emerging technologies and practices: perioperative genomics. J Am Coll Cardiol. 2005;46(11):1965–75.

Myocardial Infarction

2

Hanjo Ko

CASE

78M with history of heavy asbestos exposure who presented with new onset of dyspnea and was found to have significant right pleural thickening concerning for mesothelioma one month ago. He is scheduled for diagnostic bronchoscopy and mediastinoscopy with biopsy for cancer staging.

In the preoperative area, he complains of chest pain radiating to his jaw and left arm that started 30 min ago and has only started to subside now after he managed to get back in bed with the help of his wife.

Medications:

Metoprolol 100 mg daily
Isosorbide mononitrate 60 mg daily
Lisinopril 10 mg daily
Aspirin 81 mg daily
Atorvastatin 80 mg daily
Clopidogrel 75 mg daily (held for 7 days)
Lantus 35 units daily and aspart 5 units with meals

Allergies: NKDA

Past Medical History:

CHF—EF 55–60% with moderate MR on prior TTE obtained one year ago

CAD with MI in the past— drug-eluting stents (DES) to LCx and ramus intermedius 5 years ago, DES to OM1 and RCA with balloon angioplasty to LCx 4 years ago

DM2—poorly controlled with baseline Hgb A1c of 11.6 one month ago

Physical Exam:

Vitals: HR 94, BP 178/89, RR 24, SpO2 92% on 2L NC

MP4, full range of motion, normal mouth opening, normal thyomental distance

He is in mild distress, slightly diaphoretic, but able to lie flat and finish sentences without difficulty.

Bedside EKG showed ST elevation in V1 through V4 and II, III, aVF.

1. **What is myocardial infarction (MI)?**

MI represents a disease process in which myocardial oxygen demand exceeds myocardial oxygen supply leading to myocardial ischemia and subsequent myocardial necrosis. MI typically occurs in patients with prior coronary artery disease (CAD) due to the formation of atherosclerotic plaques and progressive narrowing of the coronary arteries. Non-ST elevation MI (NSTEMI) represents subendocardial ischemia while ST elevation MI (STEMI) suggests a more devastating and serious myocardial insult that affects the full thickness of myocardium, spreading from endocardium to epicardium. STEMI is more typically caused by the sudden thrombotic occlusion of a coronary artery that was not previously severely stenotic, and unlike NSTEMI, it is considered a medical emergency and requires immediate intervention to restore blood flow in order to salvage the remaining myocardium. Given that the amount of myocardial injury occurs, not in a linear fashion, but rather curvilinear as time passes, a careful selection and timely implementation of a reperfusion strategy has become the hallmark treatment of STEMI where "time is muscle" [1].

2. **What are different types of MIs?**

In 2012, the joint ESC/ACCF/AHA/WHF Task Force for Redefinition of Myocardial Infarction published the expert consensus to redefine myocardial infarction, especially in the era where new biomarkers (such as troponin C or I) and interventions are becoming increasingly available [2]. The new definition not only allows for better characterization of the various etiologies of MI but also helps to develop more tailored treatment to a specific type of MI (see Table 2.1).

H. Ko (✉)
Department of Anesthesiology, Perioperative and Pain Medicine, Brigham and Women's Hospital, 3737 Chestnut St., Apt 2604, Philadelphia, PA 19104, USA
e-mail: hanjoko@gmail.com

© Springer International Publishing AG 2017
L.S. Aglio and R.D. Urman (eds.), *Anesthesiology*,
DOI 10.1007/978-3-319-50141-3_2

Table 2.1 Types of MI

Type 1	Spontaneous MI related to ischemia due to a primary coronary event such as plaque erosion and/or rupture, fissuring, or dissection
Type 2	MI secondary to ischemia due to either increased oxygen demand or decreased supply, e.g., coronary artery spasm, coronary embolism, anemia, arrhythmias, hypertension, or hypotension
Type 3	Sudden unexpected cardiac death, often with symptoms suggestive of myocardial ischemia
Type 4a	MI associated with percutaneous coronary intervention (PCI)
Type 4b	MI associated with stent thrombosis as documented by angiography or at autopsy
Type 4c	MI associated with PCI restenosis or >50% stenosis on coronary angiography
Type 5	MI associated with coronary artery bypass graft (CABG)

MI can also be described by size and location: microscopic (focal necrosis), small (<10% of left ventricular myocardium), moderate (10–30%), and large (>30%). Pathologically, it can be described as acute (identified by presence of polymorphonuclear leukocytes), healing (absence of polymorphonuclear leukocytes but presence of mononuclear cells and fibroblasts), or healed (scarred tissue without cellular infiltration). The entire healing process usually takes at least 5–6 weeks. One should keep in mind that the manifestation of MI may not correspond exactly with pathological findings, and the most appropriate treatment should always be based on clinical assessment of each individual patient at any given time.

3. **What is percutaneous coronary intervention (PCI)?**

Reperfusion strategy depends on the onset and duration of MI, location of occluded coronary arteries, facility capability, and patient's overall medical condition and clinical stability. One can further divide reperfusion strategy into three main categories: PCI, fibrinolytic therapy, and surgical graft revascularization. Primary PCI consists of balloon angioplasty (with or without stenting), without the previous administration of fibrinolytic therapy or platelet glycoprotein IIb/IIIa inhibitors, to open the culprit coronary artery that's responsible for clinical MI [3].

Under fluoroscopic guidance, a culprit vessel is identified and a metal wire is past beyond the thrombosis. A balloon catheter (with or without stent) is then inflated at the site of occlusion to mechanically restore distal blood flow. When anatomically feasible and appropriate, PCI is the preferred mode of reperfusion as long as it can be accomplished in a timely fashion (typically defined as "door-to-balloon" time $\leq$ 90 min) by an experienced operator in a facility that is capable of providing additional surgical assistance and/or transferring patients to a tertiary care center where such support exists. The "door-to-balloon" time can be extended beyond 90 min in those patients with the following [4–7]:

- contraindication to fibrinolytic therapy
- high risk of bleeding with fibrinolytic therapy, including patients >75 years old due to increased risk of intracranial hemorrhage
- clinical evidence suggesting a high risk of an infarct-related mortality such as hypotension or pulmonary edema
- cardiogenic shock

Finally, assuming no contraindications and that the culprit lesion is anatomically feasible for stent deployment, stents (drug-eluting stents preferred over bare-metal stents) have better outcomes than balloon angioplasty in terms of frequency of recurrent angina, rates of restenosis, and the need for repeat revascularization procedures [8, 9].

4. **What is fibrinolytic therapy?**

There is reasonable amount of discussion on the topic of when and/or for whom fibrinolytic therapy is preferred over PCI. In general, there are a greater number of limitations with fibrinolytic therapy compared to PCI. For example, 27% of the eligible patients have a contraindication to fibrinolysis such as recent surgery (less than 3 months prior to event) or history of cerebrovascular disease or uncontrolled systolic blood pressure >200 mmHg [10]. The utilization of systemic fibrinolytic therapy, unlike successful PCI, does not necessarily guarantee thrombolysis within the culprit vessel. Furthermore, a higher risk of reinfarction and 2-year mortality is also observed in patients receiving fibrinolytic therapy compared to PCI [11].

Nevertheless, fibrinolytic therapy still yields better clinical outcomes when compared to medical optimization without any reperfusion treatment [12]. Furthermore, there are certain conditions where fibrinolytic therapy is preferred over PCI. For example, in patients who seek medical attention less than 1 h after the onset of symptoms, fibrinolytic therapy may abort the infarction completely.

5. **How does one decide which reperfusion strategy is best suited for certain patients?**

There are certain scenarios that would favor one or the other but in general, each decision needs to be tailored to individuals' clinical conditions and needs, instead of following a simple algorithm. For example, balloon angioplasty may be preferred in patients with left main disease who are candidates of CABG within days in order to avoid administration of clopidogrel. In patients whose adherence to dual antiplatelet therapy (DAPT) might be questionable, balloon angioplasty may be more ideal than DES despite no other physiological contraindications to DES. CABG, on the other hand, typically is preferred in diabetic patients with multivessel coronary artery disease [13]. However, the presence of significant chronic kidney disease combined with history of life-threatening gastrointestinal bleeding might provide arguments for CABG in certain patients in order to avoid contrast-associated nephropathy necessitating permanent dialysis and recurrent bleeding from the need of DAPT following DES. It is therefore, imperative, that one seeks expert opinion and has a candid discussion with patients regarding risks and benefits before committing them to a certain reperfusion therapy.

After the Initial Presentation:

Even though the patient presentation does not endorse significant angina, his clinical manifestation is concerning for STEMI. Given the elective nature of his surgery, the case was canceled. He was given morphine for symptomatic relief, and an esmolol infusion was started to decrease myocardial demand by slowing his heart rate. After obtaining an emergent cardiology consultation for STEMI, this patient underwent coronary artery angiography which revealed an in-stent restenosis of his prior RCA stent and a newly >80% occluded LAD.

6. **What is in-stent restenosis (ISR)?**

It is important to distinguish ISR from stent thrombosis. ISR is the result of arterial damage with subsequent neointimal tissue proliferation that leads to >50% stenosis in the diameter [14]. The need for repeat revascularization within 30 days after the initial stent deployment most likely suggests stent thrombosis since the time frame is too short for the narrowing and/or occlusion of the targeted vessels to be caused by neointimal tissue. Stent thrombosis typically presents with MI while the incidence of MI from ISR is much lower since restenosis only implies reduction in the coronary arterial lumen diameter, instead of complete occlusion. As a result, traditionally, ISR is thought to be a relatively benign entity but more recent studies have suggested that these patients can and will frequently present with acute MI [15, 16].

The optimal treatment for DES restenosis is still under investigation given the various etiologies for ISR (neoatherosclerosis, drug resistance, stent underexpansion, residual uncovered atherosclerotic plaques, etc.). The most popular modality is repeat DES or drug-coated balloon angioplasty, provided that the anatomical features of ISR are favorable for such intervention, since they provide the best clinical and angiographic results [17, 18]. However, the success rate for retreatment differs significantly depending on the clinical scenario, and therefore, it is imperative to recognize that at some point, CABG should be considered as a treatment option, especially in complex cases (e.g., multivessel DES with multivessel diffuse ISR) [19].

This patient's STEMI is most likely from the combination his newly occluded LAD and his ISR with prior RCA stent (clopidogrel was held for 7 days). That is, he has both type 1 and type 4c MI. It is important to recognize that a patient treated with a new DES for ISR should be considered high risk, and DAPT should be continued indefinitely unless a serious complication occurs, upon which time, an expert consultation should be sought in order to balance the risk of bleeding and thrombosis.

7. **What are high-risk PCIs?**

Unfortunately, there is no universally accepted definition of high-risk PCI, and therefore limited data exist to help guide management to minimize peri-procedural complications. Nevertheless, high-risk PCIs are typically associated with significant hemodynamic instability and technical challenges with a higher possibility of requiring mechanical circulatory support and/or emergent surgical intervention. An example to further categorize high-risk PCIs is as follows [20, 21] (see Table 2.2).

One needs to bear in mind that the list above is not comprehensive, and therefore it should only serve as an example to urge clinicians to seek more detailed risk stratification after consulting expert opinion.

Follow Up of the Case:

Given the new findings, a BMS was deployed into his LAD, and balloon angioplasty to RCA was also performed. BMS was chosen to minimize the duration of DAPT given that this patient might be a candidate for pleurectomy in the near future, assuming that his clinical condition is stabilized and that he is able to undergo the initial cancer staging after one month of DAPT. He was subsequently transferred to cardiac critical care unit and discharged home after a few

Table 2.2 An example to further categorize high-risk PCIs [20, 21]

Anatomical location	Intervention to an unprotected left main coronary artery or left main equivalent
	Multivessel disease
	Distal left main bifurcation intervention
	Previous CABG, including intervention to a graft, particularly a degenerated graft
	Last remaining coronary conduit
	Duke Myocardial Jeopardy score >8
	Target vessel providing a collateral supply to an occluded second vessel that supplies >40% of the left ventricular myocardium
	Ostial stenosis
	Heavily calcified lesions
	Chronic total occlusions
	SYNTAX score >33
Hemodynamic criteria	Cardiac index <2.2 L/min/m^2
	Pulmonary capillary wedge pressure >15 mmHg
	Mean pulmonary artery pressure >50 mmHg
Clinical feature	Cardiogenic shock occurring within 24 h or at the start of coronary intervention
	Left ventricular systolic dysfunction on presentation (ejection fracture <30–40%)
	Killip class II-IV on presentation or congestive heart failure
	Coronary intervention after resuscitated cardiac arrest within 24 h
	STEMI
	Acute coronary syndrome complicated by unstable hemodynamics, dysrhythmia, or refractory angina
	Prior MI
	Age >70–80 years
	History of cerebrovascular disease, diabetes, renal dysfunction, peripheral arterial disease, or chronic lung disease

days. He was instructed to follow up with his cardiologist within a week after discharge.

8. **What is the current guideline for DAPT after PCI?**

Table 2.3 reflects the current guideline for DAPT after PCI based on 2005 ACC/AHA publication [13].

For our patient, he should continue clopidogrel 75 mg daily and increase his aspirin to 325 mg daily for at least one month given the new BMS to his LAD. The decision as to whether or not hold clopidogrel prior to his elective cancer staging surgery has to be revisited.

9. **What is the implication of DAPT in the perioperative setting?**

Since DAPT has been proven to be superior in terms of preventing cardiovascular events after PCI to either aspirin alone, or clopidogrel alone, or even combination of aspirin and warfarin, the decision to withhold DAPT needs to be made individually [26]. At the same time, despite multiple clinical practice guidelines, the management of perioperative DAPT continues to evolve [27]. The risk of major adverse cardiovascular events and stent thrombosis is highest in the first year after implantation with mortality up to 45% [28]. During that first year, the endothelialization typically takes 4–6 weeks for BMS and 6–12 months for DES [29]. Early withdraw of antiplatelet agents is the main determinant for ischemic complication and the complication rate is the highest when the stent implantation is <30 days [30]. As a result, it is recommended that elective surgery should be postponed for a minimum of 4–6 weeks after BMS and 6 months after DES (preferably 12 months).

Aspirin should be continued throughout the perioperative period. The only possible exception is closed space surgeries such as intracranial surgery, spinal surgery, and posterior eye chamber surgery. For those who require semi-elective surgery such as cancer staging or diagnosis, a delay of 12 months is not ideal. As a result, timed transfusion of platelets can be considered. For example, the last dose of aspirin and clopidogrel is given 12–24 h before surgery followed by 2 pools of platelet concentration given 1–2 h immediately before surgery. The duration of holding DAPT should be minimized and ideally, aspirin should be restarted

Table 2.3 The current guideline for DAPT after PCI based on 2005 ACC/AHA publication [13]

Aspirin	Pre-PCI: Aspirin (either 75 or 325 mg) should be continued on patients who are on chronic daily aspirin. Of note, a daily dose of 75 mg of aspirin has similar cardiovascular outcomes to 325 mg but with fewer bleeding complications [22–24]
	Pre-PCI: Aspirin (300 mg or 325 mg) should be given at least 2 h and preferably 24 h for patients who are not on chronic daily aspirin
	Post-PCI: Aspirin 325 mg daily should be given – 1 month after bare-metal stent – 3 months after sirolimus-eluting stent – 6 months after paclitaxel-eluting stent After the above-specified duration, chronic daily aspirin (75 mg to 162 mg) should be continued indefinitely
Clopidogrel	Pre-PCI: A loading dose of clopidogrel 300 mg should be given preferably at least 6 h prior to procedure if feasible [25]
	Post-PCI: Clopidogrel 75 mg should be given – at least one month after bare-metal stent (unless the patient is at increased risk for bleeding, then it should be given for a minimum of 2 weeks) – 3 months after sirolimus stent – 6 months after paclitaxel stent Ideally, the duration for clopidogrel should be extended to 12 months in patients who are not at high risk of bleeding In patients with clinical features associated with stent thrombosis (i.e., renal insufficiency, diabetes, or procedural characteristics, such as multiple stents or treatment of a bifurcation lesion), it is reasonable to extend clopidogrel beyond 1 year
	Post-PCI: In patients whose subactue thrombosis may be lethal (e.g., unprotected left main, last patent coronary vessel), it is reasonable to consider platelet aggregation study. If <50% inhibition of platelet aggregation is demonstrated, it is reasonable to increase the dose of clopidogrel to 150 mg given clopidogrel resistance is a significant problem

6 h postoperatively and clopidogrel 24–48 h (± loading dose of 300 mg) [31]. Of note, this regimen is not valid for newer antiplatelet agents such as prasugrel or ticagrelor.

In cardiac surgery, it is recommended to hold clopidogrel for at least 5 days but the data concerning non-cardiac surgery are limited and conflicting [13]. Therefore, other "bridging" therapies (such as eptifibatide) should also be considered in high-risk patients since DAPT does result in a significant increase in bleeding, transfusion, mechanical ventilation, length of hospital stay, and surgical re-exploration [28, 32–34].

Similar to clopidogrel, prasugrel also binds irreversibly to the platelet $P2Y_{12}$ receptor but with a more rapid, potent, and consistent platelet inhibition at the cost of increased risk of bleeding [35, 36]. As a result, prasugrel has a more limited use in the perioperative setting.

Unlike clopidogrel, ticagrelor binds reversibly to platelet $P2Y_{12}$ receptor and is able to achieve a greater inhibition of platelet aggregation compared to clopidogrel without significant difference in the rates of major bleeding [37, 38]. The major advantage of ticagrelor is its short half-life (6–13 h) and reversibility [39]. In the perioperative setting, one only needs to hold ticagrelor for 1 day.

References

1. Gersh BJ, Stone GW, White HD, Holmes DR Jr. Pharmacological facilitation of primary percutaneous coronary intervention for acute myocardial infarction: is the slope of the curve the shape of the future? JAMA. 2005;293:979–86.
2. Thygesen K, Alpert JS, Jaffe AS, Simoons ML, Chaitman BR, White HD. Third universal definition of myocardial infarction. J Am Coll Cardiol. 2012;60:1581–98.
3. Keely EC, Hills LD. Primary PCI for myocardial infarction with ST-segment elevation. N Eng J Med. 2007;356:47–54.
4. Antman EM, Anbe DT, Armstrong PW, Bates ER, Green LA, Hand M, et al. ACC/AHA guidelines for the management of patients with ST-elevation myocardial infarction—executive summary: a report of the American College of Cardiology/American Heart Association Task Force on Practice Guidelines. Circulation. 2004;100:588–636.
5. Ahmed S, Antman EM, Murphy SA, Giugliano RP, Cannon CP, White H, et al. Poor outcomes after fibrinolytic therapy for ST-segment elevation myocardial infarction: impact of age (a meta-analysis of a decade of trials). J Thromb Thrombolysis. 2006;21:119–29.
6. Thune JJ, Hoefsten DE, Linholm MG, Mortensen LS, Andersen HR, Nielsen TT, et al. Simple risk stratification at admission to identify patients with reduced mortality from primary angioplasty. Circulation. 2005;112:2017–21.
7. Hochman JS, Sleeper LA, Webb JG, Sanborn TA, White HD, Talley JD, et al. Early revascularization in acute myocardial

infarction complicated by cardiogenic shock. SHOCK investigators. Should we emergently revascularize occluded coronaries for cardiogenic shock? N Eng J Med 1999;341:625–34.
8. Grines CL, Cox DA, Stone GW, Garcia E, Mattos LA, Giambartolomei A, et al. Coronary angioplasty with our without stent implantation for acute myocardial infarction. Stent primary angioplasty in myocardial infarction study Group. N Eng J Med 1999;341:1949–56.
9. Stone GW, Grines CL, Cox DA, Garcia E, Tcheng JE, Griffin JJ, et al. Comparison of angioplasty with stenting, with or without abciximab, in acute myocardial infarction. N Eng J Med. 2002;346:957–66.
10. Juliard JM, Himbert D, Folmard JL, Aubry P, Karrillon GJ, Boccara A, et al. Can we provide reperfusion therapy to all unselected patients admitted with acute myocardial infarction? J Am Coll Cardiol. 1997;30:157–64.
11. Gibson CM, Karha J, Murphy SA, James D, Morrow DA, Cannon CP, et al. Early and long-term clinical outcomes associated with reinfarction following fibrinolytic administration in the Thrombolysis in Myocardial Infarction trials. J Am Coll Cardiol. 2003;42:7–16.
12. Fibrinolytic Therapy Trialists (FFT) Collaborative Group. Indications for fibrinolytic therapy in suspected acute myocardial infarction: collaborative overview of early mortality and major morbidity results from all randomized trials of more than 1000 patients. Lancet. 1994;343:311022.
13. Smith SC Jr, Feldman TE, Hirshfield JW, Jacobs AK, Kern MJ, King SB, et al. ACC/AHA/SCAI guideline update for percutaneous coronary intervention. Circulation. 2006;113:156–75.
14. Mehran R, Dangas G, Abizaid AS, Mintz GS, Lansky AJ, Satler LF, et al. Angiographic patterns of in-stent restenosis: classification and implications for long-term outcome. Circulation. 1999;100:1872–8.
15. Cassese S, Byrne RA, Tada T, Pinieck S, Joner M, Ibrahim T, et al. Incidence and predictors of restenosis after coronary stenting in 10,004 patients with surveillance angiography. Heart. 2014;100: 153–9.
16. Chen MS, John JM, Chew DP, Lee DS, Ellis SG, Bhatt DL. Bare metal stent restenosis is not a benign clinical entity. Am Heart J. 2006;151:1260–4.
17. Alfonso F, Byrne RA, Rivero F, Kastrati A. Current treatment of in-stent restenosis. J Am Coll Cardiol. 2014;63:2659–73.
18. Indermuehle A, Bahl R, Lansky AJ, Froehlich GM, Knapp G, Timmis A, et al. Drug-eluting balloon angioplasty for in-stent restenosis: a systematic review and meta-analysis of randomized control trials. Heart. 2013;99:327–33.
19. Dangas GD, Claessen BE, Caixeta A, Sanidas EA, Mintz GS, Mehran R. In-stent restenosis in the drug-eluting stent era. J Am Coll Cardiol. 2010;56:1897–907.
20. Myat A, Patel N, Tehrani S, Banning AP, Redwood SR, Bhatt DL. Percutaneous circulatory assist devices for high-risk coronary intervention. JACC. 2015;8:229–44.
21. Rihal CS, Naidu SS, Givertz MM, Szeto WY, Burke JA, Kapur NK, et al. 2015 SCA/ACC/HFSA/STS clinical expert consensus statement on the use of percutaneous mechanical circulatory support devices in cardiovascular care. J Card Fail. 2015;21:499–518.
22. Yusuf S, Zhao F, Mehta SR, Chrolavicius S, Tognoni G, Fox KK. Effects of clopidogrel in addition to aspirin in patients with acute coronary syndromes without ST-segment elevation. N Engl J Med. 2001;345:494–502.
23. Mehta SR, Yusuf S, Peters RJ, et al. Effects of pretreatment with clopidogrel and aspirin followed by long-term therapy in patients undergoing percutaneous coronary intervention: the PCI-CURE study. Lancet. 2001;358:527–33.
24. Steinhubl SR, Berger PB, Mann JT III, et al. Early and sustained dual oral antiplatelet therapy following percutaneous coronary intervention: a randomized controlled trial. JAMA. 2002;288: 2411–20.
25. Patti G, Colonna G, Pasceri V, Pepe LL, Montinaro A, Di SG. Randomized trial of high loading dose of clopidogrel for reduction of periprocedural myocardial infarction in patients undergoing coronary intervention: results from the ARMYDA-2 (Antiplatelet therapy for Reduction of Myocardial Damage during Angioplasty) study. Circulation. 2005;111:2099–106.
26. Leon MB, Baim DS, Popma JJ, Gordon PC, Cutlip DE, Ho KK, et al. Stent anticoagulation restenosis study investigators. A clinical trial comparing three antithrombotic-drug regimens after coronary-artery stenting. N Engl J Med. 1998;339:1665–71.
27. Darvish-Kazem S, Gandhi M, Marcucci M, Douketis JD. Perioperative management of antiplatelet therapy in patients with a coronary stent who need noncardiac surgery: a systematic review of clinical practice guidelines. Chest. 2013;144:1848–56.
28. Abualsaud AO, Eisenberg MJ. Perioperative management of patients with drug-eluting stents. JACC Cardiovasc Interv. 2010;3: 131–42.
29. Tsimikas S. Drug-eluting stents and late adverse clinical outcomes lessons learned, lessons awaited. J Am Coll Cardiol. 2006;47: 2112–5.
30. Iakovou I, Schmidt T, Bonizzoni E, Ge L, Sangiorgi GM, Stankovic G, et al. Incidence, predictors, and outcome of thrombosis after successful implantation of drug-eluting stents. JAMA. 2005;293:2126–30.
31. Thiele T, Sümnig A, Hron G, Müller C, Althaus K, Schroeder HW, et al. Platelet transfusion for reversal of dual antiplatelet therapy in patients requiring urgent surgery: a pilot study. J Thromb Haemost. 2012;10:968–71.
32. Purkayastha S, Athanasiou T, Malinovski V, Tekkis P, Foale R, Casula R, et al. Does clopidogrel affect outcome after coronary artery bypass grafting? A meta-analysis. Heart. 2006;92:531–2.
33. Yende S, Wunderink RG. Effect of clopidogrel on bleeding after coronary artery bypass surgery. Crit Care Med. 2001;29:2271–5.
34. Leong JY, Baker RA, Shah PJ, Cherian VK, Knight JL. Clopidogrel and bleeding after coronary artery bypass graft surgery. Ann Thorac Surg. 2005;80:928–33.
35. Wiviott SD, Braunwald E, McCabe CH, Montalescot G, Ruzyllo W, Gottlieb S, et al. Prasugrel versus clopidogrel in patients with acute coronary syndromes. N Engl J Med. 2007;357: 2001–15.
36. Wiviott SD, Trenk D, Frelinger AL, O'Donoghue M, Neumann FJ, Michelson AD, et al. Prasugrel compared with high loading- and maintenance-dose clopidogrel in patients with planned percutaneous coronary intervention: the Prasugrel in Comparison to Clopidogrel for Inhibition of Platelet Activation and Aggregation-Thrombolysis in Myocardial Infarction 44 trial. Circulation. 2007;116:2923–32.
37. Cannon CP, Husted S, Harrington RA, Scirica BM, Emanuelsson H, Peters G, et al. Safety, tolerability, and initial efficacy of AZD6140, the first reversible oral adenosine diphosphate receptor antagonist, compared with clopidogrel, in patients with non-ST-segment elevation acute coronary syndrome: primary results of the DISPERSE-2 trial. J Am Coll Cardiol. 2007;50: 1844–51.
38. Storey RF, Husted S, Harrington RA, Heptinstall S, Wilcox RG, et al. Inhibition of platelet aggregation by AZD6140, a reversible oral P2Y12 receptor antagonist, compared with clopidogrel in patients with acute coronary syndromes. J Am Coll Cardiol. 2007;50:1852–6.
39. Angiolillo DJ, Capranzano P. Pharmacology of emerging novel platelet inhibitors. Am Heart J. 2008;156:S10–5.

Heart Failure

3

Dirk J. Varelmann

Case

A 57-year-old male with shortness of breath and chest pain on exertion is presenting for hip replacement.

Past medical history:

- Congestive Heart Failure (CHF)
- Hypertension
- Diabetes mellitus, insulin-dependent
- Obesity
- GERD.

Medication:

- Metoprolol 25 mg qid
- Acetylsalicylic acid (ASA) 81 mg/d
- Lisinopril 20 mg/d
- Lasix 40 mg BID
- Atorvastatin 80 mg/d
- Lantus (insulin-glargine)/Novolog (insulin-aspart)
- Omeprazole.

Vital signs:

BP 150/80 mmHg	HR 65/min	RR 20/min	SpO_2 95%
Weight 105 kg	Height 172 cm		

Physical Exam:

Neuro:	nonfocal exam
Cardiac:	regular, normal S1/S2, S3 audible, no rubs/murmurs
Pulmonary:	slightly diminished breath sounds at both bases, bibasilar fine crackles.

Bilateral lower extremity pitting edema noted.

Patient reports shortness of breath (SOB) after climbing one half flight of stairs or walking three blocks on flat surface, as well as nocturia, getting worse over the past 2 weeks. He was able to carry two bags of groceries up two flights of stairs until 2 weeks ago.

What Are the Clinical Signs of Heart Failure?

- decreased exercise tolerance
- basilar crackles on auscultation from interstitial pulmonary edema, and/or diminished bibasilar breath sounds secondary to pleural effusions
- S3 sound on cardiac auscultation
- peripheral edema, usually on the dependent limbs
- anasarca
- increased jugular venous pressure (JVP), >10 cm above sternal angle
- hepatic enlargement if concomitant right heart failure exists
- nocturia
- paroxysmal nocturnal dyspnea (PND).

As heart failure can present without signs of volume overload, the term "heart failure" (HF) is preferred over the term "congestive heart failure." Heart failure is a clinical syndrome, resulting from structural or functional cardiac disorders that impair the ability of the ventricle to fill with or eject blood [1]. The diagnosis of heart failure is primarily based on the aforementioned clinical signs and a careful patient history.

D.J. Varelmann (✉)
Department of Anesthesiology, Perioperative and Pain Medicine, Harvard Medical School, Brigham and Women's Hospital, 75 Francis St., CWN-L1, Boston, MA 02115, USA
e-mail: dvarelmann@partners.org

© Springer International Publishing AG 2017
L.S. Aglio and R.D. Urman (eds.), *Anesthesiology*,
DOI 10.1007/978-3-319-50141-3_3

What Are the Signs of Acutely Decompensated Heart Failure?

Patient presents with the abovementioned and following symptoms:

- dyspnea/orthopnea (pulmonary edema), hypoxemia
- recent weight gain secondary to edema
- coughing/wheezing, pink frothy pulmonary secretions
- "fluffy" infiltrates on chest radiography (CXR)
- increased central venous pressure, jugular vein distension
- Cardiomegaly on CXR
- Patient can be hypertensive; hypotension is an ominous sign.

How Can Heart Failure Be Classified/Graded?

Multiple grading classifications exist. One of the most common is the New York Heart Association (NYHA) functional classification (Table 3.1) [2]. The patients are assigned to the respective NYHA classes by subjective symptoms, but for an individual patient the NYHA functional class can be used to estimate exercise capacity. Goldman et al. developed a specific activity scale based on metabolic costs (METS) of specific activities to categorize the degree of cardiovascular disability (Table 3.1) [3], with 1 MET defined as 3.5 mL/min/kg O2 uptake. A poor functional status is considered the inability to climb two flight of stairs or walk four blocks on even surface[4, 5].

Is There a Difference in Anesthetic Perioperative Risk Between Acute/New Onset Versus Chronic/Compensated Heart Failure?

Patients with HF undergoing major non-cardiac surgery have a mortality of 8%, which is a >60% greater risk of operative mortality compared to patients without HF or CAD. The presence of coronary artery disease (CAD) in patients with HF poses no additional risk of mortality or readmission, indicating that HF is most relevant in those patients. The procedures with the highest risk noted are above and below knee amputations, colon cancer resection, open abdominal aortic aneurysm repair, open cholecystectomy, and pulmonary cancer resections [6]. Patients with decompensated HF are at a very high risk for developing major adverse cardiac events (MACE), including cardiac arrest and death. Patients with stable HF undergoing elective non-cardiac surgery who are appropriately managed have a comparable perioperative mortality to a control group (propensity-matched groups), although the hospital stay is prolonged and the long-term mortality rate is increased in the HF group [7].

Urgent Versus Emergent Procedures: Define Urgency and Low-Risk Versus Elevated Risk. What Are the Implications?

The American College of Cardiology (ACC)/American Heart Association (AHA) suggest the following classification of urgency by consensus, but individual institutions may use different definitions (Table 3.2) [8].

Table 3.1 New York heart association functional classification

Class	NYHA class [2]	Spec. activity scale [3]
I	Patients with cardiac disease but without resulting limitations of physical activity. Ordinary physical activity does not cause undue fatigue, palpitations, dyspnea, or angina pain	Patient can perform to completion activities requiring ≥7 METS, e.g., do outdoor work (shovel snow), or do recreational activities (skiing, basketball, squash, handball)
II	Patients with cardiac disease resulting in slight limitation of physical activity. They are comfortable at rest. Ordinary physical activity results in fatigue, palpitation, dyspnea, or angina pain	Patient can perform to completion any activities requiring ≥5, but <7 METS, e.g., carry anything up a flight of 8 stairs, walk on level ground at 4 mph
III	Patients with cardiac disease resulting in marked limitation of physical activity. They are comfortable at rest. Less than ordinary physical activity causes fatigue, palpitation, dyspnea, or angina pain	Patient can perform to completion any activity requiring ≥2, but <5, e.g., shower without stopping, strip/make bed, clean windows, walk on level ground at 2.5 mph, play golf, dress without stopping
IV	Patients with cardiac disease resulting in inability to carry on any physical activity without discomfort. Symptoms of cardiac insufficiency such as angina may be present even at rest. If any physical activity is undertaken, discomfort is increased	Patient cannot or does not perform to completion activities requiring ≥2 METS, cannot carry out activities listed above

Table 3.2 Classification and description of urgency, and the timeframe within surgery should occur

Classification of urgency	Time frame within which surgery has to occur	Description of urgency
Emergent	Within <6 h	Life or limb is threatened if not in the operating room. No or very limited time for clinical evaluation
Urgent	6–24 h	Life or limb is threatened if not in the operating room within 6–24 h. There may be time for a limited evaluation
Time-sensitive	<1 week	A delay of surgery >1 week for evaluation will negatively affect outcome, e.g., oncologic procedures
Elective	1 week–1 year	Procedure can be delayed up to one year

Risk categories for surgical procedures:

- Low risk: <1% for developing MACE/death
- Elevated risk: ≥1% for developing MACE/death

Risk Assessment Based on Left Ventricular Ejection Fraction

A decreased left ventricular ejection fraction (LVEF) is an independent prognostic factor of unfavorable outcome after major non-cardiac surgery. Patients with a LVEF <30% have significantly higher mortality than those with a LVEF ≥30%, although the mortality rate with HF and a preserved LVEF (≥40%) is still high [9–11].

What Work-up Is Desired or Required in Patients with HF?

Whereas algorithms exist on how to manage patients with CAD, those algorithms may not apply for patients with HF. As HF is mainly a clinical diagnosis, a thorough history and physical examination is mandatory.

Laboratory Work

Obtaining a basic metabolic panel (serum Na, K, Cl, CO_2, BUN, Cr) is reasonable to exclude diuretic-induced electrolyte imbalances, as well as renal insufficiency secondary to cardiorenal syndrome. Biomarkers of heart failure (BNP: brain natriuretic peptide, NT-proBNP: N-terminal probrain natriuretic peptide) may provide incremental predictive value, but there is a lack of data suggesting targeting these biomarkers for treatment of HF will reduce postoperative risk. Therefore, measurement of BNP/NT-proBNP cannot be routinely recommended.

EKG

Preoperative resting 12-lead EKG is reasonable for patients with known CAD, significant arrhythmias, peripheral arterial disease (PAD), cerebrovascular disease, or other significant structural heart disease, except for those undergoing low-risk surgery. EKG may be considered for asymptomatic patients without known CAD, except for low-risk surgery. EKG is not useful in asymptomatic patients undergoing low-risk surgical procedures.

Chest Radiography

A chest radiograph (CXR) should be obtained in patients with acutely decompensated HF (look for pulmonary edema, pulmonary vascular congestion). However, changes may be absent as adaptation processes can occur over time.

Assessment of LV Function

It is reasonable for patients with dyspnea of unknown origin or patients with HF with worsening dyspnea to undergo preoperative evaluation of left ventricular (LV) function. Reassessment of LV function in clinically stable patients with previously documented LV dysfunction may be considered if there has been no assessment within a year; however, routine preoperative evaluation is not recommended.

In patients with signs and symptoms of new or worsening HF, echocardiography may help to establish the etiology. It can also help to guide intraoperative management, as it can differentiate between systolic and diastolic dysfunction.

Noninvasive exercise testing: stress echocardiography or exercise testing may add predictive value in HF patients in whom the functional capacity is poor, but screening is not recommended.

Which Medication Should Be Continued/Discontinued Through the Perioperative Period?

Patients with chronic HF are usually on multiple medications, mostly for heart rate control (BRB: beta receptor blockers, CCB: calcium channel blockers, digoxin, amiodarone, class 1A-C antiarrhythmic agents), blood pressure control (ACEI: angiotensin-converting enzyme inhibitors, ARB: angiotensin receptor blockers, etc.), diuretics, anticoagulants, and various other medications. The most important drugs, considered to be the mainstay of HF therapy, are listed below.

BRB

Beta blockers should be continued if the patient is on BRBs chronically. Most of the data regarding beta blockers derives from patients with CAD. It is unclear whether the results of these studies can be extrapolated to the HF population. If bradycardia/hypotension occurs, BRBs may need to be temporarily discontinued. Uncompensated HF is a relative contraindication to BRBs and patients may be at an increased risk for stroke. If BRBs are about to be started, they should *not* be started on the day of surgery. 2–7 days before surgery is preferred time line to start BRBs; however, some studies suggest to initiate therapy >30 days prior to surgery.

CCB

These agents have significant negative inotropic properties and may precipitate or worsen HF in patients with a depressed LVEF or apparent HF. Therefore, these agents are not commonly used in patients with HF. In patients who take CCB as a part of their home medication regimen, CCB frequently have to be held preoperatively.

Digoxin

Data regarding digoxin in the perioperative period is very limited. Postoperative supraventricular arrhythmias are less frequent if digoxin is continued, but the anesthesiologist must be prepared to treat digoxin-induced arrhythmias (e.g., bradyarrhythmias/sinus bradycardia, tachyarrhythmias, ventricular ectopy, SA nodal block, and arrest).

ACEI/ARB

ACEI/ARB should be continued in HF patients throughout the perioperative period, if the blood pressure permits. If they are held, they should be restarted as soon as the clinical situation allows. About 50% of patients on ACEI/ARB temporarily experience intraoperative hypotension that may require treatment with volume expansion, vasopressors, or inotropic agents.

Aldosterone Antagonists

Hyperkalemia is a potential side-effect; therefore, a preoperative serum potassium level check is warranted.

Diuretics

Hypovolemia and hypokalemia are the most common side-effects of loop diuretics. Electrolytes should be checked preoperatively, as well as intraoperatively with the occurrence of large volume shifts/diuretic administration.

Anticoagulants

The risk of surgical bleeding has to be weighed against the benefits of anticoagulation (e.g., the development of cerebrovascular accidents, pulmonary embolism, and deep venous thrombosis). Bridging from anticoagulants with a long half-life to shorter acting agents (e.g., intravenous heparin/bivalirudin) may be necessary.

Your Patient Has an Implantable Cardioverter-Defibrillator (ICD). How Would You Manage It Intraoperatively? Would You Use a Magnet? Would You Call an Electrophysiologist to Deactivate the Device?

Patients with advanced heart failure often have an implantable cardioverter–defibrillator (ICD) for primary or secondary prevention of sudden cardiac death, or a biventricular pacemaker for cardiac resynchronization therapy (CRT) implanted. The various modes of pacing and resynchronization therapy are beyond the scope of this chapter.

Monopolar electrocautery can cause interference with ICDs and pacemakers or cause damage to the device. ICDs may interpret electrocautery as tachycardia and deliver antitachycardia pacing or inappropriate shocks. The pacemaker can be inhibited by electrocautery and stop pacing the heart, which is deleterious for patients who are pacemaker-dependent.

Applying a magnet over a pacemaker will temporarily switch the pacemaker to asynchronous ventricular pacing (VOO mode). If the preprogrammed rate is too slow, the symptoms of heart failure might get worse and the pacemaker/electrophysiology service should be consulted to reprogram the pacemaker to a higher rate.

The response of an ICD to the placement of a magnet on top of the device is different. ICD therapy will be suspended, but pacing function and mode are unaffected. An external defibrillator has to be immediately available, ideally with hands-off pads attached. If the patient is pacemaker-dependent, the ICD has to be temporarily reprogrammed to an asynchronous mode, as it might be inhibited by electrocautery when programmed to a mode that includes sensing of the patient's underlying rhythm (DDD(R), VVI, etc.).

Bipolar electrocautery offers the advantage of less interference with ICDs and pacemakers. If monopolar cautery is to be used, the current return pad should be placed in a fashion so that the current does not pass through or nearby the pulse generator and leads, although this might not completely avoid interference [12].

What Problems Can You Anticipate When You Induce a Patient with HF?

The patient is at risk for.

- Hypotension
- Hypertension
- Arrhythmia.

Discuss the Reasons Why the Patient May Become Hypotensive

- The patient may have a limited contractile reserve. Most anesthetic agents, including most volatile agents, have negative inotropic properties. If the patient lacks the ability to increase the heart rate (e.g., secondary to beta receptor blockade), the cardiac output (CO) will fall with a concomitant drop in blood pressure.
- The systemic vascular resistance (SVR) may drop with induction of anesthesia. In patients with chronically reduced cardiac output, the SVR is typically elevated in order to maintain a blood pressure (BP) that is sufficient for organ perfusion.
- Remember: MAP = CO × SVR.
- Most patients with advanced heart failure are on high doses of diuretics and may present with intravascular volume depletion.
- The filling of the left ventricle in the failing heart and in a heart with diastolic dysfunction becomes increasingly dependent on atrial systole ("atrial kick"). Heart failure itself puts the patient at risk for developing atrial fibrillation, by mechanisms such as atrial stretch, electrolyte imbalances, and possible neurohumoral factors (release of norepinephrine, stress of surgery, and inflammatory mediators).

What Are the Determinants of Cardiac Output?

- Heart rate and rhythm
- Preload
- Afterload
- Myocardial contractility (inotropy)
- Myocardial relaxation (lusitropy).

Cardiac output CO = (stroke volume [SV]) × (heart rate [HR]).

The stroke volume is mainly determined by preload (i.e., ventricular filling), contractility, duration of contraction, and afterload. With increasing preload, the contractility increases, therefore increasing stroke volume, up to a certain point, when a plateau is achieved and a further increase in preload does not lead to an improvement in stroke volume (the "flat part" of the Frank-Starling relationship).

What Anesthetic Technique Would You Choose for the Hip Replacement? Discuss the Options in Terms of Hemodynamic Sequelae

This procedure can be performed under regional, neuraxial, or general anesthesia. All the anesthetic modalities are acceptable and the choice is primarily guided by the type of surgery, contraindications to the specific technique, and the patient's preference. Regional anesthesia has the benefit of offering preemptive postoperative analgesia and avoidance of respiratory complications.

Hypotension is a possible side effect from neuraxial anesthesia, especially in patients with advanced heart failure on high doses of diuretics. Possible contraindications to neuraxial techniques in this specific patient population are the use of anticoagulants, the inability of the patient to tolerate positioning for the procedure, and patient refusal.

How Would You Perform Neuraxial Anesthesia?

Sympathectomy from neuraxial anesthesia can lead to profound hypotension in patients with advanced heart failure who are intravascularly volume depleted. Careful fluid administration may restore the blood pressure, as patients with HF are preload-dependent, especially in patients with diastolic dysfunction. However, volume overload with all its consequences (pulmonary edema) has to be avoided. Instead of large amounts of fluid, the use of alpha-1 agonists (phenylephrine, norepinephrine) and/or inotropes (ephedrine) is preferred. Instead of single shot spinal anesthesia, a combined spinal–epidural technique can be used. The intrathecal local anesthetic dose should be reduced. Intrathecal opioids may be added, and the epidural anesthetic should be titrated to the surgically desired level. Another option would be plain epidural anesthesia with careful titration of local anesthetic.

How Would You Induce General Anesthesia in This Patient?

Patients with HF often are unable to lie flat because of dyspnea/orthopnea. Furthermore, these patients are prone to developing hypotension after induction, as anesthetic agents often decrease contractility, heart rate, preload, and afterload. Several induction agents with different properties can be used; the choice also depends on patient characteristics, and provider preference. The ideal induction agent would have a quick onset, without producing hypotension or other side effects. Rapid organ independent clearance would be another ideal feature. In general, a moderate dose of an opioid (fentanyl 1–2 mcg/kg, sufentanil 0.1–0.2 mcg/kg), in combination with either ketamine (1–3 mg/kg), etomidate (0.2–0.3 mg/kg), or propofol (0.5–2 mg/kg) will induce an anesthetic state and blunt the hemodynamic response to intubation. A muscle relaxant with a quick onset can be used to facilitate intubation.

What Agents Would You Use for Maintenance of Anesthesia?

Both total intravenous anesthesia and the use of volatile anesthetics, are reasonable. A dose reduction may be necessary to avoid cardiovascular compromise. Supplementation with opioids and benzodiazepines can help reduce the need for volatile anesthetic agents/IV anesthetic agents and improve hemodynamic stability.

How Would You Monitor Hemodynamic Parameters Intraoperatively?

The monitoring standards of the American Society of Anesthesiology (ASA) apply in this patient population: EKG, blood pressure, oxygen saturation, circulatory function, temperature, inspired and expired gas concentration (during general anesthesia). Additionally, the following monitoring should be considered, depending on the patient status.

Continuous Invasive Blood Pressure

Continuous blood pressure monitoring via an arterial line ("a-line") is crucial in patients with advanced heart failure who are undergoing procedures with anticipated significant hemodynamic alterations. Frequent blood gas samples can be drawn from the arterial line. In patients with pre-anesthesia hemodynamic compromise, the arterial line may be placed pre-induction.

Central Venous Catheter (CVL)

A central venous line allows the administration of vasoactive drugs, as well as monitoring of the central venous pressure and analysis of the waveform. The absolute value of the central venous pressure (CVP) may not reveal the patient's volume status, but changes can indicate hemodynamic deterioration or acute decompensation (e.g., sudden increase in CVP as a consequence of acute right heart failure). The waveform can also give additional information about cardiac function (e.g., tall c-v waves as a sign of functional tricuspid regurgitation secondary to acute RV dilatation, or loss of the y-wave in cardiac tamponade).

Whether a central line needs to be placed depends on the patient's baseline hemodynamic status, the anticipated fluid shifts, and the likelihood of requiring vasopressors/inotropes.

Pulmonary Artery Catheters (PAC)

Placement of a PAC is not routinely recommended, as the current data does not suggest an improved outcome. However, in selected patients the insertion of a PAC is reasonable, especially in patients with severe/decompensated HF with expected large fluid shifts or pulmonary hypertension. PACs allow continuous cardiac output monitoring, but placement and interpretation of the obtained values require expertise.

Transesophageal Echocardiography (TEE)

Monitoring with TEE is useful in patients with severe left and/or right ventricular dysfunction. New wall motion abnormalities can be detected with high sensitivity. Rescue TEE may provide insight into the etiology of intraoperative hemodynamic instability (e.g., from hypovolemia, decreased LV/RV function, tamponade, new regional wall motion abnormalities, increased pulmonary artery pressure, pulmonary emboli, valvular regurgitation/stenosis, etc.).

Discuss the Hemodynamic Management. What Vasopressor, or Inotropes, Would You Use?

Vasopressors

The most commonly used vasopressors are phenylephrine, dopamine, norepinephrine, and vasopressin. They are used to increase blood pressure for maintaining organ perfusion, although an increased afterload in patients with HF may decrease the cardiac output.

Dopamine is a dose-dependent inotrope and vasopressor, with vasoconstrictive effects through alpha-1 receptors dominating in doses >10 mcg/kg/min. Arrhythmia and tachycardia are caused by the beta-1 effects. The use of dopamine in patients in cardiogenic shock has been associated with an increased mortality compared to norepinephrine [13].

Norepinephrine produces vasoconstriction by stimulation alpha-1 receptors, and inotropy through stimulation of the beta-1 receptors. As a result the blood pressure increases, without a drop in cardiac output (can even increase CO).

Vasopressin is a pure vasopressor. It is used in patients with shock refractory to other medication, but also in patients with low SVR caused by ACEI therapy. It does not increase pulmonary vascular resistance (PVR) and is preferred in patients requiring pharmacologic support of the right ventricle with concomitant inodilator use, to treat the decrease in systemic vascular resistance without increasing right ventricular afterload.

Inotropic Agents

Epinephrine is both a dose-dependent vasopressor and inotrope. With doses >5 mcg/min the vasopressor effect mediated through alpha-1 receptors dominates. Epinephrine has pro-arrhythmogenic properties.

Dobutamine is an inotrope with predominantly beta-1 synergistic effects. Because of the lack of alpha-1 agonistic properties it only increases the cardiac output (contractility and chronotropy), and the use of dobutamine in some patients may lead to a small reduction in blood pressure. However, in HF patients the cardiac output is usually low and an increase in cardiac output most often leads to an increase in blood pressure.

Vasodilators/Inodilators

Nitroglycerin at low doses dilates mainly the venous capacitance vessels, leading to a decrease in preload. At higher doses it leads to arterial dilation, including the large epicardial arteries, thereby improving myocardial perfusion without inducing a steal phenomenon.

Nitroprusside is a nitric oxide (NO) donor that dilates arterial vessels more than veins, thereby mainly decreasing afterload. It has a fast onset and wears off quickly. Prolonged infusion or infusion at higher doses leads to cyanide toxicity.

Nicardipine/Clevidipine are calcium antagonists of the dihydropyridine type. They act selectively on the smooth muscles of the arteries, thereby reducing afterload. Clevidipine has a half-life of 1 min and it is broken down by blood and tissue esterases, making it an attractive alternative to nitroprusside.

Milrinone is a phosphodiesterase (PDE 3) inhibitor that increases myocardial contractility and decreases left ventricular afterload by reducing the systemic vascular resistance. It is less arrhythmogenic than dobutamine and is effective in patients with heart failure with downregulated beta-adrenergic receptors. Its usability is limited by the fact that it can induce severe hypotension, especially if administered as a bolus.

What Are Common Arrhythmias Seen with HF?

Ventricular fibrillation (VF) or **ventricular tachycardia (VT)** usually requires immediate defibrillation or cardioversion. Slow VT is sometimes tolerated for a brief period, but cardioversion should be done for the patient as soon as possible. Even after successful cardioversion the patient may go back into VT/VF, therefore it is prudent to start an antiarrhythmic agent.

Atrial fibrillation (AF) is a common arrhythmia in HF patients. Hemodynamically unstable patients usually require cardioversion, whereas the treatment goal in stable patients is rate control. In the acute setting of new onset AF, it is reasonable to initiate antiarrhythmic therapy with short acting agents (diltiazem, esmolol), although amiodarone offers the advantage of less hypotension, especially when given as an infusion. Digoxin has been used as an antiarrhythmic agent, but it usually takes hours to take effect, even with a rapid dosing regimen.

Bradycardia is usually not well-tolerated in patients with HF, as it leads to systemic hypoperfusion, especially in patients with severely decreased LVEF. Atropine/glycopyrrolate are treatment options, although atropine can cause prolonged tachycardia and crosses the blood–brain barrier, which can lead to unwanted side effects in elderly patients (confusion, agitation, etc.). Dobutamine, dopamine, isoproterenol, and epinephrine have positive chronotropic properties and offer the advantage of having a shorter half-life than atropine/glycopyrrolate. In some cases, transcutaneous (pacing pads) or transvenous pacing may be necessary.

What Are Your Therapeutic Options in Patients with Advanced HF Refractory to Inotropic and Vasodilator/Vasoconstrictor Therapy?

Therapeutic options in instances where pharmacologic therapy of HF does not lead to improvement or in acutely decompeted HF, it may be necessary to consider initiation of therapy with cardiocirculatory assist devices (e.g., intra-aortic balloon counter-pulsation: IABP, left or biventricular assist devices, venoarterial extracorporeal membrane oxygenation: VA-ECMO). All of these invasive treatment options require the involvement of interventional cardiologists and/or cardiac surgeons.

How Would You Treat Right Ventricular Failure?

Patients with HF are prone to developing right ventricular (RV) failure, either secondary to ischemia, tachycardia/bradycardia, or tricuspid regurgitation. The RV is not able to pump blood against a high pulmonary vascular resistance, and is usually dependent on preload; therefore, hypovolemia can lead to decreased RV output and as a consequence to decreased LV output. In the failing heart the RV may not be able to deal with hypervolemia and the RV can acutely dilate and decompensate. Severe tricuspid regurgitation can also lead to RV volume overload. Functional tricuspid valve insufficiency can arise from RV dilation, as this leads to tricuspid annular dilation reducing the coaptation reserve of the tricuspid valve leaflets.

The treatment of RV failure consists of optimizing preload and afterload, as well as increasing RV contractility.

Pre-/afterload optimization:

- avoidance of high airway pressure (e.g., intrinsic PEEP)
- inhaled nitric oxide/prostanoids to decrease pulmonary vascular resistance (PVR)
- avoidance of hypercarbia, acidosis
- avoidance of hypoxemia.

Increasing contractility:

- inotropes and inodilators: milrinone, epinephrine, dobutamine
- vasopressors for hypotension that don't increase PVR: vasopressin
- mechanical support (right ventricular assist device, VA-ECMO).

With the Knowledge of How to Diagnose and Treat Heart Failure, How Would You Proceed with the Patient?

The patient has a history of heart failure which is treated with a beta receptor blocker, an angiotensin-converting enzyme inhibitor, and a diuretic. However, the patient's functional status has recently declined; he has dyspnea with minimal exertion (NYHA III from a previous NYHA II). The patient qualifies for further work-up (ECG, TTE) and preoperative optimization before undergoing an elective procedure with significant blood loss.

References

1. Hunt SA, Abraham WT, Chin MH, Feldman AM, Francis GS, Ganiats TG, et al. 2009 focused update incorporated into the ACC/AHA 2005 guidelines for the diagnosis and management of heart failure in adults. J Am Coll Cardiol. 2009;53(15):e1–90.
2. The Criteria of the New York Heart Association. Nomenclature and criteria for diagnosis of diseases of the heart and great vessels. 9th ed. Boston, MA: Little, Brown & Co.; 1994. p. 253–6.
3. Goldman L, Hashimoto B, Cook EF, Loscalzo A. Comparative reproducibility and validity of systems for assessing cardiovascular functional class: advantages of a new specific activity scale. Circulation. 1981;64(6):1227–34.
4. Reilly DF, McNeely MJ, Doerner D, Greenberg DL, Staiger TO, Geist MJ, et al. Self-reported exercise tolerance and the risk of serious perioperative complications. Arch Intern Med. 1999;159 (18):2185–92.
5. Girish M, Trayner E, Dammann O, Pinto-Plata V, Celli B. Symptom-limited stair climbing as a predictor of postoperative cardiopulmonary complications after high-risk surgery. Chest. 2001;120(4):1147–51.
6. Hammill BG, Curtis LH, Bennett-Guerrero E, O'Connor CM, Jollis JG, Schulman KA, et al. Impact of heart failure on patients undergoing major noncardiac surgery. Anesthesiology. 2008;108 (4):559–67.
7. Xu-Cai YO, Brotman DJ, Phillips CO, Michota FA, Tang WHW, Whinney CM, et al. Outcomes of patients with stable heart failure undergoing elective noncardiac surgery. Mayo Clin Proc. 2008;83 (3):280–8.
8. Fleisher LA, Fleischmann KE, Auerbach AD, Barnason SA, Beckman JA, Bozkurt B, et al. 2014 ACC/AHA guideline on

perioperative cardiovascular evaluation and management of patients undergoing noncardiac surgery. J Am Coll Cardiol. 2014;64(22):e77–137.
9. Healy KO, Waksmonski CA, Altman RK, Stetson PD, Reyentovich A, Maurer MS. Perioperative outcome and long-term mortality for heart failure patients undergoing intermediate- and high-risk noncardiac surgery: impact of left ventricular ejection fraction. Congest Heart Fail. 2010;16(2):45–9.
10. Kazmers A, Cerqueira MD, Zierler RE. Perioperative and late outcome in patients with left ventricular ejection fraction of 35% or less who require major vascular surgery. J Vasc Surg. 1988;8(3):307–15.
11. Meta-analysis Global Group in Chronic Heart Failure (MAGGIC). The survival of patients with heart failure with preserved or reduced left ventricular ejection fraction: an individual patient data meta-analysis. Eur Heart J. 2012;33(14):1750–7.
12. American Society of Anesthesiologists. Practice advisory for the perioperative management of patients with cardiac implantable electronic devices: pacemakers and implantable cardioverter-defibrillators. Anesthesiology. 2011;114(2):247–61.
13. De Backer D, Biston P, Devriendt J, Madl C, Chochrad D, Aldecoa C, et al. Comparison of dopamine and norepinephrine in the treatment of shock. N Engl J Med. 2010;362(9):779–89.

Hypothermia

4

Dirk J. Varelmann

1. **What is the definition of hypothermia?**

The definition of hypothermia can vary. Experts from various fields define mild, moderate, deep, and profound hypothermia differently. For patients after cardiac arrest, a temperature range of 32–34° is often referred to as "therapeutic hypothermia".

The Collaborative Research (CORE) Group suggested in a consensus paper on hypothermia in aortic arch surgery the following classification [1]:

- mild: 28.1–34 °C
- moderate: 20.1–28 °C
- deep: 14.1–20 °C
- profound: ≤14 °C

The temperature was assessed in the nasopharynx.

2. **What are the effects of hypothermia on cerebral metabolism?**

The cerebral metabolism decreases by 6–10% for each 1 °C reduction in body temperature. Therefore at 32 °C, the cerebral metabolic rate is reduced to half of the normal value [2].

3. **List other metabolic changes associated with hypothermia**

   - increased fat metabolism with release of glycerol, free fatty acids, lactate
   - decreased insulin secretion
   - insulin resistance
   - increased blood oxygen levels as a result of decreased extraction
   - hypocarbia, if ventilator settings are not adjusted to the decreased CO_2 production.

D.J. Varelmann (✉)
Department of Anesthesiology, Perioperative and Pain Medicine, Harvard Medical School, Brigham and Women's Hospital, 75 Francis St CWN-L1, Boston, MA 02115, USA
e-mail: dvarelmann@partners.org

© Springer International Publishing AG 2017
L.S. Aglio and R.D. Urman (eds.), *Anesthesiology*,
DOI 10.1007/978-3-319-50141-3_4

What other protective mechanisms of hypothermia are known?

- interruption of apoptotic pathways (caspase mediated)
- prevention of mitochondrial dysfunction
- mitigation of the destructive processes of the neuroexcitatory cascade (accumulation of glutamate, intracellular calcium influx)
- inhibition of ischemia-induced inflammatory reactions
- decreased production of nitric oxide (NO)
- reduced generation of oxygen free radicals
- reduction of ischemia-reperfusion induced vascular permeability
- improved tolerance for ischemia.

What are the three phases of hypothermia treatment?

1. Induction phase: start of cooling, for post-cardiac arrest the temperature goal is 34 °C, which should be achieved as quickly as possible
2. Maintenance phase: maintain the temperature with only minimal fluctuations
3. Rewarming (or decooling) phase: slow controlled warming (0.2–0.5 °C/h for cardiac arrest patients)

Name the most common side effects of hypothermia during the induction (cooling) phase

- hypovolemia
- hyperglycemia

- electrolyte disorders
- shivering
- cutaneous vasoconstriction [3, 4]

Frequent adjustments have to be made in ventilator settings, insulin dose, vasoactive substances, sedation, and electrolyte substitution.

The patient stabilizes during the maintenance phase. The risk for hypovolemia, shivering, and electrolyte shifts is greatly reduced. Shivering dramatically increases the metabolic rate, the work of breathing, and myocardial oxygen consumption. Shivering can be suppressed by sedatives, anesthetics, and some other drugs (magnesium, clonidine, meperidine, ketanserin, and bupropion). In extreme cases, paralysis may be required [5].

During mild hypothermia, the systolic function of the heart improves, but some mild diastolic dysfunction can develop. The cardiac output decreases, as well as the heart rate. However, oxygen supply and demand are still matched, as the oxygen consumption decreases. Deep hypothermia (Temp <30 °C) will lead to a decrease in contractility [6].

Rewarming (or: decooling) should be performed slowly, with a rise in temperature of 0.2–0.5 °C/h. Rapid rewarming can cause electrolyte shifts, with hyperkalemia being the most dangerous. The patient's sensitivity to insulin increases with rising temperatures, and the insulin dose has to be adjusted accordingly. Potassium that has been sequestered intracellularly during hypothermia is released during rewarming leading to hyperkalemia. The effect can be ameliorated by slow rewarming or with renal replacement therapy. Rapid rewarming can lead to significant decreases in jugular venous oxygen saturation. After rewarming, normothermia has to be maintained, as hyperthermia can negate the positive effects achieved by hypothermia [7].

What is the temperature goal for therapeutic hypothermia after cardiac arrest?

The Hypothermia After Cardiac Arrest Study Group ("HACA") included 275 patients, with the therapeutic hypothermia group cooled to a goal temperature of 32–34 °C. These data have been the basis for most guidelines and recommendations. Recently a large study randomized 950 unconscious patients after cardiac arrest with presumed cardiac etiology to a targeted temperature management of either 33 or 36 °C. Both groups scored similarly on the modified Rankin scale as a parameter for neurologic outcome [8]. It is worth mentioning that the patients in the latter study had active temperature management in place for 72 h after cardiac arrest to avoid fever and hyperthermia.

Briefly explain the mechanism of hypothermia leading to hypovolemia during hypothermia

The combination of several factors lead to so-called cold diuresis [9]:

- increased venous return from vasoconstriction from activation of the sympathetic system with secretion of norepinephrine
- activation of atrial natriuretic peptide (ANP)
- decreased level of antidiuretic hormone (ADH)
- renal tubular dysfunction

The at times brisk diuresis can lead to electrolyte imbalances and hypotension from hypovolemia.

What are the heart rhythm and rate changes expected with hypothermia?

Changes in heart rate and rhythm are temperature dependent. The initial increase in venous return with hypothermia can lead to sinus tachycardia, which is usually mild. Sinus bradycardia develops at temperatures <35.5 °C. Action potentials and spontaneous depolarization are prolonged, and the conduction velocity is decreased, resulting in prolonged PR and QT intervals, as well as widening of the QRS complex. A J-wave (Osborn wave) is sometimes observed. Whereas mild hypothermia decreases arrhythmias, severe hypothermia (<28 °C) will increase the risk of arrhythmias and make the treatment more challenging. Development of atrial fibrillation at temperatures <30 °C is a warning sign and should prompt rewarming to >30 °C. Other arrhythmias that can be seen with temperatures <28 °C are ventricular tachycardia (VT) and ventricular fibrillation (VF).

What are the effects of hypothermia on coronary perfusion?

With mild hypothermia the oxygen demand versus supply balance shifts in favor of the myocardium: the metabolic rate of oxygen consumption decreases in patients without coronary artery disease and the coronary perfusion increases. In severely atherosclerotic coronary arteries, hypothermia can induce vasoconstriction [10]. It is important to avoid shivering, as this may increase the metabolic rate by 40–400% [11, 12].

Will hypothermia lead to severe bleeding?

Platelet dysfunction occurs at temperatures <34 °C. Once the temperature drops below 33 °C, the function as well as the synthesis of clotting factors will be affected [13]. The risk of severe bleeding, however, with therapeutic mild hypothermia is relatively small.

Does hypothermia increase the risk of infection?

Intra- and postoperative hypothermia have been linked with an increase in wound infections and pneumonia. With therapeutic cooling, the risk of infections increases with prolonged duration (>24 h), although there seems to be no increase in mortality [14]. The beneficial effects (decreased synthesis of proinflammatory cytokines causing neuroinflammation) outweigh the risk imposed by infection. The physician needs to be vigilant about infections during induced hypothermia.

What is the impact of intraoperative hypothermia on patient morbidity?

Several studies have reported an increased cardiac morbidity, coagulopathy, and an increase in surgical site infections (SSI) with hypothermia [15–18]. Intraoperative normothermia (end of case temperature ≥36 °C without a warming device or the documented use of forced-air device intraoperatively) is part of the Surgical Care Improvement Project (SCIP) since 2006. However, the 36 °C threshold set by SCIP and below which complications are more likely to occur is somewhat arbitrary [19]. The most practical and well-studied way to keep patients warm intraoperatively is by using forced-air warming devices.

How fast should the patient be rewarmed after being cooled for cardiac/vascular surgery?

Fast rewarming rates during cardiopulmonary bypass can lead to high cerebral temperatures offsetting the potential neuroprotective benefits. The actual brain temperature may be higher than the temperature measured at other sites (e.g., pulmonary artery, nasopharyngeal, esophageal, rectum, and bladder). The rewarming rate on cardiopulmonary bypass is limited by the pump flow, the patient's characteristics (weight), and the blood temperature at the arterial (outflow) cannula. As high blood temperature can lead to cerebral hyperthermia and all its sequelae, an early and slower rewarming is preferred, with the CPB perfusate temperature kept at or below 37.0 °C [20, 21].

What is the best compartment/site to measure the temperature when rewarming on cardiopulmonary bypass?

The organ that is most susceptible to injury from hyperthermia is the brain. Unfortunately the cerebral temperature is not accessible for direct temperature measurement. Although the jugular bulb temperature underestimates the cerebral temperature, it most closely reflects the actual brain temperature compared to temperatures measured in other compartments [20, 22]. The bladder and rectal temperatures underestimate brain temperature by 2–4 °C when rewarming the patient to 37 °C. The nasopharyngeal and esophageal sites perform better than rectal or bladder sites [20].

References

1. Yan TD, Bannon PG, Bavaria J, et al. Consensus on hypothermia in aortic arch surgery. Ann Cardiothorac Surg. 2013;2:163–8.
2. Erecinska M, Thoresen M, Silver IA. Effects of hypothermia on energy metabolism in mammalian central nervous system. J Cereb Blood Flow Metab. 2003; 513–30.
3. Polderman KH. Application of therapeutic hypothermia in the intensive care unit. Opportunities and pitfalls of a promising treatment modality–Part 2: practical aspects and side effects [Internet]. Intensive Care Med. 2004; 30:757–69 Available from: http://www.ncbi.nlm.nih.gov/entrez/query.fcgi?cmd=Retrieve&db=PubMed&dopt=Citation&list_uids=14767590.
4. Polderman KH, Peerdeman SM, Girbes AR. Hypophosphatemia and hypomagnesemia induced by cooling in patients with severe head injury. J Neurosurg. 2001;94:697–705.
5. Sessler DI. Thermoregulatory defense mechanisms. Crit Care Med. 2009;37:S203–10.
6. Lewis ME, Al-Khalidi A-H, Townend JN, et al. The effects of hypothermia on human left ventricular contractile function during cardiac surgery. JACC. 2002;39:102–8.
7. Polderman KH. Induced hypothermia and fever control for prevention and treatment of neurological injuries. Lancet. 2008;371:1955–69.
8. Nielsen N, Wetterslev J, Cronberg T, et al. Targeted temperature management at 33 °C versus 36 °C after cardiac arrest. N Engl J Med. 2013;369:2197–206.
9. Stocks JM, Taylor NAS, Tipton MJ, et al. Human physiological responses to cold exposure. Aviat Space Environ Med. 2004;75:444–57.
10. Nabel EG, Ganz P, Gordon JB, et al. Dilation of normal and constriction of atherosclerotic coronary arteries caused by the cold pressor test. Circulation. 1988;77:43–52.
11. Frank SM, Fleisher LA, Olson KF, et al. Multivariate determinants of early postoperative oxygen consumption in elderly patients. Effects of shivering, body temperature, and gender. Anesthesiology. 1995;83:241–9.
12. Bay J, Nunn JF, Prys-Roberts C. Factors influencing arterial PO_2 during recovery from anaesthesia. Br J Anaesth. 1968;40:398–407.
13. Johnston TD, Chen Y, Reed RL. Functional equivalence of hypothermia to specific clotting factor deficiencies. J Trauma. 1994;37:413–7.
14. Kuchena A, Merkel MJ, Hutchens MP. Postcardiac arrest temperature management. Curr Opin Crit Care. 2014;20:507–15.
15. Frank SM, Fleisher LA, Breslow MJ, et al. Perioperative maintenance of normothermia reduces the incidence of morbid cardiac events. A randomized clinical trial. JAMA. 1997;277:1127–34.
16. Schmied H, Kurz A, Sessler DI, et al. Mild hypothermia increases blood loss and transfusion requirements during total hip arthroplasty. Lancet. 1996;347:289–92.

17. Kurz A, Sessler DI, Lenhardt R. Perioperative normothermia to reduce the incidence of surgical-wound infection and shorten hospitalization. Study of wound infection and temperature group. N Engl J Med. 1996;334:1209–15.
18. Mahoney CB, Odom J. Maintaining intraoperative normothermia: a meta-analysis of outcomes with costs. AANA J. 1999;67: 155–63.
19. Leeds IL, Wick EC, Melton GB. Advances in surgery. Adv Surg. 2014;48:65–76.
20. Nussmeier NA, Cheng W, Marino M, et al. Temperature during cardiopulmonary bypass: the discrepancies between monitored sites. Anesth Analg. 2006;103:1373–9.
21. Grigore AM, Grocott HP, Mathew JP, et al. The rewarming rate and increased peak temperature alter neurocognitive outcome after cardiac surgery. Anesth Analg. 2002;94:4–10.
22. Grocott HP, Newman MF, Croughwell ND, et al. Continuous jugular venous versus nasopharyngeal temperature monitoring during hypothermic cardiopulmonary bypass for cardiac surgery. J Clin Anesth. 1997;9:312–6.

5 Anesthetic Considerations in Patients with Valvular Heart Disease

Heather L. Lander and Martin Zammert

Case

A 70-year-old female presents with a shortness of breath on exertion and chest pain. She describes that she thought she would pass out from lightheadedness

Medications:

Toprol XL 100 mg daily
Aspirin 81 mg daily
Calcium 1 tab daily

NKDA

Physical Exam: BP: 130/70, HR: 85, RR: 16, O_2 Sat: 99% on RA. There is an audible systolic murmur at the left sternal border and concomitant holosystolic murmur at the apex with radiation to the axilla.

1. What are possible etiologies of aortic stenosis?

The etiologies for aortic stenosis can be divided into two categories:

(1) Congenital
   a. Unicuspid/Bicuspid
   b. Metabolic disease (Fabry's)
(2) Acquired
   a. Calcific disease
   b. Rheumatic disease
   c. Systemic Lupus Erythematosus (SLE)
   d. Endocarditis

2. What are possible etiologies for mitral regurgitation?

The etiologies for mitral regurgitation can be divided into two categories:

(1) Acute
   a. Papillary muscle rupture
   b. Endocarditis
(2) Chronic
   a. Myxomatous degeneration
   b. Ischemic heart disease
   c. Mitral annular dilatation
   d. Cardiomyopathy
   e. Rheumatic disease
   f. Connective Tissue Disorders

3. What are the different grades of aortic stenosis? (Table 5.1) [1]

4. What are the different grades for mitral regurgitation? (Table 5.2) [1]

5. What is the natural progression of aortic stenosis?

Aortic stenosis is the most common valvular lesion in the United States. Aortic stenosis is classically associated with a prolonged asymptomatic period followed by rapid development of symptoms. The three primary symptoms are angina, syncope and dyspnea on exertion (symptom of heart failure). Without intervention, these correlate with an average life expectancy of two to five years.

Risk factors for developing aortic stenosis include: increased age, male gender, dyslipidemia, diabetes, hypertension, smoking, renal insufficiency, or abnormal valve substrate. In high-risk patients, persistent inflammation, shear stress and pro-calcific stimuli ultimately result in

H.L. Lander · M. Zammert (✉)
Department of Anesthesiology, Perioperative and Pain Medicine, Brigham and Women's Hospital, 75 Francis Street, Boston, MA 02115, USA
e-mail: mzammert@partners.org

H.L. Lander
e-mail: hlander@partners.org

© Springer International Publishing AG 2017
L.S. Aglio and R.D. Urman (eds.), *Anesthesiology*,
DOI 10.1007/978-3-319-50141-3_5

Table 5.1 Different grades of aortic stenosis

	Valve area (cm^2)	Maximal aortic velocity (m/s)	Mean pressure gradient (mmHg)
Mild	>1.5	<3.0	<25
Moderate	1.0–1.5	3.0–4.0	25–40
Severe	0.6–0.9	>4.0	>40
Critical	<0.6	>4.0	>70

Table 5.2 Different grades for mitral regurgitation

	Mild	Moderate	Severe
Angiographic grade	1+	2+	3+–4+
Color Doppler jet area	Small, central jet <4 cm^2 or <20% of left atrial size	Signs of MR greater than mild, but not severe	Vena contracta width >0.7 cm^2 with large central jet (area >40% of left atrium) or with a wall-impinging jet swirling in left atrium
Doppler Vena contracta width (cm)	<0.3	0.3 – 0.69	≥0.7
Regurgitant volume (ml/beat)	<30	30-59	≥60
Regurgitant fraction (%)	<30	30-49	≥50
Regurgitant orifice area (cm^2)	<0.2	0.2–0.39	≥0.4
Left atrial size	Normal, unless other causes of left atrial dilation	Normal or dilated	Dilated, except acute MR
Left ventricular size	Normal, unless other causes of left ventricular dilation	Normal or dilated	Dilated, except acute MR
Mitral leaflets or support apparatus	Normal or abnormal	Normal of abnormal	Abnormal/flail leaflet, ruptured papillary muscle

valvular obstruction, decreased left ventricular ejection fraction and onset of symptoms. [2].

6. What is the natural progression of mitral regurgitation

Mitral regurgitation most commonly develops gradually because the left atrium and left ventricle are initially able to compensate for regurgitant flow. The left atrium accom modates the regurgitant volume by dilating, while the left ventricle undergoes remodeling and hypertrophy to maintain adequate forward flow. However, with an increasing regurgitant volume, the myocardial demand exceeds supply and results in decreased forward stroke volume, reduced cardiac output and subsequently decompensated heart failure.

In instances of acute mitral regurgitation, there is an abrupt increase in left atrial pressure without any time for left atrial or ventricular compensation; thus, the patient often develops acute pulmonary edema, decompensated heart failure, and cardiogenic shock.

7. How does aortic stenosis change the physiology of the heart?

The primary physiologic change in aortic stenosis is left ventricular outflow obstruction. Left ventricular outflow obstruction leads to an increased left ventricular systolic pressure and a prolonged ejection time in order to maintain cardiac output. To meet demand, the left ventricle undergoes concentric hypertrophy. With the reduction in LV compliance, the stroke volume becomes fixed. Myocardial oxygen demand increases in the presence of a hypertrophied left ventricle; however, coronary oxygen supply can be limited secondary due to the myocardial hypertrophy. The result is left ventricular dysfunction, myocardial ischemia and, without intervention, left ventricular failure.

8. How does mitral regurgitation change the physiology of the heart?

The primary physiologic change in mitral regurgitation is decreased forward flow. During systole, a portion of the left ventricular end diastolic volume regurgitates back into the left atrium, resulting in decreased forward flow, and left atrial volume overload. Over time, the left atrium dilates which can lead to arrhythmia such as atrial fibrillation.

9. What are surgical indications for aortic valve surgery?

- Severe high-grade aortic stenosis ($V_{max} \geq 4$ m/s and $\Delta P_{mean} \geq 40$ mmHg) with symptoms by history or on exercise testing.
- Asymptomatic patients with severe high-grade aortic stenosis ($V_{max} \geq 4$ m/s and $\Delta P_{mean} \geq 40$ mmHg) and left ventricular ejection fraction <50%.
- Asymptomatic patients with severe high-grade aortic stenosis ($V_{max} \geq 4$ m/s and $\Delta P_{mean} \geq 40$ mmHg) who undergo other cardiac surgery [3].

10. What surgical treatment options can be offered to this patient?

This patient is likely a candidate for open aortic valve replacement, given her symptomatic, severe, high-grade aortic stenosis. Given her advanced age, a bio-prosthetic valve is the most likely choice as this avoids the need for life-long anti-coagulation. Further investigation into her comorbidities is required to determine her surgical risk, as percutaneous valve replacement procedures are also an option.

11. What are the indications of a transcatheter aortic valve replacement (TAVR)?

Transcatheter aortic valve replacement is a minimally invasive procedure that was developed for patients with symptomatic, severe aortic stenosis who are poor surgical candidates or who have structural (either congenital or acquired) abnormalities that prevent successful surgery. There are three primary approaches from which a TAVR can be performed: transfemoral, transapical, and transaortic.

12. What are the hemodynamic goals during induction of general anesthesia in patients with severe aortic stenosis?

The hemodynamic goals for patients with severe aortic stenosis include:

- Maintain normal sinus rhythm: Cardiac output is dependent on an appropriately timed atrial contraction to ensure maximal left ventricular end diastolic volume. Ventricular filling is important as the stroke volume is fixed in severe aortic stenosis due to a reduced LV compliance.
- Avoid hypotension: Hypotension decreases coronary perfusion and can result in decreased left ventricular function and, consequently, decreased cardiac output.
- Avoid bradycardia and tachycardia: Heart rate is a major determinant of left ventricular filling. Bradycardia increases left ventricular filling time and can result in over distension of the left ventricle. Tachycardia, on the other hand, decreases left ventricular filling time and decreases left ventricular end diastolic volume resulting in reduced cardiac output. Tachycardia also increases the oxygen demand of the hypertrophic myocardium and oxygen supply can be reduced due to decreased coronary perfusion time.

13. What is the approach for induction of anesthesia in patients with multiple valvular pathologies?

In patients with multiple valvular pathologies, the leading lesion should take priority with regard to induction goals. In this case, the patient has severe aortic stenosis with concomitant mitral regurgitation. Induction should be planned according to the goals for optimizing aortic stenosis.

14. What drugs should be avoided in patients with severe aortic stenosis?

Medications to avoid include:

- Ketamine: Given that heart rate is a major determinant of left ventricular filling and oxygen demand, the sympathetic stimulation and tachycardia associated with ketamine makes it a poor choice.
- Medications that decrease SVR: Decreasing SVR results in decreased cardiac output and an increased risk of myocardial ischemia.

15. How should a patient with severe aortic stenosis undergoing heart surgery be monitored?

Prior to induction, standard ASA monitors (EKG, NIBP, temperature, oxygen saturation, and capnography) and an arterial line should be placed for hemodynamic monitoring during induction. Following induction, central venous access and transesophageal echocardiography are appropriate for intraoperative monitoring and delivery of medications. In specific situations, a pulmonary artery catheter may be indicated to help inform specific clinical decision-making.

16. Would a pulmonary artery catheter be indicated during aortic valve surgery?

To date, no study has demonstrated improved outcomes in critically ill patients monitored with pulmonary artery catheters versus non-invasive or clinical assessment. Additionally, complications related to insertion and maintenance of pulmonary artery catheters can result in serious adverse outcomes for the patient. Such complications include: arrhythmias, pneumothorax, massive hemorrhage (secondary to perforation of superior vena cava or right ventricle), and infection.

The decision to place a pulmonary artery catheter should be made on an individual basis, where a specific patient management question cannot be answered by non-invasive methods or clinical assessment. Specific situations where pulmonary artery catheter monitoring may provide helpful information include: severe pulmonary hypertension, right ventricular failure, severe lung disease, and tricuspid regurgitation [4].

17. What is the role of transesophageal echocardiography during aortic valve replacement surgery?

Transesophageal echocardiography is used during aortic valve replacement to guide appropriate selection of prosthesis size, confirm prosthesis seating and assess perivalvular leak and pre/post-procedural valvular function.

In the case of aortic valve replacement surgery, transesophageal echocardiography does not improve the surgical outcome of the patient.

18. What are the guidelines for antibiotic prophylaxis in patients with structural heart disease?

- According to the 2008 updated AHA guidelines for recommended endocarditis prophylaxis, the following patient populations should received antibiotic prophylaxis for dental procedures involving manipulation of gingival tissue, invasive procedures on the respiratory tract requiring biopsy or incision of respiratory mucosa and with surgical procedures involving infected skin or musculoskeletal tissue.

  Patients with:

- Prosthetic heart valves
- History of infective endocarditis
- Unrepaired congenital heart defect (including palliative shunts/conduits)
- Completely repaired congenital heart defects during the first 6 months after the corrective procedure
- Repaired congenital heart disease with residual defect at or adjacent to the site of prosthetic material, complex repairs
- Cardiac transplantation recipients with cardiac valvular disease.

It is important to mention the AHA does not recommend prophylaxis for patients having procedures involving the gastrointestinal, genitourinary, or reproductive system [5].

19. What regional and neuraxial anesthetic techniques can be used in patients with severe aortic stenosis undergoing non-cardiac surgery?

Neuraxial anesthetic techniques available to patients with severe aortic stenosis include epidural and continuous spinal anesthesia. Both allow for slow onset of anesthesia and close titration of medication in order to avoid hypotension.

Regional techniques are another option for specific non-cardiac cases as these also avoid induction and the stimulus of intubation, which both can lead to hemodynamic instability.

References

1. Bonow R, Carabello B, Chatterjee K, de Leon A, Faxon D, Freed M, et al. 2008 focused update incorporated into the ACC/AHA 2006 guidelines for the management of patients with valvular heart disease: a report of the American college of cardiology/American heart association task force on practice guidelines (writing committee to revise the 1998 guidelines for the management of patients with valvular heart disease): endorsed by the society of cardiovascular anesthesiologists, society for cardiovascular angiography and interventions, and society of thoracic surgeons. Circulation. 2008;118(15):e523–661.
2. Leon M, Smith C, Mack M, Miller D, Moses J, Svensson L, et al. Transcatheter aortic-valve implantation for aortic stenosis in patients who cannot undergo surgery. N Engl J Med. 2010;363(17):1597–607.
3. Nishimura R, Otto C, Bonow R, Carabello B, Erwin J, Guyton R, et al. 2014 AHA/ACC guideline for the management of patients with valvular heart disease: executive summary: a report of the American college of cardiology/American heart association task force on practice guidelines. Circulation. 2014;129(23):2440–92.
4. Binanay C, Califf RM, Hasselblad V, O'Connor CM, Shah MR, Sopko G, Stevenson LW, Francis GS, Leier CV, Miller LW. Evaluation study of congestive heart failure and pulmonary artery catheterization effectiveness: the ESCAPE trial. JAMA. 2005;294(13):1625–33.
5. Wilson W, Taubert K, Gewitz M, Lockhart P, Baddour L, Levison M, et al. Prevention of infective endocarditis: guidelines from the American heart association: a guideline from the American heart association rheumatic fever, endocarditis, and Kawasaki disease committee, council on cardiovascular disease in the young, and the council on clinical cardiology, council on cardiovascular surgery and anesthesia, and the quality of care and outcomes research interdisciplinary working group. Circulation. 2007;116(15):1736–54.

Mitral Stenosis

6

Agnieszka Trzcinka

CASE

A 52-year-old man presents with progressively worsening shortness of breath at rest and dyspnea on exertion. Echocardiography reveals evidence of mitral stenosis and pulmonary hypertension. Patient presents for mitral valve surgery.

Medications:	Atorvastatin 80 mg daily, metoprolol 100 mg daily, aspirin 81 mg daily
Allergies:	NKDA
Past medical history:	Chronic renal insufficiency
Physical exam:	
Vital signs:	HR: 84 BP: 124/62 RR: 14 oxygen saturation: 98% on room air

Patient is in no acute distress, but reports shortness of breath when walking down the hallway. Lungs are clear to auscultation bilaterally. 3/6 diastolic murmur is present.

Questions

1. **What is the definition of mitral stenosis?**

Mitral stenosis refers to a decreased mitral valve orifice area resulting in obstruction of blood flow from the left atrium into the left ventricle during diastole. The orifice area of a normal mitral valve is 4–6 cm^2. Patients become symptomatic during increased physical activity when the mitral valve area decreases to less than 2.5 cm^2. Symptoms may occur at rest when the mitral valve orifice area is less than 1.5 cm^2 [1–3].

2. **What is the most common cause of mitral stenosis?**

Rheumatic heart disease is the leading cause of mitral stenosis worldwide. This disease process leads to thickening of the mitral valve leaflets, thickening and fusion of subvalvular chordae as well as fusion of commissures. Less commonly, mitral stenosis is associated with carcinoid syndrome, mitral annular calcification, left atrial neoplasm, systemic lupus erythematosus, cor triatriatum and congenital abnormalities, such as parachute mitral valve [4–7].

3. **What are typical symptoms associated with mitral stenosis?**

Patients most often report symptoms of dyspnea on exertion that may progress to shortness of breath at rest. This symptom stems from progressively increased left atrial pressure from obstructed blood flow through small mitral valve. This leads to elevated pulmonary venous and pulmonary arterial pressure. Pulmonary hypertension may result in hemoptysis.

Patients may also experience palpitations. Elevated left atrial pressure leads to left atrial enlargement, which may result in new-onset atrial fibrillation. This places patients at a higher risk for thrombus formation and stroke.

Long-standing pulmonary hypertension contributes to right ventricular failure, which may result in significant peripheral edema [8].

4. **How is mitral stenosis managed conservatively?**

The most recent recommendations from the American Heart Association include anticoagulation therapy for patients with mitral stenosis and a history of any of the following:

(1) Embolic event in the past
(2) Atrial fibrillation (paroxysmal or persistent)
(3) Evidence of thrombus in left atrium.

A. Trzcinka (✉)
Department of Anesthesiology, Perioperative and Pain Medicine, Harvard Medical School, Brigham and Women's Hospital, 75 Francis Street, Boston, MA 02115, USA
e-mail: atrzcinka@partners.org

© Springer International Publishing AG 2017
L.S. Aglio and R.D. Urman (eds.), *Anesthesiology*,
DOI 10.1007/978-3-319-50141-3_6

Additionally, heart rate should be controlled in patients with mitral stenosis who develop atrial fibrillation (i.e., treatment with beta-blockers) [9, 10].

5. **What echo findings are consistent with mitral stenosis?**

In patients with mitral stenosis stemming from rheumatic heart disease, valve leaflets appear thickened with varying degree of valvular and subvalvular calcification. Depending on the duration and severity of the mitral stenosis, echocardiography reveals an increased transmitral pressure gradient and left atrial enlargement. Long-standing pulmonary hypertension associated with mitral stenosis results in dilatation of the right ventricle and subsequent right ventricular failure. Up to 30% of patients with mitral stenosis may have left ventricular dysfunction [11, 12].

6. **How is mitral stenosis severity graded?**

Echocardiography is the recommended tool to grade mitral stenosis, which can be evaluated using: pressure gradient, mitral valve area planimetry, pressure half-time, and the continuity equation. The grading of mitral stenosis is based mainly on the direct measurement or calculation of the mitral valve area (mean pressure gradient and pulmonary artery pressure values are only supportive findings). MVA of more than 1.5 cm^2 corresponds to mild mitral stenosis, MVA between 1.0 and 1.5 cm^2 corresponds to moderate mitral stenosis, and MVA of less than 1.0 cm^2 is classified as severe mitral stenosis [11, 12].

7. **What physical exam findings are consistent with diagnosis of mitral stenosis?**

Auscultation reveals a diastolic murmur that is appreciated best at the apex with the patient resting on left side. Often, there is an opening snap heard after S2 [13].

8. **How do you define pulmonary hypertension?**

The definition of pulmonary hypertension includes a mean pulmonary artery pressure above 25 mmHg and a pulmonary artery occlusion pressure below 15 mmHg on repeated measurements [14].

9. **What is the current classification of pulmonary hypertension?**

According to World Health Organization, pulmonary hypertension can be classified as:

(1) Pulmonary arterial hypertension
(2) Pulmonary hypertension associated with left heart disease
(3) Pulmonary hypertension related to lung disease and/or hypoxemia
(4) Pulmonary hypertension associated with chronic thromboembolic disease
(5) Pulmonary hypertension associated with miscellaneous disorders, such as sarcoidosis and lymphangiomatosis [15].

10. **What are your main anesthetic management considerations in the patient with mitral stenosis?**

(1) Maintain normal heart rate and rhythm: increased heart rate leads to shorter diastole and an elevated trans-mitral pressure gradient
(2) Prevent worsening of pulmonary hypertension which would contribute to decreased right ventricular function
(3) Provide adequate preload [16].

11. **What factors contribute to worsening pulmonary hypertension during the perioperative period?**

Hypoxemia, hypercarbia, and acidosis may worsen the patient's pulmonary hypertension. It is important to avoid heavy preoperative sedation in patients with mitral stenosis and administer supplemental oxygen if small doses of premedication are given.

12. **What monitors are needed for this patient?**

Placement of an arterial line will help anesthesiologist with early recognition and treatment of BP changes during the perioperative period as well as frequent arterial blood gas evaluations. Since induction of anesthesia may be associated with marked hemodynamic instability in patients with mitral stenosis, the arterial line should be placed before induction. Transesophageal echocardiography (TEE) will be used in this patient scheduled for mitral valve surgery to further assess valvular pathology. TEE is also a useful tool to evaluate left and right ventricular function as well as ventricular filling. The anesthesiologist may consider placement of a pulmonary artery catheter taking into consideration that pulmonary artery pressure values may not accurately reflect left ventricular filling in patients with mitral stenosis and pulmonary hypertension [16].

13. **How are you going to induce anesthesia in this patient?**

It is important to avoid tachycardia during the perioperative period and the patient should continue his current beta-blocker treatment preoperatively. Heart rate may still be difficult to control during laryngoscopy. The anesthesiologist may choose to use a large dose of opioid during induction to blunt the tachycardia response during laryngoscopy. Beta-blockers should be readily available to treat tachycardia as well.

14. **How will you treat hypotension that occurs shortly after induction?**

The goal is to optimize cardiac output when addressing hypotension in the setting of mitral stenosis. Fluid may be needed to provide adequate preload, but the anesthesiologist must monitor for possible signs of acute pulmonary edema that may develop in a patient with severe mitral stenosis. Phenylephrine (alpha-1 agonist effect) may be needed to treat vasodilation after induction and will increase afterload to maintain coronary perfusion. The anesthesiologist must also evaluate the EKG to assess for normal sinus rhythm and avoid tachycardia.

15. **How are you going to treat new acute-onset atrial fibrillation with rapid ventricular response intra-operatively?**

Tachycardia is detrimental to a patient with mitral stenosis and results in an elevated trans-mitral pressure gradient. Additionally, atrial fibrillation (especially atrial fibrillation with rapid ventricular response) would contribute to further hemodynamic instability due to decreased left ventricular filling with loss of atrial kick. Therefore, the patient would need cardioversion.

16. **Would you administer antibiotic prophylaxis before a dental procedure for prevention of infective endocarditis in patients with severe mitral stenosis?**

No. Patients with mitral stenosis do not need infective endocarditis prophylaxis. Patients in need of such therapy include those with: a history of endocarditis, prosthetic intracardiac valves, unrepaired cyanotic congenital heart disease, repaired congenital heart disease with prosthetic material for the first 6 months following the repair, s/p heart transplantation with valvular pathology, and repaired congenital heart disease with remaining defect [9, 17].

References

1. Gorlin WB, Gorlin R. A generalized formulation of the Gorlin formula for calculating the area of the stenotic mitral valve and other stenotic cardiac valves. J Am Coll Cardiol. 1990;15(1):246–7.
2. Bruce CJ, Nishimura RA. Clinical assessment and management of mitral stenosis. Cardiol Clin. 1998;16(3):375–403.
3. Rapaport E. Natural history of aortic and mitral valve disease. Am J Cardiol. 1975;35(2):221–7.
4. Iung B, Baron G, Butchart EG, Delahaye F, Gohlke-Barwolf C, Levang OW, et al. A prospective survey of patients with valvular heart disease in Europe: The Euro Heart Survey on Valvular Heart Disease. Eur Heart J. 2003;24(13):1231–43.
5. Horstkotte D, Niehues R, Strauer BE. Pathomorphological aspects, aetiology and natural history of acquired mitral valve stenosis. Eur Heart J. 1991;12 Suppl B:55–60. PubMed PMID: 1936027.
6. Akram MR, Chan T, McAuliffe S, Chenzbraun A. Non-rheumatic annular mitral stenosis: prevalence and characteristics. Eur J Echocardiogr: J Working Group Echocardiogr Eur Soc Cardiol. 2009;10(1):103–5.
7. Pressman GS, Agarwal A, Braitman LE, Muddassir SM. Mitral annular calcium causing mitral stenosis. Am J Cardiol. 2010;105(3):389–91.
8. Levy S. Factors predisposing to the development of atrial fibrillation. Pacing Clin Electrophysiol: PACE. 1997;20(10 Pt 2): 2670–4.
9. Nishimura RA, Otto CM, Bonow RO, Carabello BA, Erwin JP 3rd, Guyton RA, et al. 2014 AHA/ACC guideline for the management of patients with valvular heart disease: executive summary: a report of the American College of Cardiology/ American Heart Association Task Force on Practice Guidelines. J Am Coll Cardiol. 2014;63(22):2438–88.
10. Bruce CJ, Nishimura RA. Newer advances in the diagnosis and treatment of mitral stenosis. Curr Probl Cardiol. 1998;23(3): 125–92.
11. Baumgartner H, Hung J, Bermejo J, Chambers JB, Evangelista A, Griffin BP, et al. Echocardiographic assessment of valve stenosis: EAE/ASE recommendations for clinical practice. Eur J Echocardiogr: J Working Group Echocardiogr Eur Soc Cardiol. 2009;10(1):1–25.
12. Klein AJ, Carroll JD. Left ventricular dysfunction and mitral stenosis. Heart Failure Clin. 2006;2(4):443–52.
13. Bickley LS, ed. Bates' guide to physical examination and history taking. 11th ed. Philadelphia: Lippincott Williams & Wilkins; 2013:401.
14. Fischer SP, Bader AM, Sweiter BJ. Preoperative evaluation. In: Miller RD, Eriksson LI, Fleisher LA, Wiener-Kronish JP, Young WL, editors. Miller's Anesthesia. 7th ed. Philadelphia: Churchill Livingstone, Elsevier; 2010:1001–1066.
15. McLaughlin VV, Archer SL, Badesch DB, Barst RJ, Farber HW, Lindner JR, et al. ACCF/AHA 2009 expert consensus document on pulmonary hypertension a report of the American College of Cardiology Foundation Task Force on Expert Consensus Documents and the American Heart Association developed in collaboration with the American College of Chest Physicians; American Thoracic Society, Inc.; and the Pulmonary Hypertension Association. J Am Coll Cardiol. 2009;53(17):1573–619.
16. Cook DJ, Housmans PR, Rehfeldt. Valvular heart disease. In: Kaplan JA, Reich DL, Savino JS, editors. Kaplan's Cardiac Anesthesia: the echo era. 6th ed. Elsevier; 2011:570–614.
17. Wilson W, Taubert KA, Gewitz M, Lockhart PB, Baddour LM, Levison M, et al. Prevention of infective endocarditis: guidelines from the American Heart Association: a guideline from the American Heart Association Rheumatic Fever, Endocarditis, and Kawasaki Disease Committee, Council on Cardiovascular Disease in the Young, and the Council on Clinical Cardiology, Council on Cardiovascular Surgery and Anesthesia, and the Quality of Care and Outcomes Research Interdisciplinary Working Group. Circulation. 2007;116(15):1736–54.

7 Eisenmenger Syndrome

Marilyn Diane Michelow

CASE:

A 37-year-old woman who immigrated to the United States in her late 20s presents to the emergency department with three days of right upper quadrant pain, low grade fevers, nausea, and vomiting. She is diagnosed with acute cholecystitis by ultrasound and scheduled for urgent cholecystectomy. Her medical history is significant for a large ventricular septal defect that was not corrected in childhood. She has a diagnosis of Eisenmenger's syndrome and is followed by an adult congenital heart disease specialist. She states her baseline oxygen saturation is 88% on room air.

Medications:

Furosemide 40 mg oral twice daily
Sildenafil 10 mg oral three times per day
Bosentan 125 mg oral twice daily
Allergies: No known drug allergies

Past Medical History:

Cardiac: Uncorrected large ventricular septal defect, recent right heart catheterization documenting right ventricular systolic pressures >100 mmHg and a right to left shunt.
No history of arrhythmias or endocarditis
Pulmonary: Documented pulmonary hypertension secondary to Eisenmenger's syndrome. Baseline oxygen saturation is 88% on room air. One episode of hemoptysis three years ago that resolved spontaneously.
Renal: Chronic renal impairment with elevated creatinine, gout

M.D. Michelow (✉)
Department of Anesthesiology, Perioperative and Pain Medicine, Brigham and Women's Hospital, 75 Francis St., Boston, MA 02115, USA
e-mail: marilyn.michelow@ucsf.edu

© Springer International Publishing AG 2017
L.S. Aglio and R.D. Urman (eds.), *Anesthesiology*,
DOI 10.1007/978-3-319-50141-3_7

Physical Exam:
Vital signs: Blood pressure 110/90 Heart rate 90, sinus rhythm Respiratory rate 18 Oxygen Saturation 87% room air
General: The patient is visibly cyanotic, no acute distress
Cardiovascular: Regular rate and rhythm. Heart is enlarged. Holosystolic murmur audible throughout
Pulmonary: Lung sounds are clear to auscultation bilaterally
Abdominal: Right upper quadrant tenderness to palpation with positive Murphy's sign
Extremities: 1+ pitting edema bilaterally, hypertrophic osteoarthropathy, peripheral cyanosis
Laboratory studies:
Na 138 K4.7 Cl 108 HCO3 22 BUN 40 Cr 1.9
WBC 14 K Hematocrit 65% Platelets 90
Liver function tests notable for total bilirubin 3.6 with elevated alkaline phosphatase. AST and ALT are normal
Coagulation studies are pending

1. **What is Eisenmenger's Syndrome?**

Eisenmenger's Syndrome is characterized by *irreversible pulmonary hypertension* resulting from an uncorrected congenital cardiac anomaly. Patients with Eisenmenger's syndrome have a longstanding left to right shunt (through an intracardiac or aortopulmonary congenital lesion, such as a ventricular septal defect, atrial septal defect, or patent ductus arteriosus) that over time causes endothelial changes in the pulmonary vasculature leading to pulmonary hypertension. As right-sided pressures approach systemic pressures, the shunt is reversed, right to left or bidirectional. As a result of their reversed shunt, these patients have arteriovenous mixing and chronic cyanosis, with baseline arterial saturations of 70–95% on room air.

At the 5th World Symposium on Pulmonary Hypertension held in 2013, Eisenmenger's syndrome was classified as Group 1 Pulmonary Hypertension [1].

2. **Discuss the common complications of Eisenmenger's syndrome by system (see Table 7.1).**

3. **What is the predicted perioperative mortality for patients with Eisenmenger's syndrome undergoing noncardiac surgery?**

There is a range in the reported literature, but generally perioperative mortality is high. 7–18% in one large study, but higher for emergent procedures. One recent study found a 25–30% perioperative mortality rate for patients with Eisenmenger's syndrome undergoing major surgery or labor [2].

4. **What are the predictors of poor post-operative function in a patient with Eisenmenger's syndrome?**
   - Low baseline functional status
   - Clinical signs of heart failure
   - History of arrhythmia or current arrhythmia
   - Elevated right atrial pressure
   - Right ventricular hypertrophy or other repolarization abnormalities on EKG
   - Complex cardiac anatomy

5. **Describe the factors that will increase pulmonary vascular resistance**
   - Hypoxia
   - Hypercarbia
   - Metabolic acidosis
   - Hypothermia
   - Agitation
   - Pain
   - Tracheal suctioning

6. **How do you calculate pulmonary vascular resistance (PVR)? What are the normal values? What can you expect PVR to be in this patient?**

((mean pulmonary artery pressure − pulmonary capillary wedge pressure)*80)/Cardiac output (L) = PVR in dyne*s*cm^{-5}

Normal values for PVR are approximately <250 dyne*s*cm^{-5}, but can be >800 in patients with Eisenmenger's syndrome.

7. **Discuss the major targeted therapies available for pulmonary hypertension (Table 7.2)**

8. **What is the appropriate preoperative testing for a patient with Eisenmenger's syndrome?**
   - Recent echocardiogram to assess right ventricular (RV) function
   - Recent right heart catheterization for measurement of pulmonary and right ventricular pressures (in an emergent situation, estimation of pulmonary artery systolic pressures using the TR jet on echocardiogram would be reasonable instead of catheterization)
   - Pulmonary function tests, especially for thoracic surgical procedures
   - Labs including CBC (looking for baseline hematocrit, platelets), CMP (electrolyte abnormalities from diuretics, renal dysfunction, hyperbilirubinemia, hyperuricemia), coagulation studies including fibrinogen (clotting factor deficiencies, hypofibrinogenemia), BNP if this has been serially followed
   - Electrocardiogram looking for arrhythmias and repolarization abnormalities
   - Referral to a pulmonary hypertension specialist to optimize the perioperative pulmonary hypertension regimen
   - Assessment of functional status [1]

9. **Discuss the hemodynamic considerations for an anesthetic in a patient with Eisenmenger's syndrome. What parameters are you particularly concerned about maintaining? What will happen if the patient does have a drop or rise in systemic vascular resistance (SVR) or cardiac output (CO)?**

The principle anesthetic goals are to avoid increases in pulmonary vascular resistance and to avoid right ventricular

Table 7.1 Common complications of eisenmenger's syndrome by system[a]

System	Common complications
Cardiac	Right ventricular failure/infarction, congestive heart failure, dysrhythmias (atrial fibrillation, supraventricular tachycardia most common), infective endocarditis, cardiac syncope, sudden death
Respiratory	Hemoptysis, pulmonary hemorrhage, chronic pulmonary emboli, pulmonary infarction, hypoxia
Neurologic	Brain abscess, embolic strokes, intracerebral hemorrhage, TIA
Hematologic	Hyperviscosity syndrome, thrombosis, platelet dysfunction, clotting factor deficiencies (vWF deficiency in particular), hypofibrinogenemia
Hepatobiliary	Hyperbilirubinemia, pigment gallstones
Renal	Chronic renal disease with decreased glomerular filtration rate, hyperuricemia leading to gout, nephrolithiasis
Skeletal	Hypertrophic osteoarthropathy

[a]Adapted from [1], Copyright 2014 Springer Science+Business Media

Table 7.2 Major targeted therapies available for pulmonary hypertension

Medication class	Mechanism of action	Available drugs	Route of administration	Major side effects
Nitric oxide pathway	Inhibit PDE-5 to decrease c-GMP breakdown NO increases c-GMP production to cause pulmonary vasodilation	Sildenafil Taldalafil iNO	PO PO (once daily dosing) Continuous inhaled	Flushing, headache, hypotension
Prostanoids	Augment endogenous prostacyclin to cause pulmonary vasodilation	Epoprostenol Treprostinil Iloprost	Cont IV/Inhaled Cont SQ/IV, Int inhaled, PO Int Inhaled	Flushing, headache, diarrhea, cough. Rebound pulmonary hypertensive crisis if stopped suddenly
Endothelin receptor antagonists	Inhibit endothelin-1, a potent pulmonary vasoconstrictor	Bosentan Ambrisentan Macitentan	PO PO PO	LFT elevations, headache, anemia, contraindicated in pregnancy

Reference [3, 6]

failure. This can be done by maintaining systemic vascular resistance (SVR), avoiding decreases in cardiac output, and avoiding insults that increase PVR (see question #5).

A drop in SVR is dangerous for three reasons:

1. A drop in SVR will increase the R -> L shunt, leading to worsening hypoxemia and subsequent decrease in the oxygen delivery to tissues (particularly the heart and brain).
2. Worsening hypoxemia is a trigger for pulmonary arterial vasoconstriction, increasing pulmonary vascular resistance
3. A drop in SVR will lead to decreased coronary perfusion, which (combined with increased pulmonary vascular resistance and hypoxemia) will lead to RV ischemia, RV failure, and, if untreated, a very rapid spiral of pulmonary hypertensive crisis leading to cardiac arrest.

On the other hand, an increase in SVR can cause RV overload and lead to heart failure.

10. **Discuss the risks related to perioperative arrhythmia in Eisenmenger's syndrome patients:**

Perioperative arrhythmias are very common in patients with Eisenmenger's syndrome. There is up to a 30% incidence of perioperative arrhythmia. Most common arrhythmias include rapid atrial fibrillation (often new onset), SVT, or even VT/VF. Arrhythmias are a major cause of perioperative morbidity and mortality because a rapid rhythm can lead to a drop in cardiac output and the spiral of pulmonary hypertension and RV failure leading to sudden cardiac death.

Do everything you can to maintain sinus rhythm and promptly treat arrhythmias!

11. **Discuss the perioperative concerns relating to the hematologic abnormalities seen in Eisenmenger's syndrome.**

<u>Elevated hematocrit</u>

The physiologic response to chronic cyanosis is to increase erythropoietin production leading to an elevated hematocrit to maintain tissue oxygenation. At a hematocrit greater than 65%, some patients experience a *hyperviscosity syndrome* of increasing cardiac load, headaches, dizziness, fatigue, myalgias, and weakness.

As an outpatient this is treated with isovolemic phlebotomy, only if the patient is symptomatic.

*Perioperatively, many practitioners will perform isovolemic phlebotomy to a hematocrit of 65% so that blood for autologous donation is available for surgery.

<u>Coagulation Abnormalities</u>

Patients with Eisenmenger's syndrome generally have a bleeding diathesis, but are also prone to thromboembolism leading to DVT/PE and CVA.

- Platelets—both a qualitative and quantitative deficiency
- Abnormalities of the clotting cascade, particularly deficiency of the vitamin K dependent factors (II, VII, IX, X)
- Acquired von Willibrand's factor (vWF) deficiency

Measurement of PT and PTT may be inaccurate if not properly corrected for the elevated hematocrit. In addition, many patients with Eisenmenger's syndrome are on chronic anticoagulation for atrial fibrillation, pulmonary emboli, or strokes, which further complicates the coagulopathy picture.

*Anesthesiologists can consider giving desmopressin or factor VIII to control bleeding if acquired vWF syndrome is suspected.

*Exercise caution when considering regional anesthesia. Use of peripheral nerve blocks and epidural anesthesia is described, but spinal anesthesia is relatively contraindicated in these patients (both because of the bleeding risk and the potential drop in SVR).

Abnormal Vasogenesis

Chronic hypoxemia produces abnormal vasogenesis and operative bleeding may be higher due to increased vascularity. Pulmonary hemorrhage is a known and sometimes fatal complication for patients with Eisenmenger's syndrome.

Eisenmenger's syndrome patients DO not tolerate hypovolemia or hypervolemia well so bleeding should be closely monitored and volume replaced promptly [1, 3, 4].

12. **What kind of invasive monitoring will you need for this patient? What are the pros and cons of these monitoring techniques?**

An arterial line is indicated and helpful for close hemodynamic monitoring in this patient.

Central lines carry considerable risk in patients with right to left shunt: air or thrombus has a high chance of paradoxical embolization, and can cause a stroke or brain abscess.

PA lines carry an additional danger of pulmonary artery rupture and may also induce arrhythmias. A PA line may be helpful in a very sick patient, but is probably not indicated in this case.

A TEE evaluation can be helpful to guide volume management if a large blood loss or extensive fluid shifts are expected intraoperatively.

13. **Preparing for this case, what special medications and equipment will you want to have immediately available?**

In addition to a standard general anesthetic setup and an arterial line as discussed above, consider:

- Air filters for all lines
- Availability of TEE and a provider who can immediately perform the exam
- Ability to initiate rapid inhaled or IV pulmonary vasodilator therapies such as iNO, IV or inhaled epoprostenol [3].

14. **What is your induction strategy?**
    - Preinduction arterial line, check an arterial blood gas and correct hypoxemia and acidosis before surgery.
    - Target euvolemia before induction
    - Preinduction, consider starting an agent to reduce PVR, such as epoprostenol, milrinone, nitroglycerin, or iNO. It is reasonable in volume replete patients with Eisenmenger's syndrome to have milrinone infusing prior to induction.
    - Pre-oxygenation with 100% O_2 to get arterial sat >90%.
    - Consider a rapid sequence induction to minimize apnea time which may lead to respiratory acidosis.
    - An ideal induction agent will not drop SVR. Most providers would use an opioid, benzodiazepine and either etomidate or ketamine combination for induction to minimize the changes in SVR. Unless titrating very carefully, it is best to avoid propofol and thiopental. Inhalational induction is also possible, though again caution is advised as it will likely be accompanied by a drop in SVR [1, 3–5].

15. **What effect does this patient's right to left shunt have on the speed of anesthetic induction?**
    - IV induction may be more rapid as blood bypasses the lungs and travels more rapidly to the brain
    - Inhalational induction will be slower, especially for highly insoluble agents because less anesthetic is absorbed in the lungs and venous mixing will further decrease the arterial concentration of blood going to the brain.

16. **What is your plan for maintenance of anesthesia in this patient? Ventilator settings?**

Foremost, whatever maintenance agent you use the overarching goal is to avoid hypotension and anything that increases pulmonary vascular resistance (hypoxia, hypercarbia, hypothermia, acidosis, hypovolemia).

- It is important to provide adequate pain control without going so far as to lead to significant post-operative hypercarbia.
- It is best to avoid nitrous oxide as it is a pulmonary vasoconstrictor and can increase PVR.
- Keep the patient warm, use a Bair hugger or underbody warmer, and warmed fluids.
- This will likely be a laparoscopic procedure and minute ventilation should be adjusted accordingly to avoid hypercarbia.
- Abdominal insufflation may also lead to decreased venous return and you may need to ask the surgeons to lower the insufflation pressure, or convert to an open procedure if the patient is not tolerating pneumoperitoneum.

- Avoid high tidal volumes and high PEEP with mechanical ventilation so as not to compromise venous return [1, 3].

17. **Intraoperatively, your patient develops sudden hypotension. PVR has also doubled. What medications do you reach for?**
    1. Stabilize arterial blood pressure with a pressor (norepinepherine, epinephrine, vasopressin or dopamine are reasonable). Consider an IABP if you are worried about impending heart failure.
    2. Start pulmonary vasodilator therapy: milrinone if the patient's arterial pressure stabilizes, or iNO, inhaled or IV epoprostenol.
    3. Correct causes of pulmonary hypertension if possible (metabolic acidosis, hypovolemia, hypothermia, hypercarbia).
    4. Consider ECMO early if the cycle does not appear to be breaking. These patients can go into cardiogenic shock very quickly.

18. **What are the considerations for post-op recovery in the PACU and subsequently on the floor?**
    - Avoiding hypoxemia/hypercarbia, counterbalanced by;
    - Effective but cautious pain control
    - Avoiding NSAIDs, as the majority of adult Eisenmenger's syndrome patients have renal dysfunction
    - Removing central venous catheters as soon as possible, given the risk for paradoxical emboli
    - Careful weaning of any medications being administered for pulmonary hypertension to avoid rebound pulmonary hypertension
    - Early mobilization given risk for thromboembolism (and particularly paradoxical stroke) [3]

19. **In patients with Eisenmenger's syndrome, should you in general (not in this case) consider regional anesthesia? Why or why not?**

There is a debate about the use of regional anesthesia in Eisenmenger's syndrome due to the high incidence of platelet dysfunction and coagulation factor abnormalities. Each case should be evaluated individually. Generally, it is reasonable to avoid spinal anesthesia because of the rapid drop in SVR that can be seen with administration of intrathecal anesthetics. For labor, epidural anesthesia is thought to be safe, but always avoid it in a patient who is on anticoagulation or otherwise has a bleeding diathesis. When possible, peripheral regional techniques and avoidance of GA and sedation altogether may be ideal. However, exercise extreme caution with the use of a regional anesthetic combined with monitored anesthesia care, as there is a great risk of over-sedation leading to hypercarbia [2].

20. **What are the special considerations for the parturient with Eisenmenger's syndrome?**

Individuals with Eisenmenger's syndrome who fall pregnant have an estimated 30% mortality rate during pregnancy. The majority of this mortality is seen during and immediately after delivery. Eisenmenger's syndrome is considered an absolute contraindication to pregnancy, but you may still see it! SVR is decreased in pregnancy. In the patient with Eisenmenger's syndrome, the decrease in SVR increases the right to left shunt fraction, which in turn worsens arterial hypoxemia. At delivery, blood loss further drops SVR and increases the shunt fraction. This combined with acute anemia decreasing oxygen carrying capacity can lead to a fatal spiral of hypoxemia, pulmonary hypertension, and RV failure.

The successful use of epidural anesthesia has been reported for both vaginal delivery and cesarean section. However, some centers advocate that mothers be on thromboembolism prophylaxis during pregnancy because of the high risk of DVT/PE in this population.

Babies born to mothers with Eisenmenger's syndrome often have severe intrauterine growth restriction as a result of chronic hypoxia, as well as many fetal anomalies [5].

21. **Why are outcomes generally better for patients with Eisenmenger's syndrome than for those with primary pulmonary hypertension?**

The presence of a right to left shunt functions essentially as a 'pop off valve' for the right ventricle, resulting in lower RV pressures, which preserves right ventricular function longer and maintains systemic cardiac output in the presence of worsening pulmonary hypertension (albeit at the expense of arterial O2 saturation) [1].

22. **What is the only definitive management of Eisenmenger's Syndrome?**

Heart and lung transplantation.

References

1. Das BB. Perioperative care of children with eisenmenger syndrome undergoing non-cardiac surgery. Pediatr Cardiol. 2015;36(6):1120–8.
2. Martin JT, Tautz TJ, Antognini JF. Safety of Regional Anesthesia in Eisenmenger's Syndrome. Reg Anesth Pain Med. 2002 Sept–Oct;27(5):509–513.

3. Minai OA, Yared JP, Kaw R, Subramaniam K, Hill NS. Perioperative risk and management in patients with pulmonary hypertension. Chest. 2013;144(1):329–405.
4. Oechslin E, Mebus S, Schulze-Neick I, Niwa K, Trindade PT, Eicken A, et al. The adult patient with eisenmenger syndrome: a medical update after dana point Part III: specific management and surgical aspects. Curr Cardiol Rev. 2010;6(4):363–72.
5. Bennett JM, Ehrenfeld JM, Markham L, Eagle SS. Anesthetic management and outcomes for patients with pulmonary hypertension and intracardiac shunts and Eisenmenger syndrome: a review of institutional experience. J Clin Anesth. 2014;26(4):286–93.
6. McLaughlin VV, Shah SJ, Souza R, Humbert M. Management of pulmonary arterial hypertension. J Amer Coll Cardiol. 2015;65(18):1976–97.

8 Subacute Bacterial Endocarditis Prophylaxis

Marilyn Diane Michelow

Case

A 37-year-old woman with a ventricular septal defect (VSD) is scheduled for an upper endoscopy to evaluate for Barrett's esophagus in the setting of longstanding gastrointestinal reflux disease.

1. **Should this patient receive antibiotic prophylaxis against infective endocarditis for the endoscopy? Why or why not?**

No—according to the 2008 ACC/AHA guidelines on Infective Endocarditis in Valvular Heart Disease, this patient does not require endocarditis prophylaxis for a routine noninvasive gastrointestinal procedure [1].

2. **What are the major causative organisms of subacute bacterial endocarditis?**

Viridans Streptococci account for somewhere between 25 and 50% of subacute bacterial endocarditis cases. These organisms are found in normal human oral flora.

Streptococcus bovis is the most common nonviridans streptococcal species to cause subacute infective endocarditis and is found in the lower GI tract, most commonly associated with colonic polyps and cancer.

Other causes of subacute bacterial endocarditis include the gram negative bacilli, HACEK organisms (*Haemophilus spp*., *Actinobacillus*, *Cardiobacterium*, *Eikenella*, *Kingella*).

For completeness, common causes of acute bacterial endocarditis (with a more fulminant presentation) include *Staphylococcus aureus* (about 1/3 of cases, very common in injecting drug users and healthcare associated endocarditis), enterococci, and gram negative bacteria such as *Pseudomonas aeruginosa* and enterics like *Escherichia coli*, *Proteus*, *Klebsiella*, etc. [2].

3. **Under the current (2008) ACC/AHA guidelines, review the circumstances when endocarditis prophylaxis would be indicated for patients with valvular heart disease.**

The 2008 ACC/AHA guidelines on endocarditis prophylaxis for patients with valvular heart disease represented a significant change from prior accepted practice.

Antibiotic prophylaxis is no longer recommended for patients with valvular heart disease at risk for infective endocarditis who undergo procedures of the respiratory, upper or lower GI or GU tract (i.e., bronchoscopy, TEE, endoscopy, colonoscopy, cystoscopy) in the absence of active infection.

The ACC/AHA guidelines do recommend antibiotic prophylaxis against infective endocarditis for dental procedures that involve perforation of the oral mucosa or manipulation of the gingival tissue in the following patients: those with prosthetic cardiac valves, previous episodes of infective endocarditis, heart transplant recipients who have a regurgitant valve lesion, patients with significant congenital heart disease and those with recently repaired congenital heart disease (within 6 months) [1].

4. **What are the NICE guidelines, and how do they differ from the ACC/AHA guidelines?**

The NICE guidelines on antibiotic prophylaxis against infective endocarditis were published by the United Kingdom's National Institute for Health and Clinical Excellence in 2008.

These guidelines do not recommend antibiotic prophylaxis against infective endocarditis in any patient for routine dental, GI, GU, or respiratory tract procedures. They do recommend prophylaxis with antibiotics that would cover

M.D. Michelow (✉)
Department of Anesthesiology, Perioperative and Pain Medicine, Brigham and Women's Hospital, 75 Francis St., Boston, MA 02115, USA
e-mail: marilyn.michelow@ucsf.edu

© Springer International Publishing AG 2017
L.S. Aglio and R.D. Urman (eds.), *Anesthesiology*,
DOI 10.1007/978-3-319-50141-3_8

the causative organisms of infective endocarditis *if* the above procedures are being performed to treat an active infection.

It has been suggested that the transient bacteremia from daily tooth brushing poses a greater risk of infective endocarditis than any single dental procedure. Furthermore, a 2 year follow up study after the NICE guidelines were published did not find any increase in infective endocarditis attributable to the change in practice despite widespread adoption of the guidelines in the United Kingdom [3, 4].

5. **If you are going to provide endocarditis prophylaxis to this patient for an invasive dental procedure, what antibiotic dosing regimen would be indicated?**

Single dose oral amoxicillin 3 g or clindamycin 600 mg [4].

References

1. Nishimura RA, Carabello BA, Faxon DP, Freed MD, Lytle BW, O'Gara PT, et al. ACC/AHA 2008 guideline update on valvular heart disease: focused update on infective endocarditis: a report of the American college of cardiology/American heart association task force on practice guidelines: endorsed by the society of cardiovascular anesthesiologists, society for cardiovascular angiography and interventions, and society of thoracic surgeons. Circulation. 2008;118(8):887–96.
2. McDonald JR. Acute infective endocarditis. Infect Dis Clin North Am. 2009;23(3):643–64.
3. Richey R, Wray D, Stokes T. Prophylaxis against infective endocarditis: summary of NICE guidance. BMJ. 2008;336(7647):770–1.
4. Thornhill MH, Dayer MJ, Forde JM, Corey GR, Chu VH, Couper DJ, et al. Impact of the NICE guideline recommending cessation of antibiotic prophylaxis for prevention of infective endocarditis: before and after study. BMJ. 2011;342:d2392.

Hypertrophic Cardiomyopathy (HCM)

9

Pingping Song

Case

A 33-year-old-male presents with a 2-year history of dyspnea and presyncope on strenuous exertion. Over the past two months, his symptoms progressively worsened until he was unable to carry out his daily job as a construction worker without having significant chest pain or dyspnea. On physical exam, vital signs are within normal limits. A grade 3/6 systolic murmur is noted at the apex, and its intensity increases with Valsalva maneuver. He is not on any medications. Past medical history is unremarkable. Family history reveals that his father died of a heart attack at 38 years of age, and his paternal uncle died as the driver in a single-car accident at 25 years of age. The patient's echocardiogram reveals a septal thickness of 24 mm and a left ventricular outflow tract (LVOT) peak gradient of 80 mmHg. Coronary angiogram shows no significant flow obstruction.

1. **What is the definition of hypertrophic cardiomyopathy (HCM)?**

Hypertrophic cardiomyopathy (HCM) is a genetic cardiac disorder caused by a missense mutation in one of at least ten genes that encode the proteins of the cardiac sarcomere. It is defined by left ventricular hypertrophy (LVH) without LV dilation (maximal LV wall thickness ≥15 mm at any segment, but typically involving the interventricular septum) [1, 2]. LVH cannot be explained by other cardiac or systemic conditions (such as aortic stenosis or other valvular lesion, restrictive cardiomyopathy, systemic hypertension, etc.). HCM is also referred to as idiopathic hypertrophic subaortic stenosis (IHSS), or hypertrophic obstructive cardiomyopathy (HOCM) [3, 4].

2. **What is the pathophysiology of HCM?**

The pathophysiology of HCM involves four interrelated processes [4–6]:

(1) Dynamic left ventricular outflow tract (LVOT) obstruction and systolic anterior motion of the mitral valve (SAM) (Fig. 9.1). The LVOT is narrowed by the hypertrophic interventricular septum and the anteriorly displaced papillary muscles. This narrowed LVOT creates flow acceleration during systole, dragging the anterior mitral leaflet into the LVOT, and contacting the septum (Venturi effect), subsequently causing LVOT obstruction. The obstruction can be subaortic or mid-ventricular. The LVOT obstruction in HCM patients is dynamic, characterized by spontaneous variability and influenced by factors that alter myocardial contractility and loading conditions. With increased contractility, decreased preload or decreased afterload, the LVOT obstruction becomes more severe.
(2) Diastolic dysfunction: due to impaired ventricular relaxation and decreased ventricular compliance (increased chamber stiffness). This leads to impaired ventricular diastolic filling.
(3) Myocardial ischemia: often occurs without artherosclerotic coronary artery disease. The postulated mechanisms include: ventricular hypertrophy causing obliteration of septal perforators; inadequate number of capillaries for the degree of LV mass; impaired coronary filling due to impaired relaxation.
(4) Mitral regurgitation (MR): systolic anterior motion of mitral valve (SAM) results in varying degrees of MR due to incomplete coaptation of mitral leaflets. The severity of MR is directly proportional to the degree of LVOT obstruction.

P. Song (✉)
Department of Anesthesiology, Perioperative and Pain Medicine, Brigham and Women's Hospital, 75 Francis St, Boston, MA, USA
e-mail: psong4@partners.org

© Springer International Publishing AG 2017
L.S. Aglio and R.D. Urman (eds.), *Anesthesiology*,
DOI 10.1007/978-3-319-50141-3_9

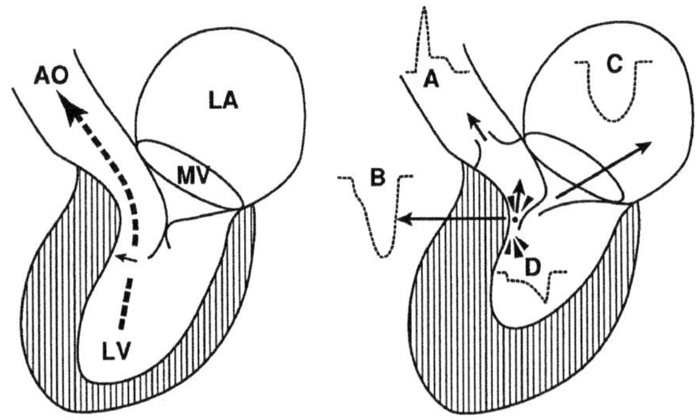

Fig. 9.1 Mechanism of LVOT obstruction and mitral regurgitation (MR) in patients with HCM. In early systole (*left*): The left ventricular outflow tract (LVOT) is narrowed by the hypertrophic interventricular septum and the anteriorly displaced papillary muscle. This creates flow acceleration during systole, dragging the anterior mitral leaflet into the LVOT and contacting the septum (Venturi effect), causing LVOT obstruction in late systole (*right*). The systolic anterior motion of the anterior leaflet (SAM) results in a failure of coaptation of the mitral leaflets and the onset of mitral regurgitation (MR). In most cases of HCM, the MR jet is directed posterior into the left atrium. Reproduced from [3], with permission of Wolters Kluwer

3. **What is the genetic background of HCM?**

HCM is inherited in an autosomal dominant Mendelian pattern with variable expression and age-related penetrance. The most common mutation in HCM is a missense mutation (a single normal amino acid is replaced for another) in the genes encoding the cardiac sarcomere. There is no clear relationship between the genotype and phenotype in HCM. It is impossible to predict the extent of expression or clinical outcome based on individual mutations [7–9].

4. **What are the common symptoms of HCM?**

(1) Dyspnea on exertion: most common symptom of HCM, occurring in over 90% of symptomatic patients. Dyspnea can result from diastolic dysfunction, mitral regurgitation, or impaired LV emptying and poor cardiac output due to LVOT obstruction.
(2) Chest pain: occurs in 25–30% of symptomatic HCM patients, usually in the setting of a normal coronary angiogram.
(3) Syncope and presyncope: occurs in about 20–25% of symptomatic HCM patients. Multiple mechanisms include arrhythmia, severe LVOT obstruction with exertion or myocardial ischemia.
(4) Sudden cardiac death: occurs in about 15% of symptomatic HCM patients. HCM is the most common cause of sudden death in otherwise apparently healthy athletes [10].
(5) Arrhythmia: supraventricular arrhythmias, most commonly atrial fibrillation; ventricular arrhythmias can also occur.
(6) Signs of advanced congestive heart failure are uncommon in HCM patients but may include orthopnea, paroxysmal dyspnea, and edema.

Physical exam is most commonly notable for systolic murmur on auscultation. A harsh systolic murmur can be best heard at the apex, caused by LVOT obstruction and/or mitral regurgitation. This murmur is dynamic in nature, and its intensity varies with changes in cardiac loading conditions and contractility. Maneuvers that decrease LV preload (e.g., changing to upright position from supine, Valsalva maneuver), enhance LV contractility and decrease LV afterload will all lead to worsening LVOT obstruction, thus increase the murmur intensity.

Other signs on physical exam are nonspecific, such as a brisk upstroke and bifid carotid pulse, resulting from sudden deceleration of blood due to LVOT obstruction.

5. **How to diagnose HCM?**

Besides clinical history, the following diagnostic methods are often used for diagnosis:

(1) Electrocardiography (ECG): over 90% of HCM patients have an abnormal ECG. Typically ECG shows localized or widespread repolarization changes. Patients may have abnormal Q waves, especially in the inferior or lateral leads. These changes reflect septal depolarization of the hypertrophied myocardium. Signs of LV hypertrophy (LVH) also exist, resulting in left axis deviation and ST-T wave abnormalities (horizontal or downsloping ST segment and T wave inversions).
(2) Echocardiography: transthoracic echocardiography (TTE) should be performed in all patients suspected of having HCM. A clinical diagnosis of HCM is confirmed when LV wall thickness ≥15 mm without LV dilation, in the absence of any identifiable cause such as hypertension or valve disease. The most common location of LV hypertrophy is the basal anterior septum in continuity with the anterior free wall. Other important TTE findings of HCM include: systolic anterior motion of mitral valve (SAM) and dynamic LVOT obstruction (see Fig. 1). For patients who do not have LVOT obstruction (LVOT gradient ≤30 mm Hg) at rest, provoking maneuvers should be performed to evaluate the gradient between the LVOT and aorta. Exercise stress echo is the preferred method [11].
(3) Exercise stress test: is recommended for all patients with known or suspected HCM as part of the risk

stratification and to assess the degree of LVOT obstruction. Positive findings during exercise testing include symptoms of dyspnea or angina, an increase or development of LVOT peak instantaneous gradient ≥30 mm Hg, an increase or development of mitral regurgitation, ST segment depression, and failure of the BP to increase appropriately with exercise [1, 2, 11].

(4) Cardiac MRI: provides superior spatial resolution compared to TTE. It can demonstrate myocardial scarring or thickening in segments which are difficult to assess via echocardiography. Cardiac MRI can be considered for patients suspected of having HCM but the diagnosis remains uncertain after TTE.

(5) Genetic testing: routine genetic testing is not recommended for diagnostic purposes due to the poor correlation between genotype, clinical presentation and outcome.

6. **What is the pharmacological treatment of HCM?**

The goal of managing HCM is to minimize LVOT obstruction by decreasing myocardial contractility, reducing heart rate, improving diastolic function, and ultimately optimizing ventricular filling. The most commonly used drugs are:

(1) Beta blockers: most effective in blunting the LVOT gradient provoked with exercise;
(2) Non-dihydropyridine calcium channel blockers, the most common drug of choice is verapamil [12, 13];
(3) Disopyramide: a potent negative inotropic agent, needs to be used with concomitant beta blockade, most reliable for reducing the LVOT gradient at rest [14].

Diuretics should be used very judiciously in patients presenting heart failure symptoms, balancing the benefit of decreasing edema and the risk of compromising LV preload and thus worsening LVOT obstruction.

7. **What are the non-pharmacological management options of HCM?**

For patients who have persistent heart failure symptoms (NYHA class III/IV) despite maximal medical therapy, or patients who have recurrent syncope from LVOT obstruction, and LVOT gradient ≥50 mm Hg at rest or with provocation, surgical myectomy should be considered. Alcohol septal ablation is another option for poor surgical candidates, such as patients of advanced age, with significant medical comorbidity, or possessing a strong desire to avoid open heart surgery [1, 2, 15, 16].

The advantages of surgical myectomy include: better symptom and LVOT gradient improvement in patients <65 years of age; opportunities to address other causes of LVOT obstruction besides septal thickening, such as abnormal papillary muscle attachment or intrinsic mitral valve disease.

The risks of alcohol ablation include complete heart block requiring permanent pacemaker implantation, and repeated procedures due to persistent obstruction.

Lastly, implantable cardioverter-defibrillator (ICD) therapy is recommended in patients who have prior cardiac arrest or sustained ventricular tachycardia (VT), in those with marked LVOT obstruction and a family history of sudden cardiac death as a first-degree relative, and in patients with a history of unexplained syncope or hypotensive response to exercise stress test [1, 2, 17].

8. **What are the hemodynamic goals whilst anesthetizing a HCM patient for non-cardiac surgery?**

Maximize effort to decrease LVOT obstruction and maintain adequate cardiac output. The principles are:

(1) Maintain intravascular volume (preload);
(2) Maintain afterload or systemic vascular resistance (SVR), avoid profound vasodilation;
(3) Decrease myocardial contractility, avoid inotropes;
(4) Maintain normal sinus rhythm and avoid tachycardia: if a patient develops atrial fibrillation or ventricular tachycardia, there should be very low threshold to cardiovert instead of rate control alone. The thickened LV is heavily dependent on the atrial contraction to maintain adequate preload;
(5) Blunt sympathetic responses during laryngoscopy and surgical stimulation.

9. **What kind of monitoring techniques will you choose for a HCM patient undergoing non-cardiac surgery?**

Besides the standard ASA monitors, placement of an invasive intravascular blood pressure monitor before induction should be considered. There is high risk of potentially rapid changes in blood pressure during induction secondary to the changes of myocardial loading conditions. The decision to place central venous pressure and pulmonary artery pressure monitoring lines is made on individual basis, taking into account the disease severity (e.g., peak LVOT gradient, signs of end-stage CHF) and complexity of the operation.

Defibrillation pads may be considered before induction if the patient does not have an AICD in place, due to the potential risk of malignant arrhythmia.

Transesophageal echocardiography (TEE) may be considered in a patient with severe LVOT obstruction or mitral regurgitation. Rescue TEE should be considered for a patient who acutely decompensates intraoperatively and fails to respond to maximal hemodynamic support.

10. **What kind of preoperative evaluation data is required?**

Clinical history: functional status, history of syncope or presyncope;

TTE data: degree of LVOT obstruction (peak instantaneous gradient); presence of SAM and MR; ventricular function;

Exercise stress testing: signs of worsening LVOT gradient, paradoxical BP response.

If patients are taking beta blockers, calcium channel blockers, or disopyramide, these medications should be continued throughout the perioperative period.

11. **What are the induction agents of choice for patients with HCM?**

The primary goal for the induction of a patient with HCM is to sufficiently blunt the sympathetic response to laryngoscopy while achieving optimal intubation conditions. Beta blockers (such as metoprolol or esmolol) can be given before induction to further decrease the risk of tachycardia [18].

An intravenous fluid bolus before induction may be considered to maintain preload, anticipating the vasodilatory effect of induction agents on blood pressure.

A combination of opioid (fentanyl or remifentanil), hypnotic agents (propofol, midazolam or etomidate) and muscle relaxant can be used. The key is to slowly titrate the hypnotic agent and opioid to avoid large fluctuations in the loading conditions and cardiac output.

Choice of vasopressors: a selective alpha-1 agonist such as phenylephrine is a good choice to augment perfusion pressure, devoid of inotropic and chronotropic effects. An alpha-1 agonist is preferred over ephedrine to control intraoperative hypotension. Inotropes such as dopamine, epinephrine, and milrinone should be avoided [19]. Norepinephrine or vasopressin can be considered as an alternative or additional agent when the dose of phenylephrine is approaching maximal.

12. **What are the maintenance techniques?**

Both volatile agents and intravenous agents can be used for anesthetic maintenance. Neuraxial technique is beneficial for blunting the sympathetic responses to painful stimulation, however careful titration is necessary to balance the risk of vasodilation and decrease in preload.

13. **What are the things to consider during emergence?**

The same considerations and hemodynamic goals guiding the preoperative and intraoperative management apply during emergence and the postoperative period. Meticulous attention to pain control is crucial. If tachycardia persists despite adequate pain control, a beta blocker should be administered, such as metoprolol.

References

1. Gersh BJ, Maron BJ, et al. ACCF/AHA guideline for the diagnosis and treatment of hypertrophic cardiomyopathy. J Am Coll Cardiol 2011;58:e212.
2. Gersh BJ, Maron BJ, et al. ACCF/AHA guideline for the diagnosis and treatment of hypertrophic cardiomyopathy: executive summary. Circulation. 2011;124:2761–96.
3. Wigle ED, Rakowski H, Kimball BP, Williams WG. Hypertrophic cardiomyopathy. Clinical spectrum and treatment. Circulation 1995;92:1680.
4. Nishimura RA, Holmes DR Jr. Clinical practice. Hypertrophic obstructive cardiomyopathy. N Engl J Med 2004;350:1320.
5. Maron MS, Olivotto I, Zenovich AG, et al. Hypertrophic cardiomyopathy is predominantly a disease of left ventricular outflow tract obstruction. Circulation 2006;114:2232.
6. Nishimura RA, et al. Hypertrophic cardiomyopathy: the search for obstruction. Circulation. 2006;114:2200–2.
7. Maron BJ, Maron MS, Semsarian C. Genetics of hypertrophic cardiomyopathy after 20 years: clinical perspectives. J Am Coll Cardiol 2012;60:705.
8. Ackerman MJ, VanDriest SL, et al. Prevalence and age-dependence of malignant mutations in the beta-myosin heavy chain and troponin T genes in hypertrophic cardiomyopathy: a comprehensive outpatient perspective [see comment]. J Am Coll Cardiol. 2002;39:2042–8.
9. Maron BJ et al. Hypertrophic cardiomyopathy: present and future, with translation into contemporary cardiovascular medicine. J Am Coll Cardiol. 2014;64(1):83–99. doi:10.1016/j.jacc.2014.05.003.
10. Spirito P, Autore C, Rapezzi C, et al. Syncope and risk of sudden death in hypertrophic cardiomyopathy. Circulation. 2009;119:1703.
11. Sherrid MV, Chaudhry FA, Swistel DG. Obstructive hypertrophic cardiomyopathy: echocardiography, pathophysiology, and the continuing evolution of surgery for obstruction. Ann Thorac Surg, 2003;75:620–32.
12. Spoladore R, Maron MS, D'Amato R, et al. Pharmacological treatment options for hypertrophic cardiomyopathy: high time for evidence. Eur Heart J. 2012;33:1724.
13. Sherrid MV, Shetty A, Winson G, et al. Treatment of obstructive hypertrophic cardiomyopathy symptoms and gradient resistant to first-line therapy with β-blockade or verapamil. Circ Heart Fail. 2013;6:694.
14. Sherrid MV, Barac I, McKenna WJ, et al. Multicenter study of the efficacy and safety of disopyramide in obstructive hypertrophic cardiomyopathy. J Am Coll Cardiol. 2005;45:1251.
15. Spirito P, Autore C. Management of hypertrophic cardiomyopathy. BMJ. 2006;332:1251.
16. Maron BJ. Surgery for hypertrophic obstructive cardiomyopathy: alive and quite well. Circulation. 2005;111:2016.

17. Auerbach A, et al. Assessing and reducing the cardiac risk of noncardiac surgery. Circulation. 2006;113:1361–76.
18. Haering JM, et al. Cardiac risk of noncardiac surgery in patients with asymmetric septal hypertrophy. Anesthesiology. 1996;85:254–9.
19. Sherrid MV, et al. Mechanism of benefit of negative inotropes in obstructive hypertrophic cardiomyopathy. Circulation. 1998;97:41–7.

10 Pacemakers and Implantable Cardioverter Defibrillators

Ciorsti J. MacIntyre

Key Points

Pacemakers

1. A magnet placed over a pacemaker will generally result in asynchronous pacing
2. Oversensing leads to under pacing
3. Undersensing leads to over pacing

Implantable Cardioverter Defibrillators

1. A magnet placed over an ICD will result in suspension of tachycardia detections/therapies
2. A magnet placed over an ICD will not affect pacing mode or rate

Case

A 58-year-old man presents with left hip pain in the setting of a fall secondary to syncope. Imaging studies reveal a left intertrochanteric fracture. He is therefore brought to the operating room for urgent intramedullary nail.

Past Medical History:

1. Hypertension
2. Dyslipidemia
3. Myocardial infarction s/p drug eluting stent of the LAD
4. Left ventricular systolic dysfunction with EF 30%

Medications:

1. Aspirin 81 mg daily
2. Rosuvastatin 40 mg daily
3. Bisoprolol 5 mg daily
4. Perindopril 4 mg daily

Allergies: None known

Physical Examination (ED): HR 70/BP 140/80 mmHg/RR 18–22/SpO_2 98% on RA

Airway exam: Mallampati II, thyromental distance >3 finger breadths, good mouth opening, no limitation to neck extension, normal dentition.

Cardiovascular Exam: Normal pulse volume and contour. Normal JVP. Normal S1, S2. S3 present. No S4. No murmurs or extra sounds. No peripheral edema. Prepectoral inspection significant for the presence of a cardiac implantable electrical device.

ECG: Sinus rhythm at 70/min with ventricular pacing.

1. **What kind of device does this patient have?**

Appropriate management of the cardiac implantable electrical device (CIED) patient requires accurate identification of the device type. This is particularly relevant for the management of device patients in the perioperative setting. There are multiple methods available to determine device type. Patients may be able to provide this information. Alternatively, they are asked to carry an up-to-date device identification card with them at all times. If a device interrogation is required to assess function or to change programming, it is also necessary to identify the device manufacturer. Failing this, the chest X-ray can provide a significant amount of useful information. The chest X-ray allows for identification of the device type (pacemaker, defibrillator, cardiac resynchronization device, subcutaneous defibrillator, etc.). The chest X-ray also allows for the identification of the chambers paced, the location and number of leads, and the device manufacturer. It can also provide information about hardware abnormalities such as lead fracture or changes in lead position.

C.J. MacIntyre (✉)
Arrhythmia Service, Harvard School of Medicine, Brigham and Women's Hospital, 75 Francis Street, Boston, MA 02115, USA
e-mail: ciorstij.macintyre@nshealth.ca

© Springer International Publishing AG 2017
L.S. Aglio and R.D. Urman (eds.), *Anesthesiology*,
DOI 10.1007/978-3-319-50141-3_10

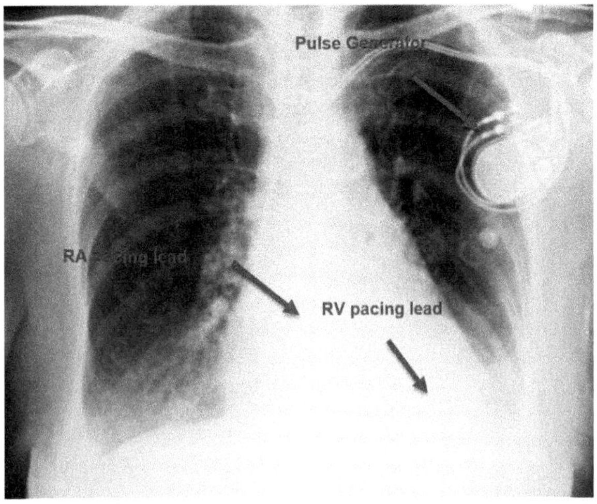

Fig. 10.1 Dual-chamber pacemaker

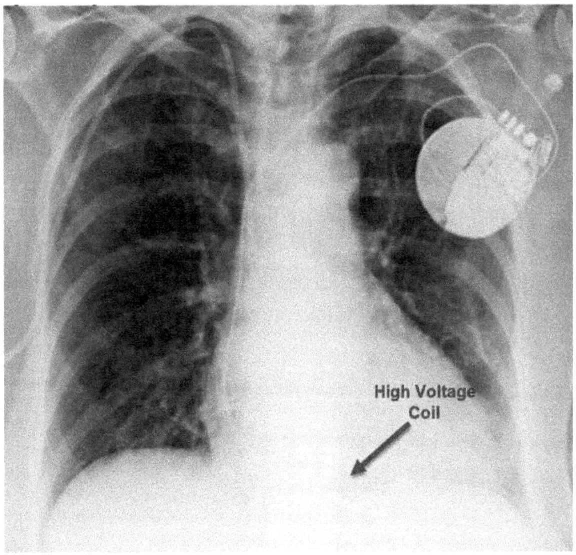

Fig. 10.2 Single-chamber ICD

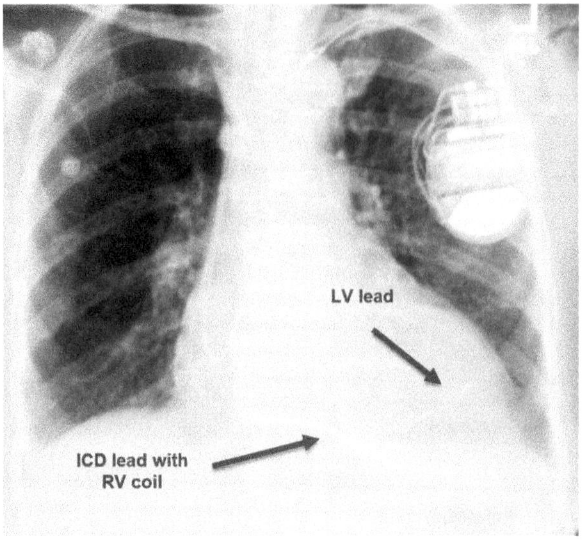

Fig. 10.3 CRT-D

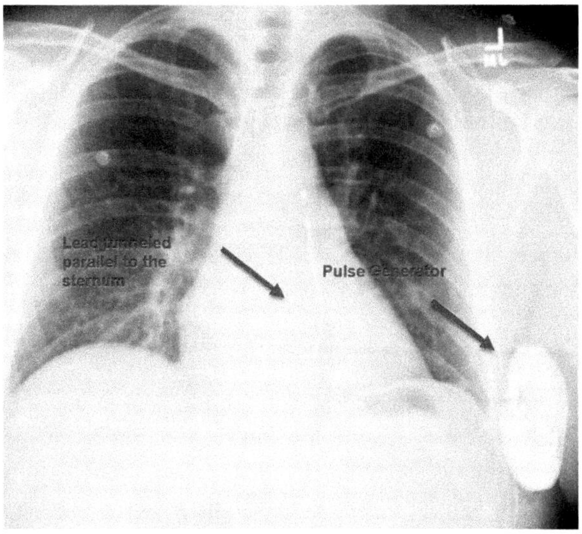

Fig. 10.4 Subcutaneous ICD

A transvenous pacemaker (Fig. 10.1) can be differentiated from an ICD by the absence of a shocking coil on the right ventricular lead (Fig. 10.2). The most common location of an atrial lead is the right atrial appendage. The most common location of a right ventricular lead is the right ventricular apex. A transvenous LV lead enters the coronary sinus from the right atrium and terminates in a branch of the great cardiac vein. On the frontal X-ray this will be superior to the RV lead (Fig. 10.3). On a lateral film, the LV lead should be located posteriorly.

A transvenous CIED will generally have a pulse generator located in the prepectoral region. An epicardial system may have an abdominal pulse generator. Alternatively, the leads may be tunneled to the right or left prepectoral region. A subcutaneous ICD will have a distinct radiographic appearance (Fig. 10.4). The generator is implanted at the mid-axillary line at the 5th to 6th intercostal space and the lead is tunneled such that it runs parallel to the sternum.

2. **What are the components of a cardiac implantable electrical device?**

All pacemakers are composed of two components: the pulse generator and the lead(s). The pulse generator is responsible for generating the electrical impulse that depolarizes the myocardium resulting in contraction of a cardiac chamber. Two types of lead systems exist: unipolar and bipolar. In a unipolar system, the lead in contact with the endocardium is the cathode and the pulse generator is the anode. In a bipolar lead, the lead tip is the cathode and the lead ring is the anode. Voltage in a unipolar lead is detected over a larger distance and as such, the pacing spike on an electrocardiogram is larger than with a bipolar lead. Types of leads include active fixation leads which are screwed into the myocardium and passive fixation which are held in place with fins.

The implantable cardioverter defibrillator (ICD) has two main components: the pulse generator and the leads. The pulse generator itself consists of a battery, a capacitor which facilitates charging and discharging, and circuits to monitor, analyze, and guide arrhythmia therapies. Cardioversion or defibrillation is delivered via a biphasic waveform between the shocking coil and the ICD pulse generator and then the reverse.

3. **Describe the code used to describe the function of pacing devices.**

The North American Society of Pacing and Electrophysiology and the British Pacing and Electrophysiology Group (NASPE/BPEG) created the five position NBG pacemaker code to describe pacemaker functions (see Table 10.1).

Position I indicates the chamber (or chambers) paced. A device used to pace in only one chamber will be represented by either the letter A (atrial) or V (ventricle). Devices that can pace in both chambers are represented by the letter D (dual). When pacing is off, position I coding is O (off).

Position II represents the chamber sensed for intrinsic signals. The letters are the same as those for the first position with A (atrium), V (ventricle), and D (dual). An O in position II indicates the absence of sensing. Programmed in this mode, the device will pace asynchronously at a specified rate, ignoring any intrinsic rhythm.

Position III represents the response to a sensed event. "I" indicates that a sensed event inhibits the output pulse. "T" indicates that an output pulse is triggered in response to a sensed event. D indicates that there are dual modes of response. This is restricted to dual-chamber systems. For example, an event sensed in the atrium inhibits atrial output but triggers ventricular output. If the ventricular lead senses an intrinsic ventricular signal during the programmed delay, it will inhibit ventricular output. O indicates no response to a sensed input.

Position IV reflects rate modulation, which is also known as rate responsiveness. R indicates that the pacemaker has rate modulation and will use sensor data to adjust its programmed paced heart rate in response to patient activity. O indicates that rate modulation is either unavailable or disabled. O is often omitted from the fourth position (i.e., DDD is the same as DDDO).

Position V indicates whether multisite pacing is present in (O) none of the cardiac chambers, one or both atria (A), in one or both ventricles (V) or (D) any combination of A or V. Multisite pacing may also refer to more than one stimulation site in a particular chamber. The fifth position of the code is rarely reported.

The first three positions of the code are always required. When a code includes only three or four characters, it can be assumed that the positions omitted are "O" or absent.

4. **Describe the pacing modes available in cardiac implantable electrical devices.**

Single-Chamber Pacing

VVI(R) pacing: Ventricular paced, ventricular sensed, and pacemaker inhibited in response to a sensed beat. This mode protects a patient from significant bradycardia of any etiology. This mode cannot maintain AV synchrony, which can lead to the pacemaker syndrome.

Ideal patient: Chronic atrial fibrillation with slow ventricular response

AAI(R) pacing: Atrial paced, atrial sensed, and pacemaker inhibited in response to a sensed atrial beat. This can be considered in patients with sinus node dysfunction with intact AV node function. This mode, however, will not protect patients from ventricular bradyarrhythmias due to AV block.

Table 10.1 The revised NASPE/BPEG generic code for antibradycardia pacing

Position I chamber(s) paced	Position II chamber (s) sensed	Position III response to sensing	Position IV rate modulation	Position V multisite pacing
O = None	O = None	O = None	O = None	O = None
A = Atrium	A = Atrium	T = Triggered	R = Rate modulation	A = Atrium
V = Ventricle	V = Ventricle	I = Inhibited		V = Ventricle
D = Dual (A + V)	D = Dual (A + V)	D = Dual (T + I)		D = Dual (A + V)
S[a] = Single (A or V)	S[a] = Single (A or V)			

[a]Manufacturers' designation (previously published) from Bernstein et al. [1]. With permission of Wiley

Ideal patient: The patient with sinus node dysfunction with normal AV node function

Dual-Chamber Pacing

DDD(R) pacing: This mode has sensing and pacing capabilities in both the atrium and the ventricle and provides physiologic pacing. Four different rhythms may be seen with this mode. These include normal sinus rhythm, atrial pacing with native QRS, AV sequential pacing, and atrial sensing with ventricular pacing.

Ideal patient: The ideal patient for DDD is the individual with normal sinus node function with AV block. The ideal patient for DDDR pacing is one with sinus node dysfunction with or without AV nodal dysfunction.

DDI(R) pacing: In this mode there is atrial sensing and pacing and ventricular sensing and pacing. The pacemaker will not track intrinsic atrial activity. When there is a sensed native atrial rate, the pacemaker will inhibit atrial and ventricular output thereby promoting native conduction to the ventricle. If AV block develops, ventricular pacing will occur at the lower pacing limit; however, it will not be synchronized with the atrium. If the sinus rate is below the programmed rate, there will be AV sequential pacing.

Ideal patient: The patient with atrial tachyarrhythmias. Mode switching is an alternative strategy for this issue.

Asynchronous Pacing

When programmed in an asynchronous mode, pacemakers are programmed to pace at a fixed rate without an attempt to sense native cardiac activity. The atrium (**AOO**), the ventricle (**VOO**), or both (**DOO**) are paced in the absence of sensing capability. Such modes are rarely used long term and are most frequently used for patients undergoing a surgical procedure if the patient is pacemaker-dependent so as to avoid pacing inhibition due to oversensing of noise from electrocautery. Asynchronous pacing may be associated with competition between the native and paced rhythms. As such, there is a small risk of a paced impulse during a native T wave, which can result in ventricular fibrillation. This risk is further reduced by programming a higher rate (≥80/min).

5. **Differentiate sensing and capture.**

Pacemakers have two primary functions: pacing and sensing.

Capture refers to cardiac depolarization and contraction of a cardiac chamber in response to a pacemaker stimulus. Capture threshold is the minimum amount of energy needed to consistently capture the myocardium.

Sensing is the ability of the pacemaker to sense an intrinsic electrical signal. The programmed sensitivity indicates the minimum intracardiac signal that will be sensed by the pacemaker to initiate a response. When programming sensitivity, as you raise the number (sensitivity) you make the pacemaker less sensitive (i.e., the pacemaker can see less). Conversely, as you decrease the number (sensitivity) you make the pacemaker more sensitive (i.e., the pacemaker can see more).

6. **Review types of pacemaker malfunction.**

Oversensing causes under pacing

Oversensing refers to the sensing of physiologic or non-physiologic events that should not be sensed. This may lead to inappropriate inhibition of pacemaker output. In a pacemaker-dependent patient, this can have severe consequences. Physiologic causes of oversensing include far-field P waves, widened QRS duration, T wave oversensing, and myopotentials. Making the device less sensitive may resolve the issue. Non-physiologic causes of oversensing include hardware issues such as loose setscrew, lead dislodgment, or lead fracture. Such etiologies will typically require lead revision. Electromagnetic interference (EMI) may also cause oversensing.

Undersensing causes over pacing

Undersensing occurs when the pacemaker fails to see the underlying rhythm. As a result the pacemaker generates an output even when it is not needed leading to "over pacing." Undersensing may be caused by hardware failure or by physiologic changes. Examples of hardware failure include lead dislodgment, perforation, or fracture. Anti-arrhythmic medications, myocardial infarction, and metabolic abnormalities may transiently or permanently alter electrogram amplitude.

Non-capture

Non-capture occurs when the electrical impulse emitted by the device fails to capture the myocardium. On the 12-lead ECG, this will be represented by a pacing stimulus that is not followed by an evoked potential. This can be intermittent or permanent. This may occur when the capture threshold is higher than the programmed device output. This may be seen in the setting of post-implantation inflammatory changes. This can be overcome by increasing the pacemaker output. Exit block occurs when the capture threshold exceeds the maximum programmable output. Other causes of rising capture threshold include fibrosis or infarction at the site of the delivered pacing stimulus and metabolic abnormalities. Hardware issues such as lead dislodgment, perforation, and fracture and battery depletion may also result in non-capture.

7. **What is an Implantable Cardioverter Defibrillator?**

The primary purpose of the implantable cardioverter defibrillator (ICD) is to detect malignant ventricular arrhythmias (VT and VF) and then terminate these arrhythmias with effective defibrillation. Post-defibrillation bradycardia is common. Similarly, patients may also have a concomitant pacing requirement. As such, all current ICDs also have pacing capabilities.

8. **What are the considerations in a patient with a pacemaker or ICD who requires cardioversion or external defibrillation?**

In the event of cardiac arrest or an unstable arrhythmia in a patient with a CIED, standard resuscitation protocols should be followed. External defibrillation or cardioversion can result in permanent damage to the device. Anterior–posterior electrode placement is preferred when performing external cardioversion or defibrillation on the CIED patient to minimize this risk. Similarly, the electrodes should be placed greater than 8 cm away from the pulse generator. Other risks include device reprogramming and acute rise in pacemaker threshold due to myocardial damage at the lead–endocardium interface. As such, cardiac devices should be interrogated following cardioversion to ensure appropriate function and programming.

9. **How do pacemakers and defibrillators respond to application of a magnet?**

Application of a standard doughnut magnet can be used in the perioperative period to change the behavior of CIEDs. Application of a magnet to a **pacemaker** will generally cause asynchronous pacing via closure of a magnetic switch. Application of a magnet to an **ICD**, however, will disable tachycardia detections without having an effect on pacing mode or rate. Tachycardia therapies can also be disabled in a subcutaneous ICD with magnet application.

10. **Describe situations in which a magnet should and should not be used.**

There are many situations in which a pacemaker needs to be made asynchronous or when ICD therapies should be disabled. As such, consideration must be given to magnet application or temporary device reprogramming. The primary advantage of reprogramming is that the team does not need to be concerned about the location of the magnet. The primary disadvantage, however, is that such changes are not immediately reversible. There is also a risk that the necessary programming changes to return the device back to baseline settings may not occur. This could leave an ICD patient unprotected from malignant ventricular arrhythmias. A magnet, however, can be quickly removed thereby immediately returning the device to the baseline settings. Of note, a patient who has tachycardia therapies disabled requires continuous telemetry monitoring.

Examples of situations in which a magnet should be applied:

- Radiofrequency ablation (RFA) **above** the umbilicus in a **pacemaker-dependent** patient to cause asynchronous pacing ***
- To inhibit tachycardia detections/therapies in all patients with an **ICD** receiving monopolar electrocautery
- If RFA **below** the umbilicus results in pacing inhibition
- If a patient is receiving **inappropriate ICD shocks.**

Examples of situations in which a magnet should not be applied:

- When patient positioning prevents stable magnet positioning (e.g., prone patients). These patients require reprogramming.

*** Magnet application will **not** cause an ICD to pace asynchronously. As such, pacemaker-dependent patients with an ICD requiring electrocautery above the umbilicus require reprogramming to an asynchronous pacing mode.

11. **Are there considerations for central venous access?**

There are multiple considerations when a patient with a pacemaker or ICD receives central venous access. Ipsilateral access can result in lead damage from needle puncture, lead dislodgement, and inappropriate ICD therapies. When possible, central venous access should only be attempted contralateral to the device. Of note, central venous access can also lead to central venous stenosis, which can prevent lead placement using a subclavian approach.

Suggested Reading

1. Bernstein AD, Daubert JC, Fletcher RD. The revised NASPE/BPEG generic code for antibradycardia, adaptive-rate, and multisite pacing. J Pacing Clin Electrophysiol. 2002;25(2):260–4.

2. Costelloe CM, Murphy WA, Gladish GW, Rozner MA. Radiography of pacemakers and implantable cardioverter defibrillators. Am J Roentgenol. 2012;199:1252–8.
3. Crossley GH, Poole JE, Rozner MA, Asirvatham SJ, Cheng A, Chung MK, Ferfuson TB, Gallagher JD, Gold MR, Hyot RH, Irefin S, Kusumoto FM, Moorman LP, Thompson A. The Heart Rhythm Society (HRS)/American Society of Anesthesiologists (ASA) expert consensus statement on the perioperative management of patients with implantable defibrillators, pcemakers and arrhythmia monitors: facilities and patient management. Heart Rhythm. 2011;8(7):1114–54.
4. Epstein AE, DiMarco JP, Ellenbogen KA, Estes NAM, Freedman RA, Gettes LS, Gillinov AM, Gregoratos G, Hammill SC, Hayes DL, Hlatky MA, Newby LK, Page RL, Schoenfield MH, Silka MJ, Stevenson LW, Sweeney MO. ACC/AHA/HRS 2008 guidelines for device-based therapy of cardiac rhythm abnormalities: a report of the American College of Cardiology/American Heart Association Task Force on Practice Guidelines (Writing Committee to Revise the ACC/AHA/NASPE 2002 Guideline Update for Implantation of Cardiac Pacemakers and Antiarrhythmia Devices. J Am Coll Cardiol. 2008;41(21):e1–62.

11 Pericardial Tamponade

Kate Mitchell Liberman

Patient Scenario

A 37-year old man presents to his primary care physician concerned about multiple episodes of dizziness associated with palpitations. He is unable to exert himself in his activities of daily living. His past medical history is significant for hyperlipidemia, anxiety, gastroesophageal reflux disease, occasional migraines, lower back pain, and constipation. He had an appendectomy at age 12, but otherwise, no surgical history. He has an allergy to bananas and latex. His medications include simvastatin, lorazepam, esomeprazole, naproxen, and colace. He smokes one pack of cigarettes per day. He does not consume alcohol and has never tried taking recreational drugs. On physical exam he is found to be bradycardic at 42 beats per minute. His blood pressure is 110/65, respiratory rate 16 breaths per minute, and oxygen saturation 98% on room air. His lungs exam is remarkable for mild rales at the bases bilaterally and he has 2+ edema in his lower extremities. His ECG shows complete heart block. After medical optimization of his heart failure symptoms, he presents to an interventional cardiologist for pacemaker placement. During the pacemaker placement, which was performed under sedation, the patient moves on the procedure table as the first lead was being placed. He then becomes suddenly dyspneic and increasingly hypotensive. His blood pressure is 80/45, heart rate 110 beats per minute, respiratory rate 25 breaths per minute and pulse oximetry 98%. Pericardial tamponade is suspected.

K.M. Liberman (✉)
Department of Anesthesiology, Perioperative and Pain Medicine, Brigham and Women's Hospital, 75 Francis Street, Boston, MA 02115, USA
e-mail: KLiberman@partners.org

© Springer International Publishing AG 2017
L.S. Aglio and R.D. Urman (eds.), *Anesthesiology*,
DOI 10.1007/978-3-319-50141-3_11

Questions

What is the definition of pericardial tamponade?

Cardiac tamponade is defined as pathologic fluid in the pericardial space leading to a restriction in ventricular filling and subsequently a decrease in cardiac output. Normally, the pericardial sac contains 20–50 mL of serous fluid that mitigates the force of friction on the epicardium. Cardiac tamponade occurs when the reserve volume of the pericardial sac is exceeded by filling with blood, clot, gas, fluid, or pus [1]. The physiology of cardiac tamponade is less a function of the effusion's composition and more a function of the rate at which it accumulates. There are four generally accepted categories of cardiac tamponade. Acute cardiac tamponade usually occurs within minutes and is most often secondary to hemopericardium from trauma. It occurs when blood accumulates more rapidly than the pericardial sac can accommodate. In severe cases, this can lead to complete collapse of the right atrium and/or the right ventricle. Subacute cardiac tamponade most often occurs over days to weeks due to large effusions, which accumulate more slowly, often from idiopathic or neoplastic causes. Low pressure cardiac tamponade is a special case when pericardial effusion and hypovolemic shock coexist. Due to the fact that ventricular pressures are low, the pressure gradient across the myocardium may be large even with relatively low pericardial pressures [2]. Finally, regional tamponade develops when a loculated effusion or hematoma exerts pressure across the myocardium. This is more difficult to diagnose on physical exam because typical findings are absent due to a focal source of compression [3].

What are the causes of tamponade?

Cardiac tamponade arises from a number of causes including infectious, noninfectious and autoimmune origins. While acute idiopathic pericarditis is the leading cause of tamponade worldwide, it is proportionately much more common in patients with tuberculous, neoplastic, or purulent pericarditis [4]. A large prospective series evaluated the etiologies of primary acute pericarditis [5]. Nearly half had acute idiopathic pericarditis, and the remaining patients commonly had metastatic disease and tuberculous pericarditis. Infectious causes of tamponade can be divided into viral, bacterial, fungal and parasitic causes. Coxsackie, echovirus and adenovirus are common viral causes, while Staphylococcus, Streptococcus, pneumococcus, and tuberculosis are the most common bacterial causes [6]. Fungal causes include Histoplasmosis, aspergillosis, and coccidioidomycosis, and the most common parasitic causes are echinococcus and toxoplasmosis. Metastatic lung and breast cancer, Hodgkin's lymphoma and melanoma are the most common sources of malignant effusions. Primary cardiac causes are comprised of early infarction pericarditis, post-pericardiotomy syndrome, dissecting aneurysms and myocarditis. Tamponade can be induced by blunt and penetrating trauma like, and it can occur as a complication of cardiac catheterization and pacemaker placement. Rheumatologic causes, include SLE and vasculitis, and occur secondary to inflammation. Uremia is a common metabolic cause. Any process which leads to an effusion, particularly if large or rapidly accumulating, can induce tamponade physiology.

What are the physical exam findings of a patient who has pericardial tamponade?

Physical exam findings of a patient with pericardial tamponade are sinus tachycardia, jugular venous distension, and pulsus paradoxus. Secondary signs of pericarditis include muffled heart sounds and rub. Dyspnea (sensitivity 87–89%), tachycardia (sensitivity 77%), pulsus paradoxus (sensitivity 82%), and elevated JVP (sensitivity 76%) are most useful in their negative predictive value [7]. That is, they are useful for ruling out tamponade when absent. If a patient has pulsus paradoxus, the odds of having tamponade increase threefold, and if absent, the odds of having tamponade are reduced 30-fold.

What is pulsus paradoxus?

Pulsus paradoxus is an exaggeration of a normal decrease in systolic blood pressure, which occurs during inspiration [8]. Under conditions of increased pericardial pressures, changes in right and left ventricular volume inevitably affect each other, as there is no additional reserve volume in the pericardial sac. At least three mechanisms have been proposed to explain this phenomenon [9]. With inspiration, increased negative pressure in the intrathoracic cavity increases venous return to the right side of the heart. The increased preload, in turn, causes bulging of the septal wall into the left ventricle, decreasing end-diastolic left ventricular volume. This exemplifies ventricular interdependence. Increased compliance of pulmonary vasculature also occurs during inspiration, leading to pooling in the pulmonary circulation. Finally, the increase in negative intrathoracic pressure opposes contraction of the left side of the heart, leading to increased afterload. These three forces conspire to decrease systolic blood pressure. Kussmaul's sign describes the disappearance of the peripheral pulse with inspiration, which is caused by the drop in blood pressure described above.

What are the diagnostic criteria for pericardial tamponade?

The diagnostic criteria for cardiac tamponade are not well defined. It is generally diagnosed when both a pericardial effusion and hemodynamic compromise are present. Another commonly used definition is one which can only be made retrospectively: the presence of a pericardial effusion as seen by either transthoracic or transesophageal echocardiography and hemodynamic compromise that is relieved by pericardial fluid drainage [10].

What noninvasive and invasive testing will help establish a diagnosis of tamponade?

While many techniques may be helpful in diagnosing pericardial effusion, establishing the diagnosis of tamponade physiology on the basis of noninvasive testing is challenging. EKG is the first test often performed. PR segment depression, low voltage QRS complex, and electrical alternans are EKG findings that are specific but not sensitive for pericardial effusion [11]. Overall, EKG has a low sensitivity for diagnosing pericardial effusion and cardiac tamponade.

Transthoracic echocardiogram (TTE) clearly demonstrates the presence or absence of effusion. A study by Merce et al. prospectively assessed patients with moderate to large pericardial effusions over a 2-year period for tamponade [12]. They found that collapse of one or more right cardiac chambers was highly sensitive for tamponade, while abnormal venous flow pattern by Doppler was more specific —systolic over diastolic predominance, respiratory accentuation of this difference and expiration inversion of the diastolic component. Other TTE signs of tamponade include exaggerated inspiratory variation of the right and left ventricle, collapse of any chamber, IVC plethora and abnormal reduction in flow across the mitral and aortic valves during inspiration [13].

Invasive measurements, such as Swan Ganz catheter measurements generally reveal pulmonary hypertension in tamponade with pulmonary artery systolic pressures ranging between 35 and 50 mmHg. Cardiac catheterization, though not necessary for diagnosis, may reveal equilibration of average intracardiac diastolic pressures. An arterial line tracing will show a narrow pulse pressure and a low mean arterial pressure.

What vascular access would you obtain prior to treating pericardial tamponade?

If pericardial tamponade is present, or highly suspected, prior to the induction of anesthesia, placing an arterial line and a central venous line (CVL) are of great use. An arterial line will offer beat-to-beat blood pressure readings, while the CVL will permit reliable titration of pressors prior to drainage of the effusion and provide central venous pressure readings. Further, after the tamponade is relieved, there can sometimes be a catecholamine surge marked by increased blood pressure and heart rate that will be quickly recognized with an arterial line. Given, the critical nature of this condition, with compromised cardiac output and the possibility of PEA arrest, decompression of the tamponade should not be delayed by placing invasive monitors. Due to the risk of significant bleeding during or after evacuation of the pericardial collection, large bore intravenous access is also necessary for resuscitation.

What are the hemodynamic goals for patients with tamponade?

For patients with cardiac tamponade, the hemodynamic goals are to maintain preload, chronotropy, afterload, and inotropy. Colloquially speaking, the goals are to keep a patient "full, fast and tight." Patients with acute tamponade are preload dependent. Increased venous return can overcome the pericardial pressure and restore the gradient between the chambers. So, it is important to administer intravenous fluids and avoid hypovolemia. Given that stroke volume is relatively fixed, cardiac output is dependent upon heart rate. Bradycardia is rarely tolerated. Patients with tamponade physiology require both inotropic support and an increase in systemic vascular resistance (SVR). Given that the heart is constricted externally from filling, a decrease in contractility is poorly tolerated. Increasing the SVR is the best way to ensure coronary perfusion. Norepinepherine and vasopressin, therefore, are the preferred pressors for patients with tamponade physiology. Epinephrine also addresses each of the hemodynamic goals [14].

Another obstacle in caring for a patient with tamponade is ventilation. The effect of positive pressure ventilation is detrimental to cardiac filling. This is generally overcome by maintaining low peak pressures, low PEEP as well as low tidal volumes. Minute ventilation is maintained by increasing the respiratory rate. Given these restrictions, ventilation may not be adequate, and P_aCO_2 may rise. Permissive hypercapnia may be tolerated on an individual basis but can lead to RV failure.

What are the medical treatments for pericardial effusion?

Patients with stable pericardial effusions may be managed medically by treating the underlying cause of the effusion. Inflammatory causes of pericarditis may be treated with NSAIDs. Aspirin, indomethacin and ibuprofen are the first-line therapy. Ibuprofen, has the lowest complication rate and has a favorable effect on coronary blood flow [15]. However, in post-infarction pericarditis, aspirin is favored. Colchicine may also be added for its impact on acute pericarditis and efficacy in preventing recurrences. Systemic steroids are reserved for patients with pericarditis caused by autoimmune disease or uremia. For long-term prevention of pericarditis, intracardiac steroids have shown some efficacy with almost 80% symptom-free remission at one year [16].

Which anesthetic agents would you choose for sedation and general anesthesia in a patient with tamponade physiology?

In hemodynamically unstable patients, the use of local anesthetics and a subhypnotic doses of midazolam, ketamine or fentanyl are appropriate in preparation for a subxiphoid pericardial drainage procedure [17, 18]. These agents have minimal effect on heart rate, contractility, and SVR, making them ideal for a patient with tamponade. For critically compromised patients ultimately requiring a pericardial window, the anesthetic may begin with sedation until a bridging pericardiocentesis is completed. After the tamponade is relieved, general anesthesia may be induced. The heart is then able to fill and contract normally and the negative inotropic effects of propofol and inhaled anesthetics will be less detrimental to the patient's hemodynamics.

In patients who require general anesthesia for a pericardial window, it is essential to choose an induction agent, which has minimal impact on inotropy and vasomotor tone, such as etomidate or ketamine [19]. Aggressive fluid resuscitation is important prior to the induction of anesthesia. Additionally, the use of infusions or boluses of norepinephrine, vasopressin, or epinephrine may be necessary during induction.

When would you choose to do a pericardiocentesis versus a pericardial window with a drain?

For patients with cardiac tamponade and hemodynamic instability, quick drainage is essential. The indications for either pericardiocentesis or surgical drainage are (1) overt clinical tamponade in patients with purulent pericarditis or large, idiopathic or chronic pericardial effusion and (2) either unresolved or relapsing tamponade after pericadiocentesis and persistent active illness three weeks after hospital admission [20]. Both percutaneous and surgical drainage are highly effective at alleviating symptoms and hypotension. During percutaneous drainage, a catheter is placed under echocardiographic guidance into the pericardial sac and left in place until there is no further drainage from the site. Surgical drainage is preferred for loculated effusions, re-accumulation of fluid, when pericardial biopsy is required, or in cases of coagulopathy—for ultimate control of the surgical field in the event of severe bleeding. In nearly every situation, coagulation studies should be obtained before the procedure, and correction of coagulopathy should be achieved prior to the intervention. It is important to drain fluid in no larger than 1 L increments, as rapid removal can cause acute right ventricular dilation [15]. Major complications from pericardiocentesis occur in only about 1% of cases [21]. Surgical drainage bares a higher risk mainly because it requires general anesthesia, which can induce hypotension when the effusion has not first been drained. Percutaneous pericardiocentesis carries fewer complications when compared to surgical drainage [22]. In cases of traumatic hemopericardium or a dissecting aortic aneurysm, surgical intervention is generally preferred because relief of tamponade does not address the cause of the effusion and may allow further bleeding.

What are the complications of percutaneous pericardiocentesis and the creation of a pericardial window?

The main complications of pericardiocentesis are related to bleeding into the pericardial sac, however, when a drain is left in place, this is unlikely to present as a problem. Other complications include acute left ventricular failure with pulmonary edema because of sudden increases in systemic venous return. Cardiac perforations are rare events, but may be life-threatening. Arrhythmias, arterial perforation, pneumothorax, vagal response, pleuropericardial fistulas, and infection have all been reported [23]. In past studies of surgical drainage, mortality has been as high as 20%, although these findings could have been confounded by underlying disease [24]. Recent data reveal reported lower rates [25]. In a large study of patients undergoing echo-guided pericardiocentesis, the effusion recurrence rate for simple pericardiocentesis was 27%, and for those who underwent surgical drainage 14% [21]. The main predictors of recurrence were the lack of extended drainage, malignancy, positive cytology, large effusion, and renal failure.

References

1. Spodick D. Acute cardiac tamponade. N Engl J Med. 2003. http://www.nejm.org/doi/full/10.1056/NEJMra022643. Accessed 23 July 2015.
2. Sagrista-Sauleda J, Angel J, Sambola A, Alguersuari J, Permanyer-Miralda G, Soler-Soler J. Low-pressure cardiac tamponade: clinical and hemodynamic profile. Circulation. 2006;114(9):945–52. doi:10.1161/CIRCULATIONAHA.106.634584.
3. Chuttani K, Pandian N, Mohanty P. Left ventricular diastolic collapse. An echocardiographic sign of regional cardiac tamponade. Circulation. 1991. http://circ.ahajournals.org/content/83/6/1999.short. Accessed 23 July 2015.
4. Permanyer-Miralda G. Acute pericardial disease: approach to the aetiologic diagnosis. Heart. 2004. http://heart.bmj.com/content/90/3/252.short. Accessed 23 July 2015.
5. Permanyer-Miralda G. Primary acute pericardial disease: a prospective series of 231 consecutive patients. *Am J ....* 1985. http://www.sciencedirect.com/science/article/pii/0002914985910239. Accessed 23 July 2015.
6. Shabetai R. Diseases of the pericardium. In: Schlant RC AR, editor. Hurst's the heart. Vol 8th ed.; 1994.
7. Roy CL, Minor MA, Brookhart MA, Choudhry NK. Does this patient with a pericardial effusion have cardiac tamponade? JAMA. 2007;297(16):1810–8. doi:10.1001/jama.297.16.1810.
8. Guntheroth W, Morgan B. Effect of Respiration on Venous Return and Stroke Volume in Cardiac Tamponade Mechanism Of Pulsus Paradoxus. Circ .... 1967. http://circres.ahajournals.org/content/20/4/381.short. Accessed 23 July 2015.
9. Reddy P, Curtiss E, Uretsky B. Spectrum of hemodynamic changes in cardiac tamponade. Am J Cardiol. 1990. http://www.sciencedirect.com/science/article/pii/000291499090540H. Accessed 23 July 2015.
10. Fowler N. Cardiac tamponade. A clinical or an echocardiographic diagnosis? Circulation. 1993. http://circ.ahajournals.org/content/87/5/1738.short. Accessed 23 July 2015.
11. Eisenberg M. The diagnosis of pericardial effusion and cardiac tamponade by 12-lead ECG: a technology assessment. CHEST .... 1996. http://journal.publications.chestnet.org/article.aspx?articleid=1069876. Accessed 23 July 2015.
12. Mercé J, Sagristà-Sauleda J. Between clinical and Doppler echocardiographic findings in patients with moderate and large pericardial effusion: implications for the diagnosis of cardiac tamponade. Am Hear .... 1999. http://www.sciencedirect.com/science/article/pii/S0002870399701936. Accessed 23 July 2015.
13. Pepi M, Muratori M. Echocardiography in the diagnosis and management of pericardial disease. J Cardiovasc Med (Hagerstown). 2006;7(7):533–44. doi:10.2459/01.JCM.0000234772.73454.57.
14. Grocott HP, Gulati H, Srinathan S, Mackensen GB. Anesthesia and the patient with pericardial disease. Can J Anesth. 2011;58(10):952–66. doi:10.1007/s12630-011-9557-8.
15. Maisch B, Seferović PM, Ristić AD, et al. Guidelines on the diagnosis and management of pericardial diseases executive summary; The Task force on the diagnosis and management of pericardial diseases of the European society of cardiology. Eur Heart J. 2004;25(7):587–610. doi:10.1016/j.ehj.2004.02.002.

16. Maisch B, Ristic D, Pankuweit S. Intrapericardial treatment of autoreactive pericardial effusion with triamcinolone. Eur Hear J. 2002. http://eurheartj.oxfordjournals.org/content/ehj/23/19/1503.full.pdf. Accessed 26 July 2015.
17. Trigt P Van, Douglas J, Smith P. A prospective trial of subxiphoid pericardiotomy in the diagnosis and treatment of large pericardial effusion. A follow-up report. Ann .... 1993. http://www.ncbi.nlm.nih.gov/pmc/articles/PMC1243074/. Accessed 27 July 2015.
18. Webster JA, Self DD. Anesthesia for pericardial window in a pregnant patient with cardiac tamponade and mediastinal mass. Can J Anaesth. 2003;50(8):815–8. doi:10.1007/BF03019378.
19. O'Connor CJ, Tuman KJ. The intraoperative management of patients with pericardial tamponade. Anesthesiol Clin. 2010;28(1):87–96. doi:10.1016/j.anclin.2010.01.011.
20. Cardiology G. Management of pericardial e V usion. 2001:235–240.
21. Tsang T, Enriquez-Sarano M. Consecutive 1127 therapeutic echocardiographically guided pericardiocenteses: clinical profile, practice patterns, and outcomes spanning 21 years. Mayo Clin .... 2002. http://www.sciencedirect.com/science/article/pii/S0025619611622118. Accessed 26 July 2015.
22. Gumrukcuoglu H, Odabasi D. Management of cardiac tamponade: a comperative study between echo-guided pericardiocentesis and surgery—a report of 100 patients. Cardiol Res .... 2011. http://www.hindawi.com/journals/crp/2011/197838/abs/. Accessed 26 July 2015.
23. Duvernoy O, Borowiec J, Helmius G, Erikson U. Complications of percutaneous pericardiocentesis under fluoroscopic guidance. Acta Radiol. 1992;33(4):309–13. doi:10.1177/028418519203300405.
24. Piehler J, Pluth J. Surgical management of effusive pericardial disease. Influence of extent of pericardial resection on clinical course. J .... 1985. http://europepmc.org/abstract/med/4046619. Accessed 27 July 2015.
25. Andrade-Alegre R, Mon L. Subxiphoid pericardial window in the diagnosis of penetrating cardiac trauma. Ann Thorac Surg. 1994;58(4):1139–41. doi:10.1016/0003-4975(94)90473-1.

Non-cardiac Surgery After Heart Transplantation

12

Elliott Woodward

Case

A 63-year-old man with a past medical history significant for orthotopic heart transplantation 18 months prior presents for open reduction and internal fixation of an unstable left lower extremity bimalleolar ankle fracture. The patient sustained the injury as a passenger in a car involved in a low-speed motor vehicle accident, and subsequent workup in the emergency department was negative for the presence of additional injuries. He reports that he has been on a stable immunosuppressive regimen for the past 6 months and denies any recent chest pain, palpitations, weight gain, leg swelling, orthopnea, fevers, chills, or malaise. Prior to his accident, he reports being able to climb two flights of stairs without chest discomfort or shortness of breath.

Medications:

Aspirin 80 mg daily
Tacrolimus 5 mg PO BID
Mycophenolate Mofetil 1000 mg PO BID
Prednisone 10 mg BID
Diltiazem 60 mg PO TID
Pravastatin 40 mg daily

Allergies: NKA

Past Medical History:

Cardiac:

Nonischemic cardiomyopathy status post orthotopic heart transplant 18 months prior
Hypertension
Hypercholesterolemia

Endocrine:

Diet controlled diabetes mellitus

Physical Exam:

Vital Signs: BP 145/92, HR 95, RR 20, oxygen saturation 99% on room air

Cardiac: Regular tachycardia without murmurs, rub, or gallop. JVP 3 cm. Left leg bandaged but no pedal edema on right leg

Respiratory: Lungs clear to auscultation bilaterally

Otherwise: Insignificant

An EKG that was performed in the ED is notable for the presence of two distinct P waves and right bundle branch block.

1. **How do the two branches of the autonomic nervous system influence cardiac function in the normal human heart**?

Autonomic regulation of cardiac chronotropy (heart rate) and dromotropy (conduction velocity) is achieved through a balance of sympathetic and parasympathetic signaling to cardiac pacemaker tissue. Autonomic control of cardiac inotropy (contraction) and lusitropy (relaxation), on the other hand, is primarily mediated through sympathetic signaling to cardiac myocytes [1, 2].

2. **Which neurotransmitters and receptors play a central role in cardiac autonomic signaling**?

When activated, *preganglionic* neurons of both the sympathetic and parasympathetic nervous system release acetylcholine from their nerve terminals in the autonomic ganglia. Acetylcholine then diffuses across the synaptic cleft where it binds to nicotinic acetylcholine receptors located on the postsynaptic neurons, ultimately promoting depolarization and signal propagation in these cells. In the *parasympathetic* system, stimulated *postganglionic* fibers release acetylcholine which binds to muscarinic acetylcholine receptors on the heart. In the *sympathetic* system, stimulated *postganglionic* fibers release norepinephrine which binds to cardiac adrenergic receptors.

E. Woodward (✉)
Department of Anesthesiology, Perioperative and Pain Medicine, Brigham and Women's Hospital, 22 Fleet St., Apt 8, Boston, MA 02113, USA
e-mail: elwoodward@partners.org

© Springer International Publishing AG 2017
L.S. Aglio and R.D. Urman (eds.), *Anesthesiology*,
DOI 10.1007/978-3-319-50141-3_12

3. **What effect does the autonomic nervous system have on the transplanted heart?**

Autonomic nerves are transected in the process of transplantation, disrupting autonomic influence on cardiac function in the early postoperative period. Autonomic reinnervation of the transplanted heart can occur over time, but its extent and time course are highly variable and therefore unpredictable [3–10].

4. **Why is the resting heart rate frequently elevated in patients who have previously undergone heart transplantation?**

In the healthy, resting individual both sympathetic and parasympathetic nerve fibers regulate automaticity in the pacemaker cells of the sinus node [1, 2]. Usually in adults, vagal parasympathetic influence predominates, resulting in an overall slowing of the rate of depolarization of these cells and therefore slowing of the resting heart rate. Disruption of autonomic signaling to the heart during the process of transplantation attenuates this parasympathetic-heavy influence, often leading to a significant elevation in resting heart rate. Resting rates of 80–110 are common, though rates as high as 130 or greater have been reported [3, 7, 9–11].

5. **How might an anesthesiologist's ability to detect intraoperative awareness be altered by the loss of cardiac autonomic innervation?**

Though neither sensitive nor specific, alterations in hemodynamic parameters such as heart rate and blood pressure due to sympathetic nervous system activation can serve as an indicator of insufficient anesthetic depth. In patients who have undergone heart transplant, this sympathetic response may be blunted or absent, highlighting the importance of having a heightened awareness of anesthetic depth in this patient population [6].

6. **Why is maintenance of preload especially important in patients who have previously undergone cardiac transplantation?**

Cardiac output is equal to the product of heart rate and stroke volume. Accordingly, decreases in stroke volume must be corrected or accompanied by a proportional increase in heart rate in order to maintain stable cardiac output. Reflex signaling through the autonomic nervous system plays a central role in this compensatory response, increasing heart rate and/or contractility when required to maintain cardiac output. This reflex signaling is disrupted in the denervated heart leaving only intrinsic adaptive cardiac responses such as the Frank–Starling mechanism intact [3, 7]. This mechanism describes the heart's ability to increase contractility in response to increased cardiac muscle stretch due to increased filling, i.e., preload.

7. **How is the hemodynamic response to medications different in individuals who have undergone heart transplantation?**

Drugs that produce hemodynamic changes through modification of vascular tone such as phenylephrine and nitroglycerin will produce relatively normal, dose-dependent alterations in preload and systemic vascular resistance. The compensatory bradycardia or tachycardia that would typically be seen with use of these medications, on the other hand, is largely dependent on the autonomic nervous system and may be disrupted [2]. Overall, the hemodynamic effect of these drugs will be preserved if not slightly augmented via loss of these compensatory changes. Similarly, drugs such as atropine that exert their effect indirectly by altering autonomic signaling will typically be less efficacious or completely ineffectual depending on the level of autonomic reinnervation that has occurred post-transplantation [7, 10]. Hemodynamic effects of drugs like epinephrine that directly binds to receptors on cardiac tissues will not only be maintained but may be exaggerated [7, 9, 10, 12, 13]. Finally, drugs with mixed direct and indirect activity such as ephedrine will typically retain only their direct effects.

8. **What does this mean for the management of intraoperative arrhythmias?**

In the denervated heart, bradycardia typically would not respond to the indirect effects of atropine and glycopyrrolate, so the provider must be prepared to treat with pacing or direct acting medications such as isoproterenol or epinephrine. The denervated heart's response to adenosine, however, is exaggerated and so use of an alternate medication such as amiodarone is preferred when treating tachyarrhythmias [9, 10].

9. **Why is it common for heart transplant patients to have pacemakers and ICDs?**

While disruption of autonomic input most commonly results in elevation of the resting heart rate in individuals who have undergone cardiac transplantation, factors such as sinus node tissue injury related to graft ischemia, surgical trauma or reperfusion injury occasionally cause post-transplant bradycardia [7, 9]. Treatment with a permanent pacemaker is typically only undertaken when symptomatic bradycardia is persistent, with rates of pacemaker placement for this indication most commonly reported at <10% [3, 9]. While there are no clear guidelines surrounding the implantation of ICDs in these patients, common reasons for placement include unexplained syncope, frequent nonsustained ventricular arrhythmia, graft failure, and graft vasculopathy with associated left ventricular dysfunction [9, 14].

10. **Why are two distinct P waves sometimes seen on the EKG in patients who have a transplanted heart?**

Two of the most common surgical approaches to cardiac transplantation include the atrial to atrial cuff technique and the bicaval technique. In the atrial to atrial cuff technique, a part of the recipient's right and left atria remains in situ and is sutured to the atria of the donor heart. This may leave the recipient with active sinus node tissue from both their native heart as well as their newly transplanted heart. While these suture lines serve as a barrier to prevent widespread conduction of pacemaker potentials originating in retained recipient sinus nodal tissue, this electrical activity can still be seen on an EKG as a second P wave [3, 6, 9, 15]. A lower rate of pacemaker implantation and a slight mortality benefit have been shown with the bicaval technique and thus most centers have moved away from the atrial to atrial cuff technique when possible [16]. Despite this fact, this phenomenon can still be seen in the operating room in patients who had their transplant prior to the more recent shift in practice. Additionally, technical limitations occasionally prohibit the use of the bicaval approach necessitating use of the atrial to atrial cuff technique.

11. **What other atrial arrhythmias are commonly seen in patients after cardiac transplant?**

First degree AV block, right bundle branch block and atrial flutter are common [3, 9, 10, 17].

12. **What is the significance of right bundle branch block in these patients?**

Isolated, stable right bundle branch block is likely of little clinical significance. Higher rates of sudden cardiac death, however, have been noted in the setting of progression of bundle branch block on serial EKGs [9].

13. **What should be done if an otherwise stable patient with a heart transplant is found to have atrial flutter, atrial fibrillation, or frequent ventricular arrhythmias preoperatively?**

Development of one of these arrhythmias in a patient with a transplanted heart may be a marker for significant underlying cardiac pathology such as rejection, LV dysfunction, or cardiac allograft vasculopathy. Identification of these arrhythmias should prompt a full workup to evaluate for the presence of these serious conditions and to ensure that cardiac function is optimized before the patient is taken to the operating room [9]. From a treatment standpoint, use of beta-blockers and calcium channel blockers for rate control may be limited by the risk of bradycardia and interactions with immunosuppressive medication. Despite the fact that amiodarone also has the potential to interfere with pharmacokinetic processing of certain immunosuppressants, it is frequently the drug of choice for treatment of atrial tachyarrhythmia in this patient population [9, 10]. Radiofrequency ablation may also be used to treat sustained arrhythmias.

14. **What is cardiac allograft vasculopathy?**

Cardiac allograft vasculopathy is the result of endothelial damage from both immune and nonimmune factors. It causes diffuse vascular remodeling, which can result in progressive and potentially rapid occlusion of affected vessels [4, 18].

15. **How common is this disease?**

Prevalence of this disease increases with time after heart transplantation with recent reports suggesting that more than half of patients alive ten years post-transplantation are affected [2, 4, 19]. It contributes significantly to post-transplant mortality and, along with neoplasia, represents one of the two leading causes for late mortality [19].

16. **How do patients with this disease present and how is the disease diagnosed and monitored?**

Denervation of the transplanted heart can complicate clinical detection of cardiac allograft vasculopathy. Typical symptoms of cardiac ischemia secondary to vasculopathy such as chest and shoulder discomfort may be absent and signs/symptoms of disease may instead present very late with silent myocardial infarction, ischemia-related arrhythmia, syncope, heart failure, or sudden cardiac death [4, 8, 18, 19]. While multiple methods for disease detection and monitoring such as ultrasound and optical coherence tomography have been proposed, current guidelines advocate for the use of coronary angiography in conjunction with functional assessments of graft activity [2, 4, 20].

17. **How is this disease treated?**

Cardiac allograft vasculopathy is primarily treated with percutaneous coronary intervention (PCI), surgical revascularization, or retransplantation. PCI is used in the majority of cases. Notably, the diffuse nature of this disease can limit the utility of treatment by PCI, particularly in disease affecting distal vasculature [3, 18]. For this reason, special attention should be paid to intraoperative coronary perfusion pressure in patients with known distal cardiac allograft vasculopathy in order to prevent ischemia.

18. **What is the role of endomyocardial biopsy (EMB) in the care of patients after they receive a heart transplant and how does this affect vascular access strategies during subsequent surgical procedures**?

Endomyocardial biopsy in conjunction with assessment of clinical signs and symptoms remains the gold standard for detection of graft rejection. It is currently the standard of care to have periodic endomyocardial biopsies performed as part of a rejection surveillance program throughout the first year after cardiac transplantation. Further, biopsies beyond this period may be performed as part of an ongoing surveillance program, if suspicion for graft rejection develops or to assess the clinical response to changes in a patient's immunosuppressive regimen. These biopsies are typically performed via the right internal jugular vein (IJ), and so when possible, cannulation of this vein should be avoided in order to preserve it for this function [3, 10, 21, 22].

19. **What are some of the clinical signs/symptoms of rejection**?

The clinical presentation of graft rejection may include development of fever, fatigue, new onset arrhythmia, new onset heart failure, and/or derangement in functional tests of the transplanted heart [3, 6, 9, 17].

20. **Why should further investigation into the possibility of rejection be carried out preoperatively if one of the above signs/symptoms is present**?

Some studies have shown that morbidity is higher in patients that have surgery in the middle of a rejection episode, suggesting that rejection should be ruled out and/or treated whenever possible prior to going to the operating room [6]. If surgery is required urgently or emergently, the risk associated with delaying the case to complete the workup must be balanced against the risk of proceeding in the presence of potential rejection.

21. **What three classes of drugs serve as the backbone for most patients' maintenance immunosuppressant regimen after heart transplantation**?

A typical maintenance immunosuppressive regimen after heart transplant is comprised of a calcineurin inhibitor (e.g., cyclosporine or tacrolimus), a steroid (e.g., prednisone) and an antimetabolite (e.g., mycophenolate). Deviations from this regimen sometimes occur in an effort to minimize morbidity related to the side-effects [7, 21].

22. **What are some of the most important cardiovascular, hematologic, endocrine, renal, and musculoskeletal side-effects of immunosuppressants from an anesthetic standpoint?**

- Cardiovascular: hypertension, hypercholesterolemia
- Hematologic: bone marrow suppression with associated anemia, leukopenia, and thrombocytopenia
- Endocrine: hyperglycemia, adrenal suppression
- Renal: renal insufficiency and electrolyte disturbances such as hyperkalemia and hypomagnesemia
- Musculoskeletal: osteoporosis [3, 6, 7, 15, 19].

23. **Should these medications be given during the perioperative period**?

Despite their side-effects, immunosuppressant medications should not be held without first consulting with the patient's transplant team. Occasionally, a single dose calcineurin inhibitor may be skipped on the morning of surgery to minimize development of perioperative renal dysfunction in the setting of dehydration. The remaining immunosuppressive medications are typically continued throughout the perioperative period [10]. Intraoperatively, dose adjustments may be necessary because of potential drug interactions or because of dilution by intraoperative fluid administration or blood loss [6]. Medications should be converted to and given IV if they cannot be given orally.

24. **Can NSAIDs be used in these patients**?

NSAIDs may worsen the nephrotoxicity that is associated with calcineurin inhibitor administration, limiting their use in transplant patients [6].

25. **Why must one have a heightened suspicion for the presence of infection in these patients**?

Use of immunosuppressive medications significantly increases the risk of infection which remains a major source of post-transplant morbidity and mortality [7, 23]. High rates of infection-related morbidity and mortality may in part be attributable to the fact that infections go unrecognized because the typical signs and symptoms are often absent in patients with compromised immune function [24].

26. **Should antibiotics be given as infective endocarditis prophylaxis in patients with a heart transplant prior to dental procedures?**

While the utility of perioperative antibiotic administration in preventing infective endocarditis after dental procedures in this patient population has not been clearly shown, the 2008 ACC/AHA guidelines recommend prophylaxis against infective endocarditis in cardiac transplant recipients who have a regurgitant valve lesion [25, 26].

27. **Are there any antibiotics that shouldn't be given to patients who have a heart transplant?**

Erythromycin and aminoglycoside antibiotics are often avoided as they may both exacerbate renal dysfunction related to calcineurin inhibitor use [10].

28. **How else might one's intraoperative anesthetic plan need to be adjusted in order to accommodate the increased risk of infection in heart transplant patients?**

Maintenance of sterility during placement of invasive lines and catheters is especially important as well as early removal of these devices. Avoidance of nasal intubation to prevent spread of nasal flora, early extubation, and aggressive pulmonary toilet may help to avoid the development of pulmonary infectious complications. If blood products are required, irradiated, leukocyte reduced, CMV negative products must be given through filters to minimize not only the risk of infection but also the risk of graft versus host disease [3, 10, 15].

29. **What effect does cyclosporine have on the activity of neuromuscular blocking drugs?**

Cyclosporine can augment the paralytic effect of some nondepolarizing neuromuscular blocking drugs [6].

30. **Why must one be cautious when reversing neuromuscular blockade in patients who have previously undergone heart transplantation?**

In normal individuals, neostigmine causes bradycardia by increasing acetylcholine-mediated parasympathetic signaling. This side-effect is usually prevented through the coadministration of an anticholinergic medication such as glycopyrrolate or atropine. *Theoretically*, denervation associated with heart transplantation renders the heart resistant to these parasympathetic effects, obviating the need for the use of an anticholinergic for this purpose. In practice, this is *not* the case and transplanted patients may instead demonstrate *heightened* sensitivity to the bradycardic effects of acetylcholinesterase inhibitors such as neostigmine [7, 27–29]. As the time from transplantation increases, it appears that the incidence of this sensitivity also increases, suggesting reinnervation may play an important role in this response [27]. This sensitivity can be profound and has caused asystole in patients despite coadministration of anticholinergics [28]. Accordingly, one should consider avoidance of neuromuscular blockade with nondepolarizing agents in patients that are more than a few months post-transplant when possible. If use of these agents is required, reversal should be done carefully with concomitant use of anticholinergic medications and with direct acting beta-agonists such as isoproterenol or epinephrine readily available to treat bradycardia if it does develop.

31. **Why might patients who have undergone cardiac transplantation be at a higher risk for complication from neuraxial/regional anesthesia?**
    - Bleeding: Thrombocytopenia may develop secondary to immunosuppressant medication use, and thus a platelet count should be obtained when a neuraxial or regional anesthesia is being considered.
    - Infection: Chronic immunosuppression puts patients at increased risk of infection. This risk should be discussed with the patient prior to use of neuraxial/regional anesthesia. Block and catheter placement should only be performed under strictly sterile conditions and early removal of any indwelling catheters that are placed may be important in minimizing risk.
    - Hemodynamic compromise: Denervation of the transplanted heart may leave it poorly equipped to manage the decrease in preload that may accompany neuraxial anesthesia. However, neuraxial anesthesia has proven to be safe and efficacious in this patient population when performed carefully, with special attention to and correction of hemodynamic abnormalities [30, 31].

32. **What are some of the basic considerations when it comes to airway management after cardiac transplantation?**

Nasal intubation should be avoided when possible to prevent the spread of nasal flora in an immunosuppressed patient. Immunosuppressive medications such as cyclosporine can also cause to gingival hyperplasia and can leave soft tissues of the upper airway more susceptible to bleeding, potentially complicating the placement of both endotracheal tubes and laryngeal mask airways [3]. Additionally, there is an increased incidence of lymphoproliferative disease in cardiac transplant recipients which has the potential to precipitate severe airway obstruction at the time of induction of anesthesia [1, 6].

References

1. Hasan W. Autonomic cardiac innervation: development and adult plasticity. Organogenesis. 2013;9(3):176–93.
2. Lymperopoulos A. Physiology and pharmacology of the cardiovascular adrenergic system. Front Physiol. 2013;4:240.
3. Blasco LM, Parameshwar J, Vuylsteke A. Anaesthesia for noncardiac surgery in the heart transplant recipient. Curr Opin Anaesthesiol. 2009;22(1):109–13.
4. Delgado JF, Manito N, Segovia J, Almenar L, Arizón JM, Campreciós M, et al. The use of proliferation signal inhibitors in the prevention and treatment of allograft vasculopathy in heart transplantation. Transplant Rev (Orlando). 2009;23(2):69–79.
5. Dipchand AI, Manlhiot C, Russell JL, Gurofsky R, Kantor PF, McCrindle BW. Exercise capacity improves with time in pediatric heart transplant recipients. J Heart Lung Transplant. 2009;28 (6):585–90.
6. Kostopanagiotou G, Smyrniotis V, Arkadopoulos N, Theodoraki K, Papadimitriou L, Papadimitriou J. Anesthetic and perioperative management of adult transplant recipients in nontransplant surgery. Anesth Analg. 1999;89(3):613–22.
7. Ramakrishna H, Rehfeldt KH, Pajaro OE. Anesthetic pharmacology and perioperative considerations for heart transplantation. Curr Clin Pharmacol. 2015;10(1):3–21.
8. Stark RP, McGinn AL, Wilson RF. Chest pain in cardiac-transplant recipients. Evidence of sensory reinnervation after cardiac transplantation. N Engl J Med. 1991;324(25):1791–4.
9. Thajudeen A, Stecker EC, Shehata M, Patel J, Wang X, McAnulty JH, et al. Arrhythmias after heart transplantation: mechanisms and management. J Am Heart Assoc. 2012;1(2):e001461.
10. Costanzo MR, Dipchand A, Starling R, Anderson A, Chan M, Desai S, et al. The international society of heart and lung transplantation guidelines for the care of heart transplant recipients. J Heart Lung Transplant. 2010;29(8):914–56.
11. Wilson RF, Johnson TH, Haidet GC, Kubo SH, Mianuelli M. Sympathetic reinnervation of the sinus node and exercise hemodynamics after cardiac transplantation. Circulation. 2000;101 (23):2727–33.
12. Chester MR, Madden B, Barnett D, Yacoub M. The effect of orthotopic transplantation on total, beta 1- and beta 2-adrenoceptors in the human heart. Br J Clin Pharmacol. 1992;33(4):417–22.
13. Gilbert EM, Eiswirth CC, Mealey PC, Larrabee P, Herrick CM, Bristow MR. Beta-adrenergic supersensitivity of the transplanted human heart is presynaptic in origin. Circulation. 1989;79(2):344–9.
14. Tsai VW, Cooper J, Garan H, Natale A, Ptaszek LM, Ellinor PT, et al. The efficacy of implantable cardioverter-defibrillators in heart transplant recipients: results from a multicenter registry. Circ Heart Fail. 2009;2(3):197–201.
15. Poston RS, Griffith BP. Heart transplantation. J Intensive Care Med. 2004;19(1):3–12.
16. Davies RR, Russo MJ, Morgan JA, Sorabella RA, Naka Y, Chen JM. Standard versus bicaval techniques for orthotopic heart transplantation: an analysis of the united network for organ sharing database. J Thorac Cardiovasc Surg. 2010;140(3):700–8 8.e1–2.
17. Vaseghi M, Boyle NG, Kedia R, Patel JK, Cesario DA, Wiener I, et al. Supraventricular tachycardia after orthotopic cardiac transplantation. J Am Coll Cardiol. 2008;51(23):2241–9.
18. Bhama JK, Nguyen DQ, Scolieri S, Teuteberg JJ, Toyoda Y, Kormos RL, et al. Surgical revascularization for cardiac allograft vasculopathy: is it still an option? J Thorac Cardiovasc Surg. 2009;137(6):1488–92.
19. Francis GS, Greenberg BH, Hsu DT, Jaski BE, Jessup M, LeWinter MM, et al. ACCF/AHA/ACP/HFSA/ISHLT 2010 clinical competence statement on management of patients with advanced heart failure and cardiac transplant: a report of the ACCF/AHA/ACP task force on clinical competence and training. J Am Coll Cardiol. 2010;56(5):424–53.
20. Salvadori M, Bertoni E. What's new in clinical solid organ transplantation by 2013. World J Transplant. 2014;4(4):243–66.
21. Singh D, Taylor DO. Advances in the understanding and management of heart transplantation. F1000Prime Rep. 2015;7:52.
22. Stehlik J, Starling RC, Movsesian MA, Fang JC, Brown RN, Hess ML, et al. Utility of long-term surveillance endomyocardial biopsy: a multi-institutional analysis. J Heart Lung Transplant. 2006;25(12):1402–9.
23. Humar A, Michaels M, AIWGoID. American Society of Transplantation recommendations for screening, monitoring and reporting of infectious complications in immunosuppression trials in recipients of organ transplantation. Am J Transplant. 2006;6 (2):262–74.
24. Fishman JA. Infection in solid-organ transplant recipients. N Engl J Med. 2007;357(25):2601–14.
25. Nishimura RA, Carabello BA, Faxon DP, Freed MD, Lytle BW, O'Gara PT, et al. ACC/AHA 2008 guideline update on valvular heart disease: focused update on infective endocarditis: a report of the American college of cardiology/American heart association task force on practice guidelines: endorsed by the society of cardiovascular anesthesiologists, society for cardiovascular angiography and interventions, and society of thoracic surgeons. Circulation. 2008;118(8):887–96.
26. Wilson W, Taubert KA, Gewitz M, Lockhart PB, Baddour LM, Levison M, et al. Prevention of infective endocarditis: guidelines from the American heart association: a guideline from the American heart association rheumatic fever, endocarditis, and Kawasaki disease committee, council on cardiovascular disease in the young, and the council on clinical cardiology, council on cardiovascular surgery and anesthesia, and the quality of care and outcomes research interdisciplinary working group. Circulation. 2007;116(15):1736–54.
27. Backman SB, Fox GS, Stein RD, Ralley FE. Neostigmine decreases heart rate in heart transplant patients. Can J Anaesth. 1996;43(4):373–8.
28. Bjerke RJ, Mangione MP. Asystole after intravenous neostigmine in a heart transplant recipient. Can J Anaesth. 2001;48(3):305–7.
29. Gómez-Ríos M. Anaesthesia for non-cardiac surgery in a cardiac transplant recipient. Indian J Anaesth. 2012;56(1):88–9.
30. Allard R, Hatzakorzian R, Deschamps A, Backman SB. Decreased heart rate and blood pressure in a recent cardiac transplant patient after spinal anesthesia. Can J Anaesth. 2004;51(8):829–33.
31. Cheng DC, Ong DD. Anaesthesia for non-cardiac surgery in heart-transplanted patients. Can J Anaesth. 1993;40(10):981–6.

Anesthesia for Coronary Artery Bypass Graft (CABG) 13

Jamahal Luxford and Levi Bassin

A 53 y/o man presents with an episode of intractable chest pain and dyspnea after shoveling snow, and a 3-month history of worsening dyspnea on exertion.

Medications:	Simvastatin 20 mg oral daily
	ACE-I
	Heparin drip—started as inpatient
	Nitroglycerin drip—started as inpatient
	Aspirin 81 mg oral daily—started as inpatient
Allergies:	Nil Known
Past Medical History:	
Cardiac:	Hypertension
	Hypercholesterolemia
Physical Exam:	
Vital Signs:	BP 125/81 HR 80 RR 16 Oxygen saturation: 98%
Coronary Angiogram:	
80% stenosis of the Proximal Left Anterior Descending Artery (LAD)	
90% stenosis of the Right Coronary Artery (RCA)	
70% stenosis of the Left Circumflex Artery (LCx)	
Right dominant circulation	
LV gram suggests a diminished ejection fraction	
Transthoracic Echocardiogram summary report:	
Normal thickness of left ventricular wall	
Normal size left ventricle	
Diminished left ventricular ejection fraction—estimated 35–40%	
Hypokinesis in the inferior wall and anterior, anterolateral and anteroseptal walls	
Normal appearance and function of the right ventricle	
Trace to mild tricuspid regurgitation. Otherwise normal valves	
No pericardial effusion	

1. **What are the indications for non-emergent CABG?**

The AHA/ACC guidelines indicate the level of evidence for CABG surgery. The following are considered Class 1 indications for surgery in stable CAD [1]:

- CABG to improve survival is recommended for patients with significant (>50% diameter stenosis) left main coronary artery disease. (*Level of Evidence: B*)
- CABG to improve survival is beneficial in patients with significant (>70% diameter) stenosis in 3 main coronary arteries (with or without involvement of the proximal LAD artery) or in the proximal LAD plus 1 other major coronary artery. (*Level of Evidence: B*)

Other indications for CABG or PCI include improving survival in patients who survive sudden cardiac death with presumed ischemia mediated VT, or to improve symptoms in patients with persistent angina despite goal-directed medical therapy. Both of these indications relate to a significant (>70% diameter) stenosis in a major coronary artery.

CABG is also recommended in patients undergoing non-coronary cardiac surgery with greater than or equal to 50% luminal diameter narrowing of the left main coronary artery or greater than or equal to 70% luminal narrowing of other major coronary arteries. (*Level of Evidence: C*)

The indications for emergency CABG are different to those for the elective situation.

J. Luxford (✉)
Department of Anesthesiology, Perioperative and Pain Medicine, Brigham and Women's Hospital, 75 Francis St, Boston, MA, USA
e-mail: jamahal@hotmail.com

L. Bassin
Cardiac Surgery, Brigham and Women's Hospital, 75 Francis St, 02445 Boston, MA, USA
e-mail: levi.bassin@gmail.com

© Springer International Publishing AG 2017
L.S. Aglio and R.D. Urman (eds.), *Anesthesiology*, DOI 10.1007/978-3-319-50141-3_13

2. **What are the important features to note on the coronary angiogram?**

The coronary angiogram will demonstrate the location and severity of coronary artery disease and will often also have a left ventriculogram. This gives an assessment of LV function and the degree of MR, if present. The degree of coronary disease may guide the conduct of anesthesia and whether an Intra Aortic Balloon Pump (IABP) will be required.

Patients undergoing CABG usually have significant involvement of the LAD and multi-vessel disease not amenable to PCI. Anatomical considerations include:

- Where is the disease and what is the extent of the disease?
- Is there left main stenosis? (>50% stenosis of the left main)
- Is there left main equivalent stenosis (>70% stenosis of the proximal LAD and LCx)
- Are any vessels completely occluded? (These will be supplied by collaterals and are more pressure dependent)

Coronary anatomy from angiography that should raise concern for the induction of anesthesia include the following:

- Severe left main (>90%) or left main equivalent disease
- Chronic obstruction of 2 vessels (e.g., RCA and LAD. This results in the majority of myocardium being supplied by the remaining vessel, in this scenario the LCx)

Also, if the patient is having active rest angina or ECG changes despite maximal medical management, regardless of anatomy, this is obviously of concern.

3. **What scoring systems are used for determining the predicted risk of mortality (PROM)?**

Several scoring systems exist and are all based on large databases of patients having undergone cardiac surgery. These scores utilize a variety of preoperative factors (such as age, LV function, renal dysfunction, etc.), to estimate a patient's 30-day PROM.

These have better predictive power for lower risk patients:

- EuroSCORE
  - European System for Cardiac Operative Risk Evaluation. First published in 1999, and predominantly a score for CABG alone [2].
- EuroSCORE II
  - Updated EuroSCORE in 2012. Based on a much larger database of contemporary surgical outcomes.
- STS score
  - Society of Thoracic Surgeons. Provides PROM for CABG, valve, or combined CABG/valve procedures [3].

4. **What factors may significantly increase the risk of cardiac surgery?**

The following are some factors which may increase the risk of cardiac surgery:

- Age
- Co-morbidities
  - LV dysfunction, renal dysfunction, pulmonary hypertension, hepatic dysfunction, active endocarditis
- Frailty (difficult to measure)
  - The American College of Surgeons suggests use of the Fried or Robinson scales [4]
- Urgency status
  - Active ischemia/failure, preoperative inotropes/mechanical support (VAD/IABP)
- Technical factors
  - Redo cardiac surgery, poor coronary targets (i.e., difficult to graft/incomplete revascularization), aortic calcification (difficult to cannulate/cross clamp).

5. **What are generally accepted rates of complications for elective CABG in a patient with normal LV function?**

Mortality	1–2%
Stroke	1–2%
Perioperative MI	2–5%
Early graft dysfunction	1–5%
Deep sternal wound infection	1% (up to 3% if bilateral IMA)
Transfusion of RBC	20–50%
Renal failure requiring dialysis	1–2%
Prolonged ventilation	1–5%

These may increase with age, LV impairment, urgent status, previous neurological event, renal impairment, and airways disease.

6. **How long should antiplatelet/anticoagulants be withheld prior to surgery?**

This depends on both the urgency of the operation and the pharmacology of the drug involved.

- Aspirin (irreversible platelet inhibitor—blocks platelet cyclo-oxygenase):
  - Can safely continue low dose aspirin (81 mg daily; this is an AHA class I recommendation.
- Clopidogrel (irreversible thienopyridine platelet inhibitor —blocks ADP):
  - Should wait 5 days, but can operate if necessary, accepting a higher risk of bleeding.
- Prasugrel (more potent irreversible thienopyridine than clopidogrel):
  - Should wait 7 days and should not operate unless absolutely required in the first 3 days.
- Ticagralor (potent reversible thienopyridine):
  - Ideally should wait 5 days, but can operate if necessary with higher risk of bleeding.
- Abciximab—reversible platelet inhibitor—(monoclonal antibody against GPIIb/IIIa):
  - Is often used in PCI and in unstable angina with critical coronary anatomy.
  - Plasma half-life of 30 min with significant platelet dysfunction for 48 h.
  - Stopping the drug 12 h prior to surgery will limit blood loss with surgery.
- Unfractionated Heparin (UFH):
  - It produces its major anticoagulant effect by inactivating thrombin and activated factor X (factor Xa) through an antithrombin III-dependent mechanism; half-life is 1–2 h.
  - Is usually ceased 6 h prior to surgery unless the patient is suffering from unstable angina/acute coronary syndrome, in which case it can be continued to the OR.
- Low Molecular Weight Heparins (LMWH):
  - Much longer half-life and dosing depends on renal function.
  - If on therapeutic LMWH, ideally should wait 24 h from the previous dose, longer if abnormal renal function.
  - The patient should ideally be switched to UFH 48 h prior to surgery.
- Bivalirudin:
  - A reversible direct thrombin inhibitor with a half-life of 25 min. Should be stopped 6 h prior to surgery.
- Coumadin (warfarin):
  - Cease 5 days prior and bridge with LMWH or UFH depending on the clinical requirement for anticoagulation.
- Novel oral anticoagulants (NOACs):
  - These include the direct thrombin inhibitor dabigatran (Pradaxa®) and the Xa inhibitors rivaroxoban (Xarelto®) and apixiban (Eliquis®).
  - These have a shorter effective half-life than Coumadin but should be stopped at least 4 days prior to cardiac surgery and bridged with LMWH/UFH as required.

7. **Should this patient have investigation of the carotid arteries performed?**

The AHA recommends carotid artery duplex in a patient with the following high risk features (Class IIa recommendation. *Level of Evidence: C*) [5]:

- >65 years of age
- Left main coronary stenosis
- Peripheral arterial disease
- History of cerebrovascular disease (stroke/TIA)
- Hypertension
- Smoking
- Diabetes mellitus

The key findings are internal carotid artery (ICA) stenosis and vertebral artery flow. This will guide perfusion management on cardiopulmonary bypass (CPB), whether cerebral oximetry monitoring may be required intraoperatively, and whether concomitant carotid intervention is warranted.

8. **When is intervention for carotid artery disease indicated in the setting of CABG?**

Concomitant carotid intervention (either pre-CABG, during, or post-CABG) is suggested for:

- ICA stenosis 50–99% with a history of stroke or TIA (Class IIa)
- Bilateral ICA stenosis 70–99% if asymptomatic (Class IIb)
- Unilateral ICA stenosis 70–99% with contralateral occlusion (Class IIb).

All of these recommendations have a *Level of Evidence: C*

The ideal timing of concomitant carotid intervention is unclear from the evidence. Preoperative carotid intervention carries a higher perioperative MI risk, postoperative carries a higher stroke risk for the CABG, and carotid/CABG in the same setting carries a higher risk of stroke [6].

9. **Are all patients presenting for an isolated CABG procedure required to have a TTE performed prior to surgery?**

Most patients in the modern era have had a TTE performed preoperatively. A select group may be able to proceed to CABG without a TTE:

- If clinical exam shows no evidence of valvular disease, and
- If the left heart catheterization showed normal LV function, and
- No MR on LV gram, and
- If they will have a TEE intraoperatively.

The important things to note on a preoperative TTE include the following:

- LV function and size
- RV function and size
- Valvular pathology
- Pulmonary pressures (estimated from the TR jet velocity)
- Presence of a pericardial effusion
- Aortic dimensions (looking for aneurysm).

10. **When is a myocardial viability test indicated in the preoperative work-up for planned CABG surgery?**

The aim of CABG is for both a survival benefit and to reduce the symptoms of debilitating and refractory angina. Patients with significant myocardial scar will not see these benefits, as revascularization will not improve the scarred territory. Furthermore patients with anatomical three vessel disease with a large LAD territory scar are not considered to have *clinical LAD* disease and these patients may not see the survival benefit of CABG over PCI.

There are 4 states of ventricular myocardium [7]:

(1) Normal contractility—viable
(2) Hibernating—reversible ischemic hypocontractility with **hypoperfusion**
(3) Stunned—transient post-ischemic hypocontractility with **normal perfusion**
(4) Scar

Viability testing is utilized to determine what is viable myocardium and would be expected to benefit from revascularization. These studies include the following:

- MRI:
  - Late gadolinium enhancement >50% of the LV wall thickness indicates nonviability.
- Nuclear imaging:
  - Technetium sestamibi or Thallium. The radioisotopes are taken up by viable myocardium.
- PET:
  - Viable myocardium will have FDG (fluorodeoxyglucose) uptake.
- Stress echocardiography:
  - With exercise or dobutamine (to 20 mcg/kg/min)
  - Viable territories should improve with dobutamine [8].

11. **What conduits are available for bypasses and what factors influence the decision to use a particular conduit?**

The most common conduits used for CABG include: the internal mammary arteries (left and right, referred to as LIMA and RIMA), the long saphenous vein, and the radial arteries. Other less commonly used vessels include the short saphenous vein, the right gastroepiploic artery, and the cephalic vein in the forearm.

Long-term patency of the grafts depends on the quality of the conduit as well as the quality of the target vessel. The LIMA has proven to be the most durable conduit with a 10-year patency of 95% when grafted to the LAD. A LIMA to the LAD is associated with improved survival compared with vein to the LAD, PCI, or medical therapy alone.

Saphenous vein grafts are immediately available, are not prone to spasm, and are not prone to competition with the native flow as opposed to arterial conduits (IMA and radial artery). However, the saphenous vein generally develops a thickened intima with associated obstructive disease as the vein becomes 'arterialized.' The 10-year patency of vein grafts to the RCA or LCX is approximately 70%.

The radial artery is particularly prone to spasm due to its thick and muscular media. Spasm is reduced by using topical and intra-luminal vasodilators (verapamil, nitroglycerin) and by grafting it to a coronary artery that has a high grade stenosis so that the native flow does not "compete" with the radial artery.

The nondominant arm is usually used and there should be clear communication preoperatively between the anesthesia and surgical teams so that a radial arterial line is not inserted into the artery that is to be harvested.

The risks of radial artery harvest include: hand ischemia (if the deep and superficial palmar arches are incomplete), and paresthesia from injury to the superficial radial nerve (on the lateral aspect of the dorsum of the hand). Postoperative hand weakness is uncommon.

An Allen's test is performed to test whether the ulnar artery can adequately supply the hand by way of intact palmar arches.

12. **What is the evidence for an Allen's Test?**

Although there is little evidence that it is a particularly predictive test, it is commonly performed in the preoperative assessment [9].

13. **Should CABG be performed "on-pump" or "off-pump"? What are some of the supposed benefits of avoiding CPB?**

On-pump CABG is the most common method of performing CABG in the USA. This refers to performing the bypasses with the heart arrested using cardiopulmonary bypass. This enables accurate visualization and performance of the coronary anastomosis in a still and bloodless field. However, this comes at the cost of the effects of CPB with possible neurological injury, renal injury, anemia, platelet dysfunction, and systemic inflammatory response.

Off-pump CABG (OPCAB) entails performing the bypasses on a beating heart without the use of CPB and is technically more difficult. There has been a lot of controversy regarding the benefits of either technique and there has been a resurgence of on-pump CABG in the USA. Two large randomized trials (ROOBY and CORONARY) failed to show a benefit of off-pump over on-pump at one year in terms of mortality, stroke or renal failure [10, 11].

In the ROOBY trial, off-pump was also found to be associated with significantly worse graft patency at one year.

14. **What are some of the issues faced by the anesthetist associated with performing OPCAB?**

Issues include the following:

- Thermoregulation (usually managed with assistance of the heart-lung machine)
- The need for scrupulous management of hemodynamics by the anesthesiologist throughout the procedure
- Changes in the utility and appearance of monitoring (ECG, TEE) during portions of the procedure
- Management of ischemia during performance of the anastomoses
- Manipulation of the heart rapidly alters loading conditions, which may also lead to arrhythmias and large swings in hemodynamics [12]

An awareness of the surgical requirements at various stages of the operation, when regional ischemia may be induced, and the cardiac manipulations performed are all required. Subsequently communication with the surgical team is even more critical than with conventional CABG.

15. **The patient says he is concerned about the anesthesia as his father had a CABG in his seventies and didn't seem "quite right" for some time after. What would you tell him?**

Neurological injury is one the most feared complications responsible for morbidity and mortality after cardiac surgery. It exists on a spectrum from definitive cerebrovascular accident (stroke) to subtle neurocognitive effects [13].

Stroke

There is a strong association between the burden of atherosclerotic disease and neurocognitive morbidity. If a patient is found to have high grade of atherosclerosis, or mobile plaque in the ascending aorta, then the operative technique may be altered in the hope of minimizing plaque mobilization.

Postoperative Cognitive Dysfunction (POCD)

Subtle neurocognitive dysfunction has been recognized to occur after cardiac surgery. Potential etiological factors have included CPB itself, inflammatory processes and embolic complications. More recent research suggests the degree of POCD after 3 months is unrelated to the type of surgery [14]. This is supported by the findings that the incidence of POCD is no different between OPCAB and conventional CABG [15].

16. **Is this patient, having cardiac surgery, at higher than average risk of awareness or is this only of historical concern?**

Cardiac surgery has classically been considered high risk for awareness. However, this occurred with older, high opiate regimes using little volatile or other amnestic, resulting in incidences of awareness >10% [16].

The cause of awareness under anesthesia is an imbalance between the requirements of the patient needed to avoid consciousness and what is administered.

- A patient with **normal** anesthesia requirements, who cannot tolerate the necessary anesthesia, i.e., due to diminished ejection fraction or hemodynamic compromise
- A patient with **normal** anesthesia requirements, who receives too little, often by error
- A patient with **higher** than normal requirements, who receives a normal amount

The largest study of intraoperative awareness to date suggested an incidence of 1:10,000 in cardiac surgery, higher than the overall incidence [16]. As conceptualized above, most episodes of awareness involved either brief interruptions of drug delivery, by human error or technical problems, or the use of intentionally low doses of anesthetic in high risk patients.

During low stimulation parts of CABG surgery, such as harvesting of the LIMA, relative hypotension is not uncommon. While it may be tempting to reduce the concentration of volatile delivered, it is important to remember awareness is still possible at this point. Relatively high doses of opiate agents and the prevalence of beta blocker usage in these patients may mask the hemodynamic changes sometimes used as surrogate measures with light anesthesia.

In routine cardiac surgery clear communication with perfusion staff is essential to ensure adequate anesthesia agent is continued on CPB and the use of some depth of anesthesia monitor is suggested. Circulating volume changes and alterations in drug concentrations are associated with the commencement and cessation of CPB, representing vulnerable times for awareness. In sicker cardiac patients (i.e., reduced EF or disease requiring tightly controlled hemodynamics) vigilance must be maintained to ensure adequate anesthesia for amnesia is administered.

17. **What is "Fast Track" cardiac surgery? Is this patient suitable?**

Although no firm definition exists, this refers to anesthesia and postoperative processes for cardiac surgical patients which encourage comfortable and safe extubation <6 h after surgery and minimizing both the duration of ICU and overall length of stay [17].

As with any general anesthetic, areas that require attention are: hemodynamic stability, thermoregulation, control of nausea and vomiting, and adequate analgesia without excessive respiratory depression from opiates (or sedatives). Attention to the appropriate management of neuromuscular blockade, and avoidance of long acting agents is also required.

A successful "fast track" process also requires appropriate patient selection and operative list management as well as adequate staffing and skill mix in the postoperative environment, so that patients may be safely extubated when clinically indicated regardless of the time of day. As with many aspects of cardiac anesthesia, the success of such goals depends on attention to teamwork and communication.

18. **What would be the utility of a Pulmonary Artery Catheter (PAC) in this patient?**

The Pulmonary Artery or Swan Ganz Catheter is a monitoring tool which is still frequently utilized within cardiac surgery. The catheter itself has a number of lumens which can be used like a conventional central venous catheter, however it also has a balloon directed tip that allows for the transduction of pulmonary artery pressures. The PAC can also continuously monitor central venous oxygen saturations, whilst specialized variants allow for pacing of the heart.

Although many studies have failed to demonstrate benefit from the routine use of the PAC, and some even suggested the potential for harm, its use in many centers for cardiac surgery is routine [18]. Some centers use it in a more pragmatic manner for only higher risk patients, or those having more complex surgery, however evidence for benefit in these situations is also limited.

19. **Should this patient have a Transesophageal Echo (TEE) performed intraoperatively?**

The use of TEE in CABG has only a Class IIa (*Level of Evidence: B*) recommendation [5]:

- Intraoperative TEE is reasonable for monitoring of hemodynamic status, ventricular function, regional wall motion, and valvular function in patients undergoing CABG

Despite this, TEE is commonly utilized in routine CABG surgery, as is PAC in some centers. In regard to this patient, given the diminished EF, a stronger case could be made for the use of intraoperative TEE on the balance of potential risks and benefits.

As an example of the breadth of anesthetic practice in what would be considered to be a highly standardized procedure (CABG), an otherwise well patient with a maintained EF presenting for CABG could have *both* a PAC and TEE, one or the other, or potentially neither (only a conventional CVC), depending on the institute and practice of the anesthesiologists and surgeons involved.

The benefits of TEE over PAC include the following:

- Better delineation of loading conditions and RWMA
- Ability to examine for additional cardiac pathology

In a situation where TEE is to be avoided, additional information can be gained through the use of epiaortic/epicardial echocardiography. If TEE is not used initially but needed as a "rescue" later, should hemodynamic or operative complications arise, it is important to be cognizant that the patient will likely be fully heparinized at this time of probe placement.

20. **What are the potential risks of TEE or PAC placement?**

TEE

Although often considered as a reasonably "non-invasive" instrument, TEE comes with its own unique risks. There are a number of absolute and relative contraindications [19] (Table 1).

The overall complication of TEE placement and intraoperative usage is 0.2%. Incidence of complications are shown in Table 2 [20]:

Table 1 Absolute and relative contraindications for TEE placement

Absolute contraindications	Relative contraindications
Perforated viscus	History of radiation to neck and mediastinum
Esophageal stricture	History of GI surgery
Esophageal tumor	Recent upper GI bleed
Esophageal perforation, laceration	Barrett's esophagus
Esophageal diverticulum	History of dysphagia
Active upper GI bleed	Restriction of neck mobility (severe cervical arthritis, atlantoaxial joint disease)
	Symptomatic hiatal hernia
	Esophageal varices
	Coagulopathy, thrombocytopenia
	Active esophagitis
	Active peptic ulcer disease

Table 2 Incidence of complications from TEE placement

Mortality	0%
Major morbidity	0–1.2%
Major bleeding	0.03–0.8%
Esophageal perforation	0–0.3%
Minor pharyngeal bleeding	0.01%
Severe odynophagia	0.1%
Dental injury and ETT malposition	Both 0.035%

Pulmonary Artery Catheter

Complications of PAC can be classified as those related to the following:

- Placement of central venous access
- In vivo presence of catheter and potential for arrhythmias
- Interpretation of hemodynamic information obtained

The most feared complication of PAC use is pulmonary artery rupture, with an incidence of 0.03–0.2% of cases, with a mortality of 41–70%. Factors which may increase this include the following: hypothermia, anticoagulation, advanced age and potentially pulmonary hypertension [21].

Attention must be paid to ensuring the PAC is not "over-wedged," having migrated distally or impacted against the vessel wall.

21. **What other monitors should be utilized during cardiac surgery?**

In addition to the routine monitors required for any general anesthetic as laid out by the standards for basic anesthetic monitoring, an arterial line and temperature monitoring should be used. As usual, temperature may be monitored at many locations, however a central site, such are bladder (utilizing a specialized urinary catheter) and a naso or oropharyngeal site are often used. This aids monitoring of the adequacy of rewarming post CPB. Oropharyngeal temperature monitoring may be preferred as it avoids the potential for nasal mucosa injury in a fully heparinized patient.

In some cardiac surgery, cerebral oximetry monitoring may be utilized, but this is unlikely for routine CABG with normal carotid arteries. Given the previous discussion on the increased risk for awareness, some form of processed EEG monitoring (BIS or similar) is often used.

A report by the ASA task force on intraoperative awareness could not come to firm consensus on the use of awareness monitoring. The consultants were equivocal regarding the use of brain electrical monitoring for cardiac surgery, whereas the ASA members agree with their use [22].

22. **Should this patient be administered an antifibrinolytic? Briefly what was the concern in relation to the use of Aprotinin in cardiac surgery?**

A large percentage of patients presenting for cardiac surgery will require a blood transfusion. Whilst this is dependent on a number of patient and surgical variables, there are standardized processes which may help to reduce transfusion rates. One of these relates to the utilization of antifibrinolytic drugs.

The Society of Thoracic Surgeons Blood Conservation Clinical Practice Guidelines gives the use of Lysine analogues (epsilon-aminocaproic acid and tranexamic acid) a Class 1 recommendation (*Level of Evidence: A*). These agents reduce total blood loss and decrease the number of patients who require blood transfusion during cardiac procedures and are indicated for the purposes of blood conservation [23].

The serine protease inhibitor aprotinin is another antifibrinolytic agent. Concerns about its potential for renal dysfunction led to the BART trial which compared the use of various antifibrinolytic agents in patients undergoing high risk cardiac surgery. The study was terminated due to an excess of cardiac deaths within the aprotinin group [24].

The STS guideline gives both high and low dose regimes of aprotonin a Class III recommendation (Evidence for Harm, should not be used).

23. **What is "coronary steal" and how is it related to the practice of cardiac anesthesia?**

Coronary steal refers to the redistribution of blood flow to non-ischemic myocardium at the expense of decreased flow to an area of collateral dependent ischemic myocardium. In the practice of cardiac surgery early concern existed about the potential for isoflurane to lead to vasodilation of coronary arterial vessels, diverting ("stealing") blood flow from a vessel with a fixed obstruction, worsening the already existing ischemia [25, 26].

Despite a good theoretical scientific basis, in the modern practice of "balanced anesthesia" with low inspired concentrations of volatile, it is of little practical clinical concern and isoflurane is commonly utilized for cardiac surgery.

This is not to diminish the role or existence of coronary steal as an entity. It is exactly this mechanism that is utilized in noninvasive cardiac testing with agents such as dipyridamole.

24. **What is ischemic preconditioning and how does it relate to surgery and anesthesia for CABG?**

Myocardium which has previously been exposed to brief intermittent episodes of ischemia appear to be protected against subsequent episodes of more significant ischemia. This concept is known as "ischemic preconditioning" and meaningful ways to utilize this in cardiac surgery is the subject of ongoing research [27]. "Remote preconditioning" (utilizing induced ischemia in muscle distant from myocardium) has shown beneficial effects in experimental models.

Volatile anesthetic agents (desflurane and sevoflurane) administered during cardiac surgery induce protective effects on myocardium in a similar manner to ischemic preconditioning [5]. However, this has a complex and inconsistent effect, with uncertain clinical significance, where ongoing research is required.

25. **What analgesic regime should be utilized for this patient? Should any agent in particular be avoided?**

Although midline sternotomy is a significant nociceptive stimulus, the analgesic regimes utilized are usually simple and effective. Baseline acetaminophen and some form of intermediate duration opiate is often all that is required. An opiate infusion is commonly utilized whilst the patient remains intubated in ICU, and then PRN opiate or PCA in the first few days postoperatively. Adequate analgesia is required to ensure patients can undertake chest physiotherapy in addition to other routine postoperative activities.

NSAID in the form of aspirin is often continued post operatively for its antiplatelet effect more than analgesia. Other NSAIDs are generally avoided both for their additional (and potentially unwanted) antiplatelet effects and other complications such as nephrotoxicity and effect on gastric mucosa. Particularly the COX-2 specific agents were found to have pro-thrombotic complications and subsequently removed from use in cardiac surgical patients [28].

26. **Could an epidural be beneficial in this case?**

Neuraxial analgesia (epidural) may seem attractive in cardiac surgery due to the potential for excellent analgesia in the area of incision, potentially beneficial sympatholysis of the coronary vessels and other perceived benefits of epidurals such as reduced respiratory complications. However, the logistics and risk/benefit balance of placing a high thoracic epidural in patients, many of whom are already on antiplatelet or anticoagulant medication, for an operation where they will be fully heparinized means it is not commonly performed. Although very unlikely, and not even well quantified, the potential for catastrophic cervical/high thoracic epidural hematoma prevents routine utilization [29, 30].

It is feasible to perform OPCAB surgery with a non-general anesthesia technique utilizing high epidural (C7-T2 region) and even a concurrent femoral nerve block for SVG harvesting. These techniques are even less commonly utilized than epidural in conjunction with on-pump CABG [31].

27. **After uneventful induction of anesthesia, ST segment elevation is noted after the sternum is opened. How should this be managed?**

This requires both further investigation of the likely etiology and appropriate management.

Detection

Monitors include: ECG, echocardiography, and PAC.

- 5 lead ECG is usually utilized.
  - It is important to observe the full leads of the monitor at baseline, so that any changes may be noted.
- Echocardiography. Intraoperative TEE:
  - Is a sensitive marker of myocardial ischemia. Although not a continuous monitor of ischemia it can be used to compare current with baseline appearance.
  - TEE views which show the myocardium supplied by all coronary arteries (such as the TG SAX view) may be used as a rapid method to examine for myocardial dysfunction.
- PAC:
  - Particular waveforms and hemodynamic information in the PAC tracing can be examined as markers for myocardial ischemia.
- Direct visualization.
  - With the sternum and pericardium opened, the function of the heart can be viewed and general qualitative comments about its function made by experienced clinicians.
- *Management*

Immediate management will be directed at improving the balance of myocardial oxygen demand and delivery. Reduction of tachycardia or elevated heart rate, reducing excessive afterload and treatment of any arrhythmia should be undertaken. Appropriate pharmacotherapy includes, but is not limited to: analgesia, deepening anesthesia, beta blockade, antiarrhythmics (if arrhythmia is involved), and nitroglycerin.

If refractory to this management, the anesthetist should discuss with the surgeon and perfusionist other options, including IABP or the commencement of CPB.

28. **What is the role of an intra-aortic balloon pump (IABP) for CABG?**

An IABP is positioned in the descending aorta, distal the left subclavian artery. It is usually inserted via the femoral artery but can also be placed via the subclavian artery or the aorta directly. It inflates during diastole and deflates just prior to the onset of systole to increase coronary perfusion (in diastole) and to reduce LV afterload and wall tension (during systole) thus increasing myocardial oxygen supply and decreasing demand.

Indications for use include cardiogenic shock, acute myocardial ischemia or prophylaxis for very high grade coronary disease (to reduce ischemic events during induction and prior to revascularization) or prophylaxis for severe LV dysfunction. The evidence for prophylaxis is controversial with some studies showing a benefit, and some showing harm.

There was no survival benefit of IABP in patients with cardiogenic shock in the IABP-SHOCK II trial where 600 patients with cardiogenic shock from acute coronary syndrome were randomized to IABP or conventional therapy [32].

29. **After successful management and resolution of the ST elevation, surgery is continued. How does the anesthetist provide the surgeon with better access to the Internal Mammary Artery?**

The most common conduit for CABG is the LIMA. Positive pressure ventilation can impede the surgeon's access and visualization especially in patients who are obese or have a chest with a large anterior–posterior diameter. The proximal portion of the LIMA is particularly difficult to see during ventilation with normal tidal volumes. Visibility for the surgeon during this portion of the operation may be improved by lowering the tidal volume (and increasing respiratory rate), as well as minimizing the amount of PEEP.

The LIMA traverses the left pleural cavity and usually enters the pericardial cavity at the level of the main pulmonary artery and is therefore at risk of being put under tension by the left upper lobe. For this reason when the collapsed lungs are being reinflated prior to the termination of CPB the anesthesiologist must manually ventilate and watch carefully (in conjunction with the surgeon) that the LIMA is not caught on top of the left upper lobe. More than one anesthesiologist has had the misfortune of tearing the LIMA anastomosis off the LAD with injudicious ventilation at this stage.

30. **How is CABG surgery performed?**

The general principle of CABG is to bypass the stenosis by anastomosing a piece of vascular conduit (IMA, saphenous vein, radial artery) with a new inflow distal to the stenosis. The key philosophical difference between CABG and PCI is that for CABG, progression of the native disease proximal to the graft will not result in an MI whilst for PCI, only the discrete portion of stenotic lesion is treated.

The new inflow is usually from the ascending aorta for saphenous veins or radial arteries, whilst the IMA has its own separate supply from the subclavian artery. Other combinations include connecting a radial artery to the side of an IMA to create a 'T' or 'Y' graft which has the benefit of reducing the aortic manipulation and thus reducing the risk of stroke.

The distal anastomoses are usually performed first followed by the proximals to the ascending aorta. For on-pump surgery the proximals can be performed when the heart is arrested or when the heart is beating with the use of a partial clamp on the ascending aorta (although this may incur a higher stroke risk).

Graft patency can be assessed by injecting the graft with a handheld syringe and feeling the resistance (before the proximals are complete, and not applicable to the in situ IMA); by placing a doppler flow probe around the graft; and by watching the run-off into the distal part of the vessel when releasing a clamp on the graft.

31. **What is epiaortic scanning and what may be its role in CABG surgery?**

Neurological injury in the perioperative period may be related to cannulation and cross-clamping of the ascending aorta with the associated embolization of debris from the injured intima [33]. Mills and Everson classified 3 aortic pathologies:

1. Medial calcification (circumferential), or the 'porcelain aorta' which is easiest to recognize;
2. Diffuse intimal thickening where palpation can be normal; and
3. Liquid intramural debris.

One method to mitigate this risk is to plan the cannulation strategy based on palpation and epiaortic ultrasound (US), an approach supported by a Class IIa AHA recommendation for routine use in CABG [34]. A technique is to place a high-frequency probe in a sterile cover and fill the pericardium with warm saline. Echocardiography is used to assess the sites of planned aortic cannulation and cross clamp sites for atheroma.

Short axis views of the ascending aorta should be obtained at 3 levels:

- Proximal to the right PA
- At the level of the right PA, and
- Distal to the right PA.

The aorta must be assessed for the following:

i. Atheroma thickness
ii. Location of atheroma (level, anterior/posterior) and
iii. Presence of any mobile components.

Many scoring systems exist for the degree of atheroma, including those of Katz or Royse.

Epiaortic scanning can be used to determine the optimal sites for cannulation and cross clamp of the aorta. However, if the ascending aorta is deemed unsafe for cannulation or clamping, an alternative site can be used for cannulation (axillary artery/femoral artery) and a non-cross clamp technique can be used.

32. **What factors influence the target blood pressure whilst on CPB?**

During cardiopulmonary bypass with non-pulsatile flow the mean perfusion pressure (MAP—CVP) should be at least 50 mm Hg. In fact it is the only "blood pressure"; there is no systolic or diastolic pressure. Lower pressures can be tolerated during periods of hypothermia and higher pressures may be required in patients with cerebrovascular disease or renal disease, although this is largely empiric.

33. **What is conduit spasm? How is it identified and treated?**

Conduit spasm refers to the vasoconstriction of an arterial graft (IMA or radial artery) although the radial artery is much more susceptible due to its thicker and more muscular media. Spasm can be due to trauma, systemic vasoconstrictors, or competitive flow from the native coronary. When it occurs it is manifest as a falling cardiac output, increasing vasoconstrictor requirements, new RWMA, and ischemic ECG changes.

It should be suspected if there is a new RWMA or ECG changes in a territory supplied by an arterial conduit (especially if there is a low grade native stenosis in the vessel being bypassed—more likely to result in competition). Treatment includes raising the MAP >80 mm Hg, adding a vasodilator (nitrate or calcium channel blocker) and ultimately coronary catheterization for diagnosis as well as therapy with an intra-arterial vasodilator.

34. **How do you manage a new regional wall motion abnormality following CABG whilst in the OR?**

- Assess and stabilize the hemodynamics—are the inotropic requirements increasing?

- Which coronary graft distribution is associated with this RWMA?
- A flow probe can be placed around the conduit to assess for flow rate and characteristics.
- If the patient is unstable, the safest thing to do is to initiate CPB and redo the graft.
- If the patient is in a hybrid room and is stable, a diagnostic angiogram will identify the culprit.
- There are some circumstances where acute PCI can salvage the myocardium with a lower risk than going back on bypass and prolonging the operation.

35. **What is the role for temporary pacing following CABG?**

For a routine CABG, temporary pacing wires are not as important as for aortic/mitral/tricuspid valve surgery where the AV node is inherently at risk. However, there is still a chance for AV nodal dysfunction any time the heart is arrested.

Atrial and ventricular pacing wires should be considered particularly for:

- Poor LV function whether systolic or diastolic (LVH) dysfunction to increase the rate with AV synchrony
- Nodal or junctional arrhythmias
- AV block
- Relative bradycardia

Ventricular pacing alone should not be used for AV nodal block or bradycardia unless the patient is in chronic AF.

Appendix: Conduct of a Standard On-Pump CABG

- Obtain large IV access and arterial pressure monitoring
- Attach standard and any additional monitors
- Perform appropriate safety checklists and check-in procedures
- Central venous access (can be obtained prior to or after induction as appropriate)
- Induction of anesthesia
- Commencement of surgery
- Initial TEE examination if being utilized
- Sternotomy
- Conduit harvest—LIMA, saphenous vein, radial artery
- Heparinization and confirmation of adequate ACT
- SBP <100 mm Hg for aortic cannulation
- Cannulation of the right atrium and aorta
- Initiate CPB
- Once full CPB flows are confirmed, cease ventilation, infusions, alarms, and empty urine
- Ensure volatile is being delivered in CPB pump
- Systemic cooling (30–35 °C—institution specific)
- Cross clamp of aorta and delivery of cardioplegia to obtain diastolic cardiac arrest
- Perform distal and proximal coronary grafts
- Intermittent antegrade ± retrograde cardioplegia every 20 min
- Commence rewarming via heart-lung machine when the last graft is started
- Give "rewarming" anesthetic agents as appropriate
- Cross clamp removed after performing all grafts, checking that there is no bleeding from the anastomoses
- Reperfusion of myocardium and internal cardioversion if the patient is in VT/VF
- Place atrial and ventricular pacing wires—test capture and thresholds
- Reinflate the lungs (recruitment) taking care for the LIMA
- Recommence mechanical ventilation and monitor alarms
- Can start to wean from CPB once the following confirmed:
  - Adequate oxygenation, warm, a perfusing cardiac rhythm, not bleeding/coagulopathic, adequate hematocrit, appropriate potassium and acid–base balance.
- TEE can be used to assist the process of weaning CPB, confirming adequate revascularization, examining function of the heart, and excluding any potential complications
- Remove venous drainage cannula
- Turn off all pump-suckers and vents (to prevent protamine getting into the pump)
- Can transfuse blood volume from the pump via the aortic cannula
- Give "test dose" protamine 10 mg (then wait 3 min)
- Remove aortic cannula (again requires a SBP<100 mm Hg)
- Continue protamine and confirm heparin completely reversed (ACT, heparinase ACT, heparin level—institute specific)
- Give remaining pump volume (either via large IV/CVC or into the right atrium)
- Check blood gas off pump
- Correct coagulopathy and anemia as required
- Place chest tubes—usually left pleural (LIMA harvest), pericardial, retrosternal
- Sternal closure
- Transfer to ICU.

References

1. Eagle KA, Guyton RA, Davidoff R, Edwards FH, Ewy GA, Gardner TJ, et al. ACC/AHA 2004 guideline update for coronary artery bypass graft surgery: a report of the American College of Cardiology/American Heart Association Task Force on Practice Guidelines (Committee to Update the 1999 Guidelines for Coronary Artery Bypass Graft Surgery). Circulation. 2004;110 (14):e340–437.
2. Nashef SA, Roques F, Michel P, Gauducheau E, Lemeshow S, Salamon R. European system for cardiac operative risk evaluation (EuroSCORE). Eur J Cardiothorac Surg. 1999;16(1):9–13.
3. Edwards FH, Clark RE, Schwartz M. Coronary artery bypass grafting: the Society of Thoracic Surgeons National Database experience. Ann Thorac Surg. 1994;57(1):12–9.
4. Chow WB, Rosenthal RA, Merkow RP, Ko CY, Esnaola NF, American College of Surgeons National Surgical Quality Improvement P, et al. Optimal preoperative assessment of the geriatric surgical patient: a best practices guideline from the American College of Surgeons National Surgical Quality Improvement Program and the American Geriatrics Society. J Am Coll Surg. 2012;215(4):453–66.
5. Hillis LD, Smith PK, Anderson JL, Bittl JA, Bridges CR, Byrne JG, et al. 2011 ACCF/AHA guideline for coronary artery bypass graft surgery: executive summary: a report of the American College of Cardiology Foundation/American Heart Association Task Force on Practice Guidelines. Circulation. 2011;124 (23):2610–42.
6. Naylor AR, Cuffe RL, Rothwell PM, Bell PR. A systematic review of outcomes following staged and synchronous carotid endarterectomy and coronary artery bypass. Eur J Vasc Endovasc Surg. 2003;25(5):380–9.
7. Camici PG, Prasad SK, Rimoldi OE. Stunning, hibernation, and assessment of myocardial viability. Circulation. 2008;117(1):103–14.
8. Pellikka PA, Nagueh SF, Elhendy AA, Kuehl CA, Sawada SG. American Society of E. American Society of Echocardiography recommendations for performance, interpretation, and application of stress echocardiography. J Am Soc Echocardiogr. 2007;20 (9):1021–41.
9. Jarvis MA, Jarvis CL, Jones PR, Spyt TJ. Reliability of Allen's test in selection of patients for radial artery harvest. Ann Thorac Surg. 2000;70(4):1362–5.
10. Shroyer AL, Grover FL, Hattler B, Collins JF, McDonald GO, Kozora E, et al. On-pump versus off-pump coronary-artery bypass surgery. N Engl J Med. 2009;361(19):1827–37.
11. Lamy A, Devereaux PJ, Prabhakaran D, Taggart DP, Hu S, Paolasso E, et al. Effects of off-pump and on-pump coronary-artery bypass grafting at 1 year. N Engl J Med. 2013;368(13):1179–88.
12. Chassot PG, van der Linden P, Zaugg M, Mueller XM, Spahn DR. Off-pump coronary artery bypass surgery: physiology and anaesthetic management. Br J Anaesth. 2004;92(3):400–13.
13. Selnes OA, Gottesman RF, Grega MA, Baumgartner WA, Zeger SL, McKhann GM. Cognitive and neurologic outcomes after coronary-artery bypass surgery. N Engl J Med. 2012;366 (3):250–7.
14. Evered L, Scott DA, Silbert B, Maruff P. Postoperative cognitive dysfunction is independent of type of surgery and anesthetic. Anesth Analg. 2011;112(5):1179–85.
15. van Dijk D, Spoor M, Hijman R, Nathoe HM, Borst C, Jansen EW, et al. Cognitive and cardiac outcomes 5 years after off-pump vs on-pump coronary artery bypass graft surgery. JAMA. 2007;297(7):701–8.
16. Pandit JJ, Andrade J, Bogod DG, Hitchman JM, Jonker WR, Lucas N, et al. The 5th National Audit Project (NAP5) on accidental awareness during general anaesthesia: summary of main findings and risk factors. Anaesthesia. 2014;69(10):1089–101.
17. Silbert BS, Myles PS. Is fast-track cardiac anesthesia now the global standard of care? Anesth Analg. 2009;108(3):689–91.
18. Schwann NM, Hillel Z, Hoeft A, Barash P, Mohnle P, Miao Y, et al. Lack of effectiveness of the pulmonary artery catheter in cardiac surgery. Anesth Analg. 2011;113(5):994–1002.
19. Hahn RT, Abraham T, Adams MS, Bruce CJ, Glas KE, Lang RM, et al. Guidelines for performing a comprehensive transesophageal echocardiographic examination: recommendations from the American Society of Echocardiography and the Society of Cardiovascular Anesthesiologists. J Am Soc Echocardiogr. 2013;26(9):921–64.
20. Kallmeyer IJ, Collard CD, Fox JA, Body SC, Shernan SK. The safety of intraoperative transesophageal echocardiography: a case series of 7200 cardiac surgical patients. Anesth Analg. 2001;92 (5):1126–30.
21. American Society of Anesthesiologists Task Force on Pulmonary Artery C. Practice guidelines for pulmonary artery catheterization: an updated report by the American Society of Anesthesiologists Task Force on Pulmonary Artery Catheterization. Anesthesiology. 2003;99(4):988–1014.
22. American Society of Anesthesiologists Task Force on Intraoperative A. Practice advisory for intraoperative awareness and brain function monitoring: a report by the american society of anesthesiologists task force on intraoperative awareness. Anesthesiology. 2006;104(4):847–64.
23. Society of Thoracic Surgeons Blood Conservation Guideline Task F, Ferraris VA, Brown JR, Despotis GJ, Hammon JW, Reece TB, et al. 2011 update to the Society of Thoracic Surgeons and the Society of Cardiovascular Anesthesiologists blood conservation clinical practice guidelines. Ann Thorac Surg. 2011;91(3):944–82.
24. Fergusson DA, Hebert PC, Mazer CD, Fremes S, MacAdams C, Murkin JM, et al. A comparison of aprotinin and lysine analogues in high-risk cardiac surgery. N Engl J Med. 2008;358(22):2319–31.
25. Reiz S, Balfors E, Sorensen MB, Ariola S Jr, Friedman A, Truedsson H. Isoflurane—a powerful coronary vasodilator in patients with coronary artery disease. Anesthesiology. 1983;59 (2):91–7.
26. Hogue CW Jr, Pulley DD, Lappas DG. Anesthetic-induced myocardial ischemia: the isoflurane-coronary steal controversy. Coron Artery Dis. 1993;4(5):413–9.
27. Murry CE, Jennings RB, Reimer KA. Preconditioning with ischemia: a delay of lethal cell injury in ischemic myocardium. Circulation. 1986;74(5):1124–36.
28. Nussmeier NA, Whelton AA, Brown MT, Langford RM, Hoeft A, Parlow JL, et al. Complications of the COX-2 inhibitors parecoxib and valdecoxib after cardiac surgery. N Engl J Med. 2005;352 (11):1081–91.
29. Svircevic V, Nierich AP, Moons KG, Diephuis JC, Ennema JJ, Brandon Bravo Bruinsma GJ, et al. Thoracic epidural anesthesia for cardiac surgery: a randomized trial. Anesthesiology. 2011;114 (2):262–70.
30. Svircevic V, van Dijk D, Nierich AP, Passier MP, Kalkman CJ, van der Heijden GJ, et al. Meta-analysis of thoracic epidural anesthesia versus general anesthesia for cardiac surgery. Anesthesiology. 2011;114(2):271–82.
31. Chakravarthy M, Jawali V, Manohar M, Patil T, Jayaprakash K, Kolar S, et al. Conscious off pump coronary artery bypass surgery–an audit of our first 151 cases. Ann Thorac Cardiovasc Surg. 2005;11(2):93–7.
32. Thiele H, Zeymer U, Neumann FJ, Ferenc M, Olbrich HG, Hausleiter J, et al. Intraaortic balloon support for myocardial

infarction with cardiogenic shock. N Engl J Med. 2012;367 (14):1287–96.
33. Goldstein SA, Evangelista A, Abbara S, Arai A, Asch FM, Badano LP, et al. Multimodality imaging of diseases of the thoracic aorta in adults: from the American Society of Echocardiography and the European Association of Cardiovascular Imaging: endorsed by the Society of Cardiovascular Computed Tomography and Society for Cardiovascular Magnetic Resonance. J Am Soc Echocardiogr. 2015;28(2):119–82.
34. Glas KE, Swaminathan M, Reeves ST, Shanewise JS, Rubenson D, Smith PK, et al. Guidelines for the performance of a comprehensive intraoperative epiaortic ultrasonographic examination: recommendations of the American Society of Echocardiography and the Society of Cardiovascular Anesthesiologists; endorsed by the Society of Thoracic Surgeons. J Am Soc Echocardiogr. 2007;20 (11):1227–35.

Part II

The Respiratory System

Section Editor: Ju-Mei Ng

Ju-Mei Ng
Department of Anesthesiology, Perioperative
and Pain Medicine, Brigham and Women's Hospital,
Boston, MA, USA

One-Lung Ventilation

14

Thomas Hickey

CASE: One-Lung Ventilation

73-year-old man presents for left lower lobectomy. He is status post-recent bronchoscopy, endobronchial ultrasound and cervical mediastinoscopy. Pathology indicated non-small cell carcinoma, likely squamous cell carcinoma. Staging is IIB (T2bN1).

Past Medical History:	Hypertension, COPD, obesity, smoker
Medications:	Lovastatin 40 mg oral daily
	Amlodipine 10 mg daily
	Valsartan 320 mg daily
	Atenolol 25 mg daily
Allergies:	Iodinated contrast dye—anaphylaxis
Physical Exam:	
VS:	BP 144/96 HR 77 RR 11 SaO2 98% (room air) Ht 70″ Wt 300 lb (136 kg)
General:	Obese, comfortable
Airway:	MP3, thick neck, large tongue, full neck extension and mouth opening, four finger thyromental distance
Chest:	Symmetric air entry bilaterally without crackles or wheezes
Data:	PFT: PreFEV1 47%, PreFVC 71%, DLCO 50%
Exercise treadmill myocardial perfusion imaging study:	Exercised for 7:00, MPHR 90%, RPP: 21,900, terminated due to dyspnea, 9 METS, non-ischemic, post stress LVEF 60%.
Chest CT:	5 × 4 cm mass obstructing the left lower lobe bronchus. Multiple 1 cm left hilar lymph nodes. Moderate to severe bilateral upper lobe predominant emphysema.

T. Hickey (✉)
Department of Anesthesiology, VA Connecticut Healthcare System, Yale University School of Medicine, 950 Campbell Avenue, West Haven, CT 06511, USA
e-mail: Thomas_hickey@post.harvard.edu

© Springer International Publishing AG 2017
L.S. Aglio and R.D. Urman (eds.), *Anesthesiology*,
DOI 10.1007/978-3-319-50141-3_14

1. **What is the functional anatomy of the lungs?**

The trachea forms from the lower larynx at approximately C6, is approximately 15 cm (20–25 cm from teeth to carina) in an adult male, consists of 16 to 20 cartilaginous rings, lies directly anterior to the esophagus, and bifurcates at T4. The right mainstem bronchus is shorter compared with the left (i.e., 2.5 vs. 5 cm) and descends more vertically, thus the tendency for right mainstem intubations. The right lung consists of upper, middle, and lower lobes, with three, two, and five segments, respectively. The left lung consists of upper and lower lobe, each with five segments. Each pyramidal-shaped segment receives a single branch of the pulmonary artery, which follow along the bronchi and bronchioles to perfuse the alveoli. Smaller bronchial arteries supply the conducting airway, pleura, and nodes. For the purposes of predicting postoperative predicted FEV_1 (ppo-FEV_1), a total of 42 lung subsegments are considered (RUL: 6, RML: 4, RLL: 12, LUL: 10, LLL: 10) (see Fig. 14.1).

2. **What are the concerns in preoperative risk assessment for lung resection?**

The "three legged stool" consists of (1) respiratory mechanics, (2) cardiopulmonary reserve, and (3) parenchymal function.

The main measure of respiratory mechanics is the FEV_1. A $ppoFEV_1$ can be estimated by multiplying the preoperative FEV_1 ($preFEV_1$) by the fraction of lung remaining at the conclusion of surgery. Respiratory complications are increased when $ppoFEV_1 < 40\%$, and <30% predicts high risk. In this patient, 10 of 42 subsegments will be resected, therefore

$$ppoFEV_1 = 47\% \times (32/42) = 35\%$$

Cardiopulmonary reserve is formally described by maximum oxygen consumption and approximated by stair climbing (at patient's own pace but without stopping) and 6 min walk. $VO_{2max} > 20$ cc/kg/min predicts low risk and is

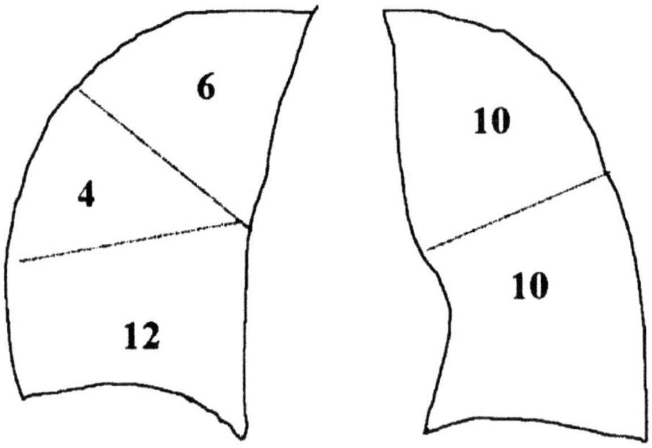

Fig. 14.1 The number of subsegments of each lobe are used to calculate the predicted postoperative (ppo) pulmonary function. There are 6, 4, and 12 subsegments in the right upper, middle, and lower lobes. There are 10 subsegments in both the left upper and the lower lobes, for a total of 42 subsegments. Following removal of a functioning right lower lobe, a patient would be expected to lose 12/42 (29%) of their respiratory reserve. If the patient has a preoperative FEV1 (or DLCO) 70% of predicted, the patient would be expected to have a ppoFEV1 = 70% (1–29/100) = 50%. Reproduced from Slinger and Darling [2]

approximated by ≥5 flights of stairs whereas the commonly used two flights of stairs correspond to a VO_{2max} of 12 cc/kg/min. A $ppoVO_{2max} < 10$ cc/kg/min predicts very high risk and is approximated by inability to climb 1 flight of stairs; this may be an absolute contradiction to lung resection. 1 MET corresponds to a VO_2 of 3.5 cc/kg/min. In this patient:

$$9\,\text{METS} \times 3.5 = 31.5\,\text{cc/kg/min}, \quad \text{thus ppoVO}_{2\text{max}} = 31.5 \times (32/42) = 24\ \text{cc/kg/min}$$

Gas exchange is estimated by DLCO, PaO_2, and $PaCO_2$. ppoDLCO < 40% predicts increased respiratory and cardiac complications, and <20% is typically considered unacceptably high risk. $PaO_2 < 60$ mmHg and $PaCO_2 > 45$ mmHg are also indicators of increased risk. In this patient:

$$\text{ppDLCO} = 51\% \times (32/42) = 39\%$$

3. **What are the additional anesthetic considerations for lung cancer patients (the "four Ms")?**

Mass effects—are there compression of heart, airway, vein, artery, or nerve?
Metabolic—is there electrolyte abnormalities (hyponatremia, hypercalcemia), or paraneoplastic syndrome such as Lambert–Eaton?
Metastases—for example, are there brain or bone lesions that might change management?
Medications—have there been chemotherapy exposures, as to bleomycin or doxorubicin, which may change management or prompt further workup? [1]

4. **Will you advise this patient to quit smoking?**

The answer should always be yes. The longer the cessation the greater the benefit, with perhaps 8 weeks being a worthwhile goal. However, even a 12 h cessation will decrease carboxyhemoglobin concentrations. And preoperative cessation predicts postoperative cessation, which has important implications for wound healing and infection.

5. **What are the indications for lung isolation? Does this case require lung isolation and OLV?**

Indications for lung isolation may be absolute or relative. Absolute indications include for the prevention of spillage of pus, blood or large volume lavage fluid from the contralateral lung; bronchopleural fistula (in which the low resistance pathway can rapidly create pneumothorax during positive pressure ventilation); large unilateral bullae prone to rupture; and during video assisted thoracoscopic surgery (VATS) procedures. Relative indications include pneumonectomy, lobectomy (especially upper), thoracic aortic aneurysm repair, and esophageal surgery. While a relative indication, lung isolation during lobectomy will provide more ideal surgical conditions.

6. **How is lung isolation achieved? What are the advantages and disadvantages of the main methods of lung isolation?**

The commonest means of lung isolation include double-lumen tubes (DLT) and bronchial blockers. DLTs are easy to insert and permit bronchoscopic evaluation and suctioning of both lungs, CPAP application to the non-ventilated lung, and easy conversion between one and two-lung ventilation. Size limitation often precludes use in pediatrics under age 12, narrower lumens increase airway resistance and make suctioning more difficult, DLTs can be malpositioned, may cause trauma to the larynx and airway, and can be unwieldy in a difficult intubation. Left-sided tubes are typically selected due to the larger margin of safety given the longer left mainstem bronchus. Right-sided tubes may be selected for distorted left mainstem anatomy (by tumor, stent, stenosis) or surgery involving the left mainstem (left pneumonectomy and left lung transplantation).

Bronchial blockers of various types are useful in critically ill intubated patients, in the difficult airway (obviating the need for multiple airway exchanges), for selective lobar blockade, and may be used via nasotracheal or tracheostomy tubes. Blockers are technically difficult to place in ETT <7 mm, dislodge more easily, limit suctioning, can be difficult to reposition, and there may be marginally slower lung collapse compared with DLTs.

7. **What is dead space? What is normal, upright ventilation and perfusion?**

Physiologic dead space includes both the anatomic dead space (that portion of inspired gas that never reaches the respiratory zone) and alveolar dead space consists of alveoli that are ventilated but not perfused (V/Q approaching infinity).

"V" is the gas that reaches the respiratory zone. "Q" is the blood that reaches the respiratory zone.

A V/Q ratio of one is the ideal, but in reality V and Q are heterogeneous especially in disease. In a healthy upright human, V/Q ratio is highest at the apex (approximately 3.5) and lowest at the base (approximately 0.6).

Blood flow is directly influenced by gravity, and thus increases from apex to bases. Ventilation similarly increases from apex to base. However, they do not increase uniformly: The classic teaching of West divides the lungs into three zones.

$$\text{In the upper third,}\quad P_A > P_a > P_v$$
$$\text{In the middle third,}\quad P_a > P_A > P_v$$
$$\text{In the lower third,}\quad P_a > P_v > P_A$$

8. **What is the most likely cause of hypoxemia in this patient?**

Malposition of the DLT, hypoventilation, low FiO_2, diffusion impairment, and shunt (V/Q = zero) are among the core causes of hypoxemia. V/Q mismatch is the commonest cause in pulmonary disease, where the heterogeneity of V/Q ratios becomes pronounced.

9. **How does V/Q matching change in the lateral decubitus position (LDP)?**

In the awake, spontaneous breathing patient in LDP, V/Q matching is maintained as perfusion increases by approximately 10% to the dependent lung due to gravity and ventilation increases due to greater excursion of the dependent hemidiaphragm. Under anesthesia, overall changes in compliance lead to V/Q mismatching, compounded by bolsters and paralysis. Once the chest is open in an anesthetized, paralyzed patient the V/Q mismatching will likely worsen further as negative pleural pressure is interrupted and tendency of the operative lung to collapse under its own elastic recoil will increase. Isolation of the operative lung leads to a large right-to-left intrapulmonary shunt, widening the A-a gradient and resulting in hypoxemia. In patients with significant lung disease, shunt due to atelectasis and V/Q mismatch due to underlying disease worsen gas exchange. Fractional blood flow changes on OLV dramatically increase the shunt fraction (see Table 14.1).

10. **What is hypoxic pulmonary vasoconstriction?**

Low alveolar oxygen tension leads to regional arteriolar vasoconstriction, profoundly reducing local blood flow and thereby matching perfusion to better ventilated lung. HPV reaches max effect in 15 min and reduces shunt fraction by 50% to approximately 20%. The effectiveness of HPV is reduced by elevated pulmonary pressures, alkalosis (acidosis actually improves it), and vasodilators.

11. **What is COPD and why is it concerning?**

Chronic obstructive pulmonary disease combines to varying degrees emphysema, chronic bronchitis, and small airways disease. PFTs show expiratory airflow obstruction with severity based largely on reduced FEV_1/FVC ratios (<70% indicates obstruction) and on the FEV_1. There are various grading systems, but generally $FEV_1 < 35\%$ is severe and >50% moderate

In COPD, the smoking history places them at increased risk for comorbidities such as cardiovascular disease, other malignancy, respiratory infection, renal disease, diabetes, peptic ulcer disease, and postoperative wound and pulmonary complications. They have baseline high $PaCO_2$ which can increase greatly intra- and postoperatively as the high FiO_2 they may require to properly oxygenate can interfere with their delicate balance of HPV (worsening V/Q matching) and also decrease hemoglobin's CO_2 affinity

Table 14.1 Approximate changes in regional blood flow, shunt fraction and PaO_2 resulting from positioning alone and from both positioning and lung isolation, assuming FiO_2 of 1.0

	Two-lung ventilation in lateral decubitus position	OLV in lateral decubitus position
Fractional blood flow, nondependent lung	40%	23%
Fractional blood flow, dependent lung	60%	77%
Shunt fraction	10%	27%
PaO_2 (mmHg)	400	150

(Haldane effect), resulting in increased $PaCO_2$. They are also simply more difficult to ventilate due to their airflow limitations; increased ventilatory pressures (and PEEP in response to hypoxemia) may lead to auto-PEEP and hemodynamic collapse. They are at risk of pulmonary hypertension and RV dysfunction and may not tolerate acute increases in pulmonary arterial pressures that are likely to occur with hypercapnea, hypoxemia, hypothermia, pain, and acidemia. Those with bullae are at risk of pneumothorax and bronchopleural fistula under positive pressure ventilation.

12. **What monitors and extra setup will you require for this patient?**

In addition to the standard ASA monitors (temperature, EKG, pulse oximeter, capnography, and noninvasive blood pressure), an arterial line (hemodynamics and blood gas monitoring) and two large peripheral IVs are recommended given the possibility of severe impairments in gas exchange, hemorrhage, and acute hypotension. A central venous line should not be required in this patient absent poor IV access.

Due to the potential for heat loss (open thorax and fluid resuscitation), measures should be taken to prevent hypothermia with fluid and body warming devices. Blood and products should be readily available, and a fiberoptic bronchoscope compatible with the chosen lung isolation technique should be in the room.

13. **Will you place an epidural?**

Excellent postoperative analgesia is essential in thoracic surgery; an important contributor to reduced pulmonary complications. Thoracic epidural analgesia (TEA) is considered the gold standard for post-thoracotomy pain control, although paravertebral blocks are becoming more widespread given the advantages of less hypotension and decreased risk of epidural hematoma. Employment of these techniques requires a committee decision involving the patient, anesthesiologist, and surgeon. In open procedures, a continuous regional technique should be employed. In addition, a multimodal analgesia strategy including opioids, NSAIDs, NMDA antagonists, and acetaminophen is advised.

14. **Shortly after placement of the DLT there is an acute rise in airway pressure. What will you do?**

The differential diagnoses for an acute rise in airway pressure soon after placement of the DLT include any kink or obstruction in the anesthesia circuit, tube and/or connectors, patient factors (bronchospasm, inadequate depth of anesthesia or paralysis, pneumothorax, and dynamic hyperinflation), or DLT malposition. The immediate steps are to take a quick scan of the monitors for the patient's hemodynamics, oxygen saturation, and capnograph, and communicate concerns to the surgical team. If there is severe hypotension, dynamic hyperinflation is likely, and treatment is to disconnect the circuit and volume load the patient. The next step would be placing the patient on 100% oxygen and assessing the capnograph pattern for a cause. Meanwhile if hemodynamics or oxygen saturation worsen, skilled assistance should be sought. Any kinks or obvious obstructions in the circuit should be quickly excluded, and the anesthetic depth or neuromuscular block deepened if this was determined to be the cause. Deflating the bronchial cuff may improve airway pressures (bronchial cuff of a left DLT herniating and obstructing the right main bronchus), but the definitive diagnosis of DLT malposition may only be made via fiberoptic bronchoscopy. Bronchoscopy and suctioning can also help with mucus plugs in the airway. Auscultation of the chest for bilateral breath sounds and wheeze will help to exclude bronchospasm and pneumothorax.

15. **Airway pressures normalize after administering bronchodilators and deepening the anesthetic. After turning lateral and initiation of one-lung ventilation, the patient soon after becomes progressively more hypoxemic. What will you do?**

Ensure delivery of 100% oxygen and scan monitors looking for other hemodynamic or respiratory derangements. After ensuring adequate ventilation of the dependent lung, look for changes in compliance or capnography suggestive of mucus plug, bronchospasm, or pneumothorax. The surgeons should be made aware of the problems with oxygenation. Meanwhile, call for skilled assistance if the saturation worsens or does not improve. If the saturation drops precipitously or if the patient is hemodynamically unstable, the surgeons should be informed of the need to return to two-lung ventilation as soon as feasible. Fiberoptic bronchoscopy will assess for DLT malposition and secretions, and auscultation of the lungs to assess for wheezing and to exclude pneumothorax. To optimize ventilation of the dependent lung, I would adjust PEEP and attempt recruitment maneuvers. If the saturation does not improve, I would discuss the application of CPAP to the nondependent lung or intermittent 2-lung ventilation with the surgeons, in order to proceed with surgery. Other strategies which may be considered include clamping of the pulmonary artery (in pneumonectomy) or inhaled nitric oxide (if there is co-existing pulmonary hypertension).

16. **What is your plan for fluid management?**

Generally a fluid sparing approach should be utilized based on the premise that "dry lungs are happy lungs." Although fluids do not cause acute lung injury, any excessive fluids exacerbate the problem when it occurs. Thus, crystalloid may be minimized with a goal to limit to less than 3L during the first 24 h, inotropes should be used to promote perfusion intra- and postoperatively, and urine output < the traditional 0.5 cc/kg/h tolerated.

17. **What is your choice of anesthetic?**

The choice of anesthetic drugs is governed by adequate anesthetic depth, protection against bronchospasm and the pursuit of earliest possible extubation. Modern volatiles at doses less than 1 MAC cause only a modest inhibition of HPV and are also bronchodilators (especially sevoflurane). There is probably no "right" anesthetic, but the trend has been to minimize or eliminate the use of volatile inhalational agents and long/intermediate acting narcotics. Total intravenous anesthesia is frequently employed for severe bullous disease.

18. **Will you extubate this patient in the OR?**

This patient has ppoFEV_1 = 35%, ppoVO_{2max} = 24 cc/kg/min, and ppDLCO = 39%. The decision for immediate extubation in the OR or delayed in the PACU/ICU depends on the operative course and the patient's hemodynamics and respiratory performance. In addition to the standard extubation criteria, ppoFEV_1 is often used to guide extubation after pulmonary resection. If standard extubation criteria are met, a patient with ppoFEV_1 > 40% should be extubated in OR. A ppoFEV_1 of 30–40% may be extubated in the OR if other postoperative predictive data are reassuring, and if ppoFEV_1 < 30% weaning ventilatory support in the ICU should be considered.

19. **What are your postoperative concerns?**

Respiratory complications are the most significant cause of perioperative morbidity and mortality following lung resection. The incidence of respiratory failure after lung resection is between 2 and 18%. Risk is predicted by preoperative respiratory function, extent of resection, age, and quality of postoperative analgesia. Immediate or early extubation, complete analgesia (TEA and multimodal strategy), aggressive and early mobilization, maintenance of lung expansion (incentive spirometry, chest physiotherapy), and continued aggressive medical management of bronchospasm are key components in preventing respiratory complications.

Reference

1. Slinger PD, Johnston MR. Preoperative assessment for pulmonary resection. J Cardiothorac Vasc Anesth. 2000;14(2):202–11.
2. Slinger P, Darling G. Preanesthetic assessment for thoracic surgery. In: Slinger P, editor. Principles and practice of anesthesia for thoracic surgery. New York: Springer; 2011. p. 11–34.

Part III

The Central Nervous System

Section Editor: Leslie C. Jameson

Leslie C. Jameson
Department of Anesthesiology,
University of Colorado, Aurora, CO, USA

Anesthesia Management for Posterior Fossa Craniotomy

15

Mihaela Podovei and Lisa Crossley

A 52-year-old female has a 5-week history of dizzyness, unstable gait, and frequent falls. She is admitted with headache, nausea, vomiting, facial nerve weakness, and palate deviation.

Past Medical History:	Breast cancer 10 years ago without known recurrence hypertension
Allergies:	None
Medications:	Linsinopril
Vital Signs:	BP 130/70, P 67 with occasional irregular beat, R 25, T 36.9
Studies:	
Cranial MRI	a 2.5 by 1.5 cm enhancing right cerebellar pontine angle tumor with compression of the 4th ventricle and hydrocephalus

Patient is admitted to the Neurosurgical ICU in preparation for a posterior fossa craniotomy for tumor resection.

1. **What is the anatomy of the posterior fossa?**

Posterior fossa is a small rigid space at the base of the skull that contains the brain stem, cranial nerves, cerebellum, and the 4th ventricle. All cranial nerves originate in the posterior fossa and all basic physiologic activities (e.g., heart rate, respirations, temperature, emetic) are regulated here. CSF circulates from the choroid plexus through the 4th ventricle into the spinal cord. Posterior fossa craniotomy can be challenging for both the neurosurgeon and the anesthesiologist. The surgeon needs good exposure to a small area, approximately 185 cm^3, dense in vital structures that are also in close proximity to noncompressible venous sinuses increasing the risk of blood loss. Tumor or vascular surgery can disrupt the physiologic functions of the posterior fossa.

2. **What are the risks of Posterior fossa procedures?**

The anesthesiologist is responsible for managing usual physiologic functions (e.g., optimal BP, ventilation, cerebral blood flow, level of anesthesia) and responding to physiologic changes that occur due to surgery in the posterior fossa (e.g., venous air embolism, paradoxical arterial air embolism (AAR), arrhythmias from cardiovascular center or cranial nerve stimulation). Additional serious neurologic complications can arise from the intersection of positioning and preexisting disease like cervical cord stretch leading to quadriplegia, optical nerve compression causing blindness, brachial, or lumbosacral nerve stretch causing permanent palsy. While not an acute complication, recognizing, usually through specialized monitoring, injury to cranial nerves IX to XII is important to safe recovery from the surgical experience. Vigilance and anticipation is critical in the prevention of unsafe situations and complications.

3. **What preoperative evaluation is necessary prior to surgery?**

Standard anesthesia evaluation should always be performed. Special attention should be placed on signs and symptoms associated with posterior fossa tumors like hearing loss, difficulty swallowing, or other cranial nerve preexisting injury.

4. **Does cardiovascular disease have increased importance in the anesthetic management?**

Chronic hypertension with or without treatment, vascular disease, especially carotid vascular disease, may increase the

M. Podovei (✉) · L. Crossley
Department of Anesthesiology, Perioperative and Pain Medicine, Harvard Medical School, Brigham and Women's Hospital, 75 Francis Street, CWN L1, Boston, MA 02115, USA
e-mail: mpodovei@partners.org

L. Crossley
e-mail: lcrossley@partners.org

© Springer International Publishing AG 2017
L.S. Aglio and R.D. Urman (eds.), *Anesthesiology*,
DOI 10.1007/978-3-319-50141-3_15

risk of hypotension if the surgeon chooses the sitting position. Presence of carotid or vertebral vascular disease increases concerns about the ability to tolerate extreme head rotation or flexion. Some centers no longer use sitting position due to the increased anesthetic management complexities and patient hypoperfusion risks. Patients with coronary disease may not tolerate the sitting position. Dysrhythmias, tachycardia, bradycardia, conduction abnormalities from brain stem traction occur regardless of position, and in individuals with preexisting arrhythmia the difficulty managing them may be increased.

5. **How would preoperative neurologic deficits alter your anesthetic management?**

Posterior fossa tumors can present clinically with evidence of cranial nerve or brain stem deficits (e.g., respiratory irregularities, chronic aspiration, altered consciousness, dysphagia). Knowledge about the presence of respiratory and upper airway dysfunction based on the involvement of cranial nerves IX and X, XI, XII is important when deciding anesthetic management.

6. **How would you assess and manage volume status prior to surgery?**

The patient scheduled for posterior fossa surgery could be hypovolemic from hypertonic treatment to decrease brain edema or ICP, or from use of diuretics. Hypovolemia could be poorly tolerated in sitting position. Vascular volume may need to be replenished with isotonic crystalloids. The use of albumin remains controversial but it is often administered. The controversy involves its use in traumatic brain injury where it is associated with higher mortality. The literature is silent in its use in other areas. In general, support of BP may require pressors and volume administration may be determined by acid base status.

7. **What are the concerns regarding central access?**

Central venous access is not routinely necessary except in patients who have limited or very difficult vascular access or the need for a right atrial catheter. Central venous catheter via the internal jugular or subclavian veins are not without risks. Internal jugular vein catheters can partially obstruct venous outflow especially with some head positions or patient attributes (e.g., short thick neck, obesity). Use of ultrasound devices has reduced placement risk. The basilic vein is primarily used for placement of the right atrial catheter. Need for right atrial catheters have decreased with the decreased use of the seated position. When considering an approach or need for a central line, the ability of the patient to tolerate Trendelenburg/head turned position should be considered. Trendelenburg position increases the venous return, and may not be well tolerated by a patient with increased ICP.

8. **What special monitoring should be considered?**

Major damage can occur to CN III-XII; neurophysiologic monitoring should be dictated by the location of the tumor. Monitoring often includes brainstem auditory evoked potentials (BAEP), somatosensory evoked potentials (SEP), electromyography (EMG) in the soft palate, tongue, vocal cords, and rarely ocular muscles.

Hemodynamic monitoring should include arterial blood pressure. If VAE or Arterial Air Embolism (AAE) is probable, precordial doppler needs to be added to end-tidal CO_2 measurement to detect right atrial air.

9. **Why is positioning a critical decision?**

Posterior fossa surgery can be done in a variety of positions, including supine with the head turned, lateral, prone, or sitting. Every position has advantages and disadvantages in regards to surgical exposure, risk of bleeding, risk of postoperative neurologic deficits, cardiovascular stability, and maintenance of cerebral perfusion pressure, risk of air embolism, and access to the patient. The decision regarding the position should involve the entire team and be individualized to the particular patient.

Independent of the position chosen, the entire team needs to be mindful of pressure points and the risk of post-op neurologic deficits (cervical cord, brachial or lumbosacral plexus injury), risk of tracheal tube dislodgment during the turns and flexion of the neck, risk of tourniquet effects from poorly applied compression stockings.

10. **What are the management considerations for the sitting position**:

The advantages of the sitting position include

- good surgical exposure
- decreased risk of bleeding
- better access to the face, tube, and extremities
- better ventilation parameters

Surgical preference and experience with a specific tumor likely determines the best position. A 1988 study suggested better outcomes in the sitting position but more recent studies show no outcome benefit in terms of neurologic complications when surgery is performed in sitting position over lateral or prone positions [1, 2].

The disadvantages of the sitting position include

- difficulty maintaining the hemodynamic stability especially in patients that are hypovolemic, have hypertension, cardiac, or peripheral vascular disease
- highest risk of air embolism
- risk of central line placement
- pneumocephalus occurs in all patient but is without clinical consequence.

11. **What are the contraindications of surgery in the sitting position**?

The contraindications to considering the sitting position includes:

- intracardiac shunts
- pulmonary AVMs
- severe hypovolemia or cachexia
- severe hydrocephalus
- highly vascular lesions, tumors, or arteriovenous malformations

12. **How do you minimize the special positioning hazards?**

If the case is going to be done in any position, the anesthesiologist needs to have a few considerations in mind. Assuring appropriate cerebral perfusion pressure is essential. To better monitor the brain perfusion, the arterial blood pressure transducer should be zeroed at the level of the base of the skull. Venous stasis and neurosurgical procedures predispose to deep vein thrombosis. Compression stockings should be used to decrease the venous pooling in the lower extremity. Hip flexion can cause lumbosacral plexus damage.

Special attention needs to be given to the position of the head. At least one inch (2 finger breaths) needs to be maintained between the chin and the chest, in order to avoid cervical cord stretching and obstruction of the venous drainage from face and tongue. Possible rare but serious complications include cervical cord damage and quadriplegia. Venous thrombosis of the tongue can preclude extubation and add to the risk of permanent damage to tongue function.

Pneumocephalus is postulated to have 100% incidence in sitting position but occurs to some degree in all positions. Most accumulations of air in the cranium are asymptomatic. Tension pneumocephalus, causing a mass effect over the underlying brain parenchyma, can be responsible for new or worsening neurologic deficits and may need to be addressed. Sometimes either aspiration of the pocket of gas or reopening of the dura is necessary to control the symptoms. Careful choice of anesthetic can help minimize risk.

13. **What are the management considerations for the prone or lateral position?**

The advantages of the prone or lateral position include

- lower (but not absent) incidence of VAE
- lower frequency of cerebral ischemia and cervical cord ischemia due to hypoperfusion
- less venous obstruction from head positioning

The disadvantages of the prone or lateral position include

- risk of ophthalmic complications such as, ischemic optic neuropathy and conjuctival edema
- increased blood loss due to increased venous pressure when prone
- pressure point injury to shoulders, hips, knees from a prolonged procedure.

14. **What is the best approach to induction?**

The use of premedication and selection of induction agents must take into consideration patient comorbidities and standard neurosurgical concerns related to increased ICP and tolerance of potential hypercarbia or hypoxia. Consequently, there are no specific drugs that are recommended based on the evidence. Principles of maintaining BP, reducing ICP, and providing good airway management are paramount. A chiari malformation or tumor involving the foramen magnum and cervical cord can produce neurologic symptoms. Prior to induction neck positioning should be checked to determine if the position aggravates neurologic symptoms, arrhythmias, respiratory, issues or causes blood pressure perturbations. These risks are present throughout the procedure. Determining benign head/neck position will be helpful both for the induction but also during positioning for the procedure. Substantial head rotation and flexion is not an unusual surgical request to improve access.

15. **What is the best approach to maintenance?**

Things to consider before choosing a maintenance technique include: need for neuromonitoring (sensory or motor evoked potentials), presence of intracranial hypertension, need for immediate neurologic exam post extubation. Total intravenous anesthesia with propofol and an opioid the advantage of providing the best conditions for neuromonitoring. Other anesthetic techniques can be adapted to give good operative conditions. There are also advocates for dexmedetomidine and volatile anesthetics. EMG monitoring of motor cranial nerves, tongue pharynx, obicularis oris/oculi, masseter and rarely ocular muscles requires no nondepolarizing muscle relaxant be continuously administered. There is no clear "best" evidence-based maintenance anesthetic.

Use of N_2O in posterior fossa surgery remains controversial N_2O has the ability to expand air bubbles. Many clinicians do not use N_2O in posterior fossa procedures particularly in the sitting position, where isolated air bubbles are much more likely to occur. There are no advantages and significant risks to the use of N_2O. N_2O use is a decision made by clinicians to serve the best interests of their patient.

Positive pressure mechanical ventilation is the standard of care. It allows for manipulation of $PaCO_2$ to change intracranial vascular volume. The vasomotor center in the medulla is in close proximity to the respiratory centers and cardiovascular signs can serve as an indicator of impending injury to both areas. Cardiovascular responses to brain stem or cranial nerve, particularly CN V, manipulation can include bradycardia, tachycardia, arrhythmias, hypo, and hypertension. Pharmacologic treatment to attenuate the cardiovascular response (long acting anti-arrhythmics, beta-blockers) can mask important warning signs and should be used with caution.

16. **What is the best approach to extubation?**

For all neurosurgical cases the ideal scenario is avoidance of hemodynamic changes particularly hypertension, coughing, and breath holding. It is also desirable to be able to perform a neurologic examination immediately after extubation in the OR. Factors like duration of the case, blood loss, face and tongue edema, hemodynamic stability, pulmonary, or cardiovascular pathology may require the patient to remain intubated until they are stable and symptoms have resolved. Criteria for extubation are the same as for all patients but the risk of inadequate respiratory and cardiac function and airway protection is greater in posterior fossa procedures. If injury to cranial nerve nuclei (particularly IX, X and XII), or postoperative swelling in the floor of the 4th ventricle is suspected, extubation may need to be postponed. There can be loss of control and patency of upper airway or impairment of the respiratory drive. Additional risks can be a result of positioning, such as a swollen tongue or airway.

17. **Discuss venous air embolism (VAE)**

The incidence of venous air embolism varies with the patient position and the detection method used. In sitting position when precordial doppler is used, VAE can be detected is nearly half of all patients. In a non-sitting position, the incidence is about 10% using doppler detection. Transesophageal Echocardiogram (TEE) for TEE is not frequently used but it detects significantly more bubbles. Detection of air bubbles is not equated with injury or symptoms.

The existence of a negative gradient between the surgical site, the right atrium and open veins predisposes to VAE. The amount of air entrained depends on the pressure gradient between the skull and the heart and the size of the open orifice. Increasing right atrial pressure reduces the risk but may also cause increased venous pressure and tumor size. All maneuvers that increase right atrial pressure increase the risk of air entering the left atrium through a patent foramen ovale, causing a paradoxical air embolism. This risk is greater in children, especially young children. Some organizations will perform a transthoracic echocardiogram to assess risk. The presence of a patent foramen ovale (PFO) increases the risk of paradoxical air embolism, and is a relative contraindication to sitting position.

The incidence of PFO in general population could be as high as 20–30%, and most patients do not know that they have a PFO. Routine PFO screening can be considered preoperatively. Transthoracic Echocardiogram (TEE) is less invasive but not as sensitive in PFO detection as TEE, but pre-op TEE usually requires a general anesthetic due to it is invasive nature. The practice of preoperative screening could be replaced by intraoperative, prepositioning contrast-enhanced TEE. If a PFO is found, position for surgery is modified and right atrial catheter placed.

18. **How do you treat VAE?**

Once venous air embolisms is identified, usually with a precordial doppler, the anesthetic management should

- prevent further air entry
  - notify the surgeon, have him/her flood the field
  - compress the jugular veins
- if the patient is sitting
  - lower their head
  - rotate into the left lateral decubitus position
- administer 100% O_2
- Attempt to aspirate the air from the right atrium through a previously placed multi-oriface catheter.

Address the cardiovascular and respiratory consequences of VAE

- Cardiovascular: dysrhythmia, systemic hypotension, pulmonary hypertension, acute right-sided failure, myocardial ischemia, cardiac arrest
- Pulmonary: hypoxemia, hypercarbia, pulmonary edema.

References

1. Black MD, et al. Outcome following posterior fossa craniectomy in patients in the sitting and horizontal positions. Anesthesiology. 1988;69:49–56.
2. Spektor S, et al. Comparison of outcomes following complex posterior fossa surgery performed in sitting versus lateral position. J Clinical Neurosci. 2015;22:705–12.

Suggested Reading

3. Cottrell JE, Patel P. Cottrell and Patel's neuroanesthesia 6th ed. Elsevier; September 2016.
4. Miller RD, Eriksson LI, Fleisher LA, Wiener-Kronish JP, Cohen NH, Young WL. Anesthesia for neurologic surgery. In: Miller's anesthesia. 8th ed. Elsevier; 2015.
5. Mirski MA, et al. Diagnosis and treatment of vascular air embolism. Anesthesiology. 2007;106:164–77.
6. Newfield P, Cottrell JE. Handbook of neuroanesthesia. 5th ed. Lippincott Williams and Wilkins; 2012.

Intracranial Aneurysm

16

Penny P. Liu

CASE:
45-year-old female presents to the emergency room with 2-day history of moderate headache, photophobia, nuchal rigidity, and nausea with vomiting.

Medications	Atenolol, Glipizide
Allergies	None
Past Medical History	Chronic hypertension, Type II Diabetes Mellitus
Physical Exam	VS: BP 148/95, HR 70, RR 20, SpO_2 98%
Mental status	The patient appears uncomfortable with nausea and photophobia. She is alert, oriented, and obeys all commands.
Studies	
EKG	Sinus rhythm, occasional PVC's, and nonspecific ST segment depression Computerized axial tomography **scan** (CT) Findings: thin layer of subarachnoid blood.
Angiogram	15 mm right middle cerebral artery aneurysm.

1. **What are the signs and symptoms of SAH?**

The most common symptom is a sudden, severe headache with the classic description "this is the worst headache of my life." Patients may have minimal symptoms from comatose and posturing to unresponsiveness. Increased intracranial pressure (ICP) can induce vomiting, syncope, neck pain and nuchal rigidity.

Although this patient has few neurologic symptoms, the risk of aneurysmal rebleeding is present. Rebleeding is a frequent cause of death and disability in patients who survive the initial hemorrhage. Rebleeding most frequently occurs in the first 3 days in about 8% of untreated patients and is initially detected by a deteriorating neurologic condition. Current surgical and endovascular treatment goals include prevent rebleeding through early diagnosis and intervention.

2. **What are some of the risk factors for SAH?**

Risk factors in aneurysmal SAH can be categorized into nonmodifiable and modifiable.

Nonmodifiable risk factors include age, gender, ethnicity, family history, and aneurysm location and size. The incidence of SAH increases with age with a peak occurring in the fifth and sixth decades of life. Subsequently, the incidence has been shown to plateau or slightly diminish with subsequent aging. SAH is more frequent in women than men. Studies have suggested hormonal and developmental factors (age of menarche and nulliparity) as contributors to the gender disparity. Studies have also suggested a higher incidence of SAH in African Americans compared to Caucasians in the United States. One of the strongest predictors of SAH is a family history of SAH. This genetic foundation has been shown across various populations and in various regions of the world [1].

The aneurysm location with the highest to lowest frequency of rupture is the anterior communicating artery (ACoA 29%), posterior communicating artery (PCoA, 19.6%), the basilar artery (14.7%), and the middle cerebral artery (MCA, 11.8%). There is a direct correlation between aneurysm size and the likelihood of aneurysm rupture, however small aneurysms are not without risk. Forget et al. [2] showed that 210 of 245 (85.7%) consecutive eighty seven percent of SAH patients presented with aneurysms smaller than 10 mm. Langham et al. [3] also supported that the majority of patients (67.3%) with aneurysmal SAH had aneurys smaller than 10 mm in size.

P.P. Liu (✉)
Department of Anesthesiology, Tufts Medical Center, 800 Washington Street, #298, Boston, MA 02111, USA
e-mail: PLiu@tuftsmedicalcenter.orgpennyliumd@gmail.com

© Springer International Publishing AG 2017
L.S. Aglio and R.D. Urman (eds.), *Anesthesiology*,
DOI 10.1007/978-3-319-50141-3_16

Certain genetic conditions have an association with intracranial aneurysms. This includes polycystic kidney disease, Marfan's syndrome, Ehler Danlos syndrome, and Type 1 neurofibromatosis.

Modifiable risk factors that increase the risk of SAH include chronic hypertension, tobacco and cocaine use. Chronic hypertension has been shown to be a strong predictor of aneurysmal SAH.

3. **What is the clinical grading of this patient's SAH?**

The World Federation of Neurological Surgeon's Grading System (WFNS) and the modified Hunt and Hess Grading System are the two most common grading schemes that provide assessment of surgical risk and prognosis.

The WFNS SAH scale has 5 grades with Grade 1 indicating the lowest neurologic injury and Grade 5 the most. It utilizes incorporates the Glasgow Coma Scale (GCS) (Table 16.1) plus the absence or presence of motor deficits for risk stratification.

The World Federation of Neurological Surgeons (WFNS) SAH Scale[1] [4] is

Grade 1: GCS 15 with no motor deficit
Grade 2: GCS between 14–13 with no motor deficit
Grade 3: GCS 14–13 *with* the presence of motor deficit
Grade 4: GCS 12–7 with *or* without motor deficit
Grade 5: GCS 6–3 with *or* without motor deficit.

- The Hunt and Hess Classification[2] [5] is

  Grade 1: asymptomatic or has a mild headache, slight nuchal rigidity
  Grade 2: moderate to severe headache, nuchal rigidity, no neurologic deficit other than cranial nerve palsy
  Grade 3: drowsy, confused, mild focal neurologic deficit
  Grade 4: stupor with moderate to severe hemiparesis
  Grade 5: coma, decerebrate posturing.

Unlike the WFNS, the most current modification of the Hunt and Hess Classification takes into account comorbid conditions such as hypertension and diabetes which when present place the patient at the next highest risk category. The current patient based on her presentation of moderate headache, nuchal rigidity would place her at an initial Hunt and Hess Grade 2. However, due to her comorbid conditions of hypertension and diabetes, her Hunt and Hess classification is now Grade 3. Her WFNS Grade is 1 based upon a Glasgow Coma Scale of 15 and no motor deficits.

4. **Describe this patient's ability for cerebral autoregulation.**

Cerebral autoregulation is the ability to maintain adequate and stable cerebral perfusion pressure over a range of mean arterial pressure (MAP). After SAH, cerebral autoregulation is frequently impaired. Focal reductions in cerebral perfusion may contribute to delayed ischemic neurological deficits (DIND). Elevated blood pressures, both transient and long term, are seen after SAH secondary to sympathetic activation. In a patient with Hunt and Hess Grade III and higher Inadequate cerebral perfusion begins at a higher MAP. Autoregulatory pressure curve is shifted toward a higher BP. In this patient with untreated chronic hypertension, the cerebral pressure curve has already been shifted to higher values but she does not have neurologic findings to suggest a further elevation in MAP is necessary.

Elevated ICP due to increased intracranial volume means a higher MAP is needed to maintain cerebral perfusion pressure (CPP). This sustained, elevated MAP increases the risk of rebleeding or secondary aneurysm rupture. Guidelines for the management of aneurysmal SAH from the onset of symptoms to aneurysm obliteration, recommend blood pressure is best controlled with a titratable agents (e.g., nicardipine, labetolol). This balances the risk of ischemic stroke, hypertension-related rebleeding, and maintenance of global cerebral perfusion pressure [6, 7]. Unfortunately, the MAP goal to achieve these often opposing goals has not been established but a maintaining systolic pressure to <160 mmHg and a MAP above 80–90 mm Hg is often suggested.

5. **What additional physiologic abnormalities are associated with SAH?**

a. **Cardiac**: Cardiac injury is usually seen after SAH. It can range from conduction abnormalities, as evident from this patient's PVC's, to actual myocardial injury which is speculated to be caused by the catecholamine release which occurs at aneurysm rupture. Autopsy studies reported micro infarctions at autopsy in patients with early mortality. The increase in troponin levels is related to both cardiovascular injury and neurologic injury associated with vasopasm. Higher values indicate poor neurologic outcome and increased likelihood of mortality. Cardiac dysfunction can last up to 6 weeks and is usually reversible.

[1]Reproduced from Teasdale GM, Drake CG, Hunt W, Kassell N, Sano K, Perulset B, De Villiers JC. A universal subarachnoid hemorrhage scale: report of a committee of the World Federation of Neurosurgical Societies. Journal of Neurology, Neurosurgery & Psychiatry 1988;51(11):1457, with permission of BMJ Publishing Group Ltd.

[2]Reproduced from Hunt WE, Hess RM. Surgical risk as related to time of intervention in the repair of intracranial aneurysms. Journal of Neurosurgery 1968;28(1):14–20, with permission of the American Association of Neurological Surgeons.

Table 16.1 Simplified Glasgow Coma Score

Glasgow coma score	
Eye opening	
Spontaneous	4
To speech	3
To pain	2
No response	1
Verbal response	
Oriented to time, place, and person	5
Confused, disoriented	4
Inappropriate words	3
Incomprehensible sounds	2
No response	1
Best motor response	
Obeys commands	6
Moves to localized pain	5
Flexion withdraws from pain	4
Abnormal flexion	3
Abnormal extension	2
No response	1
SUM	
Best score 15, worst score 3	

Sum of items in each category indicates the neurologic condition of the patient. The highest score is 15, a patient without symptoms, and the lowest is 3, a patient who is moribund. Reproduced from Teasdale G, Jennett B. Assessment of coma and impaired consciousness: A practical scale. LANCET (ii) 81–83, 1974, with permission from Elsevier

b. **Glucose metabolism**: Hyperglycemia is one factor used in predicting increased risk of vasospasm as well as a poor neurologic outcome. Whereas there is no absolute consensus target for serum glucose level, the American Diabetic Association recommends glucose between 160-100 in perioperative and critically ill patients. One study of SAH outcomes found that the likelihood of long-term cognitive dysfuntion and motor dysfunction increased with blood glucose levels <129 mg/dl and >152 mg/dl, respectively [8]. All patients but with history of diabetes require precise control of serum glucose to avoid hypoglycemia as well as hyperglycemia.

c. **Intravascular volume and hyponatremia**: Hyponatremia is frequent after SAH. Main causes are inappropriate ADH secretion (SIADH) and cerebral salt wasting syndrome. SIADH leads to diminished water excretion with normal sodium excretion. The hallmark of SIADH is hyponatremia with euvolemia or hypervolemia. Treatment requires judicious diuresis or restriction of free water intake.

   With cerebral salt wasting syndrome, the hyponatremia is the result of active urinary sodium excretion. These patients actively excrete sodium in the urine without water retention. The treatment for cerebral salt wasting syndrome is restoring intravascular volume by administering normal saline or hypertonic saline. To make the diagnosis urine sodium is determined. SIADH has normal urine sodium while cerebral salt wasting has an inappropriately high urine sodium.

   Patients with cerebral salt wasting syndrome are often hypovolemic. Restoring intravascular volume is particularly important because of the risk of vasospasm where euvolemia is a standard treatment. Overly rapid correction of serum sodium levels can cause osmotic demyelination syndrome (aka, central pontine myelinolysis). The neurologic manifestations are seizures, altered level of consciousness, gait disturbance, diminished respiratory function, dysarthria, and dysphagia. Treatment of hyponatremia requires very gradual restoration of serum sodium.

6. **Describe the treatment options for aneurysms.**

The treatment options are interventional or endovascular and surgical; the choice depends upon:

a. Anatomy and location of the aneurysm
b. Status of the aneurysm (unruptured/ruptured/bleeding)
c. Health and age of the patient

Endovascular techniques are suitable for nearly all accessible aneurysms. Often the choice, endovascular or surgical, is made by the patient or their family prior to the angiogram. Endovascular techniques are often recommended when surgical location (e.g., posterior circulation, cavernous sinus, internal carotid aneurysms) or medical difficulties (e.g., elderly, multiple comorbid conditions) increase the surgical risk. Surgical clipping is suitable when endovascular techniques have limited success (e.g., giant aneurysms (>2.5 cm in diameter), fusiform aneurysms, aneurysms with a wide neck (neck: dome ratio >0.5), and middle cerebral artery aneurysms). In younger patients (<40 years of age), surgical clipping may provide better long-term protection from rebleeding. With ongoing advancements in both microsurgical and endovascular approaches, the methods of determining the proper aneurysm characteristics and patient population for each treatment option continue to change.

When surgical treatment is chosen, a surgical clip is placed to exclude the aneurysm from the cerebral circulation without occluding the primary vessel. An endovascular option involves thrombosis of the aneurysm sac by placement of detachable platinum coils or other devices. Endovascular is an alternative and often a preferred treatment when the aneurysm anatomy and location is favorable.

Unruptured aneurysm is often electively treated. There have been no randomized trials comparing the coiling versus clipping techniques in this population. However, in a retrospective study across 429 centers in the United States, 2535 unruptured aneurysms were evaluated. The results favored endovascular coiling over surgical clipping [9].

SAH treatment is based upon characteristics of both the patient and the aneurysm. Surgical clipping or endovascular coiling of the ruptured aneurysm should be performed as early as possible to reduce the likelihood of rebleeding after SAH. It is worth noting that the International Subarachnoid Trial (ISAT) study [10, 11] was quite influential in favoring change of practice from surgical clipping to coiling. Despite some of its limitations, (small, <1 cm diameter, anterior circulation, good neurological grade), the ISAT study was the first study comparing the outcome measure of endovascular coiling with surgical clipping. Although reported in 2002, the ISAT result showed that fewer patients experienced the primary outcome, death or dependency, in the coiling group (24%) than they clipping group (31%). A strong criticism remains the surgical group contained patients who could not undergo endovascular treatment. The rate of rebleeding at 1 year was higher for the coiling group (2.6%) as compared to clipping (1%). Rebleeding may negate the advantage of the endovascular treatment [12].

7. **When should surgical treatment for SAH surgery occur?**

Rebleeding is a major cause of morbidity in SAH with mortality rates nearing 70%. Without intervention, the risk of rebleeding reaches 40% within the first month. The highest daily rate (4%) occurs within the first 24 h followed by a daily rate of 1–2% for the next 28 days. Early surgery (0–3 days) is associated with reduced frequency of rebleeding. All but the most difficult aneurysms are treated with endovascular approach at the time of diagnosis. Consequently, the difficult surgical exposure caused by local edema and blood increases risk of intraoperative bleeding and long surgery. Once secured, the ability to treat vasospasm and eliminate rebleeding improve outcomes. Late surgery (>10 days posthemorrhage) has the advantage of better surgical conditions with increased risk occurring during days 4–9.

The current standard practice is intervention as soon as the aneurysm has been diagnosed. Studies consistently support early surgery and showing its association with improved clinical outcome in low-grade as well as high-grade SAH patients. Patients who were coiled or clipped within 24 h of SAH presentation had improved clinical outcomes compared with treatment after 24 h [13]. In the Netherlands, 1500 patients from eight hospitals, found no difference in low-risk patients but better outcomes in patients with poor clinical condition on admission after early surgery [14].

8. **What is vasospasm?**

Vasospasm, a complication following SAH, is severe vasoconstriction cerebral vessels of distal from the original aneurysm. Its severity is associated with the amount of blood present on the CT scan and occurs beginning 2–3 days after SAH.

One can divide the vasospasm into (1) "clinical vasospasm" which refers to "delayed ischemic neurologic deficit" (DIND) or delayed cerebral ischemia (DCI) and (2) angiographic vasospasm, detected only on arteriogram. After surviving SAH treatment, vasospasm is a dreaded late complication. DCI can occur following SAH with or without angiographic evidence of narrowed of the cerebral vessels. Vasospasm on cerebral angiography is seen as a narrowing of the lumen of cerebral arteries. Daily studies with transcranial doppler (TCD) use increased blood flow velocity to detect narrowed arterial lumens or vasospasm in the anterior and posterior circulation. TCD changes can anticipate clinically symptomatic vasospasm.

Delayed cerebral ischemia is a clinical diagnosis that presents as confusion, depressed consciousness often with focal neurologic deficits on imaging. DCI symptoms typically begin as early as 3 days but the highest frequency is between 6 and 8 days post SAH. Seizures, hydrocephalus, cerebral edema, hypoxemia, hyponatremia, and sepsis can mimic DCI.

Persistent, untreated clinically symptomatic vasospasm is associated with increased morbidity and mortality due to cerebral ischemia and infarction. The major causes of morbidity and death in patients with aneurysmal SAH as cited by The International Cooperative Study on the timing of Aneurysm Surgery were:

(1) Cerebral infarction secondary to vasospasm—33.5%,
(2) Direct effect of hemorrhage—25.5%,
(3) Rebleeding before treatment—17.3%,
(4) Complications from treatment—8.9%,
(5) Intracerebral hematoma—4.5%, and
(6) Hydrocephalus—3%.

9. **What are the predictors of vasospasm?**

The amount of hemorrhage seen on Computed Tomography (CT) is a very powerful predictor of vasospasm. The Fisher Scale is the most well-known grading scale and provides a correlation between the amount of blood on CT and the risk of vasospasm.

Fisher Group 1: no blood on CT
Fisher Group 2: diffuse or thin layer, (<1 mm thickness)
Fisher Group 3: localized clot or thick layer, (>1 mm)
Fisher Group 4: diffuse of no SAH, but with IVH or ICH

Other predictive factors of an increase risk are systemic hypertension, age <50 years old [15], cigarette smoker, cocaine use, and female.

This patient is at low risk of vasospasm.

10. **What are the treatment options for vasospasm?**

Assuming the aneurysm has been secured, the initial treatment for vasospasm is administration of nimodipine, maintenance of euvolemia, and induced hypertension to improve cerebral perfusion [6]. Nimodipine has been shown to improve neurological outcomes but not cerebral vasospasm (Class I, Level of Evidence A). The efficacy of other calcium channel blockers, oral or IV, remains uncertain. The intravenous calcium channel blocker in widespread use is nicadipine, used for blood pressure control and vasospasm treatment [16].

Hypervolemia, hypertension, hemodilution (Triple H) therapy was historically the primary treatment of vasospasm. The theory of Triple H would enhance cerebral perfusion and blood flow to ischemic areas. However, the efficacy of HHH therapy has not been validated. There can be significant complications associated with its use (e.g., congestive heart failure, pulmonary edema, renal failure, cardiac ischemia, and sepsis) with no proven positive effect based upon review of controlled studies to date. There is support that hypertension with normovolemia is effective for mitigating clinical vasospasm. Current recommendation is to maintain euvolemia with systolic blood pressure range of 140–160 mmHg.

Magnesium therapy has been extensively studied in the treatment of cerebral vasospasm. Mg is a competitive antagonist of calcium and a noncompetitive antagonist at voltage-gated calcium channels leading to smooth muscle relaxation. Magnesium infusions may cause some reduction in delayed cerebral ischemia but the benefits have not been conclusively supported by meta-analysis or Cochrane review [17].

Statin therapy in SAH treatment is controversial. It has been proposed as a means to prevent vasospasm through cholesterol dependent as well as cholesterol independent mechanisms. Currently, initiating statin therapy is not recommended for routine use in the treatment of vasospasm and delayed ischemic neurologic deficit [18, 19].

11. **How do endovascular procedures treat vasospasm?**

Endovascular procedures are first line therapy for severe vasospasm. These endovascular interventions generally consist of balloon angioplasty for accessible lesions and intra-arterial vasodilator infusions for more distal vessels. If performed within 2 h of symptoms, balloon angioplasty has been found to be radiologically effective, no vasoconstriction observed, in 98–100% and clinically effective, reduces symptoms, in 70–80% [20]. Complications from balloon angioplasty include vessel rupture, thrombosis, and embolism.

For vessels that are unamendable to balloon angioplasty, intra-arterial infusion of vasodilatory drugs such as papaverine, verapamil, amrinone, or milrinone, distal to the vasospastic area is a common treatment. Papaverine, a nonselective, phosphodiesterase inhibitor causes transient but potent arterial vasodilation. Papaverine vasodilation is extremely transient; thus recurring vasospasm is common. The global vasodilation it causes can increase ICP. Furthermore, papaverine has been associated with neurotoxic effects, seizures, blindness, coma, and irreversible brain injury [21]. Verapamil injection does not increase the risk of

ICP elevation but can lead to hypotension and bradycardia. Amrinone and milrinone, like papaverine, are nonselective, phosphodiesterase inhibitors. Milrinone is more potent than its parent compound, amrinone. All have been used for the treatment of vasospasm [22].

12. **What are the goals of anesthetic management during the craniotomy?**

The anesthetic management goals are

- To reduce transmural pressure gradient, which can lead to aneurysm rupture.
- To maintain adequate cerebral perfusion pressure throughout the entirety of the procedure.
- To provide optimal surgical conditions by facilitating brain relaxation and reducing intracranial volume.
- To provide prompt emergence at the end of surgery for proper assessment of the patient's neurologic status.

13. **Define transmural pressure**.

The transmural pressure gradient is the difference between the pressure inside the aneurysm (estimated as MAP) and the pressure outside of the aneurysm (estimated as intracranial pressure). An unanticipated increase in mean arterial pressure can lead to aneurysm rupture. Placement of an arterial line prior to intraoperative activities that may cause significant hypo- or hypertension (e.g., induction, intubation, placement of the mayfield head holder) is extremely important. Drugs must be available to manipulate BP to maintain a consistent predetermined value.

14. **Define your goals for cerebral perfusion pressure**

Cerebral perfusion pressure (CPP) is also the difference between mean arterial pressure and the intracranial pressure. As previously stated, patients frequently have impaired cerebral autoregulation after SAH. Their lower limits of adequate cerebral perfusion now occur at a higher mean arterial pressure. Adequate cerebral perfusion pressure promotes brain oxygenation and prevents ischemia. The most current guidelines recommend minimizing the degree and duration of intraoperative hypotension during aneurysm surgery (Class IIa, Level of Evidence B) [6, 23].

15. **Describe methods used to achieve adequate brain relaxation**.

Brain relaxation is a slang term used to describe a brain that does not exhibit swelling or displacement caused by a mass, hematoma, tissue edema, or ventricular obstruction. It provides optimal surgical conditions to reduce the amount of surgical retraction and treat the surgical lesion. Brain relaxation is primarily based on decreasing interstitial fluid and CSF volume. Methods to help achieve this goal include:

(a) Mannitol or hypertonic saline
(b) Furosemide
(c) Drainage of CSF

Mannitol promotes brain relaxation by creating an osmotic pressure gradient with an intact blood–brain barrier. The dose is typically 0.5–1.0 g/kg and peak effects are seen at 30–45 min. In addition to the osmotic diuresis, it extracts interstitial fluid from tissues. In a disrupted blood–brain barrier, mannitol may cause rebound edema and increase in intracranial pressure. It should be used with caution if the serum osmolality is above 330 mOsm/L.

Hypertonic saline therapy is used to decrease interstitial fluid. There are studies primarily in intracranial tumors and head trauma that suggest benefit or no harm when compared to mannitol [24, 25].

Furosemide, a loop diuretic, can be administered alone or in combination with mannitol to provide brain relaxation. It decreases CSF production and intravascular volume. This loss of electrolytes and free water can cause hypotension and hypovolemia.

Cerebrospinal fluid drainage utilizing a lumbar or external intraventricular drain can reduce intracranial cerebral spinal fluid (CSF) volume providing brain relaxation. ICP is managed by placing the intraventricular drainage device at an appropriate level and the lumbar drainage removes small aliquots of fluid. Sudden decrease or increase in ICP can lead to reduced transmural pressure gradient and aneurysm rupture or brain herniation.

16. **What is the role of hyperventilation in brain relaxation?**

Hyperventilation improves brain relaxation and improves surgical exposure. $PaCO_2$ should be normal to slightly below normal (30 mmHg). Even transient mild hyperventilation has the potential for substantial reduction in cerebral blood flow (CBF). Several small studies in traumatic brain injury patients found hyperventilation leads to reduction in cerebral perfusion [26]. Modest hyperventilation to improving operative conditions continues to be used with caution.

17. **What anesthetic techniques can be used?**

During craniotomy for aneurysm clipping or endovascular procedures, general anesthesia can utilize inhalational agents, intravenous agents, or a combination of both.

Volatile anesthetics produce dose-dependent cerebral vasodilatation and at >1 minimum alveolar concentration (MAC) can cause enough increase cerebral blood volume to increase ICP. Nitrous oxide has also been shown to increase cerebral blood volume when used alone or in conjunction with a volatile anesthetic. These drug effects are modified by other medications and hyperventilation. Propofol-based total intravenous anesthesia (TIVA) technique can also be used. It reduces cerebral blood flow and ICP [27]. TIVA is a preferred technique when maintaining or decreasing ICP and improving operative conditions is a priority. There are no studies on long-term neurological outcome for any drug regimen. Decisions are made based on efforts to decrease ICP and improve operative conditions.

Analgesia is usually provided by a fentanyl, sufentanil, or occasionally remifentanil. The primary goal is to decrease sympathetic activity. Remifentanil has been associated with substantial hypertension during wake-up and requires postoperative increases in analgesia due to the active metabolite. The metabolite has low analgesic activity but high receptor affinity.

Nondepolarizing muscle relaxants are frequently used. Depolarizing muscle relaxants are associated with hyperkalemia in patients with SAH.

18. **What are the anesthetic management goals during temporary clip placement?**

Temporary occlusion of the aneurysmal artery decompresses the aneurysm to allow manipulation and decrease likelihood of rupture. This technique is used for large aneurysm, aneurysms in difficult locations, or aneurysms considered likely to rupture. Depending on the anatomy of the vessel, there will be either no distal blood flow producing a high risk of ischemia or reduced blood flow from collateral circulation. Mean arterial pressure should be maintained or allowed to rise to increase perfusion through collateral vessels. Ischemic time is kept to a minimum to reduce focal injury with a goal of <10 min. The temporary clip may be removed several times to achieve this goal [28]. EEG burst suppression with propofol or mild hypothermia may be requested to provide neuroprotection. Their clinical benefits have not been established. Improved outcome is not definitively supported for hypothermia or propofol [29, 30].

19. **How is intraoperative aneurysm rupture managed?**

Blood pressure management in the event of sudden, unintentional intraoperative cerebral aneurysm rupture is complex. Transient MAP reduction to 40–50 mmHg can decrease bleeding and facilitate better exposure or placement of a temporary clip on the aneurysm of primary artery. This maneuver is usually brief while the surgeon regains control of the blood vessel and aneurysm. Prolonged uncontrolled bleeding can eventually lead to hypovolemia and blood transfusion. Interventions take into consideration the size of the leak or rupture, completeness of the aneurysm dissection, and the feasibility of temporary occlusion. Effective communication is critical to improving outcome. Adenosine (0.3–0.4 mg/kg) to cause 45–60 s of asystole can facilitate a clip placement [31].

20. **Does anesthetic management differ during endovascular or surgical treatment?**

The anesthetic management goals of minimizing transmural pressure changes and maintaining adequate cerebral perfusion pressure remains the same as for craniotomy for aneurysm clipping. Endovascular intervention still requires that the patient be immobile. Although anesthesia for coiling/embolization can be performed under monitored anesthesia care with patients who are WFNS or Hunt and Hess Grade 1 and are capable of maintaining their airway, many neuro-proceduralists prefer general anesthesia. This reduces the risk of movement and allows immediate surgical intervention if necessary.

Additional considerations during endovascular approaches are the need for anticoagulation, ICU management, and the consequences of radiographic dye administration. Heparin is administered to maintain an activated clotting time (ACT) 2–3 times normal for the duration of the procedure. ACT measures are frequently monitored and heparin dosing adjusted.

To prevent contrast induced nephropathy, intravenous administration of *N*-acetylcysteine and sodium bicarbonate maybe requested. Patients with preexisting risk of renal impairment are at the highest risk of postprocedure renal insufficiency or failure. Since contrast induces a diuresis, urine output is not indicative of renal function. Close monitoring of volume status is necessary since many patients will have received osmotic drugs to control ICP prior to arrival and hypervolemia from radiographic dye administration can contribute to risk of rebleeding, congestive heart failure, and other medical complications.

References

1. Eden SV, Meurer WJ, Sanchez BN, et al. Gender and ethic differences in subarachnoid hemorrhage. Neurology. 2008;71:731.
2. Forget TR Jr, Benitez R, Veznedaroglu E, et al. A review of size and location of ruptured intracranial aneurysms. Neurosurgery. 2001;49:1322.
3. Langham J, Reeves BC, Lindsay KW, et al. Variation in outcome after subarachnoid hemorrhage: a study of neurosurgical units in UK and Ireland. Stroke. 2009;40:111.

4. Teasdale GM, Drake CG, Hunt W, Kassell N, Sano K, Pertuiset B, De Villiers JC. A universal subarachnoid hemorrhage scale: report of a committee of the World Federation of Neurosurgical Societies. J Neurol Neurosurg Psychiatry. 1988;51(11):1457.
5. Hunt WE, Hess RM. Surgical risk as related to time of intervention in the repair of intracranial aneurysms. Journal of Neurosurgery. 1968;28(1):14–20.
6. Connolly ES, Rabinstein AA, et al. Guidelines for the management of aneurysmal subarachnoid hemorrhage. Stroke. 2012;43:1711–37.
7. Pasternak JJ, Lanier WL. Neuroanesthesiology update 2014. J Neurosurg Anesthesiol. 2014;262(2):109–54.
8. Pasternak JJ, McGregor DG, Schroeder DR, et al. Hyperglycemia in patients undergoing cerebral aneurysm surgery: its association with long-term gross neurologic and neuropsychological function. Mayo Clin Proc. 2008;83:406–17.
9. Higashida RT, Lahue BJ, Torgey MT, et al. Treatment of unruptured intracranial aneurysms: a nationwide assessment of effectiveness. Am J Neuroradiol. 2007;28:146–51.
10. Molyneux AJ, Kerr RS, Stratton I, et al. International Subarachnoid Aneurysm Trial (ISAT) of neurosurgical clipping versus endovascular coiling in 2143 patients with ruptured intracranial aneurysm: a randomized trial. Lancet. 2002;360:1267–74.
11. Molyneux AJ, Kerr RS, Yu LM, et al. International Subarachnoid Aneurysm Trial (ISAT) of neurosurgical clipping versus endovascular coiling in 2143 patients with ruptured intracranial aneurysms: seizures, rebleeding, subgroups and aneurysm occlusion. Lancet. 2005;366:809–17.
12. Mitchell P, Kerr R, Mendelow AD, et al. Could late rebleeding overturn the superiority of cranial aneurysm coil embolization over clip ligation seen in the International Subarachnoid Aneurysm Trial? J Neurosurg. 2008;108:427–42.
13. Phillips TJ, Dowling RJ, Yan B, et al. Does treatment of ruptured intracranial aneurysms within 24 hours improve clinical outcome? Stroke. 2011;42:1936–45.
14. Nieuwkamp DJ, de Gans K, Algra A, et al. Timing of aneurysm surgery in subarachnoid haemorrhage-an observational study in The Netherlands. Acta Neurochir (Wein). 2005;147:815–21.
15. Kale SP, Edgell RC, Alshekhlee A, et al. Age-associated vasospasm in aneurysmal subarachnoid hemorrhage. J Stroke Cerebrovasc Dis. 2013;22(1):22–7.
16. Dorhout Mees SM, Rinkel GJ, et al. Calcium antagonists for aneurysmal subarachnoid hemorrhage. Cochrane Database Syst Rev. 2007;(3):CD00027.
17. Schmid-Elsaesser R, Kunz M, Zausinger S, et al. Intravenous magnesium versus nimodipine in the treatment of patients with aneurysmal subarachnoid hemorrhage: a randomized study. Neurosurgery. 2006;58:1054–65.
18. Kramer AH, Gurka MJ, Nathan B, et al: Statin use was not associated with less vasospasm or improved outcome after subarachnoid hemorrhage, Neurosurgery. 2008;62:422–27 (Discussion 427–430).
19. Kirkpatrick PJ, Turner CL, Smith CS, et al. Simvastatin in aneurysmal subarachnoid haemorrhage(STASH): a multicenter randomized phase 3 trial. Lancet Neurol. 2014;13(7):666–75.
20. Pandey AS, Elias AE, ChaudharyN, Thompson BG, Gemmete JJ. Endovascular treatment of cerebral vasospasm vasodilators and angioplasty. Neuroimag Clin N Am. 2013;23:593–604.
21. Smith ML, Abrahams JM, Chandela S, et al. Subarachnoid hemorrhage on computed tomography scanning and the development of cerebral vasospasm: The Fisher grade revisited. Surg Neurol. 2005;63:229–34 (Discussion 234–35).
22. Fraticelli AT, Cholley BP, Losser MR, et al. Milrinone for the treatment of cerebral vasospasm after aneurysmal subarachnoid hemorrhage. Stoke. 2008;39:893–8.
23. Steiner T, Juvela S, et al. European stroke organization guidelines for the management of intracranial aneurysms and subarachnoid haemorrhage. Cerebrovasc Dis. 2013;35(2):93–112.
24. Wu CT, Chen LC, Kuo CP, et al. A comparison of 3% hypertonic saline and mannitol for brain relaxation during elective supratentorial brain tumor surgery. Anesth Analg. 2010;110:903–7.
25. Mortazavi MM, Romeo AK, Deep A, et al. Hypertonic saline for treating raised intracranial pressure: literature review and meta-analysis. J Neurosurg. 2012;116:210–21.
26. Coles JP, Fryer TD, Coleman MR, et al. Hyperventilation following head injury: effect on ischemic burden and cerebral oxidative metabolism. Crit Care Med. 2007;35:568–78.
27. Petersen KD, Landsfeldt U, Cold GE, et al. Intracranial pressure and cerebral hemodynamic in patients with cerebral tumors: a randomized prospective study of patients subjected to craniotomy in propofol-fentanyl, or sevoflurane-fentanyl anesthesia. Anesthesiology. 2003;98:329–36.
28. Samson D, Batjer HH, Bowman G, et al. A clinical study of the parameter and effect of temporary arterial occlusion in the management of intracranial aneurysms. Neurosurgery. 1994;34:22–9.
29. Todd MM, Hindman BJ, Clarke WR, et al. Intraoperative Hypothermia for Aneurysm Surgery Trial (IHAST) Investigators. Mild intraoperative hypothermia during surgery for intracranial aneurysm. N Engl J Med. 2005;352:135–45.
30. Hindman BJ, Bayman EO, Pfisterer WK, et al. IHAST Investigators. No association between intraoperative hypothermia or supplemental protective drug and neurological outcomes in patients undergoing temporary clipping during cerebral aneurysm surgery: findings from the Intraoperative hypothermia for aneurysm surgery trial. Anesthesiology. 2010;112:86–101.
31. Bebawy JF, Gupta DK, Bendok BR, et al. Adenosine-induced flow arrest to facilitate intracranial aneurysm clip ligation: dose-response data and safety profile. Anesth Analg. 2010;110:1406–11.

Suggested Reading

32. Anderson SW, Todd MM, Hindman BJ, et al. IHAST Investigators. Effects of intraoperative hypothermia on neuropsychological outcomes after intracranial aneurysm surgery. Ann Neurol. 2006;60:518–27.
33. Buckland MR, Batjer HH, Giesecke AH. Anesthesia for cerebral aneurysm surgery: use of induced hypertensionin patients with symptomatic vasospasm. Anesthesiology. 1988;69:116–9.
34. Campi A, Ramzi N, Molyneux AJ, et al. Retreatment of ruptured cerebral aneurysms in patients randomized by coiling or clipping in the International Subarachnoid Aneurysm Trial (ISAT). Stroke. 2007;38:1538–44.
35. Colby GP, Coon AL, Tamargo RJ. Surgical management of aneurysmal subarachnoid hemorrhage. Neurosurg Clin N Am. 2010;21(2):247–61.
36. De Chazal I, Parham WM III, Liopyris P, Wijdicks EF. Delayed cardiogenic shock and acute lung injury after aneurysmal subarachnoid hemorrhage. Anesth Analg. 2005;100:1147–9.
37. Diringer MN, Bleck TP, Hemphill JC, et al. Critical care management of patients following aneurysmal subarachnoid hemorrhage: recommendations from the neurocritical care society's multidisciplinary consensus conference. Neurocrit Care. 2011;15:211–40.
38. D'souza S. Aneurysmal Subarachnoid Hemorrhage. J Neurosurg Anesthesiol. 2015;27(3):222–33.

39. Ellegala DB, Day AL. Ruptured cerebral aneurysms. N Engl J Med. 2005;352:121–4.
40. Frontera JA, Claassen J, Schmidt JM, et al. Prediction of symptomatic vasospasm after subarachnoid hemorrhage: the modified Fisher scale. Neurosurgery. 2006;59:21–7.
41. Ibrahim GM, Macdonald RL. Electrographic changes predict angiographic vasospasm after aneurysmal subarachnoid hemorrhage. Stroke. 2012;43:2102–107.
42. Ingall T, Asplund K, Mahonen M, et al. A multinational comparison of subarachnoid hemorrhage epidemiology in the WHO MONICA stroke study. Stroke. 1054;2000:31.
43. Kan P, Jahshan S, Yashar P, et al. Feasibility, safety and periprocedural complications associated with endovascular treatment of selected ruptured aneurysms under conscious sedation and local anesthesia. Neurosurgery. 2013;72:216–20.
44. Kassel NF, Torner JC, Jane JA, et al. The International cooperative study on the timing of aneurysm surgery. Part 2: surgical results. J Neurosurg. 1990;73:37–47.
45. Komotar RJ, Zacharia BE, Otten ML, et al. Controversies in the endovascular management of cerebral vasospasm after intracranial aneurysm rupture and future directions for therapeutic approaches. Neurosurgery. 2008;62:897–905 (Discussion 905–07).
46. Kruyt ND, Biessels GJ, DeVries JH, et al. Hyperglycemia in aneurysmal subarachnoid hemorrhage: a potentially modifiable risk factor for poor outcome. J Cerebral Blood Flow Metab. 2010;30(9):1577–587.
47. Lee VH, Oh JK, Mulvagh SL, et al. Mechanisms in neurogenic stress cardiomyopathy after aneurysmal subarachnoid hemorrhage.
48. Mahaney KB, Todd MM, Bayman EO, et al. Acute postoperative neurological deterioration associated with surgery for ruptured intracranial aneurysm; incidence, predictors, and outcomes. J Neurosurg. 2012;116(6):1267–78.
49. McAuliffe W, Townsend M, Eskridge JM, et al. Intracranial pressure changes induced during papaverine infusion for treatment of vasospasm. J Neurosurg. 1995;83:430–4.
50. Okamoto K, Horisawa R, Kawamura T, et al. Menstrual and reproductive factors for subarachnoid hemorrhage risk in women: a case-control study in Nagoya, Japan. Stroke. 2001;32:2841.
51. Oliver GS, Ibrahim GM, et al. Operative complications and differences in outcome after clipping and coiling of ruptured intracranial aneurysms. J Neurosurg. 2015; ahead of print, online 5 June.
52. Pearl M, Gregg L, Gailloud P. Endovascular treatment of aneurysmal subarachnoid hemorrhage. Neurosurg Clin N Am. 2010;21(2):271–80.
53. Prakash A, Matta BF. Hyperglycaemia and neurological injur. Curr Opin Anaethesiol. 2008;21:565–9.
54. Randell T, Niskanen M. Management of physiological variables in neuroanesthesia: maintaining homostasis during intracranial surgery. Curr Opin Anaesthesiol. 2006;19:492–7.
55. Schievink WI, Torres VE, Peipgras DG, et al. Saccular intracranial aneurysms in autosomal dominant polycystic kidney disease. J Am Soc of Nephrol. 1992;3:88–95.
56. Smith WS, Dowd CF, Johnson SC, et al. Neurotoxicity of intra-arterial papaverine preserved with chlorobutanol used for the treatment of cerebral vasospasm after aneurysmal subarachnoid hemorrhage. Stroke. 2004;35:2518–22.
57. Yee AH, Burns JD, Wijdicks EFM. Cerebral salt wasting: pathophysiology, diagnosis, and treatment. Neurosurg Clin N Am. 2010;21(2):339–64.

17 Carotid Endarterectomy

Reza Gorji and Lu'ay Nubani

Case

80-year-old male describes three episodes of monocular visual loss with each episode lasting longer than the prior one. On physical exam in the ER, the only neurologic finding is monocular visual loss. After a carotid ultrasonogram and a computerized tomography angiogram (CTA), he is advised that he needs treatment for carotid artery stenosis.

Past Medical History:	Hypertension, Diabetes Mellitus
Allergies:	none
Medications:	Lisinopril metoprolol, metformin
Physical Exam:	BP 150/92, P 89, R 20, T 36.7
	Carotid bruit bilateral L>R
	Heart RR, S1 S2 SEM 2
Studies:	
	Carotid Ultrasound—partial occlusion of the left Carotid artery
	CTA—75% occlusion of the Left carotid artery —Right Carotid artery 30% occlusion
	ECG—normal sinus rhythm

1. **What caused his transient monocular blindness?**

Transient monocular blindness, also called amaurosis fugax, is usually caused by retinal ischemia. In patients younger than 45 years it may be vasospasm or symptom of a migraine but in older patients or patients with atherosclerosis it is usually emboli, thrombus or plaque, giant cell arteritis or cerebrovascular ischemia that temporarily obstructs the ophthalmic artery causing symptomatic ischemia in the optic nerve and the retina. It is generally monocular and lasts for 2–30 min. Patients describe it as darkness or a gray curtain over one eye.

2. **What comorbid conditions are associated with carotid artery disease?**

Patients with carotid artery disease typically suffer from other systemic diseases like hypertension, diabetes mellitus, obesity, arteriosclerosis, and pulmonary disease from smoking. It is important to note that patients with hypertension and diabetes are also at high risk for renal disease. Morbidity and possibly mortality are increased in patients with renal disease who undergo carotid endarterectomy (CEA). There is increased risk of stroke, death, and cardiac complications in this population [1, 2].

Previous stroke or transient ischemic attack (TIA), cardiovascular disease and sickle cell disease significantly increase risk of serious complications [3]. The most consistent risk factor is age; increasing age is also associated with increasing probability of stroke. This may be related to anatomical changes in the vessel wall that occur with aging [4]. Carotid artery (CA) disease is one manifestation of atherosclerosis.

3. **How would you medically evaluate the patient?**

The preoperative evaluation must assess the patient for recognized associated comorbid conditions. Of particular importance would be the history of neurological impairment. As high as 25% of patients with CAD also have CA disease [5–7]. Stress makes these patients at risk for myocardial ischemia [8]. When planning for an elective procedure, optimizing comorbid conditions can reduce perioperative complication. When significant symptoms of cardiac ischemia are present, consultation with a cardiologist to optimize the patient's health is important.

R. Gorji (✉) · L. Nubani
Department of Anesthesiology, University Hospital, 750 East Adams Street, Syracuse, NY 13078, USA
e-mail: gorjijr@upstate.edu

L. Nubani
e-mail: nubanil@upstate.edu

© Springer International Publishing AG 2017
L.S. Aglio and R.D. Urman (eds.), *Anesthesiology*,
DOI 10.1007/978-3-319-50141-3_17

When CA therapy is elective, use of standard assessment and management protocols for each comorbid condition are recommended. For example, patients with sleep disordered breathing (obstructive sleep apnea or OSA) receive medical optimization prior to surgery followed by postoperative management.

When CA treatment is emergently required, best judgment regarding the evaluation is necessary. The 1-hour goal of event to therapy for a stroke or TIA patient requires an efficient standard protocol to prevent unnecessary delays.

The clinician must decide anesthetic management goals based on both the CA procedure and the patient's active medical problems [9].

4. **What preoperative assessment of carotid artery disease is recommended?**

Preoperative evaluation of the CA disease focuses on defining the diseased vessel. To determine the extent of the cerebrovascular disease, these diagnostic modalities are suggested

- CA duplex ultrasound
- Computer tomographic angiography
- Magnetic resonance angiography
- Cerebral angiography
- Magnetic resonance angiography

5. **What urgent medical therapies are recommended for patients with TIA or acute stroke?**

Preexisting medical therapy for these often include administration of antiplatelet/anticoagulant/antifibrinolytic agents. Aspirin [10, 11], and clopidogrel therapy [12] may be initiated prior to CA stenting or carotid endarterectomy. Statins and beta-blockers should be continued in these patients. Statins may induce vascular remodeling and regression for carotid atherosclerotic lesions [13, 14]. Statin administration use may reduce neurologic morbidity among patients undergoing carotid angioplasty and stent procedures. Long-term therapy may reduce carotid plaques in high-risk patients.

6. **Should the patient undergo a surgical or endovascular therapy for a TIA or acute stroke?**

Rapid evaluation and therapy, "Stroke Alert" requires endovascular treatment within 1 h of onset of symptoms in the adult [15]. This is an opportunity to treat a CA lesion when appropriate or establish the extent of CA disease for a surgical intervention.

7. **What type of patient will benefit the most from a CA treatment?**

Patients with carotid stenosis greater than 70% may cause cerebral hypoperfusion and patients will benefit from a CEA or endovascular intervention. Patients with stenosis between 50 and 69% will only have marginal increase in blood flow. This patient has symptoms due acute hypoperfusion and requires therapy.

Accepted indications for a therapy include the following:

- Previous TIA and TIA lasting > 1 h
- Reversible ischemic neurologic deficits with vessel stenosis >70% or an ulcerated plaque with or without stenosis
- Unstable neurologic state with concurrent anticoagulation

The benefits of CEA are seen primarily in men, patients older than 75 years of age and patients who after the onset of symptoms with "undergo surgery within <2 weeks after initial [16]."

8. **What are the options for improving CA perfusion?**

Therapy includes reducing hypercoagulability (e.g., antiplatelet drugs, systemic anticoagulation drugs, aspirin), and increase vessel diameter with surgical or endovascular management (e.g., carotid stenting and angioplasty, CEA) [17].

Procedural intervention, carotid stent placement or carotid endarterectomy is safe and effective options in patients with occlusive disease. Patients with multiple comorbid conditions may benefit more from carotid stenting and include patients with

- severe coronary artery disease or congestive heart failure
- bilateral artery stenosis or carotid artery occlusion
- contralateral laryngeal nerve palsy
- prior radiotherapy or neck surgery
- severe pulmonary dysfunction
- renal failure or insufficiency
- acute stroke

These factors are implicated in poor outcomes regardless of the technique chosen [18, 19].

Surgical treatment is more often recommended in patients

- ≤ 70 years
- female
- with a severely calcified plaque
- with a plaque involving common and internal carotid arteries
- with a tortuous internal carotid artery

9. **What premedication is indicated?**

Premedication reduces anxiety but may increase the risk of hypoventilation and delayed awakening. Use of premedication is a judgment best made by the anesthesiologist.

10. **What monitors would you use?**

Standard ASA monitors and an intra-arterial blood pressure monitor are routinely recommended. A patient with poor ventricular function may benefit from a transesophageal echocardiogram (TEE). It may complicate surgical and endovascular procedures. If a carotid artery shunt is placed emboli occur. Some organizations use transcranial Doppler to detect emboli and allow the surgeon to modify their technique. Cerebral oximetry is used to estimate adequacy of cerebral perfusion. Its efficacy is not determined [20, 21].

11. **What neuromonitoring could be used?**

Electroencephalogram (EEG), processed EEG, somatosensory evoked potentials (SSEP) are often used as a functional indicator of perfusion since they record neuronal and synaptic activity. EEG slowing indicates decreased perfusion. Administration of volatile anesthesia and TIVA increases EEG slowing in a dose dependent fashion. Slowing due to hypoperfusion may be ipsilateral only and can be treated with placement of a shunt and increasing blood pressure. Treatment may prevent neurologic injury since persistent slowing is associated with postoperative neurologic complications [22–24].

EEG measurement is limited to the electrical activity in the superficial cerebral cortex near the electrodes. EEG limitations allow false positive and false negatives interpretations. Even more limited is processed EEG; it is used by anesthesia personnel to monitor the frontal cortex; its value has not been established.

Somatosensory evoked potentials (SSEP) can detect hypoperfusion in the sensory cortex while transcranial motor evoked potentials (MEP) detect hypoperfusion in the motor cortex. MEP require modifications in anesthetic technique to obtain. SSEP and MEP indicate laterality and if adequate perfusion is present. They do not provide information about focal ischemic events [25].

12. **What additional monitoring techniques may be used?**

Carotid stump pressure is the pressure obtained by transducing the CA above the cross-clamp. It has been used as a surrogate for perfusion. Perfusion pressure presumably reflects the collateral blood flow. Stump pressure does not reliably correlate with EEG, SSEP, or changes in an awake patient's neurological exam. Stump pressure when used in conjunction with transcranial Doppler is predictive of cerebral ischemia [26].

13. **What are the consideration in choosing an anesthetic?**

Ideally, the anesthesia must maintain oxygenation, cardiovascular stability and best surgical or endovascular conditions. Both regional and general anesthesia are successfully used.

General anesthesia is the most frequently used technique in the United States. Its use is based on the clinician, surgeon, and patient preference. The major advantages of general anesthesia include

- cardiovascular stability
- patient immobility
- ventilation and airway control

The disadvantages include

- neurologic exam not available
- increased use of shunts with associated cerebral emboli
- neurological complications masked by residual anesthesia

Regional anesthesia can provide adequate anesthesia and immediate neurologic exam when minimal sedation is used. The regional can be a surgical field block but most frequently a cervical plexus block, superficial, or deep is used. The major advantages include

- real time neurologic exam
- no airway intervention
- reduction in shunt placement

The disadvantages include

- patient movement, agitation, anxiety
- hemodynamic instability which is not easily managed
- regional technique risks (e.g., cervical spinal, failed block, local anesthetic overdose)
- restricted access to patient's airway

Sedation during regional is often required increasing respiratory and cardiovascular adverse events. The neurologic advantages can be negated with sedation.

14. **Which anesthetic technique provides the best outcome?**

Anesthetic choice has no significant effect on major adverse outcomes including death, stroke and myocardial infarction (MI). General anesthesia is more common for endarterectomies and sedation for endovascular procedures. These choices reflect the different patient access in urgent situations and a different amount of stimulation.

15. **How would you maintain a general anesthetic?**

The goals of general anesthesia are to provide adequate hypnosis, analgesia, vital signs including cerebral perfusion, and surgical access. Anesthetic techniques may be a TIVA or a volatile anesthetic.

Primary induction goal is BP stability. Autoregulation begins to fail with blood pressures outside the "normal" range. This typically is a mean arterial pressure (MAP) <50 mm Hg or >150 mm Hg. Below 50 mm Hg hypoperfusion and above 150 mm Hg hyperperfusion occurs. Significant hypo or hypertension can lead to a cerebral ischemia or hemorrhagic stroke. Common induction management includes etomidate or propofol, narcotic, like fentanyl or remifentanil, and lidocaine to reduce intubation hypertension [27].

Avoiding cerebral ischemia and providing prompt emergence from anesthesia at the conclusion of the procedure are important goals. Commonly used guidelines advocate blood pressure be maintained within 20% of the preoperative value [28–30]. If EEG monitoring is used the anesthesiologist should avoid burst suppression. It will hinder detection of cerebral ischemia. No specific drug regimens are associated with improved outcomes.

16. **Describe respiratory management with general anesthesia?**

Consensus regarding respiratory management is to maintain normal $PaC0_2$ with minimal hyperventilation. $PaCO_2$ is a direct determinant of cerebral autoregulation. CBF increases about 4% per mm Hg increase in $PaCO_2$. This rule applies only to a $PaCO_2$ in the range of 20–80 mm Hg. Hypercarbia causes cerebral vasodilation and possibly redistribution of blood from preexisting dilated vessels to newly dilated vessels. It is assumed this increases the possibility of hypoperfusion in "at risk" areas of the brain [31]. Hypocarbia may vasoconstrict vessels and reduce blood flow to vulnerable areas.

17. **When do you perform regional anesthetic**?

A candidate for regional anesthesia must be cooperative and willing to be alert enough to follow commands. An obtunded patient can endanger themselves and negate the ability to monitor the patient's neurological status. Deep and superficial cervical plexus block can be performed and offer an alternative to general anesthesia [32]. Technical expertise is required for these blocks.

18. **How would you manage a patient's blood pressure during treatment for carotid artery disease?**

A patient with carotid stenosis often has ischemic areas that have hypoperfusion despite maximally dilated arteries. Perfusion in these areas is pressure dependent.

Hypotension should be avoided but the definition of hypotension is debated. Consensus is that target blood pressure should be close to patient's baseline blood pressure. Management of BP lability is critical. Some surgeons infiltrate the carotid sinus with lidocaine in order to reduce the bradycardia and hypertension that results during stimulation of the carotid sinus during surgery.

Hypotension is frequently treated with phenylephrine. It has no direct vasoconstriction effect on cerebral vasculature but increases mean arterial pressure and cerebral perfusion pressure. Hypertension is usually treated with vasodilators such nicardipine. Infusions of nitroglycerin or nitroprusside and bolus drugs like labetalol are also used. Technique is less important than providing a stable BP.

Once the plaque is removed, blood pressure goals change. Now blood pressure goals are set below patient's baseline. This reduces possibility of arteriotomy bleeding and cerebral reperfusion injury.

19. **Does reperfusion injury occur after a CEA?**

Reperfusion injury is postulated to be caused by the inability of the chronically dilated vessels to have normal autoregulation in response to a high perfusion pressure. Reperfusion injury can take the form of hemorrhage or cerebral edema. Reduction in the frequency of reperfusion injury can be achieved by keeping the blood pressure slightly below baseline pressures. Reperfusion injury can occur in any patient with carotid artery disease.

20. **This patient does not emerge from anesthesia. What could be the reason?**

Residual anesthetic drug effect as the cause of delayed recovery should be ruled out. Sequela of anesthetic drugs includes hypoventilation, hypoxia or hypercarbia, from damage to the carotid body. Patients with bilateral CEA, may be particularly vulnerable since they depend on central chemoreceptors that are depressed by opioids and residual anesthesia [33, 34].

Stroke as the cause of delayed awakening should get special consideration. Stroke and perioperative death are the major complications after carotid endarterectomy. In patients with preoperative symptoms, the perioperative stroke and death rate is 6.2% with stent placement and 3.2% after CEA. In asymptomatic patients the stroke and death rate is 2.5% and 1.4% for stent placement and CEA, respectively [25]. Patients with a previous neurological deficit or injury, whose symptoms improved/resolved, may have temporary deterioration in their function or transient reemergence of previously resolved symptoms after general anesthesia or sedation [35, 36].

Causes of stroke after CEA include cerebral ischemia during clamping of the artery, thrombosis at the endarterectomy site, embolic events, or an intracerebral hemorrhage. Emboli are the primary cause of stroke. Embolization occurs during placement and removal of the arterial clamp, and during shunt, or stent placement, and during the dissection of the CA. Statins and antiplatelet therapy are advocated to decrease risk of embolization [37, 38]. Technical problems like kinking of the artery, issues with the graft patch, or thrombosis at the arteriotomy site are associated with strokes.

The Acute Stroke protocol should be activated to identify and treat the cause of the slow or failure to awaken.

21. **How do you identify a perioperative stroke?**

A neurologic exam immediately after the procedure usually identifies a focal or global neurologic event. Activation of the stroke protocol provides information and best treatment options concerning the neurologic changes.

22. **What is the most common cause of non-stroke related death after carotid endarterectomy?**

Myocardial infarction account for 25–50% of the mortality after a carotid endarterectomy [39]. Other cardiac complications following a CEA include unstable angina, pulmonary edema and ventricular tachycardia. In a recent meta-analysis 30-day risk of MI 0.87% for CEA [40].

23. **What are common postoperative management issues after CEA?**

Hemodynamic instability postoperatively may be from loss of normal baroreceptor activity. A local hematoma can compromise the airway, requiring re-exploration. Stridor is the initial sign of airway compromise. Opening the incision and reintubation may be necessary.

24. **What cranial nerves are at risk during a CEA?**

Cranial nerve injury can be a consequence of CEA. In the Carotid Revascularization Endarterectomy versus Stenting Trial (CREST) [25], the incidence of cranial nerve injuries was 4.6% involving cranial nerves CN VII, XII, IX, X, XI. Most injuries most remain undetected or resolve. Vagus (CN X) and hypoglossal (CN XII) nerves appear the most commonly affected. Vagus nerve injury usually involves recurrent laryngeal nerve causing vocal cord paralysis and infrequently the superior laryngeal nerve causing dysphagia and aspiration. In 2.7% of patients, the hypoglossal nerve is disrupted as it crosses the carotid artery leading to ipsilateral tongue deviation or weakness. Glossopharyngeal nerve damage can be serious and impair swallowing and decreased gag reflex; this can result in aspiration. CN IX innervates the carotid body baroreceptors leading do BP lability when damaged.

25. **What is cerebral hyperperfusion syndrome?**

Cerebral hyperperfusion syndrome is a rare reperfusion phenomenon that occurs with CEA and stent placement. Several days after surgery patients experience severe unilateral headache, hypertension followed by seizures and focal neurologic defects, and rarely intracerebral hemorrhage. MRI is the most sensitive test for diagnosis. Management includes antihypertensive and seizure medications. Steroids may have role. Discontinuing antiplatelet therapy should be considered.

26. **Do patients require ICU admission after CEA?**

Patient location postoperatively depends on the surgical outcome with most patients being admitted to the standard or moderate care units where they receive frequent vital signs and neurological evaluations. Patients with unstable hemodynamics or neurological symptoms require an ICU admission. A few centers discharge patients who had a stent placement or an uncomplicated CEA home the same day after an observation period [41].

References

1. WHO. Surveillance in brief: update of noncommunicable diseases and mental health surveillance activities. WHO. 2003;5:1–5.
2. Go C, Avgerinos ED, Chaer RA, Ling J, Wazen J, Marone L, Fish L, Makaroun MS. Long-term clinical outcomes and cardiovascular events following carotid endarterectomy. Ann Vasc Surg. 2015 May 21.

3. Kochanek KD, Xu JQ, Murphy SL, Arias E. Mortality in the United States, 2013. NCHS Data Brief, No. 178. Hyattsville, MD: National Center for Health Statistics, Centers for Disease Control and Prevention, US Department of Health and Human Services; 2014.
4. Willeit J, Kiechl S. Prevalence and risk factors of asymptomatic extracranial carotid artery atherosclerosis. A population-based study. Arterioscler Thromb. 1993;13:661–8.
5. de Schryver EL, Algra A, Donders RC, van Gijn J, Kappelle LJ. Type of stroke after transient monocular blindness or retinal infarction of presumed arterial origin. J Neurol Neurosurg Psychiatry. 2006;77(6):734.
6. Department of Health and Human Services. Pub. 100–103 Medicare national coverage determination. Baltimore: Centers for Medicare and Medicaid Services; 2006.
7. Stoner MC, Abbott WM, Wong DR, Hua HT, Lamuraglia GM, Kwolek CJ, Watkins MT, Agnihotri AK, Henderson WG, Khuri S, Cambria RP. Defining the high-risk patient for carotid endarterectomy: an analysis of the prospective National Surgical Quality Improvement Program database. J Vasc Surg. 2006;43(2):285–95; discussion 295-6.
8. Fleisher LA, Beckman JA, Brown KA, Calkins H, Chaikof EL, Fleischmann KE, Freeman WK, Froehlich JB, Kasper EK, Kersten JR, Riegel B, Robb JF. 2009 ACCF/AHA focused update on perioperative beta blockade incorporated into the ACC/AHA 2007 guidelines on perioperative cardiovascular evaluation and care for noncardiac surgery: a report of the American college of cardiology foundation/American heart association task force on practice guidelines. Circulation. 2009;120(21):e169.
9. Misumida N, Kobayashi A, Saeed M, Fox JT, Kanei Y. Electrocardiographic left ventricular hypertrophy as a predictor for nonsignificant coronary artery disease in patients with non-ST-segment elevation myocardial infarction. Angiology. 2015 Mar 3.
10. International Stroke Trial Collaborative Group. The International Stroke Trial (IST): a randomised trial of aspirin, subcutaneous heparin, both, or neither among 19435 patients with acute ischaemic stroke. Lancet. 1997;349(9065):1569.
11. CAST (Chinese Acute Stroke Trial) Collaborative Group. CAST: randomised placebo-controlled trial of early aspirin use in 20,000 patients with acute ischaemic stroke. Lancet. 1997;349(9066):1641.
12. Leunissen TC, De Borst GJ, Janssen PW, ten Berg JM. The role of perioperative antiplatelet therapy and platelet reactivity testing in carotid revascularization: overview of the evidence. J Cardiovasc Surg (Torino). 2015;56(2):165–75 Epub 2015 Jan 20.
13. Corti R, Fayad ZA, Fuster V, Worthley SG, Helft G, Chesebro J, Mercuri M, Badimon JJ. Effects of lipid-lowering by simvastatin on human atherosclerotic lesions: a longitudinal study by high-resolution, noninvasive magnetic resonance imaging. Circulation. 2001;104(3):249.
14. Hart RG, Ng KH. Stroke prevention in asymptomatic carotid artery disease: revascularization of carotid stenosis is not the solution. Pol Arch Med Wewn. 2015;125(5):363–9 (Epub 17 Apr 2015).
15. In-hospital Stroke Alert Protocol: Pocket Card for Stroke Response Team Members. https://www.stroke.org/sites/default/files/homepage-slides/In-hospital-Stroke-Alert-Protocol-Card.pdf. Accessed 15 Jan 16.
16. Rerkasem K, Rothwell, PM. Carotid endarterectomy for symptomatic carotid stenosis. The Chorane Stroke Group, Apr 2011.
17. Grotta JC. Clinical practice. Carotid stenosis. N Engl J Med. 2013;369:1143.
18. Goodney PP, Likosky DS, Cronenwett JL. Vascular Study Group of Northern New England factors associated with stroke or death after carotid endarterectomy in Northern New England. J Vasc Surg. 2008;48(5):1139–45 (Epub 30 June 2008).
19. Bennett KM, Scarborough JE, Shortell CK. Predictors of 30-day postoperative stroke or death after carotid endarterectomy using the 2012 carotid endarterectomy-targeted American College of Surgeons National Surgical Quality Improvement Program database. J Vasc Surg. 2015;61(1):103–11 (Epub 24 Jul 2014).
20. La Monaca M, David A, Gaeta R, Lentini S. Near infrared spectroscopy for cerebral monitoring during cardiovascular surgery. Clin Ter. 2010;161(6):549–53.
21. Pennekamp CW, Bots ML, Kappelle LJ, Moll FL, de Borst GJ. The value of near-infrared spectroscopy measured cerebral oximetry during carotid endarterectomy in perioperative stroke prevention. A review. Eur J Vasc Endovasc Surg. 2009;38 (5):539–45.
22. Mccleary AJ, Maritati G, Gough MJ. Carotid endarterectomy; local or general anaesthesia? Eur J Vasc Endovasc Surg 2001;22:1e12.
23. Schneider JR, Novak KE. Carotid endarterectomy with routine electroencephalography and selective shunting. Semin Vasc Surg 2004;17:230–235.
24. Hans SS, Jareunpoon O. Prospective evaluation of electroencephalography, carotid artery stump pressure, and neurologic changes during 314 consecutive carotid endarterectomies performed in awake patients. J Vasc Surg. 2007;45:511–515.
25. Brott TG, Hobson RW II, Howard G, Roubin GS, Clark WM, Brooks W, Mackey A, Hill MD, Leimgruber PP, Sheffet AJ, Howard VJ, Moore WS, Voeks JH, Hopkins LN, Cutlip DE, Cohen DJ, Popma JJ, Ferguson RD, Cohen SN, Blackshear JL, Silver FL, Mohr JP, Lal BK, Meschia JF. CREST Investigators. Stenting versus endarterectomy for treatment of carotid-artery stenosis. N Engl J Med. 2010;363:11–23.
26. Guay J, Kopp S. Cerebral monitors versus regional anesthesia to detect cerebral ischemia in patients undergoing carotid endarterectomy: a meta-analysis. Can J Anaesth. 2013;60(3):266–79 (Epub 6 Feb 2013).
27. Qi DY, Wang K, Zhang H, Du BX, Xu FY, Wang L, Zou Z, Shi XY. Efficacy of intravenous lidocaine versus placebo on attenuating cardiovascular response to laryngoscopy and tracheal intubation: a systematic review of randomized controlled trials. Minerva Anestesiol. 2013;79(12):1423–35 (Epub 09 Jul 2013).
28. Stoneham MD, Warner O. Blood pressure manipulation during awake carotid surgery to reverse neurological deficit after carotid cross-clamping. Br J Anaesth. 2001;87:641–4.
29. Allain R, Marone LK, Meltzer J, Jeyabalan G. Carotid endarterectomy. Int Anesthesiol Clin. 2005;43(1):15.
30. Yastrebov K. Intraoperative management: carotid endarterectomies. Anesthesiol Clin North America. 2004;22(2):265–87, vi–vii.
31. Sundt TM Jr, Sharbrough FW, Anderson RE, Michenfelder JD. Cerebral blood flow measurements and electroencephalograms during carotid endarterectomy. J Neurosurg. 1974;41(3):310–20.
32. Spargo JR, Thomas D. Local anaesthesia for carotid endarterectomy. Cont Ed in Anaesth Crit Care Pain. 2004;4:62–5.
33. Miller RD. Anesthesia for vascular surgery (Chap. 69). In: Miller's anesthesia. 8th ed. New York: Elsevier/Churchill Livingstone, 2015. 2155. Print.
34. Barash PG, Cullen BF, Stoelting RK. Anesthesia for vascular surgery (Chap. 39). In: Clinical anesthesia. 7th ed. Philadelphia: Lippincott Williams & Wilkins, 2013. 1128. Print.
35. Thal GD et al. Exacerbation or unmasking of focal neurologic deficits by sedatives. *Anesthesiology* (1996); 85(1):21–5.
36. Lazar RM, Fitzsimmons BF, Marshall RS, Berman MF, Bustillo MA, Young WL, Mohr JP, Shah J, Robinson JV. Reemergence of stroke deficits with midazolam challenge. Stroke. 2002;33:283–5.
37. Engelter S, Lyrer P. Antiplatelet therapy for preventing stroke and other vascular events after carotid endarterectomy. Cochrane Database Syst Rev. 2003;3:CD001458.
38. Perler BA. Should statins be given routinely before carotid endarterectomy? Perspect Vasc Surg Endovasc Ther. 2007;19: 240–5.

39. Jabbour P. Extracranial atherosclerosis. Neurovascular surgical technique. 1st ed. New Delhi: Jaypee Brothers Medical, 2013. 259. Print.
40. Boulanger M, Camelière L, Felgueiras R, Berger L, Rerkasem K, Rothwell P, Touzé E. Periprocedural myocardial infarction after carotid endarterectomy and stenting systematic review and meta-analysis. Stroke. 2015;46.
41. Doberstein CE, Goldman MA, Grossberg JA, Spader HS. The safety and feasibility of outpatient carotid endarterectomy. Clin Neurol Neurosurg. 2012;114(2):108–11.

Spine Surgery and Intraoperative Monitoring 18

Fenghua Li and Reza Gorji

CASE

69-year-old man presents with pain in his neck, shoulders and arms, right-hand dexterity and difficulty walking. A MRI image of his cervical spine reveals multilevel degenerative changes and a high grade cervical stenosis with significant cord compression at C3–4. He is scheduled for a C3–7 posterior decompression with instrumented fusion from C3 to T2.

Medications:	Gabapentin	100 mg three times a day
	Tramadol	50 mg every 6 h if needed
	Hydrochlorothiazide	12.5 mg twice a day
	Metoprolol	25 mg once a day
	Losartan	50 mg once a day
	Pantoprazole	40 mg twice a day
	Crestor	10 mg twice a day
Allergies:	NKDA	
Past Medical History:		
Cardiac:	HTN, Hyperlipidemia	
Pulmonary:	Obstructive sleep apnea (OSA)	
GI:	Gastroesophageal reflux disease	
Other: Chronic Pain		

(continued)

Physical Exam:	
Vital signs:	BP 145/71, HR 56, RR 18, SpO2 95%, Weight 89.9 kg, Height 1.72 meters, BMI 30.4, obesity class 1
Airway:	Mallampati 3, limited neck extension and flexion due to pain
Neuromuscular:	Deltoid muscle weakness, positive hoffmann's bilaterally, spastic gait while walking, weakness of lower legs
EKG:	NSR, first-degree AV block, non-specific ST-T changes
Otherwise:	Insignificant

1. **Describe the anatomy of the spinal column and spinal cord**

The spinal column is comprised of 33 vertebrae: 7 cervical vertebrae, 12 thoracic vertebrae, 5 lumbar vertebrae, sacrum (5 fused vertebrae), and coccyx (4 fused vertebrae). Each vertebra, except C1, has a vertebral body, bilateral pedicles, bilateral lamina, bilateral transverse processes, a spinous process, and 4 articular processes. Vertebrae connect to each other via superior and inferior facets and inter-vertebrae disks. Two posterior lamina, two lateral pedicles and vertebra body anteriorly form the vertebral canal where the spinal cord lies. C1 (Atlas) lacks vertebrae body and consists of an anterior arch and tubercle, posterior arches, spinous process, and lateral masses. C2 (Axis) has a strong odontoid process that articulates with C1.

The spinal cord is a continuation of the medulla at the foramen magna and extends to the conus medullaris at the first or second lumbar vertebra in the vertebral canal in adults. On a cross-sectioned view, the cord is composed of gray matter and white matter. The gray matter resembles the shape of the letter H, surrounds the central canal, and contains cell bodies of neurons. It is divided into four main

F. Li (✉) · R. Gorji (✉)
Department of Anesthesiology, SUNY Upstate Medical University, 750 East Adams Street, Syracuse, NY 13210, USA
e-mail: LiF@upstate.edu

R. Gorji
e-mail: Gorjir@upstate.edu

© Springer International Publishing AG 2017
L.S. Aglio and R.D. Urman (eds.), *Anesthesiology*,
DOI 10.1007/978-3-319-50141-3_18

columns: the dorsal horn, intermediate horn, ventral horn, and lateral horn (see Fig. 18.1) [1]. The white matter contains myelinated and unmyelinated nerve fibers that carry information through the cord. The white matter is divided into the dorsal column (or funiculus), lateral column and ventral column. The cord has four regions (cervical, thoracic, lumbar and sacral) and two bulges at the cervical and lumbar region. The dorsal roots and ventral roots join together to form 31 pairs of spinal nerves that exit from spinal foramen. The spinal cord is surrounded with three meninges: pia, arachnoid, and dura.

2. **Which arteries supply blood to the spinal cord?**

The anterior spinal artery, two posterior spinal arteries, and radicular arteries are the main arteries that supply blood to the spinal cord. The vertebral arteries at the medulla level branch off to form the anterior spinal artery, which supplies the anterior two-thirds of the cord, while the posterior spinal arteries arising from either vertebral arteries or posterior inferior cerebellar arteries on the same side supply the posterior one-third. The radicular arteries that originate from the segmental arteries of aorta further augment the blood supply to spinal cord. The Artery of Adamkiewicz is the largest segmental feeder in the thoracolumbar region. Injury to those segmental arteries can cause anterior spinal cord ischemia, resulting in paralysis.

3. **How is blood flow to the spinal cord regulated?**

The spinal cord blood flow (SCBF) is autoregulated and kept relatively constant. Average SCBF is about 60 ml/100 g/min, but the blood flow to gray matter is four times higher than in white matter. SCBF is well maintained at the mean arterial blood pressure (MAP) between 60 and 120 mmHg [1]. Blood pressure that is lower than the autoregulation lower limit causes ischemia to the spinal cord. Hypoxia and hypercarbia increase SCBF, while hypocarbia reduces SCBF.

4. **What are the indications for spine surgery?**

Spine surgery is indicated for following conditions:

(1) Degenerative spine pathology resulting neurological dysfunction and pain, such as spondylosis, spondylotic myelopathy, spinal stenosis, spondylolithesis, and disk herniation;
(2) Spinal structure instability requiring stabilization, such as vertebra fracture due to trauma or other pathology;
(3) Infection of spine, such as spinal abscesses and tuberculosis;
(4) Spinal deformity, such as scoliosis;
(5) Spinal tumors, such as meningiomas and intraspinal cord tumors;
(6) Spinal hematoma that compresses the spinal cord or nerve roots;
(7) Inflammatory diseases, such as rheumatoid arthritis and ankylosing spondylitis.

5. **What is cervical spondylotic myelopathy?**

Cervical spondylotic myelopathy (CSM) is a syndrome produced by central spinal canal stenosis and compression of the spinal cord due to cervical spondylosis, a progressive degenerative process affecting the vertebral body and disk. CSM is the most common cause of myelopathy in older adults.

The common possible manifestations are summarized [2] as following:

(1) pain in the neck and subscapular or shoulder that radiates to the arms;

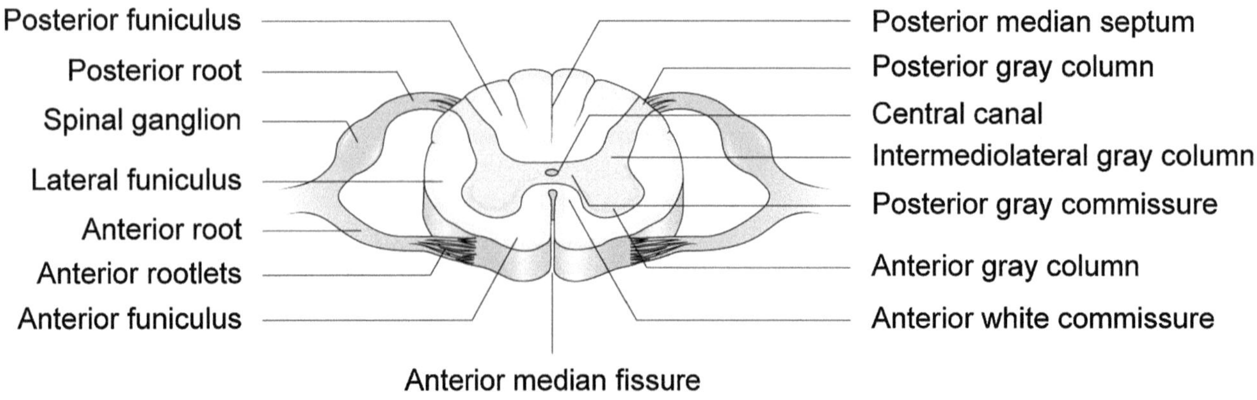

Fig. 18.1 Anatomy of spinal cord (cross-section view). Reproduced from Stier et al. [1, Figs. 20–15], with permission from Elsevier

(2) numbness, or paresthesia, in the arms;
(3) gait disturbance characterized by a spastic, scissoring quality;
(4) sensory deficits related to the dorsal column;
(5) weakness in the lower extremities with upper motor neuron characteristics (increased reflexes and muscle tone, and the presence of the Babinski sign);
(6) lower motor neuron findings (weakness in the arms and hands);
(7) bladder dysfunction;
(8) Lhermitte's sign; an electric shock-like sensation in the neck that radiates down to the spine and arms, produced by forward flexion of the neck.

Magnetic Resonance Imaging is used to confirm the diagnosis. The Nurick grading system [3] classifies the severity of CSM from the least severe, grade 1, to the most severe, grade 5 based on gait abnormality (see Table 18.1).

6. **What is central cord syndrome?**

Central Cord Syndrome (CCS) is the most common incomplete spinal cord injury and is characterized by a disproportionately greater motor impairment in the upper extremities than in lower extremities, bladder dysfunction, and various sensory losses below the level of injury. The mechanism involves the compression of the cord by osteophytes and infolded ligamentum flavum. Patients with CSM can suffer CCS after minor neck injury without evidence of spinal fracture. Hyperextension of neck should be avoided during direct laryngoscope in patients with CSM to prevent neurological damage.

7. **What is the anterior cord syndrome? What is the Brown-Sequard syndrome?**

Anterior cord syndrome (ACS) results from injury to the anterior spinal artery or compression of the anterior cord. It is characterized by variable motor impairment, pain, and temperature sensation impairment with preservation of proprioception below the level of injury.

Brown-Sequard syndrome an incomplete spinal cord injury and results from hemisection of spinal cord. It is manifested as ipsilateral loss of motor and proprioception with contralateral loss of pain and temperature sensation. It usually occurs after penetrating trauma.

8. **What is spinal shock?**

Spinal shock is a neurogenic shock caused by an interruption of sympathetic output from the spinal cord and unopposed parasympathetic activity after acute spinal cord injury (SCI). The severity of spinal shock is related to the severity and completeness of SCI. Loss of sympathetic activity below the level of injury results vasodilation and decrease in venous return, leading to hypotension. Bradycardia can occur if the SCI is above T6 level. Treatment includes fluid therapy and the use of vasopressors to support blood pressure in order to maintain MAP > 85 mmHg for the first week following the initial injury.

9. **What is the American Spinal Injury Association (ASIA) impairment scale?**

The ASIA impairment scale is used to define the severity of a spinal cord injury. It combines the sensory and motor deficits with completeness of the injury to classify the injury into five grades from Grade A to grade E. The ASIA impairment scale evaluates and scores 10 key muscle groups and 28 dermatomes for both light touch and pin prick.

Grade A: Complete injury; no motor or sensory function is preserved in sacral segments S4-S5.
Grade B: Sensory incomplete injury; sensation is preserved without motor function below the neurological level, and includes S4-S5.
Grade C: Motor incomplete injury; motor function is preserved below the neurological level, and more than half of the key muscle functions below the neurological level of injury have a muscle grade <3.
Grade D: Motor function is preserved below the neurological level; more than half of the key muscle functions below the neurological level of injury have a muscle grade ≥ 3.
Grade E: Normal.

Table 18.1 Nurick classification of cervical myelopathy based on gait abnormality

Grade	Gait abnormality
1	Spinal cord disease with no problem working
2	Slight difficulty walking and cannot work full time
3	Difficulty walking and cannot work full time
4	Can only walk with help of frame walker
5	Chair-bound or bedridden

Modified from Abd-Elsayed and Farag [9, Table 9]

10. **What is the new neurological deficit (NND) rate for spinal surgery?**

Spinal surgery poses potential risks to the spinal cord, nerve roots, caudal equina, and peripheral nerves. Although the overall incidence of NND is small, the consequence of neurological complications, such as spinal cord paralysis, could be disastrous for both patient and family. Revision surgery, spinal fusion, use of implants, and surgical approach may affect the rate of NND. The most recent data from the Scoliosis Research Society shows that the overall rates of new nerve roots, cauda equina, and spinal cord deficits for 108,419 patients were 0.61, 0.07, and 0.27% [4].

11. **What is the mortality rate of spine surgery?**

The mortality of spinal surgery is low and varies depending on the location of the procedure. Lumbar spine (range from 0.07 to 0.52%) and cervical spine surgery (range from 0.1 to 0.8%) carry lower mortality compared to thoracic spine surgery (range from 0.3 to 7.4%) [5]. Recent studies from the Scoliosis Research Society Morbidity and Mortality database showed that the overall mortality rate is 1.8–1.9 per 1000 spinal deformity procedures [6, 7]. However, mortality increases in patients over 60 years of age. High ASA scores, fusion and implants are associated with an increased mortality rate. The main causes are respiratory (respiratory failure, pneumonia, pulmonary embolism, etc.), cardiac (cardiac failure, myocardial infarction, or cardiac arrest), sepsis, multi-system organ failure, stroke, and blood loss. Although mortality due to intraoperative blood loss accounted for 4% of all mortality, it can be prevented if careful planning and intraoperative management are implemented.

12. **What are the goals of intraoperative neuromonitoring (IONM) during spine surgery?**

There are three goals of IONM during spine surgery. The principle goal of IONM is to prevent injury to the spinal cord and nerve roots by way of surgical manipulation and instrumentation. Secondly, IONM is used to prevent ischemia due to hypoperfusion to the spinal cord. The third goal is to prevent peripheral nerve injury by way of inappropriate positioning.

13. **What is the somatosensory-evoked potential (SSEP)? How does SSEP monitoring prevent spinal cord injury during spinal surgery?**

SSEPs are electric responses from peripheral nerve stimulations. It was introduced in the 1980s and is indicated for monitoring spinal cord integrity in scoliosis correction, spinal cord tumor, spinal decompression, and instrumentation surgeries. SSEPs can be recorded along sensory pathways. Cortical SSEPs are recorded from the electrodes placed on scalp according to the international 10–20 system. The most common peripheral stimulating sites are the ulnar or medium nerve for upper extremity SSEPs, and the posterior tibia nerve or common peroneal nerve for lower extremity SSEPs. SSEPs voltage is very small compared to EKG and EEG; it requires averages to obtain high quality waveforms for monitoring by reducing 60 Hz interferences. SSEP is characterized as amplitude and latency that are affected by many factors. SSEP waveforms P14 and N20 from upper extremity and N34 and P37 from lower extremity are commonly used for monitoring. The baseline SSEPs must be obtained before the surgical incision.

SSEPs are primarily mediated by the dorsal column-medial lemniscal system. The anatomy of this sensory pathway includes peripheral nerves, first-order neurons in the dorsal ganglion, second-order neurons with nucleus gracilis and cuneatus, third-order neurons in the thalamus, and sensory cortex. Peripheral nerves enter the dorsal root ganglion where primary sensory neurons receive sensory input. The central axons of sensory neurons ascend ipsilaterally within the fasciculus gracilis and fasciculus cuneatus to the caudal medulla where the neuron fibers synapse with second-order neurons within the nucleus cuneatus and nucleus gracilis. The axons of second-order neurons decussate and ascend as medial lemniscus to third-order neurons in the ventral posterior lateral nucleus of the thalamus. The third-order neurons in the thalamus project axons to the primary somatosensory cortex in the contralateral posterior gyrus. When the peripheral nerves are stimulated, action potentials propagate along the pathway and generate the SSEPs that can be recorded. Any disruption to the sensory pathway can lead to loss of SSEP production. Surgical manipulation and instrumentation during spinal surgery could result in spinal cord and nerve root injury. SSEP monitoring will alert both the surgeons and anesthesiologists for any impending spinal cord injury, thus allowing surgeons to correct reversible causes in time, while the anesthesiologists affirm physiological and anesthesia stability.

14. **What are the anesthetic effects on SSEP recording?**

Anesthetics affect cortical SSEPs but have minimal effect on subcortical SSEPs. The deeper the anesthesia is, the more SSEPs are suppressed. It is very important to keep anesthetic level steady state while SSEP's are recorded.

(1) Halogenated inhalational anesthetics such as isoflurane, sevoflurane and desflurane depress the amplitude of

SSEP's and prolong latency of SSEPs in dose dependent fashion. Those agents affect cortical SSEPs more than subcortical SSEP's because more synapses are involved in generating cortical SSEPs. In our practice, we use less than 1 MAC of inhalational agent, and the recordings of SSEPs are usually adequate for monitoring.

(2) Nitrous oxide (N_2O) produces an increase in SSEP's latency and decrease in amplitude of SSEPs. It affects cortical SSEPs more than other halogenated agents at equal potency. N_2O use should be avoided if the cortical SSEPs are desired for monitoring.

(3) Intravenous (IV) anesthetics have less effect on cortical SSEPs. In general, IV anesthetics prolong SSEP latency; all IV anesthetics, except etomidate and ketamine, decrease SSEP amplitude. Both etomidate and ketamine increase SSEP amplitude.

(4) Muscle relaxants have no effect on SSEPs. Nevertheless, paralysis improves the quality of SSEPs recordings.

15. **What are the systemic factors, other than anesthesia, that affect SSEP monitoring?**

A patient's blood pressure, temperature, hypoxia, and anemia can significantly affect SSEPs.

(1) Hypotension causes reduced blood flow to the brain, spinal cord and peripheral nerves. When blood pressure drops to below threshold, blood supply to neural structures is compromised. For example, when cerebral blood flow is less than 18 ml/100 gm/min, cortical SSEPs start to change. It is important to maintain the patient's blood pressure in line with the patient's baseline reading. The SSEPs recording is usually not affected if mean arterial pressure is kept above 80 mmHg.

(2) Hypothermia reduces nerve conduction velocity and prolongs SSEPs latency. When temperature drops below 22 °C, the SSEPs' signals begin to disappear [8]. Subcortical SSEPs are resistant to hypothermia.

(3) Hypoxia causes SSEP changes and SSEPs finally disappears.

(4) Severe anemia of hematocrit less than 15% decreases the amplitude, but can return to baseline if anemia is resolved [9].

16. **What alarm criteria are used during SSEP monitoring?**

Significant changes in SSEP responses should provide alarming to surgeons, anesthesiologists, and monitoring neurologists. A 10% increase in latency and a 50% reduction in amplitude of SSEPs from the baseline are considered to be alarming criteria. The changes in SSEP should be interpreted within clinical context; systemic contributing factors and technique problems resulting SSEP changes need to be excluded.

17. **In additional to spinal surgery, in what other clinical condition is SSEP monitoring indicated?**

There are other clinical conditions that may require SSEP monitoring.

(1) SSEPs monitoring of brain ischemia is used in cerebrovascular surgeries for aneurysm clipping, AVM resection, and carotid endarterectomy.

(2) It is used for thoracic aorta aneurysm resection to monitor spinal cord ischemia.

(3) SSEPs can be used for cortical mapping during tumor resection.

18. **What are the disadvantages of SSEP monitoring?**

SSEPs monitor the integrity of the sensory pathway from peripheral nerves to the primary sensory cortex.

(1) Injury to the motor pathway, including anterior spinal cord, cannot be detected by SSEP monitoring.

(2) Anesthesia and physiological factors affect its recording and interpretation.

19. **What are motor evoked potentials (MEPs)? Which neural structures are monitored by MEPs? Why is MEP monitoring required during spinal surgery?**

MEPs are electric responses to motor cortical stimulation. The stimulation is either transcranial or direct cortical via electric or magnetic stimulation. Transcranial electric stimulation (TES) over the motor cortex is the most common method. MEPs are recorded along the motor pathway at either the epidural site (D-wave) or at the muscle site as compound muscle action potentials (CMAPs). Muscle MEPs do not require the use of averages and are used for spinal surgery. Transcranial MEPs (TcMEPs) are recorded from the thenar, hypothenar and extensor carpi radialis muscles in the upper arms, and tibialis anterior and aductor halluces muscles in lower extremities, as well as other muscle groups.

MEPs monitor the integrity of the motor pathway, consisting of upper motor neuron system (UMN), lower motor neuron systems (LMN), and peripheral muscle group. After cortical stimulation, action potentials propagate along the corticospinal tract to the spinal cord and activate the anterior horn neurons. The signals then travel along the peripheral nerves and stimulate the muscle fibers to contraction.

The corticospinal tract is located in the dorsolateral funiculus and is supplied by the anterior spinal artery. SSEPs only monitor the sensory pathway that is located in the dorsal column. Since SSEPs do not detect spinal cord injury from the motor pathway due to surgical manipulation or ischemia, MEPs monitoring is necessary to detect potential motor pathway injury and prevent motor deficits.

20. **What are the anesthetic effects on MEPs?**

MEPs are depressed by anesthetics.

(1) Halogenated inhalational agents and N_2O can inhibit MEP responses at different sites that involve synapse transmission, especially at the level of the cerebral cortex and anterior horn cells. All inhalational anesthetics need to be avoided if MEPs are recorded. However, the MEP is recordable if less than 0.5 MAC of desflurane is used, as was shown in a recent study [10].
(2) Intravenous anesthetics such as propofol, barbiturates, dexmedetomidine, and benzodiazepines affect MEPs to a lesser extent. They can increase latency and decrease amplitude of MEPs. However, MEPs recording is optimal during total intravenous anesthesia (TIVA). Opioids, etomidate, and ketamine do not significantly affect MEPs recoding.
(3) Muscle relaxants use inhibits or eliminates CMAP, thus make MEP recording impossible.

In summary, TIVA with propofol and opioid infusion is recommended if MEPs are recorded, while inhalational anesthesia is suboptimal for MEP recording.

21. **What other factors affect MEPs recording during spine surgery?**

Blood pressure and temperature can affect MEP recordings. Blood flow to brain and spinal cord is autoregulated to keep constant CBF. When mean blood pressure (MAP) falls to the lower limits of autoregulation (LLA), spinal cord ischemia can occur. Comorbidity such as chronic hypertension and diabetes mellitus can change autoregulation mechanisms; cord perfusion may be affected by blood pressure more directly, making it more sensitive to change. Hypotension can cause generalized MEP deterioration or loss. Thus, it is important to keep a blood pressure at the patient's baseline during MEP recording. Moderate hypothermia to 31 °C significantly reduces MEP amplitude, while deep hypothermia renders MEP recordings impossible [11].

22. **What muscle MEP changes warn of a pending spinal cord injury?**

A marked amplitude reduction or acute threshold elevation more than 100 mV or loss of MEPs is a warning sign for spinal cord injury [11]. However, interpretation of muscle MEPs needs consideration from stimulus techniques and physiological effects.

23. **What are the complications and contraindications of MEP recordings?**

MEP recording is invasive and has complications if inappropriate use occurs. These complications include hazardous outputs resulting in excitotoxic injury, electrochemical injury, thermal injury to brain and scalp, bite injuries, seizures, movement-induced injury, and arrhythmia. Needle-stick injury occurs at a rate 0.34% [12] in OR staff, especially with anesthesiologists, if subdermal needle electrodes are used; so, non-needle electrode use is advocated.

Relative contraindications of TES for MEPs include seizure disorders, skull defect, cortical lesions, increased intracranial pressure, intracranial apparatus (vascular clips, shunt or electrodes), and cardiac pacemaker.

24. **What is the role of electromyography (EMG) during spinal surgery?**

Needle electrodes inserted at the motor point of the muscle monitor activation. Since MEP only activates 3.1–3.9% of lower motor units [13], the MEP does not represent the whole segmental nerve roots motor function. EMG is often used to monitor at risk nerve roots and peripheral nerves during spinal surgery.

There two types of intraoperative EMG monitoring: free-run or spontaneous EMG (EMG) and triggered EMG (tEMG). EMG is more sensitive to retraction, irrigation, and manipulation during surgery. However, EMG is not indicative of nerve root injury. EMG also provides instantaneous feedback for the surgical team. tEMG monitoring is used in the pedicle screw placement and direct nerve root stimulation using a hand held stimulator to determine if the pedicle screws have breached the pedicle wall or are in closer proximity, and thus posing a risk of injury to the existing nerve roots.

Factors affecting EMG recording include anesthesia and electrical interferences:

(1) Anesthesia effect: Muscle relaxants use may abolish the EMG activity, so deep paralysis during the EMG recording should be avoided and train of four should indicate at least of 3 out of 4 twitches for EMG to be of value;

(2) Electrical interference: Electrical interference prevents EMG recording during cauterization.

Alarm criteria [13] during EMG monitoring:

Normal EMG response is absent of activity. Relevant activities include spikes, bursts or trains. Spikes and bursts do not often represent neural insults, but significant activity patterns may indicate impending nerve injury.

This activity can be characterized as:

(1) Phasic or a burst pattern consisting of a single or nonrepetitive asynchronous potentials which are often complex and polyphasic in configuration, (2) Tonic or train activity consisting of periods of prolonged or repetitive synchronously grouped motor units discharge that last up to several minutes, and (3) The alarm threshold for tEMG varies. In general, pedicle screw placements associated with a stimulation threshold greater than 10 mA suggest the pedicle wall is intact. Direct nerve not stimulation will have an average threshold of 2.2 mA.

25. **Which IONM modalities should be chosen for spine surgery?**

The choice of monitoring techniques depends on multiple factors. First, the location of neural structure at risk is the most important consideration (Fig. 18.2). For cervical and thoracic spine surgeries, the spinal cord and nerve roots are at risk, so the combination of SSEP, MEP, and EMG monitoring is recommended. Since the spinal cord ends at L1, nerve roots are at risk of injury during lumbar sacral spinal surgery; SSEP and EMG are the most sufficient monitoring techniques.

Second, sensitivity and specificity of modality need careful consideration in choosing the monitoring technique. MEP is very sensitive and specific in detecting impending neurologic injury. SSEP monitoring for scoliosis surgery has 92% sensitivity and 98% specificity for detecting new neurological deficits [14], but some studies showed SSEPs had poor sensitivity in detecting neurological injury. In general, multimodality IONM is sensitive and specific in detecting intraoperative neurological injury during spine surgery, and it is recommended to use multimodality IONM when the spinal cord or nerve roots are at risk.

Third, the choice of IONM modality also depends on the availability of anesthetic technique. MEPs and cortical SSEP are very sensitive to anesthetics, especially when inhalational anesthetics are used; however, subcortical SSEP and EMG are relatively insensitive to general anesthesia. Muscle relaxants use deteriorates conditions for MEP and EMG recording. Anesthesiologists need to keep close communication with the IONM technologist and surgeon to choose an appropriate anesthesia technique that optimizes the acquisition IONM signals.

Fourth, availability of qualified IONM technologists is an absolute requirement. A surgeon's preferences and understanding of the IONM techniques plays a great role in the choice of monitoring modalities as well.

26. **Why is multimodality IONM used in spine surgery?**

The goal of IONM in spine surgery is to preserve neural function. Since SSEP, MEP, and EMG have their own strengths and disadvantages, a combination of the three modalities provides global assessment of functional integrity of the nervous system from the cortex to the spinal cord, nerve roots, and peripheral nerves. Multimodality IONM improves patient outcome in complex spine surgery. Use of SSEP and MEP monitoring has more than 90% sensitivity and specificity in detecting spinal cord injury and has become the standard care in scoliosis patients undergoing corrective surgery.

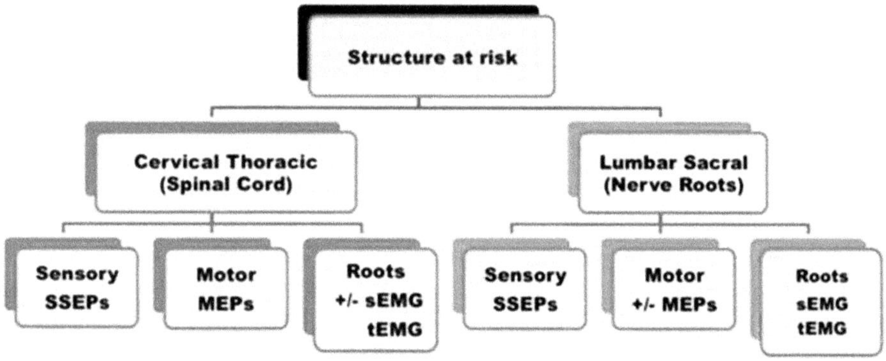

Fig. 18.2 Choices of IONM in spine surgery based on structure at risk. *SSEPs* Somatosensory-evoked potentials; *MEPs* motor evoked potentials; *sEMG* spontaneous electromyography; *tEMG* trigged electromyography. Adopted from Gonzalez et al. [25], with permission from the American Association of Neurological Surgeons

27. **What are your preoperative concerns for major spine surgery?**

Major spine surgery involves multiple spine levels and carries higher mortality and morbidity [15]. Careful pre-anesthesia evaluations should be done according to the American Society of Anesthesiologists (ASA) guideline [16] and a multidisciplinary approach is needed to optimize patients undergoing a major spine surgery.

First, a patient's comorbidities should be assessed and be optimized. The patient for major spine surgery often has many comorbidities including HTN, smoking, obesity, diabetes mellitus, renal disease and coagulation abnormality. Comorbidities increase a patient's risk in major spine surgery. Care from other specialists needs to be coordinated to ensure patient readiness.

Second, patients with a history of coagulation problems, such as a bleeding disorder, need a consultation by a hematologist; patients need to have type and crossed blood available.

Third, communication between the operative surgeon and anesthesiologist is essential. The discussion needs to include length of the procedure, expected blood loss, strategies for blood loss reduction, use of intraoperative neuromonitoring (IONM), postoperative patient care, possible staging the procedure, etc.

Fourth, screening for contraindications for intraoperative neuromonitoring should be done preoperatively. The need for an intraoperative wake-up test should be discussed with patients who are going to have major spinal surgery.

Lastly, a neurological exam related to spine disease needs to be done to document any preexisting neurological deficits.

28. **What preoperative laboratory tests would you like to order?**

The preoperative studies are dictated by findings of a patient's history and physical exams. The cardiac study should follow the 2014 AHA/ACC guideline on perioperative cardiovascular evaluation and management of patients undergoing non-cardiac surgery. Basic metabolic panels, hemoglobin/hematocrit, and coagulation panel including PT/PTT/INR, type and cross-match of blood need to be done for major spine surgery.

29. **How do you manage the airway in patients with cervical spine disease?**

The ASA difficulty airway algorithm serves as the guideline in patients with cervical spine pathology. However, preventing spinal cord injury is a paramount task in airway management for cervical spine surgical patients. Careful airway evaluation needs to determine management plans. In addition to the recommended airway exams, cervical spine stability and risk of cord injury should be considered. Raw et al. [17] defines the C-spine instability as following: (1) below C2: all anterior or posterior elements are destroyed; or there is >3.5 mm horizontal displacement of one vertebra to adjacent one on a lateral X-ray, or there is more than 11° of rotation one vertebra to adjacent one. (2) above C2: disruption of the transverse ligament of the atlas; a Jefferson burst fracture of the atlas following axial loading, which causes atlantoaxial instability; a disruption of the tectorial and alar ligaments and some occipital condylar fractures also cause atlanto-occipital instability. In patients with rheumatoid arthritis, cervical inflammatory changes result in atlantoaxial subluxation and basilar invagination.

The technique that has the least effect on cervical spine movement should be applied to avoid spinal cord compression. Studies have compared different types of airway management devices, including the video-assisted laryngeal scope. Among current techniques available, fiberoptic intubation produces the least amount of movement to the cervical spine. In patients with unstable cervical spines, such as cervical spine fracture or dislocation, awake fiberoptic intubation is required if the patient is cooperative. If awake intubation is not possible, manual in-line stabilization (MILS) is mandatory and should be applied in those patients. Awake intubation is also needed if a neurologic examination needs to be done after intubation, or use of a laryngoscope is impossible.

Central cord syndrome can occur in patients with CSM after minor injury without evidence of fracture. Avoiding hyperextension during direct laryngoscope is important to prevent cord injury.

30. **What positions are used during spine surgery?**

The position chosen for spine surgery is dependent on the location of involved spine segments and surgical approaches. Prone position is commonly used for spine surgery. Supine position with upper extremities tucked on sides is used for anterior approach surgery, such as anterior cervical decompression and fusion. Lateral decubitus is occasionally applied for spine surgery for anterior approach to thoracic and lumbar spine. Double-lumen endotracheal intubation is required for anterior thoracic spine surgery.

31. **What are physiological effects of prone position?**

The Prone position is used in posterior spine surgery and poses a huge challenge to anesthesiologists. Cardiovascular responses in prone position are reduced venous return to the heart (due to increased abdominal pressure and pooling of venous blood in the lower extremities), and increased systemic and pulmonary vascular resistance. The left ventricular ejection and cardiac index may decrease in prone position. Thus, hemodynamic instability can occur when turning patient prone from supine position. CVP is not accurate to monitor fluid status in prone position.

Respiratory effects in the prone position include restriction of the diaphragm by abdominal contents and weight against thorax, increased peak airway pressure and airway edema. Oxygenation, however, may improve with prone positioning due to improved ventilation and perfusion match. The effects of prone position on cardiovascular responses and respiratory mechanics are frame-dependent. The Jackson table provides the most stable hemodynamics and lung compliance does not increase because of abdomen freedom.

Other risks are pressure sores, blindness, air embolism (cervical spine surgery), difficulty securing endotracheal tube, and peripheral nerve injuries including brachial plexus and lateral femoral cutaneous nerve.

32. **What monitors will you choose to use in major spine surgery?**

ASA standard monitors should be applied to spine surgical patients. An arterial line pressure monitor is indicated if spinal cord perfusion pressure monitoring is desired, especially spinal cord compression or significant hemodynamic fluctuation due to blood loss is expected. Arterial pulse pressure (PPV) monitoring is indicated if goal directed fluid therapy is intended to avoid fluid overload during major spine surgery. Central venous access is required in patients without adequate peripheral intravenous access or expected significant blood loss.

33. **What anesthetic technique do you choose for this patient with IONM?**

It depends on the IONM modality chosen for monitoring. Since total intravenous anesthesia (TIVA) best facilitates cortical SSEP and MEP recordings, TIVA consisting of propofol and remifentanil, or fentanyl infusion is a common choice to maintain anesthesia during spine surgery with SSPP and MEP monitoring. If SSEP and EMG are used for monitoring, inhalational anesthetics up to 1 MAC may be used for maintenance of anesthesia. Dexmedetomidine has a minimal effect on both SSEPs and MEPs and is sometime added into the anesthesia regime to reduce total amount of propofol use.

34. **Will you use bispectral index (BIS) monitoring?**

BIS is a processed EEG device and measures the hypnosis of hypnotic drug effect that reflects anesthesia depth. BIS values range from 0 to 100. A BIS value of 100 indicates a full awake state, while a BIS 0 value indicates no brain activity. BIS 40–60 corresponds to an anesthesia state and prevents intraoperative awareness during propofol infusion. BIS guided titration of anesthesia reduces drug overdose and facilitates earlier emergence during TIVA.

35. **What are your considerations in reducing allogeneic blood transfusion (ALBT)?**

Significant blood loss can occur in major spine surgery that involves decompression, osteotomy and fusion. A high Elixhuser comorbidity score, thoracolumba fusion, and number of fusion levels are strong predictors of ALBT in spinal fusion in Unites States [18].

The methods currently used in decreasing blood transfusion in spine surgery are:

(1) Perioperative use of antifibrinolytics, such as epsilon-aminocaproic acid (EACA) and tranexamic acid (TXA). EACA 100 mg/kg loading dose followed by 10 mg/kg/hr infusion is recommended; TXA is used with a loading dose of 10 mg/kg followed by infusion of 1 mg/kg/hr till the end of case
(2) recombinant factor VII
(3) cell saver use
(4) hemodilution and preoperative autologous donation
(5) preoperative use of erythropoietin

Intraoperative application of antifibrinolytics and cell saver are common strategies in reducing blood loss and transfusion in our institution. Both EACA and TXA are equally effective.

Increased abdominal pressure is associated with increased blood loss. Positioning the patient with the abdomen free is important to reduce intraoperative blood loss.

36. **What are your considerations in fluid management during spine surgery in the prone position?**

Intraoperative fluid management is essential and can affect patient outcome when major spine surgery is done in the prone position. Cardiac index decreases in the prone position due to reduced venous return and left ventricle compliance. CVP is not accurate in the prone position; however, the ability of pulse pressure variation (PPV), a predictor of fluid responsiveness, is not affected by prone position [19]. PPV is useful in monitoring fluid status.

Crystalloids are used for fluid maintenance, with Lactate Ringer's being the preferred. Large quantities of normal saline should be avoided due to the risk of hyperchloremic metabolic acidosis. Colloids are generally used for the replacement of blood loss; Albumin is preferred to hydroxyethyl starch in major spine surgery.

Among the strategies of fluid therapy, goal direct fluid therapy is probably the best method to maintain proper intravascular volume without fluid overload. Fluid overload in major spine surgery in prone position is a major problem resulting in increased facial edema, delayed postoperative extubation, and increased length of hospital stay.

37. **After 30 min into surgery, left upper extremity SSEP amplitude reduction is detected. What should you do now?**

SSEP can detect peripheral nerve injuries secondary to inappropriate positioning. At early exposure during the surgery, changes in SSEPs should not result from spinal cord injury due to surgical manipulation; once the technical problems are excluded, the upper extremities and shoulder position need to be inspected to ensure there is no compression on the brachial plexus.

38. **The loss of MEPs is noticed immediately after rod tightening followed by decrease in SSEP amplitude. What is your management now?**

After confirming that there are no technical problems, the anesthesiologist needs to check the anesthesia level, blood pressure and temperature to rule out causes by anesthesia and physiologic events. The mean arterial blood pressure needs to be raised to more than 80 mmHg, or near 120% of the patient's baseline levels (awake). The correlation of change to surgical location and manipulation time should be validated. The surgeon has to inspect the surgical sites for possible compressing forces, instrumental positioning, implant positioning and examine the structure alignment with the X-ray. Repositioning the implant, reduction in correction force needs to be done by the surgeon if technical and physiological factors are excluded out. If the IONM alarm continues after loosening the rods, which may take several minutes to recovery, cessation of the procedure and a wake-up test should be considered to confirm the changes. Patient needs to follow verbal command to move extremities during the wake-up test.

39. **What is your plan for extubation after 7 h of surgery?**

ETT extubation should be very cautious and needs to follow the ASA difficulty airway algorithm after long duration of spinal surgery in prone position. Preoperative airway exams, intubation grade view, airway/facial edema after prone position, and effect of surgical instrumentation on c-spine motion should be considered before extubation. If facial, lip, and tongue edema are visible, a leak test may help determine the severity of trachea edema and swelling. If there is no leak around ETT after deflation of the balloon, the patient should not be extubated until airway edema recedes. The leak test has low predictive value; however, the positive air leak around of the ETT does not insure the safe extubation.

40. **What is postoperative vision loss (POVL)? What can be done to prevent it?**

POVL is a rare but devastating complication associated with spine surgery in the prone position. The incidence of POVL is about 3.09–9.4 per 10,000 in spine surgical patients [20, 21]. The main cause of POVL is ischemic optic neuropathy (ION), and other causes include central retinal artery occlusion and cortical blindness.

Decreased optic nerve perfusion due to increased interstitial fluid accumulation and venous outflow reduction in the globe may be the mechanism of ION. A POVL study group in 2012 has identified risk factors [22] that contribute to POVL in spinal surgery patients: male sex, obesity, use of Wilson frame, longer anesthesia time, greater estimated blood loss, and colloid usage as a percentage of non-blood replacement are risk factors. Anemia and hypotension were not confirmed to be risk factors of POVL in this study.

To enhance the awareness and to reduce frequency of POVL associated with spine surgery, the American Society of Anesthesiologists (ASA) published the Practice Advisory on POVL in 2006 that has been updated in 2012 [23]. Patients who undergo spine surgery while in the prone position, and those who have long procedures and experience substantial blood losses, are at high risk. High-risk patients should be identified preoperatively and POVL risk should be discussed with these patients. Intraoperatively, the patient's head should be positioned at or above the level of the heart whenever possible, and be maintained in neutral position. Direct compression of globes is avoided. Hypotension and severe anemia (HCT <28) should be avoided.

Staging procedures may be considered in patients who have experienced significant blood loss. Colloids, along with crystalloids, are recommended for fluid resuscitation. Postoperatively and in cases of high-risk patients, the anesthesiologists should check the patient's vision. An urgent ophthalmology consult should be obtained if vision concerns present while patient is being optimized. Consider MRI and CT of head to rule out any intracranial causes.

41. **How do you manage postoperative pain after major spine surgery?**

Postoperative pain management after spine surgery begins with the preoperative evaluation. Pain treatment history, analgesics (especially narcotic use) and antidepressants need a detailed review and documentation. If the patient has a history of chronic pain and narcotic use, a pain consult should be obtained for intraoperative and postoperative pain management. Multimodality pain management is recommended for patients undergoing spine surgery. Preemptive analgesia, such as preoperative gabapentin use, and local anesthetic infiltration prior to incision reduce postoperative pain. Intraoperatively, propofol anesthesia produces less postoperative pain compared to sevoflurane [24]. Use of an NMDA receptor such as ketamine has an opioid sparing effect. Postoperatively, intravenous opioids are still the main medication for postoperative pain management. Intrathecal morphine at the end of the case if feasible is safe and effective analgesic method. Non-opioids including NSAIDs, acetaminophen, antidepressants, etc., can be used to supplement pain control.

References

1. Stier GR, Gabriel CL, Cole DJ. Neurosurgical disease and trauma of the spine and spinal cord: anesthetic consideration. In: Cottrell and young's neuroanesthesia. 5th ed. PA: Mosby; 2010.
2. Levin K. Cervical spondylotic myeopathy. In: Waltham MA, editor. Uptodate, Post TW. Access 18 May 2015.
3. Abd-Elsayed AA, Farag E. Anesthesia for cervical spine surgery. In: Farag E editor. Anesthesia for spine surgery. Cambridge: Cambridge University Press; 2012.
4. Hamilton DK, Smoth JS, Sansur. Rate of new neurological deficit associated with spine surgery based on 108,419 procedures: a report of the scoliosis research society mortality and morbidity committee. Spine. 2011;36:1218–28.
5. Dekutoski MB, Norvell DC, Dettori JR. Surgeon perception and reported complications in Spine surgery. Spine. 2010;35(9 Suppl): S9–21.
6. Smith JS, Saulle D, Chen CJ. Rate and causes of mortality associated with spine surgery based on 108419 procedures: a review of the scoliosis research society morbidity and mortality. Spine. 2012;37:1975–82.
7. Divecha HM, Siddique I, Breakwell LM, et al. Complications in spinal deformity surgery in the United Kingdom: 5-year results of the annual British scoliosis society national audit of morbidity and mortality. Eur Spine J. 2014;23(suppl 1):S55–60.
8. Stecker MM, Cheung AT, Pochettina A, et al. Deep hypothermic circulatory arrest: I. Effect of cooling on electroencephalography and evoked potentials. Ann Thorac Surg. 2001;71(1):22–8.
9. Banoub M, Tetzlaff JE, Schubet A. Pharmacologic and physiologic influences affecting sensory evoked potentials: implication of perioperative monitoring. Anesthesiology. 2003;99(3):716–37.
10. Chong CT, Manninen P, Sivanaser V, et al. Direct comparison of the effect of desflurane and sevoflurane on intraoperative moto-evoked potential monitoring. J Neurosurg Anesthesiol. 2014;26(4):306–12.
11. MacDonald DB, Skinner S, Shils J, et al. Intraoperative motor evoked potential monitoring—a position statement by the American Society if neurophysiological monitoring. J Clin Neurophysiol. 2013;124:2291–316.
12. Tamjus A, Rice K. Risk of needle-stick injuries associated with the use of subdermal electrodes during intraoperative neurophysiological monitoring. J Neurosurg Anesthesiol. 2014;2691:65–8.
13. Leppanen RE. Intraoperative monitoring of segmental spinal nerve root function with free-run and function and electrically-triggered electromyography and spinal cord function with reflexes and F-responses. J Clin Monit Comput. 2005;19(6):437–61.
14. Nuwer MR, Dawson EG, Carlson LC, et al. Somatosensory evoked potential spinal cord monitoring reduces neurologic deficits after scoliosis surgery: results of a large multicenter survey. Electroencephlogr Clin Neurophysiol. 1995;96:6–11.
15. Street JT, Lenhan BJ, Dipaola CP, et al. Morbidity and mortality of major adult spinal surgery. A prospective cohort analysis of 942 consecutive patients. Spine J. 2012;12:22–34.
16. ASA Committee on Standards and Practice Parameters. Practice advisory for preanesthesia evaluation: an updated report by the American Society of anesthesiologists task force on pre-anesthesia evaluation. Anesthesiology. 2012;116:522–38.
17. Raw DA, Beattie JK, Hunter JM. Anesthesia for spine surgery in adults. Br J Anaesth. 2003;91(6):886–904.
18. Yoshihara H, Yoneoka D. Predictors of allogeneic blood transfusion in spinal fusion in the United States, 2004–2009. Spine. 2014;39(4):304–10.
19. Yang SY, Shim JK, Song Y, et al. Validation of pulse pressure variation and corrected flow time as predictors of fluid responsiveness in prone positioning. Br J Aneasth. 2013;110:713–20.
20. Shen Y, Drum M, Roth S. The prevalence of perioperative vision loss in United States: a 10 year study of spinal, orthopedic, cardiac and general surgery. Anesth Analg. 2009;109:1534–45.
21. PatilCG Lad EM, Lad SP, et al. Vision loss after spine surgery. A population-based study. Spine. 2008;33:1491–6.
22. POVL study group. Risk factors associated with ischemic optic neuropathy after spinal fusion surgery. Anesthesiology. 2012;116: 15–24.
23. ASA. Practice advisory for perioperative vision loss associated with spine surgery. Anesthesiology. 2012;116:274–85.
24. Tan T, Bhinder R, Carey M, et al. Day surgery patients anesthetized with porpofol has less postoperative pain than those anesthetized with sevoflurane. AnesthAnalg. 2010;111:83–5.
25. Gonzalez AA, Jeyanandarajan D, Hensen C et al. Intraoperative neurophysiological monitoring suring spine surgery: a review. Neurosurg Focus. 2009;27(4):E6.

Transsphenoidal Hypophysectomy

19

Saraswathy Shekar

CASE: Transsphenoidal Hypophysectomy

A 63-year-male with headaches, visual disturbances, and hoarseness of voice presents to the hospital. He reports new onset of diabetes and joint pains. His wife reports excessive snoring during sleep. His medical history includes

Medications:	Simvastatin 20 mg oral daily
	Lisinopril 20 mg oral daily
	Glyburide 10 mg oral daily
Allergies:	NKA
Past Medical History:	Hypertension
	Hyperlipidemia
	Obesity
	Recent admission with Congestive heart failure
	Remote smoker
Physical Exam:	Mandibular
	Large coarse facial features
	Airway examination: Mallampatti Class 3
	CVS S1 S2
	BP 170/100 HR 100 RR20
	Weight 140 kg, Height 6′, BMI 41.8 kg/m^2
	EKG Left ventricular hypertrophy

1. **What is the anatomy of the pituitary gland?**

The pituitary is located within the sella turcica which is the bony roof of the sphenoid sinus. It is made up of the glandular anterior adenohypophysis and posterior neurohypophysis. It is extra dural. The infundibulum, which contains the neurovascular bundle, extends from the hypothalamus to the pituitary gland.

The optic chiasma is above the pituitary gland. On either side of the pituitary are the cavernous sinuses. The cranial nerves III, IV, V, and VI and the cavernous portion of the carotid arteries are on either side of the pituitary within the cavernous sinuses (Fig. 19.1) [1].

2. **What are the hormones secreted by the pituitary?**

The anterior pituitary secretes six hormones: Adrenocorticotropic hormone (ACTH), thyroid-stimulating hormone (TSH), growth hormone (GH), follicle-stimulating hormone (FSH), luteinizing hormone (LH), and prolactin [1].

The posterior pituitary contains nerve endings, which release oxytocin and vasopressin (Antidiuretic hormone ADH), which are formed in supraoptic and paraventricular nuclei of the hypothalamus. Hypothalamic osmoreceptors and peripheral stretch receptors regulate secretion of ADH.

The hypothalamus regulates the anterior pituitary through hypothalamic-releasing factors, which travel down the portal venous system in the pituitary stalk.

3. **What are the common types of pituitary tumors?**

Pituitary adenomas are classified by size. Tumors that are greater than 1 cm are macroadenomas. Tumors less than 1 cm are microadenomas. They are also classified as functioning or non-functioning. Prolactin, ACTH, and GH secreting tumors are more common than TSH or FSH secreting tumors.

4. **What are the clinical presentations of non-functioning pituitary tumors?**

Non-functioning adenomas comprise 40% of pituitary adenomas [2].

S. Shekar (✉)
UMass Medical Center, University of Massachusetts Medical School, 55 Lake Avenue North, Worcester, Worcester, MA 01655, USA
e-mail: saraswathy.shekar@umassmemorial.org

© Springer International Publishing AG 2017
L.S. Aglio and R.D. Urman (eds.), *Anesthesiology*,
DOI 10.1007/978-3-319-50141-3_19

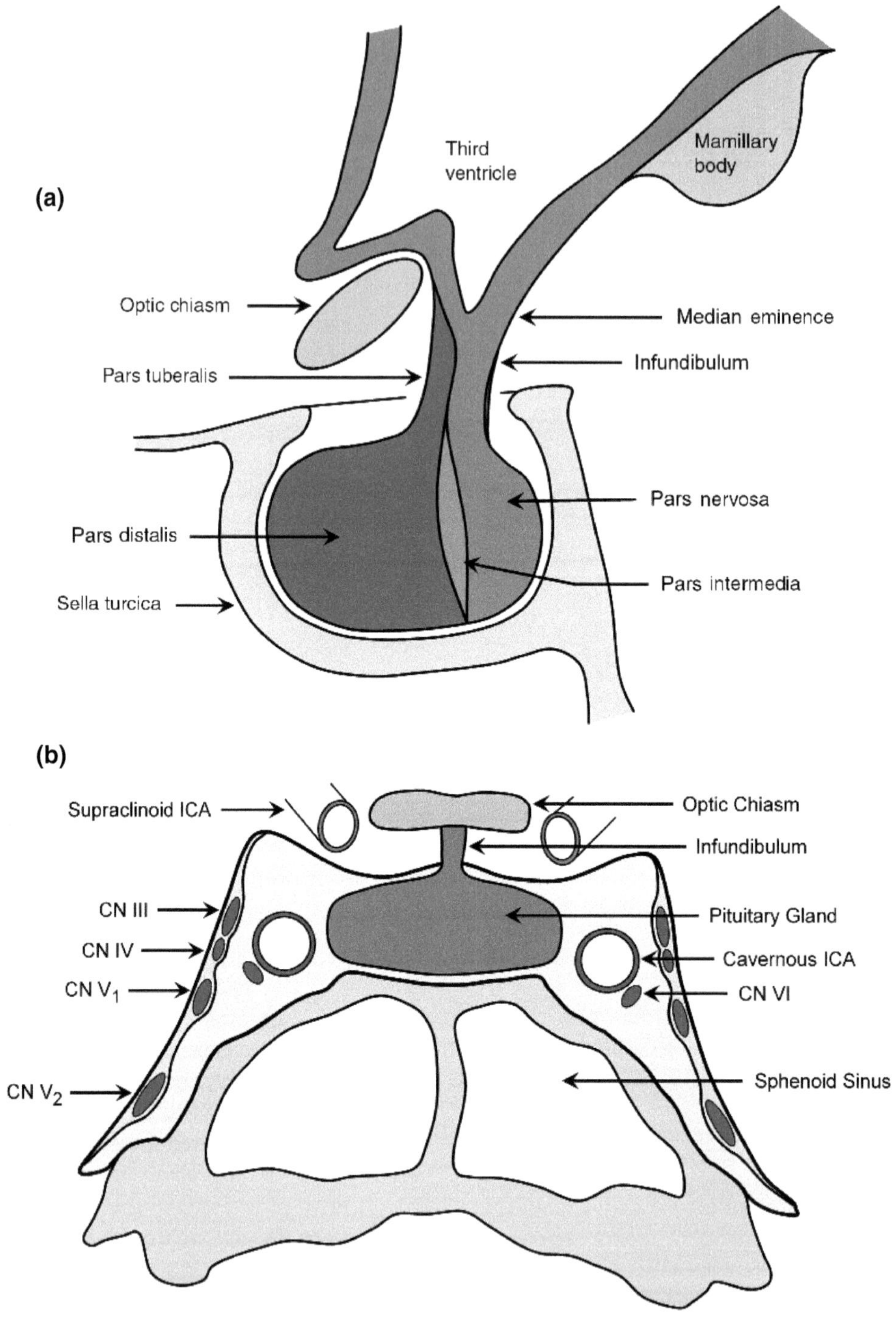

Fig. 19.1 Anatomy of the pituitary gland. **a** Schematic midline sagittal view of the sella turcica, pituitary, gland, and infundibulum. **b** Schematic coronal view of the cavernous sinuses, ICA, internal carotid artery; CN, cranial nerve. Reproduced from [8]

Examples of non-functioning adenomas include craniopharyngiomas, Rathke's cleft cyst, chromophobe adenomas, or meningiomas. About 50% of craniopharyngiomas occur in childhood.

They may present with mass effects like hypopituitarism, headaches, and visual deficits from compression of optic chiasma (typically bi-temporal hemianopia) [1, 2].

5. **What are the clinical presentations of functioning tumors?**

Functioning tumors produce excess secretion of pituitary hormones [2], hyperprolactinemia, acromegaly, Cushing disease hyperthyroidism or diabetes insipidus [2].

Either functioning or non-functioning pituitary tumors can in rare instances cause raised intracranial pressure (ICP) by directly compressing the third ventricle and the patient may present with signs of raised ICP like headache, nausea, vomiting, and papilledema [1].

Pituitary tumors may present with pituitary apoplexy due to sudden enlargement of the tumor or hemorrhage into tumor.

Extension into the cavernous sinuses can produce diplopia, ophthalmoplegia, ptosis, and facial sensory syndromes due to cranial nerve involvement [1, 2].

Hydrocephalus can occur from compression of third ventricle from suprasellar extension.

6. **What are the findings in a patient with prolactin secreting tumor?**

Prolactinomas are the most frequently occurring hyper-functioning pituitary adenoma. Hyperprolactinemia in women causes amenorrhea, loss of libido, and infertility [1].

In men it causes decreased libido, erectile dysfunction, premature ejaculation, and oligospermia

7. **What are the concerns in a patient with growth hormone secreting tumors?**

Growth hormone secreting tumors can produce gigantism in patients before epiphyseal plates are fused and Acromegaly in adults [2].

Patients with acromegaly have cardiovascular, respiratory, endocrinologic, and musculoskeletal issues, which need to be addressed [1–3].

Cardiovascular issues:

(a) Maybe from interstitial myocardial fibrosis
(b) Hypertension
(c) Cardiac hypertrophy,
(d) Diastolic dysfunction, conduction defects like bundle branch block
(e) Cardiomyopathy
(f) Congestive heart failure

Respiratory:

(a) Coarse facial features can cause difficult mask ventilation
(b) Thickening of laryngeal and pharyngeal tissues leading to reduction of glottis opening
(c) Macroglossia
(d) Prognathism and malocclusion
(e) Hypertrophy of epiglottis, aryepiglottic folds, and arytenoid cartilage
(f) All of the above contribute to obstructive sleep apnea and difficulty in airway management.

Endocrine:

(a) Diabetes is common
(b) Glucose intolerance

Musculoskeletal:

(a) Arthritis
(b) Vertebral hypertrophy
(c) Osteophyte formation of cervical spine and reduced range of motion of neck
(d) Osteoporosis
(e) Enlargement of hands and feet
(f) Carpal tunnel syndrome

8. **What is the cause of hoarseness in acromegaly?**

The causes of hoarseness in acromegaly patients can be possible laryngeal stenosis, or recurrent laryngeal nerve injury.

9. **What is the grading for airway involvement in acromegaly patients?**

Four grades of airway involvement are described [4]:

(a) Grade 1—no significant involvement
(b) Grade 2—nasal and pharyngeal mucosa hypertrophy but normal cords and glottis
(c) Grade 3—glottic involvement including glottic stenosis or vocal cord paresis
(d) Grade 4—combination of grades 2 and 3, i.e., Glottic and soft tissue abnormalities

Grade 3 and 4 may need to awake fiberoptic intubation

10. **What are the features of adrenocorticotrophic hormone (ACTH) excess?**

ACTH excess produces Cushing's disease [1, 3], which is characterized by

(a) Truncal obesity, moon face
(b) Obstructive sleep apnea
(c) Coronary artery disease
(d) Glucose intolerance
(e) Osteoporosis
(f) Myopathy, skin fragility and difficult intravenous access.
(g) Hypertension, left ventricular hypertrophy.
(h) Exophthalmos due to retro orbital fat deposition
(i) Electrolyte abnormalities like hypernatremia, hypokalemia, and alkalosis

11. **What is the preoperative work up for a patient presenting for a Transsphenoidal Hypophysectomy**?

A detailed history and physical specifically for signs and symptoms of endocrine hypo- or hyper-function [2, 5].

Endocrine tests:

(a) Adrenal axis screening—Serum Cortisol, ACTH, Dexamethasone suppression test, 24-h urinary-free cortisol, Synacthen test
(b) Serum Prolactin, LH, FSH, and testosterone levels in men
(c) Serum GH
(d) Insulin-like growth factor GF1 sensitive for acromegaly
(e) Serum TSH, free thyroxine

Serum electrolytes, Complete blood count
Radiology
MRI
Visual fields and visual acuity tests
Evaluate for presence of intracranial hypertension
Sleep studies for evaluating sleep apnea
Cardiac workup including EKG, Echocardiogram especially for patients with acromegaly and Cushing's disease

All preoperative neurologic and cranial deficits are assessed and documented.

12. **What is pituitary apoplexy and what is the management?**

A large bleed into the pituitary associated with a macroadenoma or a rapidly growing macroadenoma causes infarction and produces symptoms of pituitary apoplexy [2].

The patient presents with severe headache visual field deficits, ophthalmoplegia, shock, and altered consciousness.

Cavernous sinus compression by the tumor can cause venous stasis and pressure on any of the structures within.

This is a medical emergency and management consists of steroids, intravenous fluids, thyroxine, and neurosurgical consult for possible urgent surgical decompression.

Endocrinology should be consulted for management of panhypopituitarism. These patients are extremely sensitive to anesthetic agents and will need pressors to support blood pressure intraoperatively.

13. **What is the management of pituitary tumors?**

All patients are to be evaluated by an endocrinologist [1, 3].

Medical management:

Dopamine agonists like bromocriptine for hyperprolactinemia. Patients with hyperprolactinemia respond very well to medical management [1].

Somatostatin analogs like Octreotide and Lanreotide can be used to decrease secretion of growth hormone in patients with growth hormone producing tumors

Replacement therapy for management of hypopituitarism is with hydrocortisone and thyroxine

Patients with signs and symptoms of raised intracranial pressure have to be treated with mannitol, diuretics and steroids [1].

Surgery:

Pituitary resection can be performed through Transsphenoidal (endo nasal or sub labial) and transethmoidal approaches.

Transcranial approach is used for larger tumors or part of a staged approach

Patients with visual loss need emergent surgical decompression

Radiotherapy:

Gamma knife or brachytherapy can work for some of these tumors [1, 6].

14. **What are the indications for Transsphenoidal Hypophysectomy?**

Microadenomas and most macroadenomas are amenable to transsphenoidal hypophysectomy [6].

Tumors, which are larger or extending laterally into the cavernous sinus, may require an open bifrontal craniotomy

Some larger asymmetric tumors with suprasellar, parasellar, retrosellar, and subfrontal extension may need a staged approach. The primary procedure is performed through transsphenoidal approach and residual tumor is resected in a subsequent transcranial approach [6].

15. **What are advantages of the Transsphenoidal route?**

It is the least traumatic to the sella and avoids any brain retraction and visible scars [6].

It provides excellent visualization of pituitary gland.

It offers lower morbidity and mortality rate as compared to a transcranial procedure.

Decreased frequency of blood transfusions.

It allows for a shorter hospital stay.

16. **What is the anesthetic plan and the concerns intraoperatively for this procedure?**

This procedure requires general anesthesia with two large bore intravenous access and arterial line for invasive blood pressure monitoring. Standard monitoring like EKG, non-invasive blood pressure, end tidal carbon dioxide (ETCO2), and pulse oximetry are used.

Airway management and tracheal intubation in acromegaly may need large masks and longer laryngoscope blades.

Fiberoptic intubation should be considered in patients in whom difficult airway management is predicted [4].

The endotracheal tube is taped to the lower jaw and to the left. Reinforced endotracheal tubes maybe preferred.

The surgeon packs the nose with vasoconstrictor, usually 4% cocaine or infiltrates the nasal mucosa with lidocaine and epinephrine. This can cause hypertension, tachycardia, cardiac arrhythmias, and EKG changes like ST elevation compatible with coronary ischemia. This may be treated with boluses of labetalol or metoprolol [1, 3].

Standard general anesthetic is used with short acting narcotics like remifentanil for rapid emergence. 1. During this surgery it is important to ventilate to normocapnia because excessive hyperventilation will result in loss of brain bulk and make any suprasellar extension of the tumor less accessible from below. The surgeon will ask for a Valsalva maneuver for helping to push the suprasellar portion of the tumor into the sella [6].

A throat pack is also placed by the surgeon to absorb blood.

The abdomen is prepped for fat pad harvesting.

In patients with visual disturbances secondary to compression of optic chiasma adequate perfusion pressure must be maintained by the use of vasopressors. This can be done with an infusion of phenylephrine. Stress dose steroids are administered usually hydrocortisone.

Intraoperatively urine output and electrolytes are monitored to watch out for development of diabetes insipidus.

The surgeon may ask the anesthesiologist to perform a Valsalva maneuver at the end of tumor resection to detect cerebrospinal fluid (CSF) leak. If there is a leak, fat pad harvested from the abdomen is placed in the tumor bed [6].

A lumbar drain maybe placed to reduce CSF rhinorrhea. If there is a CSF leak there is a risk of the optic chiasma herniating into the sella.

Since the approach is through the nasopharynx, there can be bleeding which needs to be suctioned. The throat pack is removed prior to extubation. The nose is packed at the end of the procedure by the surgeon and the patient has to be warned of this preoperatively.

This procedure can rarely be complicated by carotid injury, which can be catastrophic. Blood must be readily available.

17. **How is the patient positioned in the operating room?**

The patient is supine with the head elevated, extended and turned slightly turned to the left. This promotes venous drainage. The operating table is usually turned 90 degrees away. The patient's head is placed in a Mayfield holder, which can be stimulating and may need extra analgesia such as a bolus of remifentanil or propofol. Positioning in the operating room table has to be done carefully in acromegaly and Cushing's disease patients because of osteoporosis and fragile skin. Patients with exophthalmos need to have special protection of eyes to prevent corneal abrasions. Computer-guided frameless stereotaxy may be used to guide resection [6].

18. **Describe the surgical approach of the Transsphenoidal pituitary resection**

The surgeon follows the midline of the nose, removing bone. He penetrates through the sphenoid air sinuses and removes the floor of the pituitary fossa. The tumor is then removed with an operating microscope.

19. **Why is a lumbar drain placed in some of these procedures?**

In patients with very large tumors with suprasellar extension a lumbar drain is placed to inject saline or air to push the suprasellar part of the tumor into the intrasellar operative field. This allows for more complete excision of the tumor [6].

20. **What are the postoperative concerns**?

These patients cannot undergo mask ventilation after extubation because of the danger of pneumocephalus. Therefore, it is prudent to emerge the patient completely awake with regain of spontaneous respirations Nasal airways or nasogastric tubes should not be placed. Laryngeal mask airways must be readily available if patients need brief periods of ventilation.

Acromegaly and Cushing's patients with obstructive sleep apnea need close postoperative monitoring. Continuous Positive Airway Pressure (CPAP) or Bi-level Positive Airway Pressure (BIPAP) is contraindicated after this [1, 3].

These patients need close observation to observe visual disturbances and symptoms of hypopituitarism [7].

Medications for nausea and vomiting are given prophylactically.

Preoperative hormone replacements need to be continued postoperatively. The endocrinologist follow-up is essential

21. **What are the complications of Transsphenoidal Hypophysectomy?**

(a) Cerebrospinal fluid leak is the most common complication [6].
(b) Inadvertent carotid injury
(c) Carotid cavernous fistula
(d) Injury to the cavernous sinus
(e) Cranial nerve palsy
(f) Tumor recurrence
(g) Hypopituitarism
(h) Venous air embolism
(i) Diabetes Insipidus
(j) Empty sella syndrome may present with visual impairment
(k) Hydrocephalus may follow after removal of tumors with suprasellar extension.
(l) Epistaxis, nasal septal perforation
(m) Meningitis

22. **What is Diabetes insipidus?**

Diabetes insipidus (DI) is produced when there is deficiency of ADH. It may occur intra- or postoperatively within first 24 hours in patients having pituitary surgery [6]. The patient has polyuria, accompanied by polydipsia. There is low urine osmolarity (less than 300 mosm/kg) and elevated serum osmolarity (greater than 295 mosm/kg) urine-specific gravity is less than 1.005. Serum sodium is elevated. DI maybe self-limiting and secondary to handling of the pituitary stalk (stalk effect)

Accurate recording of fluid intake and output must be done

Patient may need DDAVP, a synthetic analog of vasopressin. Early diagnosis is important to avoid hypernatremia and dehydration [6].

23. **What is Syndrome of Inappropriate ADH secretion? (SIADH)**

This syndrome is due to lesions in the region of the supraoptic and paraventricular nuclei that impair hypothalamic osmoreceptors. This results in elevated ADH release [6].

This syndrome is characterized by

(a) Hyponatremia(less than 135 meq/l)
(b) Low serum osmolarity
(c) Normal renal excretion of sodium
(d) Elevated urine osmolarity (greater than 20 mmol/l)
(e) Absence of volume depletion
(f) All other causes of non-osmotic released ADH such as hypotension, hypovolemia, positive pressure ventilation, pain, and drugs like narcotics must be ruled out.
(g) Treatment is with fluid restriction.
(h) In severe cases (Serum Sodium less than 120 meq/l) hypertonic saline (3%) is administered slowly.
(i) Rapid correction of serum sodium can lead to central pontine myelinolysis.

24. **What is Cerebral salt wasting Syndrome? (CSW)**

CSW is one of the causes of hyponatremia associated with intracranial disease [6].

It is responsive to volume and salt loading.

These patients have concentrated urine; the urine sodium [Na] usually is greater than 20 mEq/L.

Non edematous.

Normal uric acid.

Hypovolemic compared to patients with SIADH.

25. **What are causes and signs of Venous Air Embolism? (VAE)**

In this procedure there is a small risk of VAE since the head is elevated and there is entry into the air containing sphenoid sinus [7].

VAE is more common in the sitting position and posterior fossa surgery where the venous channels are open.

The greater the pressure gradient between the cerebral veins and the right atrium and lower the central venous pressure, the greater is the tendency for air to enter to enter the open venous sinuses.

The signs are tachycardia, hypotension, and sudden fall in End tidal Carbon di oxide (ETCO2) as the entrained air (about 5 ml/kg) occludes the right ventricular outflow tract, rise of end tidal Nitrogen, EKG signs of right ventricular strain, dysrhythmias, and cardiovascular collapse.

26. **How do you detect and manage VAE?**

The precordial Doppler ultrasound is the most sensitive indicator for venous air embolism but not specific or quantitative. It is cumbersome to use and has false negatives [7].

The TEE (Transesophageal echocardiogram) is the most sensitive indicator of VAE. It can detect air in left heart and aorta but needs special expertise

Management is:

(a) Increase inspired Oxygen to 100%
(b) Head down, Left lateral decubitus
(c) Stop further entrainment.
(d) Surgeon floods the field with saline.
(e) Aspirate from Right atrial catheter if present
(f) Vasopressors
(g) Intravenous fluids
(h) Cardiopulmonary resuscitation
(i) Hyperbaric oxygen therapy for cerebral embolism.

References

1. Nemergut EJ, Dumont AS, Barry UT, Laws ER. Perioperative management of patients undergoing transsphenoidal pituitary surgery. Anesth Analg. 2005;101:1170–81.
2. Greenberg MS. Handbook of neurosurgery. 7th ed. Thieme; 2010.
3. Lim M, Williams D, Maartens N. Anaesthesia for pituitary surgery. J Clin Neurosci. 2006;13(4):413–8.
4. Southwick JP, Katz J. Unusual airway difficulty in the acromegalic patient–indications for tracheostomy. Anesthesiology. 1979;51 (1):72–3.
5. Vance ML. Perioperative management of patients undergoing pituitary surgery. Endocrinol Metab Clin of N Am 07/2003; 32 (2):355–65.
6. Schwartz TH, Anand V. Endoscopic pituitary surgery. 1st ed. Thieme; 2011.
7. Cottrell JE, Young WL (editors). Cottrell and young's neuroanesthesia. 5th ed. Mosby; 2010.
8. Lysack JT, Schaefer PW. Imaging of the pituitary gland, sella, and parasellar region. In: Swearingen B and Biller BMK, editors. Contemporary endocrinology: diagnosis and management of pituitary disorders. Totowa, NJ: Humana Press; 2008. p. 45–91

Additional Reading

9. Butterworth JF, Mackey DC, Wasnick JD, Morgan & Mikhail's clinical anesthesiology. 5th ed. McGraw-Hill Education/ Medical 2013.

Part IV

The Neuromuscular System

Section Editor: Zhiling Xiong

Zhiling Xiong
Department of Anesthesiology, Perioperative and Pain Medicine,
Brigham and Women's Hospital, Boston, MA, USA

Depolarizing Neuromuscular Blocking Agents 20

Caroline S. Gross and Zhiling Xiong

CASE:

A 54-year-old female presents to the emergency department after a fall on ice. On presentation she is initially awake and oriented, reporting that she slipped on her way out of a restaurant with her husband. She struck her head against the concrete sidewalk, but otherwise has no obvious injuries. During evaluation in the ED, she becomes progressively more confused and obtunded. Head CT reveals subdural blood. She is taken to the OR for emergency evacuation of the subdural hematoma.

Medications
ASA 81 mg daily
Lisinopril 10 mg daily
Simvastatin 40 mg daily
Sertraline 100 mg daily
Coumadin 5 mg daily
Tylenol PRN
Allergies
No Known Drug Allergies
Past Medical History
Hypertension
Hyperlipidemia
Depression
DVT diagnosed 1 month ago following left knee replacement, on Coumadin
Osteoarthritis
Past Surgical History
C-section
Laparoscopic appendectomy
Left total knee replacement
Physical Exam:
Vital signs: BP 128/90 HR 70 BPM RR 18 SpO2 95% on room air
General: The patient is lying in bed, somnolent, opening eyes to voice but not following commands
Head/Ears/Eyes/Nose/Throat: abrasion over right forehead
Cardiovascular: Regular rate and rhythm, no murmurs
Pulmonary: CTA bilaterally
Abdominal: Soft, nontender, nondistended
Extremities: Mild swelling of left calf, well healed surgical scar on left knee
Neuro: Arousable, disoriented to place and time, uncooperative with exam but no obvious lateralizing exam findings
Laboratory studies:
Na 138 K 5.2 Cl 108 HCO3 22 BUN 28 Cr 1.7
WBC 8K Hematocrit 35% Platelets 180
Coagulation studies are pending

The decision is made to proceed to the operating room for emergency evacuation of subdural hematoma. Rapid sequence induction is performed with propofol, fentanyl, and succinylcholine.

1. **What is the mechanism of action of succinylcholine?**

The succinylcholine molecule consists of two acetylcholine molecules linked to each other at the acetyl portion of the molecule. This structural similarity to the endogenous acetylcholine molecule accounts for its ability to exert effects similar to acetylcholine at nicotinic acetylcholine receptors.

C.S. Gross (✉) · Z. Xiong
Department of Anesthesiology, Perioperative and Pain Medicine, Brigham and Women's Hospital, 75 Francis Street, Boston, MA 02115, USA
e-mail: csgross@partners.org

Z. Xiong
e-mail: zxiong@partners.org

© Springer International Publishing AG 2017
L.S. Aglio and R.D. Urman (eds.), *Anesthesiology*,
DOI 10.1007/978-3-319-50141-3_20

Nicotinic acetylcholine receptors exist in both neuronal and muscle forms. The receptors themselves are composed of five transmembrane subunits, which form a central cation pore. Clinically, succinylcholine acts on the muscle nicotinic acetylcholine receptors. It binds to these acetylcholine receptors at the neuromuscular junction, causing opening of the ion channel in the receptor and membrane depolarization leading to skeletal muscle fasciculations. This is followed by a rapid desensitization of the receptor and inactivation of the ion channels, preventing propagation of action potentials and manifesting clinically as flaccidity. Unlike the acetylcholine molecule, which is broken down in <1 ms, succinylcholine remains at the neuromuscular junction. This causes a neuromuscular blockade which lasts for about 5–10 min, until the succinylcholine molecule is metabolized [1].

2. **How is succinylcholine metabolized?**

Succinylcholine is normally broken down through hydrolysis by pseudocholinesterase (also known as plasma cholinesterase or butyrylcholinesterase) into succinylmonocholine and choline. Pseudocholinesterase is synthesized in the liver. There are many conditions that can lead to reduced plasma activity of this enzyme, including pregnancy, oral contraceptives, liver disease, uremia, malnutrition, or plasmapheresis. The decrease in plasma cholinesterase in these cases can lead to a slight increase in the duration of action of succinylcholine, which is generally clinically irrelevant. Obese patients have increased plasma cholinesterase activity [2].

3. **What is the onset and expected duration of action of succinylcholine?**

The peak onset of a dose of 1–2 mg/kg is achieved in less than 60 s. The time to peak onset will be longer if lower doses are used. Spontaneous respirations and diaphragmatic contraction generally will resume after about 5 min. Full recovery of neuromuscular function is dose dependent, and is about 10–12 min after a dose of 1 mg/kg [2].

4. **What is the clinical significance of abnormal plasma cholinesterase?**

Mutations in the gene that codes for plasma cholinesterase can result in abnormal enzyme activity, and therefore prolonged duration of neuromuscular blockade following succinylcholine administration. Significant prolongation of succinylcholine's activity occurs when an individual is homozygous for the abnormal allele. The incidence is estimated to be 1: 2000. More commonly, an individual may be heterozygous for the abnormal allele (incidence about 1:30). Patients who are homozygous can have a neuromuscular blockade lasting up to 2–6 h. In comparison, individuals who are heterozygous for the abnormal allele will have a slightly prolonged paralysis [3].

5. **What is the dibucaine number?**

Dibucaine is a local anesthetic that is known to inhibit normal plasma cholinesterase by 80%. In individuals who are homozygous for the atypical plasma cholinesterase, the activity of the enzyme is only inhibited 20%. In individuals who are heterozygous inhibition is about 50–60%. The dibucaine number therefore reflects the levels of normally functioning plasma cholinesterase. It will not be affected by conditions that cause a decrease in the *quantity* of normal plasma cholinesterase (i.e., liver disease, pregnancy). It is, in other words, a qualitative rather than quantitative test [3].

6. **What are some of the potential negative side effects of succinylcholine administration?**

Minor: fasciculation, myalgia, increased intragastric pressure

Major: anaphylaxis, sinus bradycardia, asystole, tachycardia, elevation in intracranial pressure, increased intraocular pressure, hyperkalemia, trismus

7. **What is the appropriate dose of succinylcholine?**

Generally, a dose of 1.0 mg/kg will yield excellent intubating conditions within 1.5 min of succinylcholine administration. It is important to remember that an increased dose may be required if the patient is pretreated with a small dose of a nondepolarizing neuromuscular blocking agent [4].

In the obese patient, it is generally recommended that succinylcholine be dosed according to total body weight. Dosing based on ideal or lean body weight has been associated with suboptimal intubating conditions. This is in part due to increased plasma cholinesterase activity in the obese patient [5].

8. **What is the incidence of anaphylaxis related to succinylcholine administration?**

The incidence of anaphylaxis related to succinylcholine administration is estimated to be between 1:5000 and 1: 10,000. It is felt to be one of the most common causes of anaphylaxis in patients receiving general anesthesia.

9. **Is there a risk of administration of succinylcholine to a patient with elevated intracranial pressure?**

There is a theoretical potential for succinylcholine to cause an elevation in intracranial pressure (ICP), which is of concern in a patient with abnormal intracranial compliance. The clinical significance of this increase is debated. While succinylcholine may cause increases in ICP, it is important to remember that both hypoxemia and hypercarbia can lead to increased cerebral blood volume and similarly cause an increase in intracranial pressure. In addition, inadequate neuromuscular blockade and depth of anesthesia at the time of intubation can also cause elevations in ICP. Some studies suggest that pretreatment with a small dose of nondepolarizing NMBA may attenuate potential increases in intracranial pressure when succinylcholine is used [2].

10. **How much can the serum potassium be expected to rise following administration of an intubating dose of succinylcholine?**

In general, serum potassium is expected to increase by about 0.1–0.5 mEq/L within a few minutes of succinylcholine administration.

11. **Is succinylcholine contraindicated in a patient with renal failure?**

The rise in serum potassium following administration of succinylcholine in patients with renal failure is not exaggerated. Succinylcholine can safely be administered to patients with renal failure, provided that serum potassium is not abnormally elevated [6].

12. **Should rapid sequence induction and intubation be performed with succinylcholine or rocuronium?**

This is not a straightforward question and should be addressed on a case-by-case basis. If there are clear contraindications to succinylcholine, then a rapid sequence intubation dose of rocuronium becomes a more obvious choice. The patient described in the case scenario above is presenting for emergency surgery and, given her NPO status and risk for aspiration of gastric contents, requires a rapid sequence intubation. However, there are some concerns about succinylcholine administration in this case. Her potassium is already somewhat elevated, and as previously stated, we expect that succinylcholine will cause a slight increase in her serum potassium. It is unlikely that her serum potassium will reach a dangerous level, given that the starting value is 5.1, but this is important to keep in mind. It is also important to avoid further elevations in intracranial pressure in a patient with abnormal intracranial compliance, and, as discussed previously, succinylcholine has the potential to cause an increase in ICP. The need to rapidly and reliably achieve optimal intubating conditions in this patient is likely more important than the theoretical transient increases in ICP. In regards to providing optimal intubating conditions, most clinicians would reach for succinylcholine. A recent Cochrane review (a meta-analysis which included 37 studies) concluded that succinylcholine produced superior intubation conditions to rocuronium. Interestingly, there was no statistical difference in intubation conditions when succinylcholine was compared to 1.2 mg/kg rocuronium. However, succinylcholine was felt to be clinically superior, particularly given its shorter duration of action [7].

13. **What patient populations are at risk for severe hyperkalemia following succinylcholine administration?**

Severe hyperkalemia, which can lead to cardiac arrest, can occur in patients with the following pathologies:

- Extensive burns
- Prolonged immobility
- Muscle trauma
- Upper motor neuron lesions (stroke or cord injury)
- Lower motor neuron lesions (i.e., Guillain-Barré)
- Myopathy (muscular dystrophies)

The mechanism of hyperkalemia is believed to be an up-regulation of skeletal muscle nicotinic acetylcholine receptors in all cases except myopathies. Hyperkalemia in patients with myopathy (i.e., Duchenne or Becker muscular dystrophy) appears to result from rhabdomyolysis [8]. In the other conditions, there is a proliferation predominantly of the fetal-type nicotinic acetylcholine receptors. These receptors differ from adult receptors in that they have a prolonged opening of the ion channel leading to an exaggeration of potassium efflux [3].

14. **What are the potential cardiac side effects of succinylcholine?**

Sinus bradycardia and junctional rhythms can occur following succinylcholine administration, particularly in the pediatric population. In addition, asystole can occur following a second dose of succinylcholine in both children and adults. The mechanism of succinylcholine-induced bradycardia is not entirely clear, but is believed to result from the action of SCh at cardiac muscarinic receptors [3].

15. **Can anything be done to prevent the fasciculation seen following administration of succinylcholine?**

A small dose of a nondepolarizing drug (10–30% of ED 95) administered 3–5 min prior to succinylcholine administration can reduce the likelihood of fasciculations and the development of myalgia. Other interventions that have been shown to decrease the incidence of fasciculations include administration of magnesium, or lidocaine. NSAIDs can also be administered to reduce the likelihood of developing myalgias. Interestingly, studies have suggested that using a slightly higher dose of succinylcholine (1.5 mg/kg rather than 1 mg/kg) is associated with a lower rate of both fasciculation and myalgias. Of note, there is not a clear association between fasciculation and myalgia. Should one choose to pretreat with a small dose of a nondepolarizing NMBA, it is important to be cognizant of potential side effects (blurry or double vision, difficulty breathing/swallowing), as well as the potential need for a slightly increased dose of succinylcholine [9].

16. **What are the characteristics of neuromuscular blockade with a depolarizing NMBA?**

Single twitch height is decreased during phase I blockade with succinylcholine. In train of four stimulation (four stimuli applied at 2 Hz every 0.5 s), four twitches will be present, but all diminished in amplitude. There should not be tetanic fade. Of note, anticholinesterase drugs augment phase I blockade. See Fig. 20.1.

17. **What is a Phase II Block?**

A phase II block occurs after exposure to a high dose of succinylcholine (e.g., an infusion, multiple doses). While the mechanism of phase II blockade is not entirely clear, it appears to occur following post-junctional membrane repolarization, but in a period when the membrane still does not respond normally to acetylcholine. It resembles the blockade of nondepolarizing neuromuscular blocking agents, in the sense that both train of four and tetanic fade develop. While a phase II blockade appears clinically similar to blockade with nondepolarizing agents, it is generally wise to avoid attempting reversal with anticholinesterase agents (i.e., neostigmine), as the response is somewhat difficult to predict. See Fig. 20.1 [10].

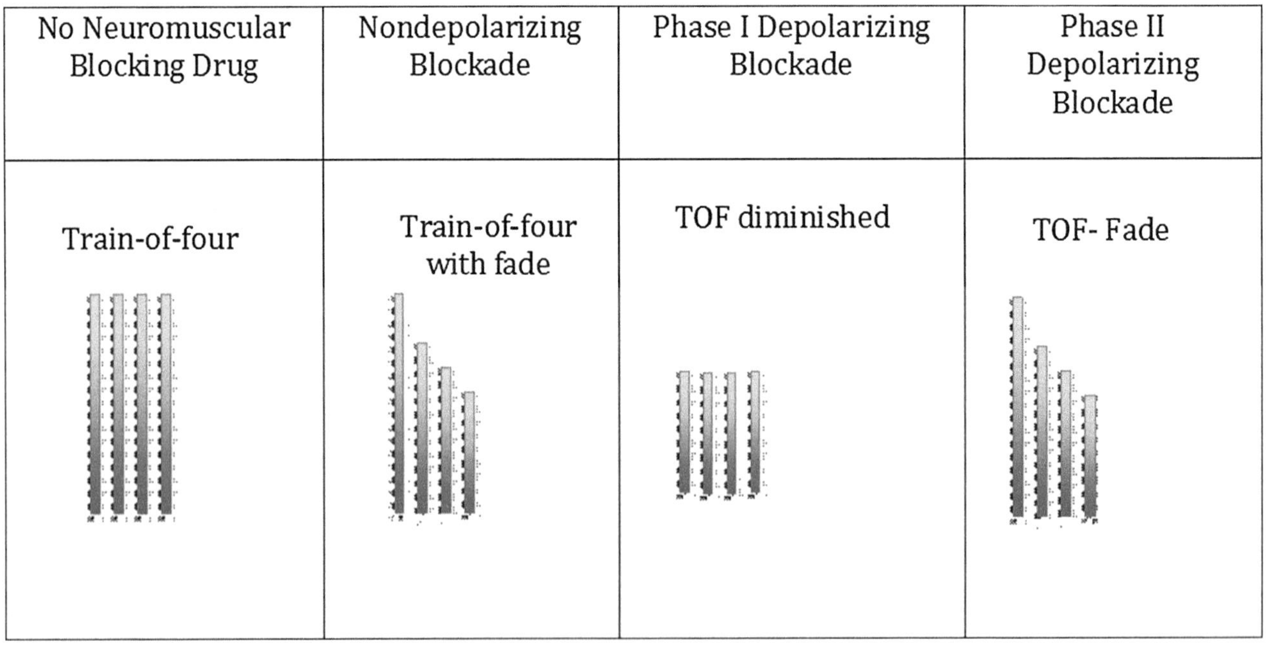

No Neuromuscular Blocking Drug
Nondepolarizing Blockade
Phase I Depolarizing Blockade
Phase II Depolarizing Blockade
Train-of-four
Train-of-four with fade
TOF diminished
TOF- Fade

Fig. 20.1 Train-of-four (TOF) stimulation is often used for intraoperative monitoring of neuromuscular blockade. It is achieved by delivering 4 electrical stimulations at 2 Hz every 0.5 s. This table provides a schematic representation of the expected twitch response to TOF stimulation in the presence of neuromuscular blockade. In the presence of nondepolarizing blockade, the TOF stimulation demonstrates fade of twitch height. In a phase I depolarizing blockade, the twitch height is diminished, but no fade is present. In a phase II depolarizing blockade, response to TOF stimulation resembles that of a nondepolarizing blockade, again with fade of twitch height

18. **What is the significance of trismus following succinylcholine administration?**

Trismus refers to spasm of the jaw muscles and can be seen following succinylcholine administration, most commonly in the pediatric population. In some cases, rigidity may be so severe that it can prevent the clinician from opening the patient's mouth. The other concern is that masseter rigidity may be the first sign of malignant hyperthermia. Succinylcholine is a well-known triggering agent of malignant hyperthermia in susceptible individuals. Masseter spasm is by no means diagnostic of malignant hyperthermia, but its occurrence should prompt the clinician to maintain a high index of suspicion for potential progression to malignant hyperthermia [10].

19. **Are there concerns about administering succinylcholine in the pediatric population?**

Succinylcholine is generally avoided in the pediatric population. There is particular concern about the use of succinylcholine in young male patients, given the potential for previously undiagnosed Duchenne-type muscular dystrophy (an X-linked hereditary disease). There have been multiple case reports of hyperkalemia, rhabdomyolysis, and cardiac arrest following administration of succinylcholine in children with muscular dystrophy [2]. Another reason to avoid succinylcholine in pediatric patients is its propensity to cause bradycardia in this patient population.

References

1. Jonsson M, Dabrowski M, Gurley DA, et al. Activation and inhibition of human muscular and neuronal nicotinic acetylcholine receptors by succinylcholine. Anesthesiology. 2006;104:724–33.
2. Donati D. Neuromuscular blocking agents. In: Barash et al., editors. Clinical anesthesia. 7th ed. Philadelphia: Lippincott Williams & Wilkins; 2013. p. 523–57.
3. Miller RD. Neuromuscular blocking drugs. In: Basics of anesthesia. 6th ed. Philadelphia: Elsevier Saunders; 2011. p. 143–61.
4. Naguib M, Samarkandi AH, El-Din ME, Abdullah K, Khaled M, Alharby SW. The dose of succinylcholine required for excellent endotracheal intubating conditions. Anesth Analg. 2006;102:151–5.
5. Lemmens HJ, Brodsky JB. The dose of succinylcholine in morbid obesity. Anesth Analg. 2006;102:438–42.
6. Thapa S, Brull SJ. Succinylcholine-induced hyperkalemia in patients with renal failure: an old question revisited. Anesth Analg. 2000;91:237–41.
7. Perry JJ, Lee JS, Sillberg V, Wells GA. Rocuronium versus succinylcholine for rapid sequence induction intubation. Cochrane Database Syst Rev. 2008;. doi:10.1002/14651858.CD002788.pub2.
8. Gronert GA. Cardiac arrest after succinylcholine: mortality greater with rhabdomyolysis than receptor upregulation. Anesthesiology. 2001;94:523–9.
9. Schreiber JU, Lysakowski C, Fuchs-Buder T, et al. Prevention of succinylcholine-induced fasciculation and myalgia: a meta-analysis of randomized trials. Anesthesiology. 2005;103: 877–84.
10. Naguib M, Lien CA, Claude M. Pharmacology of neuromuscular blocking drugs. In: Miller RD, editor. Miller's anesthesia. 8th ed. Philadelphia: Elsevier Saunders; 2015. p. 958–91.

Nondepolarizing Neuromuscular Blocking Agents

21

Erin Bettendorf and Zhiling Xiong

CASE: 27-year-old man with a history of asthma presenting with 12 h of abdominal pain, anorexia, nausea, and vomiting and found to have acute appendicitis. He is scheduled for an emergent laparoscopic appendectomy.

PMH: Asthma
PSH: Tonsillectomy and adenoidectomy, age 6
Allergies: NKDA
Medications: Albuterol, montelukast
FH: Maternal aunt "took a long time to wake up" from anesthesia

Questions

Is neuromuscular blockade beneficial in this case? Why or why not?

Muscle relaxation is useful in a variety of surgeries including laparoscopic cases such as this. When used during induction, muscle relaxants help provide optimal intubating conditions by inhibiting contraction of the muscles attached to the vocal cords, allowing for ease of passage of the endotracheal tube. Additionally, neuromuscular blockers can improve surgical conditions in many instances, facilitating the safe and efficient completion of the surgery.

Where is the site of action of neuromuscular blocking drugs?

Neuromuscular blockers act at the acetylcholine receptor, located largely in the neuromuscular junction. The receptors are composed of five subunits—two alpha subunits, one beta, one delta, and one epsilon. Acetylcholine binds to the alpha subunits, as do most neuromuscular blocking medications. There are two classes of acetylcholine receptors—nicotinic and muscarinic. Nicotinic receptors are located on skeletal muscle and autonomic ganglia and are the site of action of neuromuscular blocking medications. Muscarinic acetylcholine receptors are found throughout the body in smooth muscle, the SA and AV node in the heart and in the secretory glands.

Describe the process of normal signaling at the neuromuscular junction leading to muscle contraction.

The transmission of a signal begins with an action potential moving down a nerve causing calcium influx through voltage gated calcium channels. The sudden increase in intracellular calcium leads to the movement of acetylcholine-containing storage vesicles from the cytoplasm to the cell membrane. At the cell membrane, the vesicles fuse and release acetylcholine into the neuromuscular junction. The acetylcholine molecules cross the junction and bind to nicotinic acetylcholine receptors at the motor end plate. In order for a conformational change to occur in the nicotinic acetylcholine receptor, both alpha subunits making up the receptor must have an acetylcholine molecule bound to them. Once two acetylcholine molecules are bound, the receptor conformational change opens an ion channel, allowing sodium and calcium to move into the cell and for potassium to move out. The movement of these ions causes a change in potential across the cellular membrane. When enough receptors are triggered and a large enough potential difference exists across the perijunctional membrane,

E. Bettendorf (✉) · Z. Xiong
Department of Anesthesiology, Perioperative and Pain Medicine, Brigham and Women's Hospital, 75 Francis Street, Boston, MA 02115, USA
e-mail: ebettendorf@partners.org

Z. Xiong
e-mail: zxiong@partners.org

© Springer International Publishing AG 2017
L.S. Aglio and R.D. Urman (eds.), *Anesthesiology*,
DOI 10.1007/978-3-319-50141-3_21

depolarization occurs. This leads to opening of sodium channels on the muscle cell membrane, causing calcium to leave the sarcoplasmic reticulum. This sudden increase in intracellular calcium allows actin and myosin to interact and cause muscle contraction.

What is the difference between a mature acetylcholine receptor and an immature or fetal receptor?

The immature acetylcholine receptor is found in fetal muscle and contains a gamma instead of epsilon subunit. Immature acetylcholine receptors are also called extrajunctional receptors because they can also be located outside of the neuromuscular junction when found in adults.

How is acetylcholine metabolized?

As acetylcholine molecules diffuse away from the nicotinic receptors on the motor end plate, the molecules are rapidly broken down in the neuromuscular junction by the enzyme acetylcholinesterase into choline and acetate. The choline can then be taken up by the presynaptic membrane and converted back into acetylcholine. Acetylcholinesterase is located at the motor end plate adjacent to the acetylcholine receptors.

What are the two broad categories of neuromuscular blocking agents?

The two classes are depolarizing and nondepolarizing muscle relaxants. Succinylcholine is the only depolarizing neuromuscular blocking drug in clinical use. There are several different nondepolarizing muscle relaxants, examples of which include rocuronium, vecuronium, cisatracurium, and pancuronium.

What is the mechanism of action of depolarizing muscle relaxants?

Structurally similar to acetylcholine, depolarizing neuromuscular blockers (succinylcholine) bind at the acetylcholine binding site (alpha subunits) and cause propagation of an action potential. Unlike acetylcholine, however, depolarizing muscle relaxants are not broken down by acetylcholinesterase. This results in longer binding, leading to which increases the time until the motor end plate can repolarize and causes a short period of muscle relaxation. Thus, they are competitive agonists at the acetylcholine receptor.

How is succinylcholine metabolized?

When administered to a patient, the majority of a dose of succinylcholine is metabolized before ever reaching the neuromuscular junction. It is broken down quickly and efficiently by plasma pseudocholinesterase (also known as butyrylcholinesterase). The fraction that does reach the neuromuscular junction can then bind the acetylcholine receptor and cause its clinical effects. Subsequently, succinylcholine will redistributes from the neuromuscular junction and is rapidly broken down.

What can alter the duration of action of succinylcholine?

The normal onset of succinylcholine is 30–90 s and the duration of action is 3–5 min. However, this can be significantly lengthened in a variety of situations. Pseudocholinesterase deficiency decreases the amount of enzyme available to break down succinylcholine. For patients who are heterozygous for an atypical pseudocholinesterase gene, the duration of succinylcholine can be 20–30 min. For homozygous patients, a single dose of succinylcholine can cause paralysis for several hours.

There are several acquired forms of prolonged action of succinylcholine. Decreased activity of butyrylcholinesterase can be seen in patients with liver disease, pregnancy, kidney disease and from various medications (ex: cholinesterase inhibitors, metoclopramide, esmolol, cyclophosphamide, oral contraceptives, echothiophate). Patients with hypothermia will have prolonged duration of action. Giving a high dose of succinylcholine or an infusion can also lengthen the action of succinylcholine.

What are the side-effects of succinylcholine?

Succinylcholine has several significant and potentially severe side-effects. However, with appropriate planning and patient selection, the risk of this medication can be reduced. Histamine release can be seen in some patients, but is generally mild and transient.

Hyperkalemia occurs with succinylcholine administration as a result of efflux of potassium into the extracellular space with muscle contraction. In some patients, this hyperkalemia can cause life-threatening arrhythmias.

Fasciculations are visible muscle contractions that can be seen in many patients, indicating muscle relaxation. They often do not occur in patients with low muscle mass, elderly patients, and children. Patients may develop myalgia as a result of uncoordinated muscle contraction. Pretreatment with a nondepolarizing neuromuscular blocker will decrease fasciculations, but its effect on myalgias is controversial. Contractions of the abdominal wall can lead to increased intragastric pressure. This is offset by increased lower esophageal sphincter tone, resulting in no increased risk of aspiration. Increased intracranial pressure occurs with succinylcholine, but can be reduced if with nondepolarizer pretreatment. Increased intraocular pressure is not altered by nondepolarizing medications and is independent of fasciculations.

Succinylcholine is the only neuromuscular blocking medication that can be a trigger for malignant hyperthermia.

As a structural analog of acetylcholine, succinylcholine can bind to and effect receptors in the parasympathetic and sympathetic nervous system. Smaller doses stimulate the parasympathetic system predominantly, causing bradycardia and decreased inotropy. Larger doses can cause increased heart rate. The cardiovascular effects are often limited in adults. However, children are at increased risk for succinylcholine-induced bradycardia, which can be severe. Prior to administration of succinylcholine in children, atropine can be given prophylactically.

Which patients are at increased risk for hyperkalemia from succinylcholine administration and why?

In patients with acute nerve or tissue damage, increased production of immature acetylcholine receptors occurs at extrajunctional locations. When succinylcholine is given, these extrajunctional receptors depolarize along with the mature acetylcholine receptors at neuromuscular junctions, causing increased levels of potassium release from the intracellular compartment. In a healthy patient, potassium levels can increase by 0.5 meq/L with the administration of succinylcholine. In patients with preexisting tissue damage, this increase can be significant and potentially life-threatening. Conditions in which this increased risk exists include burn injuries, spinal cord injuries, cerebral vascular accidents, severe trauma, intracerebral or spinal cord masses, severe infections, significant metabolic acidosis, prolonged immobilization and myopathies such as Duchenne's muscular dystrophy.

Describe the mechanism of action of nondepolarizing neuromuscular blockers.

Nondepolarizing muscle relaxants bind the alpha subunit of the acetylcholine receptors at the neuromuscular junction. Hence, they are competitive inhibitors of the acetylcholine receptor. By preventing the binding of acetylcholine, the movement of ions and the change in potential across the postsynaptic membrane of the neuromuscular junction, paralysis occurs.

What are the two categories of nondepolarizing muscle blockers used in clinical practice?

One group is the benzylisoquinolines, which include the drugs mivacurium, atracurium and cisatracurium. The other group includes the steroidal medications—rocuronium, vecuronium, and pancuronium.

What are the durations of action of the various clinically available nondepolarizing muscle relaxants?

Rocuronium—at larger doses initial doses, onset is short (1–2 min) and intermediate duration of action
Vecuronium—onset in 2–3 min and intermediate to long duration
Pancuronium—onset in 2–3 min and long duration
Atracurium—onset in 2–3 min and intermediate duration
Cisatracurium—onset in 2–3 min and intermediate duration

How are the nondepolarizing muscle relaxants each metabolized and eliminated?

Rocuronium is not metabolized, only excreted. Excretion occurs primarily through the liver with a contribution from the kidneys. In patients with severe liver failure, decreased liver mass (i.e., elderly) or pregnancy, rocuronium duration of action can be prolonged.

Vecuronium undergoes partial metabolism in the liver and is eliminated via the kidneys and in bile. Renal failure can prolong its duration of action.

Pancuronium is metabolized to a limited degree in the liver and is excreted renally.

Atracurium is broken down by Hofmann degradation and ester hydrolysis. Given this significant metabolism, only a small fraction ultimately is eliminated via the kidneys and bile.

Cisatracurium is exclusively metabolized by Hofmann elimination. It is independent of kidney or renal function, giving it a consistent duration of action.

What is Hofmann Elimination?

Hofmann degradation is a nonenzymatic, spontaneous breakdown of a compound. It occurs at normal physiologic pH and temperature in vivo. Both atracurium and cisatracurium undergo Hofmann elimination.

What are the side-effects of pancuronium?

Pancuronium can increase heart rate, blood pressure and cardiac output via vagolysis. It has increased risk of arrhythmias compared to other medications in its class. It also has a long duration of action, making it less useful in many surgical settings compared to similar medications.

What are the features of mivacurium?

Mivacurium is a benzylisoquinoline derivative. It is a short acting neuromuscular blocking drug. The onset is usually 3–5 min and its duration of action is approximately 10–20 min. It is the only nondepolarizer that is metabolized by pseudocholinesterase. Thus, patients who have either atypical plasma cholinesterase or pseudocholinesterase deficiency will have a prolonged duration of action of mivacurium in a similar manner to succinylcholine.

Does neostigmine reverse the neuromuscular blockade caused by mivacurium?

Because the anticholinesterase drug neostigmine not only inhibits true cholinesterase but also the pseudocholinesterase, there is concern about the possibility that neostigmine might paradoxically prolong the duration of mivacurium action. However, most experts believe that the benefits of increasing the concentration of acetylcholine produced by neostigmine to compete for the binding sites on the nicotonic cholinergic receptor in the neuromuscular junction should outweigh the inhibition of the activity of plasma pseudocholinesterase and therefore the action of mivacurium may be reversed. Conventional wisdom says that no reversal agent is needed given the fact that mivacurium is such a short acting drug.

Which neuromuscular blocker(s) have active metabolites?

Atracurium and cisatracurium metabolism produce laudanosine. Laudanosine has been shown to cause central nervous system excitation. This excitation has the potential to cause increased minimum alveolar concentration requirements for inhalation anesthetics and may even cause seizures. Laudanosine is metabolized in the liver and excreted in urine and bile, so patients with hepatic failure are at increased risk of laudanosine toxicity.

Which nondepolarizing muscle relaxants cause histamine release?

Like succinylcholine, several nondepolarizers are capable of triggering histamine release. They are tubocurarine > metrocurine > atracurium = mivacurium. Slow administration of the medication and/or pretreatment with H_1 and H_2 antihistamine drugs reduce this side effect.

Should any of the nondepolarizing muscle relaxants be avoided in our patient? Why or why not?

Atracurium can cause bronchospasm and should be avoided in asthmatic patients. It causes a dose-dependent release of histamine. There are also reports of atracurium-induced bronchospasm in patients without asthma.

How will you gage the depth of neuromuscular blockade?

To determine the level of muscle relaxation, a peripheral nerve stimulator is commonly used at the ulnar or facial nerve, evaluating the adductor pollicis and orbicularis oculi, respectively. To determine a "train of four," four electrical stimuli of 2 Hz are given over 2 s. When four twitches are present, the ratio of the fourth twitch compared to the first twitch gives an indication of the level of residual neuromuscular blockade. A ratio of less than 0.9 is considered to be residual blockade.

Tetany involves a single stimulus that lasts at least 5 seconds. Sustained tetany is often done with 50–100 Hz.

What is post-tetanic potentiation?

After sustained tetany, there is a transient increase in twitch height, such as with a train of four, immediately afterward. The possible cause of this is increased acetylcholine in the neuromuscular junction.

Which sources of neuromuscular blockade monitoring correlate with which muscle groups?

Monitoring of the facial nerve and assessing a train of four in the orbicularis oculi correlates with return of diaphragmatic function. The adductor pollicis correlates well with the return of function of the muscles of the larynx.

How will you determine if the patient's neuromuscular blockade is reversible?

When a patient has four twitches on train of four stimulations, they are reversible. Reversal agents can take up 10–15 min or even longer in the cases of more significant muscle relaxation, to reach peak effect and to fully reverse the patient's muscle relaxation.

What will you use for reversal and why?

Reversal of neuromuscular blockade should include both a cholinesterase inhibitor and an anticholinergic agent. The most commonly used cholinesterase inhibitor is neostigmine. It is a lipid-insoluble agent that cannot cross the blood–brain barrier. Its onset is 5–7 min and duration of action is approximately 1 hour. If neostigmine is used to reverse a long-acting muscle relaxant, it is possible that its reversal effect could wear off before the neuromuscular blocking medication, resulting in recurarization.

What are potential side-effects of reversal agents?

Cholinesterase inhibitors can cause several significant side-effects through the resulting increased levels of acetylcholine stimulating muscarinic receptors. In the cardiovascular system, they cause bradycardia. They lead to bronchospasm and increased secretions in the lungs. The gastrointestinal system will have increased secretions, salivation, and intestinal spasm. Increased rates of postoperative nausea and vomiting can result from cholinesterase inhibitor administration. Constriction of the pupils is an ophthalmological side effect.

Physostigmine is a cholinesterase inhibitor that can cross the blood–brain barrier. If given to patient, it can cause cerebral excitation. The most commonly used cholinesterase inhibitor, neostigmine, does not cross the blood–brain barrier.

How can the side-effects of cholinesterase inhibitors be minimized?

The administration of anticholinergic medications helps to mitigate several side-effects of cholinesterase inhibitors such as neostigmine. Anticholinergic drugs used in combination with cholinesterase inhibitors function by acting largely at the muscarinic acetylcholine receptors (as opposed to neuromuscular blocking drugs, which are used for their effect on nicotinic acetylcholine receptors). The recommended agent to use in conjunction with neostigmine is glycopyrrolate given their similar duration of action and the fact that they do not cross the blood–brain barrier.

What is the difference between a phase I and phase II block?

In a phase I block, which occurs after a single dose of succinylcholine, peripheral nerve stimulation shows no fade with train of four monitoring or sustained tetany. There is no post-tetanic facilitation. Recovery is rapid from a phase I block. A phase II block can occur after multiple doses of succinylcholine or with an infusion. The cause of a phase II block may be a result of repolarization of the neuromuscular junction that does not respond normally to acetylcholine given the persistent presence of succinylcholine. In a phase II block, train of four and tetanic stimulation will show fade. Recovery is variable but slower than with a phase I block.

What factors could contribute to prolonged neuromuscular blockade?

Inadequate reversal of muscle relaxants, either through underdosing of reversal agents or administration of reversal medications when the patient has not sufficiently recovered from the neuromuscular blocker can contribute to weakness. Additionally, there are several possible sources for prolongation of neuromuscular blockade. Various medications can contribute to weakness including amiodarone, verapamil, some antiretrovirals (zidovudine, lamivudine), corticosteroids, statins, some antibiotics (penicillin, tetracycline, aminoglycosides, and clindamycin), sulfonamides, NSAIDs and dantrolene. Volatile anesthetics potentiate the action of muscle relaxants. Hypothermia can worsen neuromuscular blockade. Multiple electrolyte disturbances can play a role in muscle weakness, including hypophosphatemia, hypermagnesemia, hypocalcemia, and hypokalemia.

What should be done to manage a patient with prolonged neuromuscular blockade?

If a patient has delayed recovery from muscle relaxation, sedation should be continued and respiratory support provided until the neuromuscular blockade has worn off. In a sedated patient, assessing for sustained tetany of at least 5 s is recommended periodically to determine return of muscle function.

Further Reading

1. Appiah-Ankam J, Hunter JM. Pharmacology of neuromuscular blocking drugs. Contin Educ Anaesth Crit Care Pain. 2004;4(1): 2–7.
2. Bowman WC. Neuromuscular block. Br J Pharmacol. 2006;147 (Suppl 1):S277–86.
3. Butterworth JF, IV, Mackey DC, Wasnick JD. Butterworth JF, IV, Mackey DC, Wasnick JD, Butterworth, JF, IV, et al. Chapter 11. Neuromuscular blocking agents. In: Butterworth JF, IV, Mackey DC, Wasnick JD. Butterworth JF, IV, Mackey DC, Wasnick JD, Butterworth, JF, IV, et al. editors. Morgan & Mikhail's Clinical Anesthesiology, 5e. New York, NY: McGraw-Hill; 2013. http://accessmedicine.mhmedical.com.ezp-prod1.hul.harvard.edu/content.aspx?bookid=564&Sectionid=42800542. Accessed 10 July 2015.
4. Cooperman L. Succinylcholine induced hyperkalemia in neuromuscular disease. JAMA. 1970;213:1867–71.
5. Kampe S, Krombach JW, Diefenbach C. Muscle relaxants. Best Pract Res Clin Anaesthesiol. 2003;17(1):137–46.
6. Lein CA, Kopman AF. Current recommendations for monitoring depth of neuromuscular blockade. Curr Opin Anaesthesiol. 2014;27 (6):616–22.
7. Michalska-Krzanowska G. Anaphylactic reactions during anaesthesia and the perioperative period. Anaesthesiol Intensive Ther. 2012;44(2):104–11.

Myasthenia Gravis

22

Huan Wang and Zhiling Xiong

Case:
A 52-year-old male with hyperlipidemia, myasthenia gravis, and recent diagnosis of colon cancer presents for tumor resection.

Medications	Pyridostigmine 360 mg/day Simvastatin 40 mg nightly
Allergies	NKA
Past Medical History	Hyperlipidemia, Myasthenia Gravis, Colon cancer
Physical Exam	Ht: 175 cm Wt: 62 kg
VS	Temp 36.9 °C BP 115/78 h 77 RR 16 Oxygen saturation: 98% on RA
Airway Exam	Mallampati II, 2–3 fingerbreadth thyromental distance, neck full range of motion, mouth 4 fingerbreadth opening

Alert and oriented × 3, Cardiac and lung exam normal. Abdomen soft, nontender, and non-distended. Strength is normal in all major muscle groups.

1. **What is the pathophysiology for myasthenia gravis?**

Myasthenia gravis (MG) is an autoimmune disease of the skeletal muscle neuromuscular junction (NMJ). It is caused by circulating IgG autoantibodies resulting in destruction or inactivation of the α-subunit of the muscle-type nicotinic acetylcholine receptor (nAChRs), leading to decreased ability for neural transmission, and consequently muscle weakness and fatigue. Sparing of other α-subunits of neuronal-type nicotinic acetylcholine receptors likely accounts for the lack of autonomic or CNS involvement of the disease [1].

Normally, the amount of acetylcholine released by the presynaptic motor neuron decreases with repeated stimulation, known as presynaptic rundown. In MG, the coupling of presynaptic rundown and insufficient number of activated postsynaptic receptors causes the characteristic fatigability that improves with rest often described in the disease [2].

2. **What are the mechanisms by which these antibodies reduce the number of functional receptors in myasthenia gravis?**

These antibodies reduce the number of functional receptors by several mechanisms [3]:

(1) Receptor destruction by cross-linking of receptors with the IgG antibodies.
(2) The antibody—receptor complex causes direct damage to the NMJ membrane.
(3) Different antibodies target muscle-specific receptor tyrosine kinase at the NMJ, an enzyme responsible for the arrangement of nAChRs, leading to developmental malfunction.

3. **What is the epidemiology of myasthenia gravis?**

Myasthenia gravis is considered one of the most common progressive autoimmune disorders of neuromuscular transmission. The prevalence of myasthenia gravis has been cited as 50–142 cases per 1 million people [4]. Interestingly, there is a gender discrepancy by age group, wherein younger populations (20–30 years old) females are more affected than males, and in the elderly (>60 years old) males are more frequently affected.

H. Wang (✉) · Z. Xiong
Department of Anesthesiology, Perioperative and Pain Medicine, Brigham and Women's Hospital, 75 Francis Street, Boston, MA 02115, USA
e-mail: hwang37@partners.org

Z. Xiong
e-mail: zxiong@partners.org

© Springer International Publishing AG 2017
L.S. Aglio and R.D. Urman (eds.), *Anesthesiology*,
DOI 10.1007/978-3-319-50141-3_22

4. **What are the anatomical origins of myasthenia gravis?**

Due to the strong association between MG and hyperplasia of the thymus (more than 70% of MG patients have thymus hyperplasia, and 10% have thymomas), the thymus is hypothesized to be the origin of receptor-binding antibodies. It is important to note, however, that thymectomy is not curative in all patients, thus other potential sites of antibody production have been postulated as well [5].

5. **What are the classifications of myasthenia gravis?**

There are four types of MG classifications based on the skeletal muscles involved and the severity of the symptoms [6]:

Type I Ocular MG that is limited to involvement of the extraocular muscles (~10%)
- Patients with confined ocular MG for longer than 3 years are unlikely to experience progression of their disease.

Type II Skeletal muscles weakness
- ***Type IIa***—Slowly progressive, mild form
  - Spares the muscles of respiration
  - Good response to anticholinesterase drugs and corticosteroids
- ***Type IIb***—Rapidly progressive, severe form
  - Muscles of respiration may be involved
  - Poor response to pharmacotherapy

Type III Acute onset and rapid deterioration of skeletal muscle strength within 6 months
- Associated with a high mortality rate

Type IV Severe whole body generalized muscular weakness
- Results from progression of type I or type II

6. **What are the signs and symptoms of myasthenia gravis?**

MG is characterized by skeletal (voluntary) muscle weakness and progressive fatigability after repetitive use, with improvement following rest. It may be localized to specific muscle groups or may be generalized. Symptoms can vary throughout the day and have variable duration.

(a) Facial muscles weakness—ptosis and diplopia are often the initial symptoms because skeletal muscles innervated by cranial nerves (ocular, pharyngeal, and laryngeal) are the most vulnerable.
(b) Bulbar muscles weakness—dysphagia, dysarthria, and difficulty handling saliva place the patients at high risk of pulmonary aspiration.
(c) Limb weakness—proximal muscles are affected more severely than distal ones. The distribution of arm, leg, or trunk weakness can occur in any combination and is usually asymmetrical and patchy [5].
(d) Respiratory weakness—complete respiratory compromise rarely presents in isolation, but is the defining feature of *myasthenic crisis*.

7. **What is the differential diagnosis of myasthenia gravis?** (Table 22.1) [6, 7]

8. **What are the diagnostic tests for myasthenia gravis?**
- Tensilon test (administration of anticholinesterase, i.e., edrophonium)
  - Positive if strength improves with inhibition of cholinesterase. Works by increasing the amount of acetylcholine available to interact with the decreased number of postsynaptic nACRs, improving the likelihood of adequate end-plate depolarization.
  - Edrophonium is usually administered in small doses (2-8 mg), and improvement is seen within 5 min and lasts for about 10 min.
- Electromyography
  - Confirmed by the decremental response in compound muscle action potential after repetitive nerve stimulation.
- Radioimmunoassay
  - Detection of anti-acetylcholine antibodies in the serum, however, the antibodies may not be detectable or not be present in all patients.

9. **What are the treatments for myasthenia gravis?**

Treatment of MG can be categorized into medical versus surgical methods:

Medical:

- Anticholinesterase drugs—first line of treatment
  - *Mechanism*: Inhibit enzyme responsible for hydrolysis of acetylcholine, therefore increasing the amount of neurotransmitter available at the NMJ.
    Pyridostigmine (Mestinon)
    Most widely used as it is well tolerated orally, with few muscarinic side effects and has a long duration of action.

Table 22.1 Differential diagnosis of Myasthenia Gravis

Condition	Symptoms and characteristics	Comments
Drug-induced myasthenia gravis (penicillamine, nondepolarizing muscle relaxants, aminoglycosides, procainamide)	Induced weakness in normal persons by triggering autoimmune MG; exacerbation of MG	Distinguished by improvement of symptoms after discontinuation of the drug
Eaton–Lambert syndrome	Weakness improves after repetitive use; commonly seen in small cell lung cancer	Caused by antibodies to calcium channels
Grave's disease	Diplopia, exophthalmos	Thyroid-stimulating immunoglobulin present
Botulism	Generalized weakness, ophthalmoplegia, mydriasis	Incremental response on repetitive nerve stimulation
Progressive external ophthalmoplegia	Ptosis, diplopia, generalized weakness in some cases	Mitochondrial abnormalities
Intracranial mass	Ophthalmoplegia, cranial nerve weakness	Abnormalities on CT or MRI

Adapted from Stoelting's Anesthesia and Coexisting Disease [6]

Onset is around 30 min with peak effect in 2 h and overall duration around 3-6 h

Dosing-tailored to response (max dose 120 mg PO q3hrs), 30 mg PO = 1 mg IV/IM

Higher dosages may actually induce muscle weakness, leading to *cholinergic crisis*

Confirmed by onset of muscarinic side effects (salivation, miosis, bradycardia), accentuated muscle weakness after administration of edrophonium

- Although anticholinesterase drugs benefit most patients, the improvements may be incomplete and may wane after weeks or months of treatment.

- Immunosuppression—indicated when muscle weakness not adequately controlled by anticholinesterase drugs
  - *Mechanism*: Prevent the destruction of nAChRs at the motor end plate [8]

    Corticosteriods—most commonly used and most consistently effective, but also associated with the greatest likelihood of adverse effects [9]

    Azathioprine or Cyclopsorine—can be used in patients who do not respond or cannot tolerate corticosteroids [10]
- Short-Term Immunotherapy
  - *Plasmapheresis*—used for short-term symptomatic improvement in patients who are experiencing *myasthenic crisis*, respiratory compromise, or are being prepared for thymectomy [11]

    Mechanism: removes antibodies from the circulation, allowing receptors to proliferate

    Transient effects, improvement occurs over days with decreased ventilatory dependence

    Repeated treatments could lead to increased risk of infection, hypotension, and pulmonary embolism.
  - *Immunoglobulins*—same indications and mechanism as plasmapheresis

    Does not have effect on circulating concentrations of acetylcholine receptor antibodies.

Surgical:

- Thymectomy—goal is to induce remission or at least reduce the dosage of pharmacotherapy [12]
  - *Mechanism*: Speculative, hypothesized removal of antigenic stimulus by the removal of myoid cells, or alterations in immune regulation by removal of the thymus

    Acetylcholine receptor antibody titer usually decreases following successful thymectomy with clinical improvement [13]
  - *Surgical approach*:

    Median sternotomy—optimizes visualization and removal of all tissues

    Mediastinoscopy through a cervical incision – associated with a smaller incision and less postoperative pain
  - *Postoperative*:

    Decreased need for anticholinesterase medication, full benefit often delayed for months after surgery.

Preoperative

10. **How would you manage a MG patient based on their preoperative medications?**
    - Anticholinesterase—the decision to continue or hold the dose on the morning of surgery is per the discretion of the surgeon or the anesthesiologist. Some choose to hold the dose to avoid interactions with neuromuscular blocking agents [14].
    - Corticosteroids—often will require perioperative stress dose steroid coverage
    - Plasmapheresis—will require preoperatively if the patient's disease is poorly controlled [15]

- Anxiolytics/opioids—try to avoid given likely pre-existing respiratory muscles weakness.

11. **What are some of the anesthetic considerations preoperatively?**
    - Cardiovascular—MG patients have increased risk for heart disease because the culprit antibodies have a high affinity for β1 and β2 adrenergic receptors [16]. Patients often have comorbid atrial fibrillation, heart block, or cardiomyopathy.
    - Airway protection—bulbar involvement can severely compromise the patient's ability to cough and clear secretions, as well as protect or maintain a patent airway
    - Respiratory muscle strength:
      - Pulmonary function tests (PFTs)—useful for quantifying respiratory muscle strength, specifically negative inspiratory pressure and forced vital capacity (FVC).

        Optimizing strength and respiratory function—if vital capacity <2L, plasmapheresis is usually performed preoperatively to increase the likelihood for adequate pulmonary function postoperatively.

        It is important to inform the patient about the possibility of postoperative ventilator support.

        May be necessary to use as a reference to determine the optimal conditions for extubation, as well as a predictor tool for the need for postoperative mechanical ventilation [17].
      - Flow volume loops—useful if a thymoma presents as an anterior mediastinal mass, which could lead to intrathoracic airway or vascular obstruction upon the induction of anesthesia.

    - Maximal inspiratory and expiratory flow volume loops obtained with the patient in supine and upright positions will measure the extent of the respiratory impairment as well as whether the impairment is fixed or dynamic.
    - Autoimmune disease—MG is associated with other autoimmune diseases, including hypothyroidism (∼10% of patients with MG), rheumatoid arthritis, systemic lupus erythematous, and pernicious anemia.

12. **What are some risk factors for the need for mechanical ventilation during the postoperative period?**
    a. Disease duration of longer than 6 years
    b. Presence of COPD or pulmonary disease unrelated to myasthenia gravis
    c. Daily dose of pyridostigmine more than 750 mg
    d. Vital capacity of less than 2.9 L
    e. Frequent crisis

<u>**Intraoperative**</u>:

13. **Can neuraxial anesthesia be safely used in this case?**
    Neuraxial anesthesia with epidural and spinal anesthesia can safely be used in MG patients. However, it is important that muscle function and ventilation be carefully monitored perioperatively.
    - Choice of local anesthetic—Amide
      - Use reduced doses of amide to avoid high blood levels
      - Avoid ester anesthetics. They are metabolized by cholinesterase and may have prolonged elevated levels in patients on anticholinesterase drugs.
    - Local anesthetic effects—monitor for weakness
      - Be mindful that local anesthetics themselves can potentiate neuromuscular blocking agents by decreasing the sensitivity of the post-junctional membrane to acetylcholine, leading to further weakness in MG patients

14. **Can the patient be paralyzed with nondepolarizing muscle relaxants?**
    Nondepolarizing neuromuscular blockers can be used in patients with MG, however, it must be used with caution:
    - Dose—decreased dosing due to increased sensitivity
      - There is increased sensitivity to nondepolarizing anesthetics due to the decreased number of acetylcholine receptors requiring blockade
      - Drug onset is shorter, duration is longer
      - Effect of continued preoperative anticholinesterase treatment

        Higher initial dose might be needed due to increased resistance—higher amounts of acetylcholine available to outcompete nondepolarizing muscle relaxants [18]

        Prolonged recovery after reversal has been reported [19]

        Cholinesterase depletion can affect the breakdown of mivacurium, which is metabolized by pseudocholinesterase, resulting in a prolonged block
    - Monitoring—use peripheral never stimulator at baseline and throughout the case
      - Due to the unreliable nature of drug response, peripheral nerve stimulators should be used throughout the case, and the dosing of any nondepolarizing muscle relaxant should be increased in small increments corresponding to 0.1–0.2

times the 95% effective dose (ED_{95}) until the desired neuromuscular blocking effect is achieved.
- Alternatives
  - Volatile anesthetics—can try to avoid muscle relaxants by using inhaled agents for both facilitating intubation and providing relaxation for surgery
  - Regional techniques—reduce or eliminate the need for muscle relaxation for surgery

15. **What is the response to succinylcholine for patients with MG?**
Even in MG patients, succinylcholine can be used if needed for rapid tracheal intubation.
    - Increased dose is usually required in patients with MG due to resistance from the loss of functional acetylcholine receptors.
    - The ED_{95} of succinylcholine in MG patients is 2.6 times that in non-myasthenic patients (0.8 mg/kg vs. 0.3 mg/kg) [20].
    - However, the dose of succinylcholine used for rapid airway control in normal patients (1.5–2.0 mg/kg body weight) is approximately 5 times ED_{95}, which means our normal dose of 1.5–2.0 mg/kg should be adequate for most MG patients for rapid intubation as well.
    - Myasthenic patients are more likely than normal patients to develop a phase II block, particularly with repeated doses of succinylcholine [21].
    - Prolonged block—cholinesterase depletion due to plasmapheresis or inhibition caused by pyridostigmine given preoperatively may decrease the metabolism of succinylcholine causing prolonged block [22]

16. **What are the effects of volatiles anesthetics in this patient?**
    - Inhaled volatiles anesthetics provide profound muscular relaxation and can be used alternatively due to the difficulty in predicting neuromuscular blocker response in MG patients.
    - If used in conjunction, sevoflurane was shown to potentiate the effects of nondepolarizing agents to the greatest degree of all the volatile anesthetics in patients with MG [23].

17. **What are the effects of other IV drugs in patients with MG that should be considered?**
    - IV anesthetics (barbiturates, propofol, etomidate, ketamine)—all have been used without event
    - Opioids:
      - Do not appear to depress neuromuscular transmission in MG
      - Central respiratory depression could be problematic in patients with decreased pulmonary reserve, therefore their use in MG patients should always be minimized if possible
      - More desirable to use titratable short-acting opioids such as remifentanyl
    - Beta adrenergic blockers—exacerbate MG
    - Aminoglycosides antibiotics, polymyxins—prolong neuromuscular blockade

Postoperative

18. **What is the differential for weakness in MG patients after surgery?**
Weakness after surgery in MG patients is a unique scenario with a broad differential.
    - Myasthenic crisis versus Cholinergic crisis
      - Myasthenic crisis—exacerbation of the symptoms of myasthenia gravis
      - Cholinergic crisis—precipitated by excessive anticholinesterase and is characterized by increased weakness and excessive muscarinic effects including salivation, diarrhea, miosis, and bradycardia
      - Diagnosis—IV edrophonium (see "Tensilon test" from above)
        If patient's symptoms improve → myasthenic crisis
        If patient's symptoms worsen → cholinergic crisis
    - Residual effects of anesthetic drugs
    - Nonanesthetic drugs interfering with neuromuscular transmission (antibiotics, corticosteroids, etc.)

19. **What are some postoperative considerations for MG patients?**
Extubation—needs to be carefully planned based on the preoperative condition of the patient, the surgical procedure, and the residual anesthetic effects. Things to consider:
    - Patient needs to be very awake prior to extubation due to increased risk for weakness
    - Adequate postoperative pain control
    - Pulmonary toilet
    - Avoidance of drugs that interfere with neuromuscular transmission

All patients with MG should be closely monitored postoperatively in the postanesthesia care unit or the surgical intensive care unit, where respiratory support can be immediately reinstituted.

References

1. Miller RD. "Myasthenia Gravis." *Miller's Anesthesia*. New York: Elsevier/Churchill Livingstone. 2005.
2. Maselli RA. Pathophysiology of myasthenia gravis and Lambert-Eaton syndrome. Neurol Clin. 1994;12:285–303.
3. Postevka E. Anesthetic implications of Myasthenia Gravis: a case report. AANA J 2013;81(5).
4. Hirsch NP. Neuromuscular junction in health and disease. Br J Anaesth. 2007;99(1):132–8. doi:10.1093/bja/aem144.
5. Abel M, Eisenkraft JB. Anesthetic implications of myasthenia gravis. Mt Sinai J Med. 2002;69(1–2):31–7.
6. Stoeling RK, Hines RL, Marschall KE. "Myasthenia Gravis" *Stoelting's Anesthesia and co-existing disease*. 6th ed. Philadelphia, PA: Saunders/Elsevier; 2012.
7. Drachman DB. Myasthenia gravis. N Engl J Med. 1994;330: 1797–810.
8. Cornelio JF, Antozzi C, Mantegazza R, et al. Immunosuppressive treatments: their efficacy on myasthenia gravis patient's outcome and on the natural course of the disease. Ann NY Acad Sci. 1993;681:594–602.
9. Pascuzzi RM, Coslett B, Johns TR. Long-term corticosteroid treatment of myasthenia gravis: repot of 116 patients. Ann Neurol. 1984;15:291–8.
10. Schalke BCG, Kappos L, Dommasch D, et al. Cyclosporine A in the treatment of myasthenia gravis: a controlled randomized double blind trial cyclosporine A/Azathioprine-study design and first results. Muscle Nerve. 1986;9(Suppl):157.
11. Perlo VP, Shahani BT, Higgins CE, et al. Effect of plasmapheresis in myasthenia gravis. Ann N Y Acad Sci. 1981;377:709–24.
12. Kirschner PA. The history of surgery of the thymus gland. Chest Surg Clin N Am. 2000;10:153–65.
13. Vincent A, Newsome-Davids J, Newton P, et al. Acetylcholine receptor antibody and clinical response to thymectomy in myasthenia gravis. Neurology. 1983;33:1276–82.
14. Baraka A, Taha S, Yazbeck V, et al. Vecuronium block in the myasthenic patient. Influence of anticholinesterase therapy. Anaesthesia. 1993;48:588–90.
15. Howard JF. The treatment of myasthenia gravis with plasma exchange. Semin Neurol. 1982;2:273–88.
16. Narin C, Sarkilar G, Tanyeli O, Ege E, Yeniterzi M. Successful mitral valve surgery in a patient with myasthenia gravis. J Card Surg. 2009;24(2):210–2.
17. Naguib M, el Dawlatly AA, Ashour M, et al. Multivariate determinants of the need for postoperative ventilation in myasthenia gravis. Can J Anaesth. 1996;43:1006–13.
18. Tripathi M, Kaushik S, Dubey P. The effect of use of pyridostigmine and requirement of vecuronium in patients with myasthenia gravis. J Postgrad Med. 2003;49(4):311–314 (discussion 314–315).
19. Kim JM, Mangold J. Sensitivity to both vecuronium and neostigmine in a sero-negative myasthenic patient. Br J Anaesth. 1989;63:497–500.
20. Eisenkraft JB, Book WJ, Mann SM, et al. Resistance to succinylcholine in myasthenia gravis: a dose-response study. Anesthesiology. 1988;69:760–3.
21. Baraka A, Baroody M, Yazbeck V. Repeated doses of suxamethonium in the myasthenic patient. Anaesthesia. 1993;28:782–4.
22. Baraka A. Suxamethonium block in the myasthenic patient. Correlation with plasma cholinesterase. Anaesthesia. 1992;47: 217–9.
23. Nitahara K, Sugi Y, Higa K, Shono S, Hamada T. Neuromuscular effects of sevoflurane in myasthenia gravis patients. Br J Anaesth. 2007;98(3):337–41. doi:10.1093/bja/ael368.

Malignant Hyperthermia

23

Milad Sharifpour and Raheel Bengali

Case

A 17-year-old male is brought from the emergency room to the operating room for a laparoscopic appendectomy for acute appendicitis.

PMHx: The patient does not have any medical problems.

PSHx: The patient has not had any surgical procedures in the past.

Medications:
1. Occasional ibuprofen for headaches
Allergies: NKDA
Physical Examination:
Vital Signs: T: 99.1 HR: 82 RR: 17 SaO_2: 100% on RA BP: 114/73 Ht: 71" Wt: 74kg

The patient appears diaphoretic. The rest of the physical examination is only notable for RLQ pain, which worsens with deep palpation, with no other abnormalities.

Standard American Society of Anesthesiologist monitors (non-invasive blood pressure cuff, pulse oximeter, EKG leads) are placed. Rapid sequence induction is performed, using intravenous propofol and fentanyl to induce general anesthesia and succinylcholine to facilitate tracheal intubation. The trachea is intubated using a MAC 3 blade and a 7.5 endotracheal tube (ETT). Correct ETT placement is confirmed by chest rise, auscultation, and capnography. An oropharyngeal temperature probe and an upper body forced air warming blanked are subsequently placed. Two grams of cefazolin are administered before surgical incision. General anesthesia is maintained with a mixture of sevoflurane, oxygen, and air. Six milligrams of intravenous morphine is administered, in two-milligram aliquots, for analgesia.

Half way through the case, the surgeon asks for additional muscle relaxation, as the abdomen "feels tight". You notice that the patient is tachycardic (HR: 102 and regular) and has an elevated end-tidal carbon dioxide (E_TCO_2 48 mmHg) despite no changes in minute ventilation.

You notify the surgeon and page your attending for additional help.

1. **What is your differential diagnosis?**
   A. Malignant Hyperthermia
   B. Infection/fever
   C. Inadequate depth of anesthesia/analgesia
   D. Neuroleptic malignant syndrome
   E. Thyroid Storm
   F. Pheochromocytoma
   G. Anaphylaxis
   H. Hypoventilation

2. **What is Malignant Hyperthermia (MH)?**

Malignant hyperthermia is a rare and potentially deadly pharmacogenetic disorder, which presents in susceptible individuals upon exposure to triggering agents [1].

Unregulated release of calcium from the sarcoplasmic reticulum into the myoplasm, secondary to a defect in ryanodine receptor protein (RYR1), leads to a hypermetabolic state characterized by uncontrolled muscle contraction (rigidity), heat production, excess carbon dioxide (CO_2) production, acidosis, hyperkalemia, rhabdomyolysis, and myoglobinuria.

M. Sharifpour
Department of Anesthesia, Critical Care, and Pain Medicine, Massachusetts General Hospital, 55 Fruit Street, Boston, MA 02114, USA
e-mail: msharifpour@partners.org

R. Bengali (✉)
Department of Anesthesiology, Perioperative and Pain Medicine, Brigham and Women's Hospital, 75 Francis Street, Boston, MA 02115, USA
e-mail: rbengali@partners.org

© Springer International Publishing AG 2017
L.S. Aglio and R.D. Urman (eds.), *Anesthesiology*,
DOI 10.1007/978-3-319-50141-3_23

3. **What are the triggers for MH?**

Halogenated volatile anesthetics, non-depolarizing muscle relaxant succinylcholine, and in rare instances physical exertion in presence of high temperature.

4. **What are the early clinical signs of MH?** [1, 2]
   A. Sustained jaw rigidity after administration of succinylcholine
   B. Tachycardia
   C. Irregular rhythm
   D. Tachypnia
   E. Hot soda lime canister
   F. Hypercarbia

5. **What are the late clinical signs of MH?** [1, 2]
   A. Increased temperature
   B. Cyanosis
   C. Generalized muscle rigidity
   D. Dark/deoxygenated blood on the surgical field
   E. Dark urine
   F. Oliguria
   G. Disseminated intravascular coagulation

6. **What changes are seen in monitored variables?**
   A. Increased end-tidal CO_2 (early)
   B. Increased heart rate (early)
   C. Decreased SaO_2 (late)
   D. Increased body temperature (late)

7. **What laboratory abnormalities are seen in patients with MH?**
   A. Increased $PaCO_2$
   B. Decreased PaO_2
   C. Hyperkalemia
   D. Acidosis (respiratory and metabolic)
   E. Myoglobinuria
   F. Increased creatinine kinase
   G. Hemolytic anemia, thrombocytopenia

8. **How is MH diagnosed?**

In the absence of personal or family history suggestive of MH, it is impossible to identify individuals susceptible to MH. Caffeine-Halothane contracture test (or the in vitro contracture test) is the gold standard for testing individuals at risk for MH, and to confirm a clinical diagnosis of MH [1, 2].

Two grams of muscle tissue is harvested from quadriceps muscle. Muscle fascicles are exposed separately to 3% halothane, as well as increasing concentrations of caffeine, in a bath of bicarbonated Krebs-Ringer's solution. Subsequently, a supramaximal electrical current is applied to each muscle strip and a force transducer measures the resulting isometric contraction. The sensitivity of caffeine-halothane contracture test is 97% and its specificity is 78%.

Molecular genetic testing is an alternative and less invasive method to confirm MH susceptibility in individuals with appropriate personal or family history of MH. However, unlike caffeine-halothane contracture test, a negative molecular genetic test does not rule out MH susceptibility.

9. **Does a previous uneventful anesthetic rule out MH susceptibility?**

Previous uneventful anesthetic(s) do not rule out the possibility of MH susceptibility and a patient can develop an MH crisis despite previous uneventful anesthetics.

10. **What myopathies or syndromes are associated with MH?**
   A. Central core disease
   B. Multiminicore disease
   C. King-Denborough syndrome

All three conditions are associated with an RYR1 defect [1]. While a number of musculoskeletal abnormalities, such as strabismus, scoliosis, and hernias have been associated with MH susceptibility, there is no evidence to support such association.

11. **How is MH treated?**

Early recognition is the cornerstone of treating MH and is associated with improved outcomes. Dantrolene sodium is the only definitive therapy for treating MH crisis. It binds to the ryanodine receptor and prevents further release of calcium from the sarcoplasmic reticulum.

12. **How should an MH crisis be managed?**

Once the diagnosis is made, the surgeon should be notified and extra help should be requested.

Triggering agents (volatile anesthetics) should be discontinued immediately and the anesthetic should be converted to total intravenous anesthesia with non-triggering agents (propofol, opioids, benzodiazepines, ketamine). Activated charcoal filters should be placed in the inspiratory and expiratory ports of the anesthesia machine to accelerate removal of triggering anesthetic gases. The patient should be ventilated with 100% oxygen at high flows to prevent rebreathing [3, 4].

Additional intravenous lines (peripheral or central), an arterial line, and a urinary catheter should be placed, if not already in place.

Intravenous dantrolene sodium (2.5 mg/kg bolus) should be administered as soon as possible. If there is no response (decrease in temperature, decrease in heart rate, decrease in CO_2 production) within five minutes, a further 1 mg/kg bolus should be administered. This should be repeated every five minutes until there is clinical response [3, 4].

The patient should be cooled, using cooling blankets and cold intravenous fluids, and by placing ice packs in the axillae and groin.

Hyperkalemia should be treated with intravenous dextrose, insulin, and sodium bicarbonate. In case of life-threatening hyperkalemia (arrhythmias and EKG changes), calcium chloride should be administered, despite the possibility that it can exacerbate MH reaction [3, 4].

Myoglobinuria should be treated with intravenous crystalloids, bicarbonate (to alkalinize the urine), mannitol (dantrolene preparations contain mannitol), and furosemide.

Arrhythmias should be managed by treating the underlying metabolic abnormalities and hypoxemia.

Blood gases, electrolytes, and coagulation studies should be checked frequently to monitor the correction of metabolic derangements.

The MH Hotline (800) 986-4287 should be contacted for additional assistance.

The patient should be admitted to the intensive care unit for close monitoring in case of recurrence of MH symptoms and metabolic derangements.

13. **How is dantrolene prepared?**

Each vial of dantrolene sodium contains 20 mg of the drug, which is lipophilic, and 3 g of mannitol to improve water solubility. Before intravenous administration, the contents of each vial should be dissolved in 60 ml of sterile preservative free water.

This is a time consuming process and at least one member of the team should be dedicated to preparing the dantrolene.

14. **What are the common side effects of dantrolene?**
    A. Nausea
    B. Muscle weakness
    C. Dizziness
    D. Hepatic failure

15. **Given the elevated intracellular calcium, should this patient be treated with calcium channel blockers (e.g. verapamil)?**

Verapamil should be avoided as the combination of verapamil and dantrolene can have significant negative inotropic effect and cause cardiovascular collapse [4].

16. **Can muscular rigidity develop in the presence of neuromuscular blockade?**

Triggering agents directly affect the ryanodine receptor protein, which leads to release of calcium from the sarcoplasmic reticulum, without requiring action potential generation. Therefore, muscular rigidity can develop in presence of neuromuscular blocking agents. This generalized rigidity indicates depletion of ATP, which is required for muscle relaxation [4].

17. **Does MH crisis only occur in the operating room?**

No. Malignant Hyperthermia crisis can have delayed onset and occur in the postoperative period. It is imperative to have a low index of suspicion in patients who exhibit tachycardia, tachypnea, hypercapnia, and hyperpyrexia after exposure to triggering agents [1].

Similarly, there are case reports of so-called "awake MH" in MH susceptible individuals without general anesthesia, in response to viral illness, exposure to high environmental temperatures, and physical stress at the time of an awake MH event [1].

18. **How should this patient be managed in the future if he requires surgery?**

Regional anesthesia (neuraxial or peripheral nerve blocks) should be utilized when possible. If general anesthesia and controlled ventilation are indicated, a non-triggering approach, using intravenous anesthetics (propofol, ketamine, barbiturates, benzodiazepines), opioids, and non-depolarizing muscles relaxants should be used.

The anesthesia machine should be flushed with high flow oxygen to purge the system of residual volatile anesthetics. Activated charcoal filters should be placed in the inspiratory and the expiratory limbs of the machine to expedite this process.

References

1. Hopkins PM. Malignant hyperthermia: advances in clinical management and diagnosis. Br J Anaesth. 2000;85(1):118–28.
2. Glahn KPE, Ellis FR, Halsall PJ, Muller CR, Snoeck MMJ, Urwyler A, Wappler F. Recognizing and managing a malignant hyperthermia crisis: guidelines from the European malignant hyperthermia group. Br J Anaesth. 2010;105(4):417–20.
3. Hopkins PM. Malignant hyperthermia. Anaesth Intensive Care Med. 2011;12(6):263–5.
4. Schneiderbanger D, Johannsen S, Rowewer N, Schuster F. Management of malignant hyperthermia: diagnosis and treatment. Ther Clin Risk Manag. 2014;14(10):355–62.

Part V
The Endocrine System

Section Editor: Sibinka Bajic

Sibinka Bajic
Department of Anesthesiology, Perioperative and Pain Medicine,
Brigham and Women's Hospital, Boston, MA, USA

Diabetes Mellitus

24

Amit Prabhakar, Jonathan G. Ma, Anthony Woodall, and Alan D. Kaye

Case A 44-year-old obese woman presents with a 3-day history of abdominal pain, weakness, headache, polyuria, nausea, and vomiting. Upon arrival, she states that she has not taken any of her prescribed medications for the past week. She has a 5-year history of diabetes mellitus (DM) II. CT of the abdomen and pelvis reveals a perforated appendix.

Medications:	Lantus 20 units BID, HCTZ 25mg daily, Simvistatin 20 mg QHS, Lisinopril 20 mg daily.
Allergies:	Sulfa
Past Medical History:	Type 2 DM, hyperlipidemia, hypertension, obesity
Physical Exam	
Height:	60 inches
Weight:	100 kg
VS:	BP 90/50
	HR 110
	Temp 38.5
	RR 22

A. Prabhakar (✉)
Department of Anesthesiology, University Medical Center, 4621 Prytania Street, New Orleans, LA 70115, USA
e-mail: aprab1@lsuhsc.edu; aprab2@lsuhsc.edu

J.G. Ma
Louisiana State University Health and Sciences Center, 1542 Tulane Avenue, Room 659, New Orleans, LA 70112, USA
e-mail: jma@lsuhsc.edu

A. Woodall
Department of Anesthesiology, Louisiana State Hospital, 1542 Tulane Ave. Suite 653, New Orleans, LA 70112, USA
e-mail: awoo11@lsuhsc.edu

A.D. Kaye
Department of Anesthesiology, 1542 Tulane Ave., Room 659, New Orleans, LA 70112, USA
e-mail: alankaye44@hotmail.com

© Springer International Publishing AG 2017
L.S. Aglio and R.D. Urman (eds.), *Anesthesiology*,
DOI 10.1007/978-3-319-50141-3_24

1. **How is diabetes mellitus characterized and what are the most common forms?**

Hyperglycemia of DM is the consequence of relative or absolute deficiency of insulin and a relative or absolute excess of glucagon. In **Type 1 DM**, there is an absolute deficiency in insulin production and dependency on exogenous insulin to prevent lipolysis and eventually ketoacidosis. The onset of Type 1 diabetes usually occurs by adolescence, although it may occur at any age and is thought to result from to autoimmune destruction of the islets of Langerhans cells in the pancreas [1].

Type 2 DM is characterized by a relative deficiency of insulin, typically caused by insulin resistance. The onset is usually in adulthood and the specific etiology is unknown, however this form is strongly linked to obesity. **Gestational diabetes** is defined as any degree of glucose intolerance with the onset first recognized during pregnancy. These patients may have a predisposition to developing Type 2 DM later in life.

Hyperglycemia has been recognized as a major factor in the development of complications associated with diabetes. Chronic hyperglycemia leads to angiopathy and long-term complications involving the various organs. The cause of diabetic complications is multifactorial, including glycosylation of proteins and glucose reduction to sorbitol, which functions as a tissue toxin. This pathophysiologic process is associated with a decrease in myoinositol content, metabolism, and with a decrease in sodium-potassium-adenosine triphosphatase activity. Microangiopathy can cause: diabetic cardiomyopathy, nephropathy, neuropathy, retinopathy, and encephalopathy. Macroangiopathy leads to CAD, PVD, diabetic myonectosis, and stroke. Diabetes is a major risk factor for heart disease, stroke, kidney disease, blindness, and nontraumatic amputations.

2. **A medical student approaches you and asks if this patient could have Metabolic syndrome X. What is Syndrome X?**

Metabolic syndrome is also known as insulin resistance syndrome, cardiometabolic syndrome, and Reaven's syndrome. As the name implies, it is a syndrome rather than a specific disease state. The syndrome is caused by an underlying disorder of energy utilization and storage and the cause is still unknown. Diagnosis is made by co-occurrence of 3 out of 5 following medical conditions: central obesity, HTN, high fasting plasma glucose/impaired glucose tolerance, high serum triglycerides, and low HDL.

Prevalence in the USA is an estimated 34% of adult population and prevalence increases with age. The metabolic syndrome increases the risk of developing cardiovascular disease, particularly heart failure and diabetes. The hallmark of syndrome X is insulin resistance with hyperinsulinemia. The clinical significance of this condition stems from its association with multiple metabolic abnormalities, including low levels of high-density lipoprotein (HDL), increased blood pressure, and increased plasminogen activator inhibitor-1 levels. All these abnormalities have definite or possible association with coronary artery disease. Whether syndrome X and Type 2 DM are on a spectrum of disease with insulin resistance as a common denominator or are totally separate entities has yet to be clearly understood.

3. **What are some other less common causes of glucose intolerance?**

There are several rare genetic diseases that result in defects in both Beta-cell production of insulin and insulin action [2]. Other causes result from destruction of the exocrine pancreas from inflammatory processes like pancreatitis, specific viral infections such as rubella, Coxsackie B, mumps, and cytomegalovirus, and immune mediated insulin autoantibodies or insulin receptor antibodies [2].

4. **What is the prevalence of diabetes?**

Recent data suggest that the overall prevalence of diabetes in the United States is 9.3% [3]. Type 1 DM accounts for approximately 5–10% of diabetic population [1]. Type 2 DM accounts for the remaining 90–95% of patients. Gestational DM has an incidence of approximately 7% among pregnant women [1, 4]. Experts predict the overall prevalence of DM to increase by 200% in the next several decades as rates of obesity continue to climb worldwide [5, 6].

5. **What are the diagnostic criteria for diabetes mellitus?**

Current diagnostic criteria from the American Diabetes Association include one of the following findings [7]:

1. Hemoglobin $A1_c$ greater than or equal to 6.5%.
2. Fasting plasma glucose level greater than or equal to 126 mg/dL
3. Symptoms of diabetes and a random blood glucose level >200 mg/dL
4. Oral glucose tolerance test with 2 h plasma glucose level greater than or equal to 200 mg/dL

6. **What are management strategies for the different types of DM?**

Treatment of DM includes diet, oral hypoglycemic drugs, exogenous insulin, exercise, and weight reduction if warranted. Management of Type 1 DM requires administration of exogenous insulin analogues. Titration of rapid and long-acting analogues is often required to achieve euglycemia and to mimic the normal basal and postprandial insulin secretion responses. Different insulin preparations are encountered in diabetric patients being assessed for surgery, and understanding their time-action profiles and side effects is essential in clinical management.

Rapid acting insulin (*lispro/*Humalog® and *aspart/ NovoLog*®) analogues have quick onset of action (between 5 and 15 min), peak activity at 2 h after injection and their duration of action does not exceed 5 h [1].

Long-acting insulin analogues include NPH and glargine (Lantus®) which have a prolonged effect secondary to lower solubility. Lower solubility is achieved by amino acid substitution and addition of zinc to human insulin [8, 9]. This time-action profile allows for once-daily dosing and duration of action of 18–24 h.

Regular insulin is short-acting insulin best utilized intravenously for glucose control during intraoperative period.

In the past decade, newer therapies for newly diagnosed Type 1 DM have been introduced, including immunosuppression with varied successes. It is important to realize that 15% of patients with Type 1 DM have other autoimmune processes and that the elevated glucose levels are probably caused by destruction of pancreatic beta cells in these instances.

Management of Type 2 DM entails a wide array of anti-diabetic medications and lifestyle modifications that can also be supplemented by insulin analogues if needed.

An overview of the various anti-diabetic pharmacological agents currently available is described below:

Sulfonylureas (glyburide, glipizide, glimepiride): These medications act by both stimulating insulin secretion by beta cells and improving peripheral sensitivity to insulin.

Biguanides (metformin): This class of medications acts by improving skeletal muscle insulin sensitivity, decreasing hepatic gluconeogenesis, and decreasing glycogenolysis. These should be stopped 48–72 h prior to surgery to prevent an increased risk of lactic acidosis.

Thiazolidinediones (pioglitazone and rosiglitazone): These act as insulin sensitizers by increasing the efficiency of glucose transporters via altering gene transcription. Side effects include potential hepatic injury, fluid retention, and increased incidence of myocardial ischemia.

Alpha-glucosidase inhibitors (acarbose and miglitol): Glucosidase is an enzyme that is present in the brush border of the small intestine. Enzyme inhibition results in reduction of carbohydrate breakdown and subsequent delayed glucose absorption. This helps to attenuate postprandial glucose surges.

Meglitinides (repaglinide and nateglinide): These work by increasing beta-cell insulin secretion. Of note, they have a faster onset and shorter duration of action relative to Sulfonylureas.

Amylin analogues: Amylin is a pancreatic hormone that is released in conjunction with insulin. Its release induces a decrease in glucagon secretion, slower gastric emptying, and satiety. Pramlintide is an example and is administered subcutaneously.

Incretin mimetics (exenatide and liraglutide): Incretins are intestinal peptides that are secreted in response to food intake. These peptides work by decreasing glucagon secretion, hepatic glucose production, and gastric emptying subsequently resulting in appetite suppression. Their use is limited by rapid enzymatic breakdown by DPP-4.

Dipeptidyl peptidase-IV(DPP-4) inhibitors (sitagliptin and saxagliptin): DPP-4 is responsible for the rapid degradation of incretins. Thus inhibition prolongs the beneficial effects of endogenous incretins. Examples include sitagliptin and saxagliptin.

7. **Preoperatively, how would you determine patient's degree of glycemic control?**

Close monitoring of glucose levels by both the patient and physician are imperative to prevent or prolong the onset of systemic consequences. Active involvement by a motivated patient is essential to effectively manage the disease. Fingerstick blood sampling should be done one to three times daily depending on the degree of insulin deficiency. Patients should also keep a log of eating habits and daily blood glucose levels to assess the need for lifestyle and or medication modifications. Regularly scheduled checkups for onset of hypertension and hyperlipidemia are important as these can significantly increase the risk of vascular disease.

Hemoglobin A1c (HgbA1c) is a measure of glycosylated hemoglobin and is considered a marker of long-term glycemic control. HgbA1c correlates with the average blood glucose over a 3-month span, or the life span of a red blood cell. An HgbA1c of 6% indicates average blood glucose less than 120 mg/dl. An HgbA1c of 8% correlates with an average blood glucose of 180 mg/dl. An HgbA1c of 10% corresponds to average blood glucose of 240 mg/dl [5].

8. **What are complications associated with DM?**

DM is a complex disease that involves all organ systems with numerous wide-ranging complications. A summary of these are below.

Cardiovascular Disease

Chronic DM can lead to significant complications in both the micro- and macrovasculature. Diabetics are at a significantly increased risk of developing hypertension, coronary artery disease, peripheral artery disease, systolic and diastolic dysfunction, and congestive heart failure [5]. Cardiovascular pathology has been shown to be the cause of death in 80% of diabetic patients [5]. Numerous studies have shown that diabetics have a two- to threefold increase of perioperative cardiovascular morbidity and mortality compared to nondiabetics [10]. The American College of Cardiology and the American Heart Association guidelines for preoperative cardiac assessment classify diabetics as a minimum of intermediate risk if undergoing noncardiac surgery [5, 11]. Autonomic neuropathy in patients with DM can greatly impair the sensation of ischemic cardiac pain and can result in an unrecognized cardiac event or silent myocardial infarction. The Framingham study found that 39% of diabetic patients had an unrecognized myocardial infarction compared to 22% in nondiabetics [5, 12].

Hypertension and diabetic cardiomyopathy are also major concerns for diabetic patients. Echocardiographic studies have shown that 60–75% of asymptomatic, well-controlled diabetic patients have diastolic dysfunction and increased left ventricular filling pressures [13]. With time, this initial dysfunction can progress to heart failure. The onset of hypertension in diabetics closely correlates with the development of microalbuminuria and subsequent nephropathy. Trials have shown that using an angiotensin-converting enzyme inhibitor or beta-blocker for blood pressure control reduced the risk of death in diabetic patients [14].

Gastroparesis

Diabetes affects the gastrointestinal tract in several ways. First, it damages the ganglion cells of the gastrointestinal tract, inhibiting motility, which delays gastric emptying and overall transit time through the gut. Gastrointestinal system dysfunction is common in patients with DM and is closely related to vagal autonomic neuropathy. Radioisotopic studies have shown that approximately 50% of patients with long standing DM have delayed gastric emptying [15]. Radionuclide studies have shown that the rate of gastric emptying of liquids between diabetic and nondiabetic patients is similar. However, there is a significant delay in gastric emptying of solids in diabetics compared to nondiabetics [16]. Signs and symptoms of gastroparesis include anorexia, nausea, vomiting, bloating, and epigastric discomfort [5]. Thus diabetic patients are at a greater risk of aspiration when compared to nondiabetics and consideration of rapid sequence intubation should be included in your anesthetic plan. Preoperative treatment with agents that inhibit acid secretion and neutralize stomach acid is essential. Use of famotidine, metoclopramide, or a liquid antacid preoperatively can reduce the risk of aspiration. Rapid sequence induction is commonly employed to try to minimize the risk of aspiration in patients with symptoms of gastroparesis.

Autonomic Neuropathy

DM can have extensive consequences on both the autonomic and peripheral nervous systems. Diabetic autonomic neuropathy can manifest as resting tachycardia, exercise intolerance, orthostatic hypotension, constipation, gastroparesis, impaired neurovascular function, genitourinary dysfunction, and hypoglycemic autonomic failure [5]. The majority of these issues can be elucidated by a thorough history and physical exam.

Heart rate variability in response to Valsalva, deep breathing, or position changes can predict an increased likelihood of hemodynamic instability under anesthesia [17]. Autonomic dysfunction also affects the body's ability to regulate blood pressure, leading to significant orthostatic hypotension. This underlying defect is caused by a lack of baroreceptor reflex induced vasoconstriction. This denervation may also involve vagal control of the heart rate. The changes in heart rate seen with atropine and β-blockers are blunted in patients with significant autonomic dysfunction [18].

Diabetic patients may also have an impaired thermoregulatory response to anesthesia related to inappropriate regulation of peripheral vasoconstriction to conserve body heat. This predisposes diabetic patients to exaggerated hypothermia in the operating room [19]. Patients with autonomic neuropathy may also have impaired ability to sense hypoglycemia [20]. This should be taken into consideration preoperatively when patients have fasted for several hours.

Damage to the autonomic nervous system can significantly affect the choice of anesthetic technique. Patients are at significantly increased risk of hypotension caused by induction agents such as propofol. For this reason, etomidate may be a better induction agent because of its considerably lower incidence of cardiovascular side effects.

Diabetic Retinopathy

Diabetic retinopathy is the leading cause of blindness in working-aged persons in the United States [21]. The prevalence and severity of retinopathy is directly correlated with the duration and extent of hyperglycemia. Nearly all patients with Type 1 DM and approximately 60% of Type 2 DM patients will have some retinopathy after 20 years [22]. Retinopathy can be classified as either proliferative or nonproliferative. Tight control of both glucose and hypertension remains the cornerstone for prevention [23]. Presence of retinopathy in a patient preoperatively should alert the anesthesiologist to other potential hazards. Because the retina shares a common embryological origin with the central nervous system, presence of retinal microvasculature dysfunction may correlate with cerebral vasculature insufficiency. A study examining the relationship between diabetic retinopathy and postoperative cognitive dysfunction in patients undergoing cardiac surgery found that the presence of retinopathy is a predictor of postoperative cognitive dysfunction because of coexisting impaired cerebral circulation [23].

Stiff joint Syndrome

While the specific pathophysiology is unknown, Stiff joint syndrome is thought to be a result of nonenzymatic glycosylation of collagen in connective tissue resulting in abnormal cross-linkage [24]. This syndrome is characterized by stiffness of the fingers, wrists, ankles, and elbows. Involvement of the metacarpophalangeal and proximal interphalangeal joints of the fifth digit is usually implicated first [5]. Larger joints tend to be involved later in the disease process. This is of particular importance if the cervical spine, temporomandibular, and or the arytenoid joints are involved. Involvement of these joints can severely limit range of motion resulting in a potentially difficult airway. Salzarula first reported a case of difficult intubation in a patient with DM and stiff joint syndrome in 1986 [24]. A positive prayer sign may suggest the presence of systemic joint stiffness. This sign is described as the inability to completely oppose the palmer surface of the hands.

9. **What is diabetic ketoacidosis and how is it managed?**

Diabetic ketoacidosis (DKA) is a potentially fatal condition characterized by a lack of insulin and imbalance of counterregulatory hormones. DKA is defined by absolute insulin deficiency with hyperglycemia with increased lipolysis, increased ketone production, hyperketonemia, and acidosis. The incidence of DKA is between 4 and 8 per 1000 in persons with DM and is more commonly associated with Type 1 DM [25]. DKA can occur in Type 2 DM, however, it rarely occurs without a precipitating event. Onset of DKA is often triggered by a significant stress response caused by infection (e.g., UTI, pneumonis, gastroenteritis), tissue injury, missed insulin treatment or previously undiagnosed diabetes. Patients present with a history of medication noncompliance, polyuria, polydypsia, abdominal pain, nausea, vomiting, and dehydration. Lack of insulin paired with high catecholamine levels limit glucose uptake by peripheral tissues [25, 26]. Lack of intracellular glucose leads to lipolysis and proteolysis with production of ketone byproducts. Consequently, laboratory evaluation will reveal an anion gap metabolic acidosis, hyperglycemia, hyperkalemia, elevated serum ketones, and presence of ketones in the urine [27].

Treatment consists of fluid and electrolyte replacement, insulin and dextrose infusion to prevent hypoglycemia. Metabolic derangements such as hypokalemia, hypocalcemia, and hypomagnesia should be expected with resuscitation and treated aggressively. Correction of acidemia and insulin administration results in a shift of potassium intracellularly resulting in plasma hypokalemia. Patients will present with elevated serum potassium concentrations initially even though they have profound total body potassium depletion ranging from 3 to 15 mmol/kg of body weight [25, 27]. Surgery should be delayed until resolution of DKA unless DKA is propagated by a surgical condition.

10. **What is Hyperglycemic Hyperosmolar State (HHS) and how is it managed?**

HHS is complication predominantly seen in Type 2 DM in which hyperglycemia causes severe dehydration, increase in serumosmolarity and high risk of mortality and coma.

It is more common in patients with Type 2 DM because these patients have a relative deficiency of insulin. Precipitating factors include medication noncompliance, infection, or other injury that potentiates an imbalance in regulatory hormones. Overall, HHS is less prevalent than DKA with an incidence of 1 out of 1000 diabetic patients [25, 26]. However, rates of morbidity and mortality are much higher in HHS compared to DKA [25, 26]. Compared to patients with DKA, patients have more profound hyperglycemia with reported blood glucose concentrations greater than 1000 mg/dL, and absence of ketones. Patients present with many of the same symptoms as DKA and include polyuria, nausea, vomiting, dehydration, and altered mental status. Laboratory evaluation reveals metabolic derangements in potassium, sodium, calcium, and magnesium. Treatment includes rehydration, electrolyte correction, and insulin infusion.

11. **Preoperative considerations in DM patients**

In the preoperative setting, diabetic patients need to be closely evaluated to determine the extent of systemic disease. A thorough history and physical should be obtained with careful consideration for potential cardiovascular disease, nephropathy, autonomic neuropathy, risk of aspiration, and stiff joint syndrome. Like any preoperative assessment, the focus is to stratify individual perioperative risk and optimize the patient's medical status if time permits.

Preoperative testing should take into consideration the age of the patient, previous anesthetic history, current medications, and adequacy of glycemic control. Metabolic panels should be done to assess for both metabolic derangements and kidney function. An HbgA1c can be useful to evaluate adequacy of long-term glycemic control. A standard EKG can be utilized to assess baseline cardiac function and rhythm. The American College of Cardiology and American Heart Association Guidelines on Perioperative Cardiovascular Evaluation and Care for Noncardiac Surgery encourage utilization of the Revised Cardiac Risk Index [12]. This index predicts perioperative cardiovascular risk based upon the presence of diabetes, ischemic heart disease, nephropathy, cerebrovascular disease, and heart failure [12]. Patients with limited functional capacity can suggest underlying microvascular and macrovascular disease. These patients may benefit from stress echocardiography if the findings will influence the anesthetic plan.

Oral hypoglycemic medications should be withheld 24–48 h before the day of surgery to prevent excessive hypoglycemia and lactic acidosis in the setting of preoperative fasting. Poorly controlled Type 2 DM patients on only oral hypoglycemic medications should be transitioned to insulin preoperatively. Other preoperative considerations should include surgery start time and shortening duration of preoperative fasting. The use of premedication should take into consideration the patient's preexisting systemic disease, cognitive function, and risk for aspiration.

In summary, perioperative and intraoperative glycemic-control regimens depend on several factors. Differentiating Type 1 from Type 2 DM is extremely important. Patients with Type 1 DM are at risk for DKA if they are without insulin. The risk of ketosis is amplified when the patient undergoes the stress of surgery. The degree to which blood sugar levels are chronically controlled affects management. Glycosylated hemoglobin (hemoglobin $A1_c$) is the most accurate way to assess glucose control over the previous 2 to 3 months. As levels of glycosylated hemoglobin rise, so does the complication rate of DM. The amount of exogenous insulin a patient normally requires is important in deciding how blood glucose should be treated intraoperatively. The magnitude of the surgery plays an important role in determining therapy. There are many different protocols for preoperative and intraoperative insulin management, but there are limited prospective studies comparing different regimens.

12. **Intraoperative considerations in DM patient**

Standard ASA monitors should be used in all patients undergoing general anesthetics. These include pulse oximetry, continuous EKG monitoring, noninvasive blood pressure, temperature, and end tidal carbon dioxide and gas analysis. Patients deemed high risk for hemodynamic instability may require invasive arterial blood pressure monitoring.

Surgery invokes significant physiologic stress on the body. This stress results in a complex cascade of metabolic changes that are mediated by catecholamines, cortisol, insulin, and glucagon [2]. Cortisol and catecholamines prevent peripheral glucose uptake while hepatic gluconeogenesis is also ongoing increasing the risk of hyperglycemia. Serum glucose monitoring from either venous or arterial samples should be done at least every hour. Treatment of hyperglycemia includes administration of intravenous insulin via boluses or continuous infusion.

Hypoglycemic shock is due to critical hypoglycemia resulting in tissue energy failure and is characterized by hemodynamic collapse and brain injury [28]. Treatment consists of slow bolus infusion of intravenous dextrose.

13. **Postoperative considerations in DM patient?**

Postoperative management should focus on glucose control as the patient recovers from the stress response of surgery. Patients should have their blood glucose taken at least once in the postanesthesia care unit to check for either hypo- or hyperglycemia. Advancement of diet should be considered to prevent hypoglycemia. Patients should also resume their preoperative medication regiment as soon as possible. If the patient is moderately hyperglycemic in the recovery room and insulin is administered, residual stress response physiology needs to be considered to prevent sudden hypoglycemia. While tight control of blood glucose has been shown to be beneficial in the critical care setting, there is little evidence to support a similar strategy in the postoperative period [29, 30].

Insulin therapy can result in anaphylactic and anaphylactoid reactions, especially when using protamine-containing insulin preparations. Protamine-derived insulin is made from fish sperm and can cause immunologic sensitization when protamine reversal is administered after cardiopulmonary bypass or heparin reversal [31, 32]. The protamine reaction can be devastating and includes profound hypotension, pulmonary vasoconstriction, and noncardiogenic pulmonary edema.

References

1. Ahmed I, Mruthunjaya S. Anaesthetic management of diabetes. Anaesth Intensive Care Med. 2014;15(10):453–7.
2. McAnulty GR, Robertshaw HJ, Hall GM. Anaesthetic management of patients with diabetes mellitus. Br J Anaesth. 2000;85: 80–90.
3. Cowie CC, Rust KF, Byrd-Holt DD, et al. Prevalence of diabetes and impaired fasting glucose in adults in the U.S population: national health and nutrition examination survey 1999–2002. Diab Care. 2006;29:1263–8.
4. Hillier TA, Vesco KK, Pedula KL, et al. Screening for gestational diabetes mellitus: a systematic review for the U.S preventative services task force. Ann Intern Med. 2008;148:766–75.
5. Kadoi Y. Anesthetic considerations in diabetic patients. Part 1: preoperative considerations of patients with diabetes mellitus. J Anesth. 2010;24:739–47.
6. Robertshaw HJ, Hall GM. Diabetes mellitus:anaesthetic management. Anaesthesia. 2006;61:1187–90.
7. American Diabetes Association. Diagnosis and classification of diabetes mellitus. (Miscellaneous Article). Diabetes Care. 33 (20100100) (Supplement): S62, January 2010.
8. Lantus (insulin glargine) package insert. Kansas City, MO, Aventis Pharmaceuticals, April 2000.
9. Heinemann L, Linkeschova R, Rave K, et al. Time action profile of the long-acting insulin analog insulin glargine (HOE 901) in comparison with those of NPH insulin and placebo. Diab Care. 2000;23:644.
10. Gu W, Pagel PS, Warltier DC, Kersten JR. Modifying cardiovascular risks in diabetes mellitus. Anesthesiology. 2003;98:774–9.
11. Fleisher LA, Beckman JA, Brown KA, et al. ACC/AHA 2007 guidelines on perioperative cardiovascular evaluation and care for noncardiac surgery: a report of the american college of cardiology/American Heart Association task force on practice guidelines (Writing Committee to Revise the 2002 guidelines on perioperative cardiovascular evaluation for noncardiac surgery) developed in collaboration with the american society of echocardiography, american society of nuclear cardiology, heart rhythm society, society of cardiovascular anesthesiologists, society for cardiovascular angiography and interventions, society for vascular medicine and biology, and society for vascular surgery. J Am Coll Cardiol. 2007;50:1707–32.
12. Margolis JR, Kannel WS, Feinleib M, et al. Clinical features of unrecognized myocardial infarction-silent and symptomatic. Eighteen year follow-up: Framingham study. Am J Cardiol. 1973;32:1–7.
13. Boyer JK, Thanigaraj S, Schechtman KB, Perez JE. Prevalence of ventricular diastolic dysfunction in asymptomatic, normotensive patients with diabetes mellitus. Am J Cardiol. 2004;93:870–5.
14. Turner RC. The U.K. prospective diabetes study. A review. Diab Care. 1998;21(Suppl 3):C35–8.

15. Kong MF, Horowitz M, Jones KL, Wishart JM, Harding PE. Natural history of diabetic gastroparesis. Diab Care. 1999;22: 503–7.
16. Wright RA, Clemente R, Wathen R. Diabetic gastroparesis: an abnormality of gastric emptying of solids. Am J Med Sci. 1985;289:240–2.
17. Huang CJ, Kuok CH, Kuo TBJ, et al. Pre-operative measurement of heart rate variability predicts hypotension during general anestheisa. Acta Anaesthesiol Scand. 2006;50:542–8.
18. Tsueda K, Huang KC, Dumond SW, et al. Cardiac sympathetic tone in anaesthetized diabetics. Can J Anaesth. 1991;38:20.
19. Kitamura A, Hoshino T, Kon T, Ogawa R. Patients with diabetic neuropathy are at risk of a greater intraoperative reduction in core temperature. Anesthesiology. 2000;92:1311–8.
20. Bottini P, Boschetti E, Pampanelli S, Ciofetta M, et al. Contribution of autonomic neuropathy to reduced plasma adrenaline responses to hypoglycemia in IDDM: evidence for a nonselective defect. Diabetes. 1997;46:814–23.
21. US Centers for Disease Control and Prevention. National diabetes fact sheet: general information and national estimates on diabetes in the United States, 2005. Atlanta: Centers for Disease Control and Prevention; 2005.
22. Mohamed Q, Gillies MC, Wong TY. Management of diabetic retinopathy: a systematic review. JAMA. 2007;298(8):902–16.
23. Kadoi Y, Saito S, Fujita N, Goto F. Risk factors for cognitive dysfunction after coronary artery bypass graft surgery in patients with type 2 diabetes. J Thorac Cardiovasc Surg. 2005;129:576–83.
24. Salzarulo HH, Taylor LA. Diabetic "stiff joint syndrome" as a cause of difficult endotracheal intubation. Anesthesiology. 1986;64:366–8.
25. Fishbein H, Palumbo PJ. Acute metabolic complications in diabetes. In: National diabetes data group. Diabetes in America. Bethesda (MD): National Institutes of Health, National Institute of Diabetes and Digestive and Kidney Diseases;1995. p. 283–91.
26. Chiasson JL, Jilwan N, Belanger R, Bertrand S, et al. Diagnosis and treatment of diabetic ketoacidosis and the hyperglycemic hyperosmolar state. CMAJ. 2003;168:859–66.
27. Kitabchi AE, Nyenwe EA. Hyperglycemic crises in diabetes mellitus: diabetic ketoacidosis and hyperglycemic hyperosmolar state. Endocrinol Metab Clin N Am. 2006;35:725–51.
28. Dierdorf SF. Anesthesia for patients with diabetes mellitus. Curr Opin Anaesthesiol. 2002;15:351–7.
29. Gandhi GY, Nuttall GA, Abel MD, et al. Intensive intraoperative insulin therapy versus conventional glucose management during cardiac surgery. Ann Intern Med. 2007;146:233–43.
30. The NICE-SUGAR Study Investigators. Intensive versus conventional glucose control in critically ill patients. N Engl J Med. 2009;360:1283–97.
31. Park KW. Protamine and protamine reactions. Int Anesthesiol Clin. Summer 2004;42(3):135–45.
32. Stewart WJ, McSweeney SM, Kellet MA, et al. Increased risk of severe protamine reactions in NPH insulin-dependent diabetics undergoing cardiac catheterization. Circulation. 1984;70:788.

Thyrotoxicosis

25

Mark R. Jones, Rachel J. Kaye, and Alan D. Kaye

Case

52-year-old female with thyroid nodules presents for total thyroidectomy.

Thyroid masses were discovered on symptom-based physical several months ago. Patient symptoms are local pressure and difficulty swallowing. Her thyroid function is normal. Initial evaluation with ultrasound showed solid 3 cm mass in the left thyroid lobe. The rest of the thyroid had additional nodules, including the index nodule of 2 cm in the isthmus.

Medications	Simvastatin 10mg PO daily
	Albuterol 90 mcg/actuation inhaler prn
Allergies	NKA
Past Medical History	Hypercholesterolemia
	Mild asthma- dx'd one year ago, triggers: cold air
Past Surgical History	Anterior cruciate ligament repair
	Rotator cuff repair
	Tubal ligation
Review of Systems	Pertinent items are noted in HPI. On direct questioning,
	there is no coronary artery, chronic obstructive pulmonary,
	renal and GI disease

(continued)

Physical Exam	VS:BP 132/80 mmHg
	HR 78RR 14
	SaO_2 99%
	Weight: 78.926 kg
	Height: 1.626 m

Airway: Mallampati score is II. Neck ROM is full. Normal mouth opening and TM distance. Voice is clear.
Dental: *Cracked crown left upper rear*
Head and Neck: The airway is midline. Lid lag or eye prominence is not present. A visible neck mass is in the midline. To palpation, there is a well-demarcated 2 cm midline thyroid nodule and a larger, less distinct nodule on the right. Both are mobile and not fixed. There is no thyromegaly. There is no palpable adenopathy on the left. The carotid upstrokes are normal. The range of motion of the neck is normal.
Cardiovascular: The cardiovascular exam is normal. The heart rhythm is regular.
Pulmonary: The pulmonary exam is normal. Breath sounds are clear to auscultation.
Neurological: The neurological exam is normal. The patient is oriented x3. There is no tremor and the patient seems to comprehend well.
Labs: wNL

1. **What is the thyroid gland?**

The thyroid gland is a butterfly-shaped gland found slightly inferior to the cricoid cartilage and wrapping around the trachea, to which it is firmly attached, in the anterior and lateral mid-neck. It is composed of two lobes joined at the center by an isthmus, which altogether weigh approximately 20 g. As a hormone-secreting organ, the thyroid commands a significant blood supply, relying on an extensive capillary network, which is supplied by the superior and inferior thyroid arteries. The superior, middle, and inferior thyroid veins each drain

M.R. Jones
Beth Israel Deaconess Medical Center, Harvard Medical School, Resident in Anesthesiology, Boston, MA, USA
e-mail: jarkmones@gmail.com

R.J. Kaye
Bowdoin College, Brunswick, ME, USA

A.D. Kaye (✉)
Department of Anesthesiology, LSU School of Medicine, New Orleans, LA, USA
e-mail: Alankaye44@hotmail.com

© Springer International Publishing AG 2017
L.S. Aglio and R.D. Urman (eds.), *Anesthesiology*,
DOI 10.1007/978-3-319-50141-3_25

their respective portions of the thyroid gland. Adrenergic and cholinergic systems innervate the gland. The superior and recurrent laryngeal nerves (RLN), branches of the vagus nerve, innervate the larynx and thyroid. Recurrent laryngeal nerve and external motor branch of the superior laryngeal nerve travel close to the gland, which poses a risk for nerve injury during thyroid surgery. The internal and external laryngeal nerves branch off from the superior laryngeal nerve, with the former supplying sensory and autonomic innervation to the upper larynx, and the latter providing motor innervation to the cricothyroid and transverse arytenoid muscles. The remaining muscles and lower larynx are innervated with motor and sensory fibers from the recurrent laryngeal nerve. Vocal cords (VC) are innervates by RLN. It is extremely important to monitor RLN function during thyroid surgery to prevent VC paralysis postoperatively. The intraoperative laryngeal EMG testing is used introperatively to reduce the rate of recurrent laryngeal nerve injury [1].

2. **What is the function of the thyroid gland?**

Thyroid gland produces thyroid hormones: triiodothyronine (T3) and thyroxine (T4) from a thyroglobulin precursor in the thyroid follicles. Thyroglobulin, an iodinated glycoprotein, comprises the bulk of the proteinaceous colloid that fills the follicular cells of thyroid gland. Twenty to forty follicles form a lobule, and these lobules, separated by connective tissue, come together to form the thyroid gland [2].

The production of normal levels of thyroid hormones (TH) is dependent on adequate dietary iodine intake. When present, iodine is reduced to iodide in the gastrointestinal tract, absorbed into the blood, and actively transported into the thyroid follicular cell in a process known as iodide trapping. From there, in a process termed organification, iodide is oxidized and incorporated with thyroglobulin into monoiodotyrosine (MIT) and diiodotyrosine (DIT), which are precursors to the hormonally active T4 and T3. The enzyme thyroid peroxidase (TPO) subsequently catalyzes the coupling of MIT and DIT molecules into T4 or T3 [1, 2].

Both hormones are reversibly bound to circulating plasma proteins for transport to peripheral tissues. Approximately 0.02% of the total T4 remains unbound to protein in the circulation, and is known as free T4 [2]. T3 binds to receptors in target cells with 15-fold greater affinity than T4, and is proportionately more active. T3 and T4 function is to regulate cellular metabolism by increasing carbohydrate and fat metabolism, metabolic rate, minute ventilation, heart rate, contractility, all the while maintaining water and electrolyte balance, as well as the normal activity of the central nervous system. All of these systemic effects begin at the cellular level, where thyroid hormones regulate the nuclear transcription of messenger RNA. T3 bids to a DNA domain called the thyroid response element, inducing a plethora of enzymes responsible for tissue metabolism, such as the ubiquitous Na, K-ATPase. Thyroid hormones modify cellular energy consumption and basal metabolic rate can increase as much as 60–100% as a consequence of increased TH levels. It drives additional glucose to be absorbed in the gastrointestinal tract, and stimulates glycogenolysis, gluconeogenesis, and insulin secretion, all the while promoting cellular glucose uptake [3, 4].

3. **What controls thyroid function?**

The production of thyroid hormones is regulated by the hypothalamic–pituitary axis, which continuously senses the concentration of T4 and T3 in the blood. In response to low thyroid hormone (TH), the hypothalamus releases thyrotropin releasing hormone (TRH), which in turn induces the anterior pituitary gland to release thyrotropin stimulating hormone (TSH). Somatostatin is released by the hypothalamus and inhibits the release of growth hormone (GH, somatotropin) and thyroid stimulating hormone (TSH) from the anterior pituitary. As previously stated, iodine is required to manufacture TH, and hypothyroid status may develop in an iodine-deficient patient [5].

4. **What is Hyperthyroidism?**

Hyperthyroidism is condition that occurs due to excess production of TH. Thyrotoxicosis is the condition that occurs due to the presence of excess TH, and the term itself refers to any disorder of increased TH concentration of any cause and includes hyperthyroidism. Many etiologies of thyrotoxicosis exist, and Graves' disease (multinodular goiter) is the most common cause of hyperthyroidism in the United States. Graves' disease occurs more often in women with a female: male ratio of 5:1 and a population prevalence of 1–2%. Surgery in goiter cases is indicated for cosmetic reasons or for airway compromise via tracheal compression [2].

Along with Graves', toxic adenoma and toxic multinodular goiter combine to make up 99% of the cases of hyperthyroidism in this country. Other common causes include the earlier stages of Hashimoto's thyroiditis, exogenous TH abuse, and de Quervain's subacute thyroiditis. Diagnoses that present with signs and symptoms similar to hyperthyroidism is condition that occurs due to excess production of TH and include other hypermetabolic states such as malignant hyperthermia, carcinoid, choriocarcinoma, hydatidiform mole, pheochromocytoma, struma ovarii, and certain drugs such as antipsychotic agents, anticholinergic agents, serotonin antagonists, sympathomimetic agents, and strychnine poisoning. Regardless of etiology, patients with hyperthyroidism are in a hypermetabolic state and display signs and symptoms to be discussed later [6, 7].

5. **What are the signs and symptoms of hyperthyroidism?**

By system

- Cardiovascular
  - Initially, mean arterial pressure is decreased via interaction of TH with vascular smooth muscle. This activates the renin–angiotensin–aldosterone system, which increases blood volume, eventually resulting in an increase in cardiac output, heart rate, and ultimately systolic hypertension [3]. This hyperdynamic circulation may induce heart failure in 6% of patients over time; and while overt cardiac failure rarely arises from thyrotoxicosis, thyrotoxic cardiomyopathy with left ventricular dilation does occur in up to 1% of thyrotoxic individuals [8, 9].
  - Arrhythmias (sinus tachycardia, supraventricular tachycardia, and atrial fibrillation). Elderly patients who develop unexplained cardiac problems should be evaluated for thyrotoxicosis [2].
- Skin
  - Increased blood flow causes flushing
  - Excessive sweating
  - Heat intolerance
  - Pretibial myxedema classically occurs in Graves' disease and is characterized by edematous skin over the dorsum of the legs and feet
- Respiratory
  - Goiter mass effect can compress the trachea leading to dyspnea, dysphagia, cough, dysphonia, and worsening of symptoms when lying prone
  - The hypermetabolic state of thyrotoxic patients induces hypercarbia and increased oxygen consumption, resulting in a compensatory increase in minute ventilation and tidal volumes [4].
- Neurological
  - Insomnia despite complaints of extreme fatigue
  - Trouble concentrating, confusion, amnesia
  - Fine tremor, predominately in the hands
  - Hyperactive tendon reflexes
- Eyes
  - Sympathetic overstimulation results in a wide, staring gaze and lid lag
  - Exophthalmos (Graves' disease) secondary to autoimmune inflammation and edema of extraocular muscles and retro-orbital tissue [10].
- Gastrointestinal
  - Malabsorption, diarrhea, and increased frequency of bowel movements secondary to decreased gastrointestinal transit time
  - Acid secretion falls due to parietal cells antibodies in up to 30% of patients, which may affect drug absorption [4].
- Hematologic
  - Increased plasma volume results in a normochromic, normocytic anemia
- Metabolic
  - TH antagonizes insulin peripherally, resulting in hyperglycemia
  - Increased calorigenesis results in weight loss in spite of an increased appetite
- Psychological
  - Emotional instability, depression, agitation, nervousness
  - Anxiety, restlessness, hyperactivity
- Musculoskeletal
  - A Proximal limb muscle wasting and weakness
  - Increased bone turnover and osteoporosis, with resultant changes in parathyroid hormone levels
- Renal
  - Increase in tubular reabsorption and secretion, eventually producing hyperkalemia and hyponatremia
- Systemic
  - The increase in metabolism produces a proportionate increase of metabolic end products, culminating in vasodilation and enhanced tissue blood flow [4].

6. **How is hyperthyroidism diagnosed?**

To investigate any clinical suspicion for hyperthyroidism and thyrotoxicosis, there are several laboratory tests that are available. Free T4 and total T4 are commonly measured, and an elevation in either is indicative, but not confirmatory, of a hyperthyroid state. The current best test of TH action remains the TSH assay. Minute changes in thyroid function can result in dramatic swings in TSH secretion. The normal level of TSH in the body lies between 0.4 and 5.0 mU/L, and any TSH less than 0.03 mU/L accompanied by an elevation in T3 and T4 is diagnostic of overt hyperthyroidism. A thyroid storm patient, on the other hand, may experience TSH levels less than 0.01 mU/L. To contrast, the TSH of a patient with overt hypothyroidism can skyrockets to 400 mU/L or more [2].

7. **What is thyroid storm?**

Thyroid storm, the most feared complication of hyperthyroidism, is a sudden, life-threatening surge in the level of TH that overcomes a patient's metabolic, thermoregulatory, and cardiovascular compensatory mechanisms. It typically occurs in an individual with untreated hyperthyroidism under a stress of infection, trauma, or surgery. Thyroid storm precipitated by stress of surgery usually occurs 6–18 h postoperatively, rather than intraoperatively. Other causes are withdrawal of antithyroid medication therapy, radioiodine therapy, cerebrovascular accident, diabetic ketoacidosis, myocardial or bowel infarction, pulmonary embolism, and pregnancy.

Typical findings in thyroid storm involve an exaggeration of the typical symptoms of hyperthyroidism, such as tachycardia and hyperpyrexia, anxiety, disorientation, delirium, chest pain, shortness of breath, heart failure, dehydration, and shock. Thyroid storm carries a high mortality rate, ranging from 10–30%. Diagnostic criteria for thyroid storm, established in 1993 by Burch and Wartofsky, are listed in Table 25.1 [4, 11].

8. **What is the treatment for hyperthyroidism, and when is surgery indicated?**

Treatment regimens for thyrotoxicosis begin with medical management with antithyroid medications (thionamides): propylthiouracil (PTU) or methimazole (MMI). Both drugs interfere with TH synthesis through inhibition of organification and coupling. PTU also inhibits the peripheral conversion of T4 to the active T3 molecule. Antithyroid medications achieve a euthyroid state after 6–8 weeks, after which the dosage is decreased but continued for up to two years. Even after prolonged therapy with antithyroid medications, the majority of patients experience recurrences of disease [2]. Patients refractory to antithyroid medication or who experiences relapse of disease may be treated with radio-ablative iodine therapy or surgery. Surgery is highly successful and carries a lower risk of developing hypothyroidism in the future versus ablative therapy (10–30% vs. 40–70%) [2]. Common complications from thyroidectomy include hypocalcemia secondary to parathyroid gland damage (9–14%) and vocal cord paralysis (0.7–1%); but with over 150,000 thyroidectomies performed each year in the United States, the mortality rate remains low at less than 0.1% [12].

The treatment of pregnant patients with hyperthyroidism includes low-dose antithyroid medication, but PTU and MMI can cross the placenta and can cause fetal hypothyroidism. If required doses of PTU or MMI during pregnancy exceed 300 mg/day in the first trimester, subtotal thyroidectomy should be performed [2].

Cretinism, the devastating end result of fetal hypothyroidism, results in short stature and mental retardation [13].

Table 25.1 Diagnostic Criteria for Thyroid Storm*

Thermoregulatory dysfunction: temperature, F	Score	Cardiovascular dysfunction: heart rate, bpm	Score
99–99.9	5	90–109	5
100–100.9	10	110–119	10
101–101.9	15	120–129	15
102–102.9	20	130–139	20
103–103.9	25	≥140	25
≥104	30		
Central nervous system dysfunction	Score	Cardiovascular dysfunction: heart failure	Score
Absent	0	Absent	0
Mild (agitation)	10	Mild (pedal edema)	5
Moderate (delirium, psychosis, extreme lethargy)	20	Moderate (bibasilar rales)	10
Severe (seizure, coma)	30	Severe (pulmonary edema)	15
Gastrointestinal and hepatic dysfunction	Score	Cardiovascular dysfunction: atrial fibrillation	Score
Absent	0	Absent	0
Moderate (diarrhea, nausea/vomiting, abdominal pain)	10	Present	10
Severe (unexplained jaundice)	20		
Precipitant history	Score		
Absent	0		
Present	10		

A score of 45 or greater is highly suggestive of thyroid storm; 22-44 suggests an impending thyroid storm; <25 is unlikely to represent a thyroid storm

*Reproduced from Burch H. B. and Wartofsky L. [31], with permission of Elsevier

9. **What are the pre-anesthetic considerations in a patient with hyperthyroidism?**

To safely perform an elective thyroid surgery, the thyrotoxic patient must be made euthyroid prior to the procedure. Normalization and stabilization of TH may be achieved via a six to eight week regimen of the antithyroid medications described above (PTU or MMI). Iodine-containing solution can be used for treatment of thyroid storm since iodine blocks release of T4 and T3 from thyroid within hours. High concentration iodide effectively limits the release of TH from the thyroid gland, but its effects are short lived. Iodide actually increases total TH stores in the gland itself, rendering it unacceptable for long-term therapy.

Preoperative laboratory testing should include a CBC to evaluate anemia, blood glucose levels, and routine radiologic studies of the neck to evaluate the degree of upper airway compression if symptoms of it are present. In patients with severe tracheal compression, CT, MRI, multi-slice 3D CT, and high-resolution virtual laryngoscopy based on spiral CT data can provide valuable information on the extent of thyroid growth [14, 15]. In the event of a large goiter, specially invading mediastinum, where significant bleeding is possible, a blood type and screen is indicated. Patients should have eye protection applied via lubricant and eye pads, especially those with significant proptosis who are particularly vulnerable to ulceration and drying [16].

10. **What if the patient is not euthyroid?**

In emergent cases, several protocols may achieve more rapid stabilization of TH levels in the thyrotoxic individual. Intravenous beta blockers normalize the heart rate and diminish many symptoms such as anxiety and diaphoresis. The most commonly utilized beta blocker is a continuous infusion of intravenous esmolol at 50–500 ug/kg/min in order to achieve the goal heart rate of less than 85 bpm [17]. While esmolol will not affect any of the underlying pathologies of hyperthyroidism, the beta blocker propranolol has tertiary effects similar to PTU, in that it obstructs the conversion of T4 to T3 in peripheral tissue [2]. If these peripheral blocking effects are desired intravenous propranolol can be administered.

The second step in an emergent case is to administer antithyroid medication. It should be recognized that the thionamides (PTU and MMI) exert a limited effect if taken for less than two weeks, but should nonetheless be given. MMI reaches a euthyroid state more rapidly than PTU and is less associated with side effects such as agranulocytosis, hepatitis, and vasculitis [18]. Thionamides should also be administered either orally, through a nasogastric tube, or rectally, as they do not have a form compatible with intravenous delivery. Furthermore, since MMI and PTU only inhibit the synthesis of TH, iodide preparations should follow 2–3 h afterwards to block the release of TH and further diminish circulating levels.

Another essential medication for the emergent thyrotoxic patient are intravenous steroids—glucocorticoids. Dexamethasone will act to decrease TH release as well as lower peripheral T4 to T3 conversion. Finally, supportive therapies with fluid and electrolyte replacement, oxygen administration, and a cooling blanket remain vital measures in emergent surgery on hyperthyroid patient [4].

Thyrotoxicosis does not ameliorate immediately following the removal of the thyroid gland; the half-life of T4 is seven to eight days [19]. Beta blockade must be continued postoperatively throughout this period, but antithyroid medication may be halted.

11. **What if the patient has a large goiter?**

A substantial goiter should concern the anesthesiologist as it may compress, deviate, or invade and narrow the lumen of the underlying trachea. CT scan of the neck should be ordered preoperatively to determine the degree of tracheal stenosis in patients with large thyroid that shows signs and symptoms of airway compression.

Flow-volume loops, seldom helpful in a routine setting, may assist with identification of compromise in patients with tracheal compression [20]. Variable extrathoracic obstruction secondary to tumors or tracheomalacia will manifest as plateauing of the inspiratory limb of the flow-volume loop, while the expiratory phase maintains airway patency. Variable intrathoracic obstructions, most often due to vocal cord paralysis, will reveal a plateau in the expiratory phase alone. Finally, fixed upper airway lesions such as goiter will produce plateau in both the inspiratory and expiratory cycles of the flow-volume loop.

Because of its thoracic anatomical position, the superior vena cava (SVC) is vulnerable to compression as well, potentially leading to superior vena cava syndrome [4]. Venography is useful to detect SVC syndrome and the underlying anatomic delineation. In addition to sequelae such as thrombus formation, headache and vertigo, this gradual, insidious compression of the SVC may cause retrograde collateral flow and interstitial edema, resulting in swelling of the face, neck, and upper extremity.

12. **What drugs may be used for preoperative sedation?**

Slow titration of benzodiazepines with or without the addition of a narcotic, may be used to elicit the desired level of sedation and anxiolysis. Anticholinergic drugs such as atropine are not recommended as a preoperative medication due to their propensity to induce tachycardia and interfere with temperature-regulating mechanisms [2].

13. **What kind of anesthetic would you used the thyroidectomy?**

Surgery is performed with general anesthesia with endotracheal intubation; however, the use of LMA (laryngeal mask airway) is becoming popular. Propofol is currently the induction agent of choice in hyperthyroid patients. Thiopental is often preferred as it decreases the peripheral conversion of T4 to T3 secondary to its thiourylene nucleus, but its availability is currently uncertain. Drugs with sympathomimetic properties system should be avoided, including ketamine, atropine, ephedrine and epinephrine. Similarly, vagolytic drugs such as pancuronium should not be used as they may induce an increase in heart rate.

14. **How should you prepare to intubate this patient?**

If significant airway compression exists, intubation may involve advanced airway devices such as awake fiberoptic intubation techniques [21]. The anesthesiologist should pass a reinforced endotracheal tube beyond the point of compression, using minimal preoperative sedation [22]. Indeed, awake intubation may be preferred, and all parties should be aware that surgical airways can be quite difficult in these patients due to anatomic distortion and increased tissue vascularity. In patients with large airway compression, small-reinforced anode endotracheal tubes can prevent airway collapse. A rigid bronchoscope should be accessible in case of airway collapse, and the tube itself should be passed beyond the thyroid gland [2]. The anesthesiologist should anticipate a difficult intubation in roughly one out of every twenty thyroidectomies [23].

15. **What is appropriate maintenance anesthesia for patient with hyperthyroidism?**

To avoid an exaggerated sympathetic nervous system (SNS) response to surgical stimulation, it is imperative that adequate depth of anesthesia be maintained. Increased drug metabolism is a concern when dosing medications in hyperthyroid patients. Combined with infusion of remifentanyl or sufentanyl, the volatile anesthetics such as isoflurane, desflurane, and sevoflurane therefore become particularly effective owing to their capacity to quell SNS responses to surgical stimulation without sensitizing cardiac tissue to catecholamines. Larger doses of desflurane should be used with caution, however, due to transient SNS stimulation sometimes seen with sudden increases in desflurane concentration [24].

The systemic increase in metabolism associated with thyrotoxicosis may appear to require an increase in mean alveolar concentration (MAC) to adequately anesthetize the patient, but this is not the case. Controlled studies in hyperthyroid animals have shown no clinically significant increase in anesthetic requirements [25]. An increase in drug metabolism does not affect the brain partial pressure of the anesthetic needed to generate the sought after pharmacologic result. The anesthesiologist should bear in mind, however, that the occurrence of thyroid storm may indeed alter the MAC by increasing the body's temperature, about 5% for every degree above 37 °C [18]. Intraoperative electro-physiological monitoring of the recurrent laryngeal nerve (RLN) is designed to detect and prevent RLN damage during thyroid surgery. Nondepolarizing neuromuscular blocker should not be given due to the RLN monitoring. Antagonism of neuromuscular blockers should involve glycopyrrolate in combination with an acetylcholinesterase inhibitor rather than atropine in order to avoid drug-induced tachycardia, as glycopyrrolate exhibits substantially less chronotropic effect [26].

Many different RLN monitoring systems have been studies, including glottis observation, glottis pressure monitoring, endoscopically placed intramuscular vocal cord electrodes, endotracheal tube-based surface electrodes, and postcrycoid surface electrodes. Endotracheal tube-based surface electrodes represent the most common monitoring equipment format for RLN monitoring for reasons including safety, utility, and simplicity.

16. **How should thyrotoxic patients be monitored during anesthesia?**

Monitoring of the thyrotoxic patient during maintenance anesthesia should be aimed at recognizing thyroid storm as soon as possible. Blood pressure and end-tidal carbon dioxide should be set up initially; core body temperature and cardiac function via electrocardiogram should be monitored constantly in order to detect any rises in temperature or heart rate. To prevent hyperthermia, cooling mattresses and chilled crystalloid solutions are recommended, and the beta blocker esmolol is recommended to treat tachycardia. Any more invasive monitoring must be decided on a case-by-case basis. In the case of thyroid storm, two large bore peripheral intravenous lines should be placed along with an arterial line [2, 4].

17. **What are the complications of thyroid surgery and the appropriate responses?**

Thyroid storm is the most feared complication of surgery on hyperthyroid patients. The diagnosis and treatment is convoluted by the syndrome's resemblance to malignant hyperthermia, carcinoid crisis, and pheochromocytoma. To differentiate between the common culprits, malignant hyperthermia and thyroid storm, the physician should recall that many of the clinical manifestations of malignant hyperthermia are absent in thyroid storm; specifically, metabolic acidosis, profound hypercarbia, and muscle rigidity will not be present in thyroid storm [27]. Furthermore, creatine phosphokinase levels skyrocket in malignant hyperthermia, and are actually decreased to approximately half of normal in thyrotoxic etiologies. In fact, patients suffering from thyroid storm may not even experience elevations from their baseline level of TH, rendering measurement of serum TH of little use. The diagnosis carries a mortality rate of 10–20%, and there currently exists no definitive test to diagnose thyroid storm. The pathophysiology most likely involves a release of TH from its binding protein in circulation secondary to binding inhibitors. Treatment is similar to the emergent hyperthyroid patient and should begin immediately in the critical setting [7]:

- IV beta blockers to decrease HR to 85 bpm
- IV dexamethasone 2 mg q6
- Oral PTU 200–400 mg q8
- Cooling blankets, ice packs, cool humidified oxygen
- MIVF

Salicylates such as aspirin are contraindicated during thyroid storm due to their tendency to disproportionately increase free TH levels by displacing it from binding proteins [26].

18. **What are the extubation concerns?**

The patient's ability to protect their airway must be considered prior to extubation, and the endotracheal tube should remain in place if there is any concern. Postoperative tracheal collapse resulting from prolonged compression by a substantial goiter and injury to the recurrent laryngeal nerves are two notable causes of airway compromise in these cases [28]. Similar to intubation, if the patient presents with tracheomalacia or significant compression, a fiberoptic bronchoscope is recommended to directly visualize patency of the airway, as well as evaluate vocal cord movement when the bronchoscope and endotracheal tube are removed. In the event of tracheal collapse, reintubation should immediately proceed. Be prepared for this scenario with a laryngoscope, extra endotracheal tubes, and a tracheostomy set [29].

19. **What should you monitor postoperatively?**

Bilateral injury to the recurrent laryngeal leads to blateral vocal cord paralysis. This serious condition requires emergency intervention-intubation to resolve the potentially life-threatening respiratory distress. In case of bilateral RLN injury immediate revision neck surgery may help to indicate the type of RLN damage, which is a predictor of functional recovery and major factors influencing future therapeutic management. More commonly, however, the recurrent laryngeal nerve is damaged unilaterally; hoarseness and risk of aspiration are thus more common and problematic than respiratory obstruction [4]. RLN injury is more common in operations for thyroid carcinoma, hyperthyroid (toxic) goiter and recurrent goiter cases.

Other causes of postoperative respiratory compromise include hemorrhage, pneumothorax, hypocalcemia, and tracheomalacia. Formation of neck hematoma can occur rapidly and without warning, prompting emergent intervention for any sign of respiratory failure. Emergent opening of incision site and draining of hematoma has to be performed. Any sign of airway compromise should prompt emergent endotracheal intubation before edema from venous and lymph restriction compromises the airway. Corticosteroids and racemic epinephrine may decrease laryngeal edema, but should not be a substitute for intubation. Pneumothorax is possible when surgical dissection extends to the mediastinum, and in such instances must remain in the differential diagnosis of postoperative respiratory compromise. Hypocalcemia can occur in total thyroidectomies by inadvertent excision of the parathyroid glands. Circumoral and digital numbness and tingling will precede stridor and airway obstruction if calcium is not supplemented. This occurs most often within 3 days postoperatively, but rarely in the immediate postoperative period [2, 30].

References

1. Williams RH, Melmed S. Williams textbook of endocrinology. Philadelphia: Elsevier/Saunders; 2011.
2. Stoelting, R. Stoelting's anesthesia and co-existing disease (Revised/Expanded ed.). Philadelphia: Churchill Livingstone/Elsevier; 2008.
3. Brent GA. Mechanisms of thyroid hormone action. J Clin Invest. 2012;122:3035.
4. Yao FSF, Artusio JF. Yao & Artusio's anesthesiology: problem-oriented patient management. Philadelphia: Lippincott Williams & Wilkins; 2012.
5. Ain KB, Rosenthal MS. The complete thyroid book. New York: McGraw-Hill; 2005.

6. Adler SN, Gasbarra DB, Klein DA. A pocket manual of differential diagnosis. Philadelphia: Lippincott Williams & Wilkins; 2008. p. 66–67.
7. Nayak B, Burman K. Thyrotoxicosis and thyroid storm. Endocrinol Metab Clin North Am. 2006;35(4):663–86, vii.
8. Dahl P, Danzi S, Klein I. Thyrotoxic cardiac disease. Curr Heart Fail Rep. 2008;5(3):170–6.
9. Klein I, Ojamaa K. Thyroid hormone and the cardiovascular system: from theory to practice. J Clin Endocrinol Metab. 1994;78:1026.
10. Bahn RS. Graves' ophthalmopathy. N Engl J Med. 2010;362:726.
11. Sarlis NJ, Gourgiotis L. Thyroid emergencies. Rev Endocr Metab Disord. 2003;4:129.
12. Kandil E, Noureldine SI, Abbas A, Tufano RP. The impact of surgical volume on patient outcomes following thyroid surgery. Surgery. 2013;154(6):1346–52; discussion 1352–3.
13. Van Vliet G, Deladoëy J. Diagnosis, treatment and outcome of congenital hypothyroidism. Endocr Dev. 2014;26:50–9. doi:10.1159/000363155 (Epub 2014 Aug 29).
14. Barker P, Mason RA, Thorpe MH. Computerised axial tomography of the trachea. A useful investigation when a retrosternal goitre causes symptomatic tracheal compression. Anaesthesia. 1991;46:195–8.
15. Freitas JE, Freitas AE. Thyroid and parathyroid imaging. Semin Nucl Med. 1994;24:234–45.
16. Jones MR, Motejunas MW, Kaye AD. Preanesthetic assessment of the patient with hyperthyroidism. Anesthesia News, 2014; 40 (12):25–29.
17. Thome AC, Bedford RF. Esmolol for perioperative management of thyrotoxic goiter. Anesth. 1989;71:291–4.
18. Miller R. Miller's anesthesia (Revised/Expanded ed.). New York: Elsevier/Churchill Livingstone; 2005.
19. Kehlet H, Klauber PV, Weeke J. Thyrotropin, free and total triiodothyronine, and thyroxine in serum during surgery. Clin Endocrinol (Oxf). 1979;10(2):131–6.
20. Lunn W, Sheller J. Flow volume loops in the evaluation of upper airway obstruction. Otolaryngol Clin North Am. 1995;28:721–9.
21. Sandberg WS, Urman RD, Ehrenfeld JM. The MGH textbook of anesthetic equipment. Philadelphia: Elsevier/Saunders; 2011.
22. Elisha S, Boytim M, Bordi S, Heiner J, Nagelhout J, Waters E. Anesthesia case management for thyroidectomy. AANA J. 2010;78(2):151–60.
23. Bouaggad A, Nejmi SE, Bouderka MA, Abbassi O. Prediction of difficult tracheal intubation in thyroid surgery. Anesth Analg. 2004;99:603–6.
24. Pac-Soo CK, Ma D, Wang C, Chakrabarti MK, Whitwam JG. Specific actions of halothane, isoflurane, and desflurane on sympathetic activity and A delta and C somatosympathetic reflexes recorded in renal nerves in dogs. Anesthesiology. 1999;91(2):470–8.
25. Babad AA, Eger EL II. The effects of hyperthyroidism and hypothyroidism on halothane and oxygen requirements in dogs. Anesth. 1968;29:1087–93.
26. Pimental L, Hansen K. Thyroid disease in the emergency department: a clinical and laboratory review. J Emerg Med. 2005;28:201–9.
27. Peters K, Nance P, Wingard D. Malignant hyperthyroidism or malignant hyperthermia. Anesth Analg. 1981;60:613–5.
28. Green WE, Shepperd HW, Stevenson HM, Wilson W. Tracheal collapse after thyroidectomy. Br J Surg. 1979;66:554–7.
29. Geelhoed GW. Tracheomalacia from compressing goiter: management after thyroidectomy. Surgery. 1988;104:100–8.
30. Netterville J, Aly A, Ossoff R. Evaluation and treatment of complications of thyroid and parathyroid surgery. Otolayngol Clin North Am. 1990;23:529–50.
31. Burch HB, Wartofsky L. Life-threatening thyrotoxicosis. Thyroid storm. Endocrinol Metab Clin North Am. 1993;22(2):263–77.

Pheochromocytoma

26

Julie A. Gayle, Ryan Rubin, and Alan D. Kaye

CASE PRESENTATION:

A 65-year-old male with labile hypertension, episodes of angina relieved with nitroglycerin, and elevated creatinine presents for right adrenalectomy for a recently diagnosed adrenal mass on MRI. Patient has occasional palpitations and diaphoresis. Stress test revealed no signs of acute ischemia. Cardiac catheterization revealed two-vessel coronary artery disease [1].

- Medications (by mouth):
  - isosorbide mononitrate 120 mg daily
  - amlodipine besylate 5 mg daily
  - enalapril 20 mg daily
  - atorvastatin 40 mg daily
  - gemfibrozil 600 mg daily
  - aspirin 325 mg daily
  - potassium 20 meq daily
  - nitroglycerin prn
  - fluoxetine 20 mg daily
- Past medical history
  - Hypertension
  - Coronary artery disease
  - Hypercholesterolemia
  - Familial tremor
  - Depression
- No known drug allergies
- Physical exam
  - Height 5′ 11″ Weight 85 kg BMI 26
  - VS BP 180/105 (patient reports he had not yet taken his daily antihypertensive medications) HR 90 RR 18 SaO_2 98%
  - Cooperative, yet anxious appearing gentleman with a constant tremor most prominent in his hands
  - Airway exam—Mallampati class 1 with good mouth opening and thyromental distance
  - CV exam III/IV systolic murmur at the upper right sternal border with no carotid bruits
  - Lungs clear to auscultation bilaterally
- Lab/imaging of note
  - Creatinine of 1.5 mg/dL
  - Hemoglobin 13.5 mg/dL
  - EKG normal sinus rhythm with occasional premature ventricular contractions, left ventricular hypertrophy, and nonspecific ST and T wave changes
  - Transthoracic echocardiogram showed a normal ventricular function with an ejection fraction of 79%, left ventricular hypertrophy, and aortic sclerosis
  - MRI showed a large right adrenal mass 1.8 cm by 6 cm with central necrosis [1].

1. **What is a pheochromocytoma?**

Catecholamines secreting neuroendocrine tumors arising from the chromaffin cells of the sympathoadrenal system are known as pheochromocytomas. A rare and potentially lethal neuroendocrine tumor, pheochromocytomas are typically found in the adrenal gland. However, extraadrenal pheochromocytomas are tumors that originate in the ganglia of the sympathetic nervous system. More specifically, 85% of pheochromocytomas are adrenal and 15% are extraadrenal. Extraadrenal sites include cranial nerves, sympathetic ganglia in the pelvis, mediastinum or neck. The most common

J.A. Gayle (✉)
Department of Anesthesiology, Louisiana State University School of Medicine, 1542 Tulane Ave., Suite 659, New Orleans, LA 70112, USA
e-mail: jgayle477@cox.net

R. Rubin · A.D. Kaye
Department of Anesthesiology, Louisiana State University School of Medicine, 1542 Tulane Ave., Ste. 643, New Orleans, LA 70112, USA
e-mail: rrubin@lsuhsc.edu

A.D. Kaye
e-mail: alankaye44@hotmail.com

© Springer International Publishing AG 2017
L.S. Aglio and R.D. Urman (eds.), *Anesthesiology*,
DOI 10.1007/978-3-319-50141-3_26

extraadrenal site in the abdomen is at the origin of the inferior mesenteric artery called the area of Zuckerkandl [2].

2. **What is the incidence of pheochromocytoma?**

Pheochromocytoma occurs in about 0.01–0.1% of patients with hypertension [3]. The actual incidence of pheochromocytoma is difficult to report accurately due to historic inconsistencies in the precise definition of pheochromocytoma. Estimates are 500–1600 cases per year yielding a prevalence of 1:6500 to 1:2500 in the United States [4]. While pheochromocytomas may occur at any age, they are most common in the fourth to fifth decades of life. Among men and women, pheochromocytoma is equally common [5].

3. **What is the function of the adrenal gland?**

Adrenal glands have two functionally separate units contained within one capsule. The adrenal cortex and the adrenal medulla are two different units within the adrenal gland each having distinct embryologic and functional characteristics [6]. The adrenal cortex has three functional zones and secretes mineralocorticoids, glucocorticoids, and sex steroids. The adrenal medulla synthesizes and secretes catecolamines. These catecholamines include epinephrine, norepinephrine, and dopamine and modulate the body's sympathetic response to stress. Excessive secretion of epinephrine and norepinephrine from the adrenal medulla are responsible for the signs and symptoms associated with pheochromocytomas.

4. **Describe the pathophysiology of pheochromocytoma.**

The English meaning of the word pheochromocytoma as interpreted from the Greek language is "dusky-colored tumor" referring to the color these cells acquire when stained with chromium salts [7]. During embryonic development, the chromaffin cells that evolve into pheochromocytomas settle near the sympathetic ganglia, vagus nerve, paraganglia, and carotid arteries. Some of these chromaffin tissues may land in other sites such as the renal and hepatic hili, gonads, bladder wall, prostate, and rectum [8]. The effect of large amounts of catecholamines in circulation, specifically epinephrine and norepinephrine, is responsible for the pathophysiologic processes that occur in patients with pheochromocytoma.

Alpha-adrenergic and beta-adrenergic receptors mediate the actions of catecholamines. Vascular constriction is a result of alpha-1 receptor stimulation. Alpha-2 receptors mediate the presynaptic feedback inhibition of norepinephrine release. Cardiac rate and contractility is increased by beta-1 receptor activity. Beta-2 receptor receptors modulate arteriolar and venous dilation and relaxation of bronchial smooth muscle [8]. Excessive secretion of the catecholamines epinephrine, norepinephrine, and rarely dopamine into circulation leads to severe and refractory hypertension.

Some precipitants of hypertensive crisis in patients with pheochromocytoma include [9]:

- Induction of anesthesia
- Childbirth
- Certain opioids
- Dopamine antagonists (metoclopramide)
- Beta-blockers
- Cold medications
- Radiographic contrast media
- Drugs that inhibit catecholamine reuptake
  - Cocaine
  - Tricyclic antidepressants

5. **What are the signs and symptoms of pheochromocytoma?**

Although pheochromocytoma is the cause of sustained hypertension in less than 0.1% of hypertensive patients, approximately 50% of patients with pheochromocytoma have sustained hypertension. Paroxysms of palpitations, hypertension, diaphoresis, headaches, and feelings of impending doom may be present at the time of diagnosis [4]. By system:

Neurologic
Headache, diaphoresis, feelings of apprehension and anxiety, tremors, hypertensive encephalopathy, seizures

Cardiovascular/cardiopulmonary
Hypertension, palpitations, tachycardia, diaphoresis, pallor, dyspnea, orthopnea, postural hypotension (volume contraction), congestive heart failure, pulmonary edema, cardiomyopathy, tachyarrythmias

Gastrointestinal
Nausea, diarrhea, abdominal pain, malnutrition, weight loss, metabolic disturbances including impaired glucose control and insulin resistance

6. **What is the more common clinical presentation of pheochromocytoma?**

The "classic triad" of symptoms in a patient with pheochromocytoma includes episodic headache, sweating, and tachycardia. These symptoms strongly suggest a diagnosis of pheochromocytoma. Approximately 50% of patients will have paroxysmal hypertension making hypertension, paroxysmal or sustained, the most common sign of pheochromocytoma. Headaches occur in up to 90% of symptomatic patients; while up to 70% of symptomatic patients experience sweating [10, 11].

7. **How is pheochromocytoma diagnosed?**

Diagnosis is based on clinical manifestations. Once a clinical diagnosis is made, biochemical diagnostic tests to detect excessive catecholamine excretion are indicated. These tests include plasma metanephrine testing, and 24 h urine collection for catecholamines and metanephrines [12, 13].

Test selection is based on risk. Patients at high risk include those with predisposing genetic syndromes or family and/or a personal history of pheochromocytoma. When associated with multiple endocrine neoplasia type 2 (MEN2), symptoms are present in approximately 50% of patients; however, only one-third of patients have hypertension [14]. In patient populations considered high risk, plasma metanephrine testing is preferred. Urine 24 h collection for catecholamines and metanephrines is indicated in patients at lower risk.

Other biochemical tests include urinary vanillylmandellic acid (VMA) levels and clonidine suppression test. Urinary VMA level is an older and less expensive test, but it is nonspecific. Clonidine suppression test lowers plasma catecholamines in patients without tumor and has no effect on patients with pheochromocytoma [7].

Imaging studies such as abdominal CT scanning or MRI should be performed after the above testing confirms the diagnosis of pheochromocytoma.

8. **What is the treatment for pheochromocytoma?**

Treatment of choice for pheochromocytoma is surgical resection. In order to avoid high rates of mortality, optimization, and presurgical medical stabilization requires a multidisciplinary approach. A collaborative effort with experienced healthcare providers including surgeon(s), anesthesiologist(s), and an endocrinologist offers the lowest possible surgical risk to the patient.

9. **What are preoperative considerations for a patient with a pheochromocytoma?**

Adrenergic receptor blocking agents are used to reduce the risk hypertensive crisis during induction of anesthesia and tumor manipulation. Alpha-adrenergic antagonists aim to normalize blood pressure, heart rate and function and help to restore intravascular volume. Other preoperative concerns include assessment of end-organ dysfunction due to the disease process and normalization of glucose and electrolyte levels [15].

Of equal importance is knowledge and avoidance of those drugs that are contraindicated in patients with pheochromocytoma and that may provoke a hypertensive crisis [16].

TABLE: Common medications to avoid in patients with pheochromocytoma

- Opioid analgesics
  - Morphine
  - Tramadol
  - Naloxone
- Antiemetics
  - Metoclopramide
  - Prochlorperazine
- Corticosteroids
- Norepinephrine reuptake inhibitors
- Selective serotonin reuptake inhibitors
- Linezolid
- Nasal decongestants
  - Pseudoephedrine
  - Phenylpropanolamine
- Tricyclic antidepressants
- Monoamine oxidase inhibitors type A
- Intravenous glucagon
- Weight loss supplements
- Attention deficit hyperactivity medications

** lists above are examples only and not completely inclusive**

Other preoperative concerns include instructions on foods and beverages containing tyramine. Large amounts of tyramine exacerbate uncontrolled catecholamine release [16].

TABLE: Common foods to avoid in patients with pheochromocytoma

- Nuts (peanuts, brazil coconuts)
- Beers and wine
- Chocolate
- Cured and smoked meats
- Aged cheeses
- Fermented soy bean or fish products
- Certain fruits and vegetables (bananas, pineapples, avocados, fava beans, eggplant)

lists above are examples only and not completely inclusive

10. **Describe preoperative adrenergic blockade and volume preparation of a patient with pheochromocytoma presenting for surgery.**

All patients with pheochromocytoma are treated with alpha-adrenergic blockade for 1–2 weeks prior to surgery. Phenoxybenzamine, is a long acting, noncompetitive alpha antagonist. It is prescribed in an escalating dose to achieve a reduction in symptoms and blood pressure stabilization prior to surgery [15]. Because it is long acting and irreversible, phenoxybenzamine can be cause refractory hypotension following removal of the adrenal gland and into the postoperative period. Phenoxybenzamine can provoke tachycardia by blocking the alpha-2 receptors on the presynaptic membrane and subsequent increased norepinephrine release by the cardiac sympathetic nerve endings. Once alpha blockade is established, beta-blockers can be used to treat tachycardia and arrhythmias. Failure to establish alpha-adrenergic blockade prior to use of beta-blockers can result in congestive heart failure.

Doxazosin, prazosin, terazosin are selective, short-acting alpha-1 adrenergic blockers. As a group, these drugs result in less reflex tachycardia and a lower incidence of postoperative hypotension. However, use of theses short-acting, selective alpha-1 receptor blockers may not provide adequate control of perioperative hypertensive episodes. Calcium channel blockers have been used alone or in combination with selective alpha-1 receptor blockers to control blood pressure in patients with pheochromocytoma [17]. Calcium channel blockers block norepinephrine mediated calcium influx into vascular smooth muscle aiding in controlling hypertension and tachyarrythmias. Thought to be less effective than alpha adrenoreceptor blockade, calcium channel blockers may be used to supplement adrenoreceptor blockade in patients with inadequate blood pressure control [18].

Roizen criteria assess the adequacy of preoperative management of pheochromocytoma and continue to be cited as guide to reducing perioperative morbidity and mortality [19, 20]. Criteria include:

- No in-hospital blood pressure >160/90 mmHg for 24 h prior to surgery
- No orthostatic hypotension with blood pressure less than 80/45 mmHg
- No ST or T wave changes for 1 week prior to surgery
- No more than five premature ventricular contractions per minute

Recent attention has been focused on the use of magnesium sulfate, clevidipine, and vasopressin as agents effective in perioperative management of patients with pheochromocytoma. Although not new to management of pheochromocytoma, magnesium sulfate has demonstrated efficacy for hemodynamic control before tumor resection in adults, children, and other rare circumstances such as pregnancy. Clevidipine, a calcium channel blocker, provides rapid titration and precise hemodynamic control in the management of hypertensive crisis before tumor resection. Following tumor resection, vasopressin has demonstrated usefulness in managing catecholamine-resistant shock [21].

Currently, it appears that institutional preference governs whether to use alpha or specific alpha-1 adrenergic receptor blockers. Both are widely accepted for preoperative management of the patient with pheochromocytoma [18]. Weighing of risks and benefits of each drug class, severity of symptoms, therapeutic effects and side effects during the perioperative period warrants careful consideration in preparing a patient with pheochromocytoma for surgical resection.

11. **What are anesthetic considerations in a patient presenting for surgical resection of pheochromocytoma**?

General and neuraxial anesthesia in combination have been successfully used for pheochromocytoma resection. The important concept is to avoid wide swings in blood pressure. In order to promptly recognize and treat sudden extremes of blood pressure, vigilance in the form anticipating provocative events, ensuring proper monitoring including arterial line placement, and adequate intravenous access are required. Drugs should be immediately available to correct periods of hemodynamic instability. Drugs that blunt sympathetic response during times of hemodynamic stimulation including nitroglycerin, nitroprusside, nicardipine, and propofol may be useful [4].

Other drugs that are considered safe for use in patients with pheochromocytoma include benzodiazepines, etomidate, fentanyl, alfentanil, remifentanil, rocuronium, vecuronium, isoflurane, and sevoflurane. **Desflurane can cause significant sympathetic stimulation and is probably best avoided in patients with pheochromocytoma** [4].

TABLE: Predictable triggers of hemodynamic instability

- Induction and intubation
- Pneumoperitoneum during laparoscopic approach
- Surgical incision
- Tumor manipulation and abdominal exploration
- Ligation of venous drainage

Proper large bore intravenous access and monitoring in the form of invasive arterial blood pressure, central venous pressure monitoring, 5 lead EKG monitoring, pulse oximeter, end tidal CO_2, urinary catheter, blood glucose, and temperature monitoring are indicated. In patients with cardiomyopathy, cardiac output monitoring is suggested.

Avoiding drugs commonly used in the administration of anesthesia that may precipitate a hypertensive crisis is critical. Drugs that increase sympathetic tone such as **ketamine**, **ephedrine**, **pancuronium**, **metoclopramide should not be used** in patients with pheochromocytoma [22]. **Histamine provoking drugs such as morphine and atracurium should also be avoided**. **Droperidol, especially at higher**

doses, has been associated with hypertensive crisis in patients with pheochromocytoma [4].

12. **What are the intraoperative considerations for a patient with a pheochromocytoma?**

Intraoperative goals during surgical removal of pheochromocytoma are to avoid drugs and maneuvers that might produce a catecholamine surge, maintain cardiovascular stability and manage hemodynamics and volume status following tumor removal.

Specific variables are reported to predispose patients undergoing surgical resection of pheochromocytoma to increased intraoperative hypertension. These variables include a high norepinephrine production and a larger tumor size (greater than 4 cm.) Other variables include patients with a high blood pressure at presentation and after alpha-adrenergic blockade (mean arterial pressure greater than 100 mmHg). Patients with a postural drop in blood pressure greater than 10 mmHg after alpha receptor blockade also demonstrate a predisposition to develop intraoperative hypertension [23].

13. **Surgical approach and hemodynamic considerations**.

With advancements in tumor localization imaging, a laparoscopic approach to pheochromocytoma resection offers decreased postoperative pain and a quicker recovery. Pneumoperitoneum and tumor manipulation lead to excessive catecholamine secretion and sudden dramatic increases in blood pressure. In addition, insufflation with carbon dioxide gas contributes to hypercarbia leading to increased sympathetic tone. Spikes in blood pressure associated with tumor manipulation should be treated with short-acting agents such as phentolamine, esmolol, or labetalol. Background infusions of inhalational agents and vasoactive infusions such as nitroglycerin, nitroprusside, and nicardipine have been used successfully to control hypertensive episodes related to surgical manipulation of the tumor as well [4]. Review of the literature turns up mostly multidrug combinations for controlling intraoperative spikes in blood pressure. Significant hypertension should not be tolerated. To avoid significant and refractory hypotension following adrenal vein ligation and tumor removal, use of short-acting drugs that mimic expected duration of the hypertensive spikes related to tumor manipulation are recommended. The following is a list of several drug combinations that have been successfully used intraoperatively to manage significant hypertensive episodes prior to surgical removal of pheochromocytoma [4]:

- labetalol infusion
- prazosin and metoprolol
- dexmedetomidine, remifentanil, nitroprusside, and labetalol
- nitroglycerin, esmolol, and clonidine

14. **Discuss catecholamine withdrawal after venous ligation**.

A combination of factors may contribute to refractory hypotension following ligation of the adrenal veins. These include residual alpha blockade from phenoxybenzamine and a sudden drop in circulating catecholamines. Other causative factors include downregulation of adrenoreceptors, contralateral adrenal gland suppression, myocardial dysfunction, and hypovolemia from blood and fluid losses. **Volume loading** before tumor ligation is preferable to initiating vasoactive medications unless fluid boluses prove ineffective. If necessary, phenylephrine, vasopressin, and norepinephrine are acceptable [8].

15. **What are the postoperative considerations after surgical removal of a pheochromocytoma?**

In the immediate and prolonged postoperative period, complications such as hypotension, hypertension, and hypoglycemia can occur. Hypertension occurs in approximately 50% of patients for a few days. Elevated levels of catecholamines can persist up to a week after tumor resection necessitating antihypertensives. Also, pheochromocytoma tumor may still be present. Persistent hypotension may be due to residual alpha-adrenergic blockade or intra-abdominal bleeding [8]. Anecdotal reports of hypotension requiring 48 h of vasopressors can be found in current literature. Hypoglycemia resulting from excessive rebound secretion of insulin may occur after tumor removal and has been reported for up to 6 days postoperatively. Altered mental status following general anesthesia and pain medications may cloud diagnosis and prompt recognition and treatment of hypoglycemia [17].

16. **Special circumstances**:
    - *Pregnancy and pheochromocytoma*
      Pheochromocytoma is a rare and dangerous cause of hypertension during pregnancy. Clinical features of pheochromocytoma in pregnancy are similar to that of the general population. Postural changes, mechanical effects of the gravid uterus, uterine contractions, and increased fetal movements may precipitate paroxysmal attacks [24]. The supine position during pregnancy may cause tumor compression and paroxysmal supine hypertension that is absent in the sitting or standing position. Hypertension and proteinuria may be diagnosed as pre-eclampsia rather

than pheochromocytoma. Management of pheochromocytoma in pregnancy once diagnosed is similar to the general population. Phenoxybenzamine and if needed beta-adrenergic blockade are generally considered safe in pregnancy for treating pheochromocytoma. Although phenoxybenzamine crosses the placenta and may cause perinatal depression and transient hypotension [25]. Hydralazine or labetalol in combination with magnesium sulfate are also useful in treating hypertension and arrhythmias resulting from excessive catecholamine excretions during pregnancy [26]. Diagnosis of pheochromocytoma during pregnancy carries a high risk of maternal and/or fetal mortality. Cesarean section is the preferred mode of delivery. Vigorous fetal movements and labor may be associated with hypertensive crisis. Diagnosis of pheochromocytoma early in pregnancy offers a choice of surgical intervention to remove the tumor; hopefully followed by an uneventful pregnancy [27]. Diagnosis of pheochromocytoma later in pregnancy may result in conservative medical management until the fetus in nearer to term and an elective cesarean section and tumor removal can be performed [28].

- *Undiagnosed pheochromocytoma*
  The classic symptoms of pheochromocytoma are headache, palpitations, and excessive sweating in addition to paroxysmal hypertension. All three of these classic symptoms only occur in less than 50% of patients. Sustained hypertension occurs in more than 50% of patients with pheochromocytoma and may be mistakenly thought to be essential hypertension. Other symptoms associated with pheochromocytoma may also be attributed to other more common causes rather than this rare neuroendocrine tumor. Nevertheless, a patient with undiagnosed pheochromocytoma undergoing anesthesia and surgery is at risk for an unanticipated, life-threatening hypertensive crisis. Factors triggering pheochromocytoma crisis in a patient with an undiagnosed tumor include the typical sequence of events during induction of anesthesia and surgical events. Anxiety in an awake patient, light anesthesia during intubation and/or surgery, and mechanical factors including straining, scrubbing, tumor manipulation, and carbon dioxide insufflation for laparoscopy may all trigger excessive release of catecholamines from pheochromocytoma and hypertensive crisis refractory to the typical treatments [29]. If occult pheochromocytoma is suspected, judicious use of short-acting vasodilators such as phentolamine or nitroprusside may prove effective. In the event of extreme tachycardia, beta blockade should only be used after alpha blockade is adequate to avoid unopposed alpha receptor activity and subsequent vasoconstriction, hypertension, and heart failure [29]. If at all possible, aborting the surgical procedure is probably wise [27].

References

1. Myklejord DJ. Undiagnosed pheochromocytoma: the anesthesiologist nightmare. Clin Med Res. 2004;2(1):59–62.
2. Manger WM, Gifford RW. Pheochromocytoma. J Clin Hypertens. 2002;4:62–72.
3. Young WF Jr. Endocrine hypertension: then and now. Endocr Pract. 2010;16:888–902.
4. Woodrum D, Kheterpal S. Anesthetic management of pheochromocytoma. World J Endocr Surg. 2010;2(3):111–7.
5. Guerrero MA, Schreinemakers JM, Vriens MR, Suh I, Hwang J, Shen WT, Gosnell J, Clark OH, Duh QY. Clinical spectrum of pheochromocytoma. J Am Coll Surg. 2009;209(6):727.
6. Bland ML, Desanclozeaux M, Ingraham HA. Tissue growth and remodeling of the embryonic and adult adrenal gland. Ann N Y Acad Sci. 2003;989:59.
7. Sasidharan P, Johnston I. Phaeochromocytoma: Perioperative Management. Anaesthesia Tutorial of the Week 151. 14 Sep 2009.
8. Ahmed A. Perioperative management of pheochromocytoma: anaesthetic implications. J Pak Med Assoc. 2007;57(3):140–6.
9. Eisenhofer G, Rivers G, Rosas AL, Quezado Z, Manger WM, Pacak K. Adverse drug reactions in patients with pheochromocytoma: incidence, prevalence and management. Drug Saf. 2007;30 (11):1031–62.
10. Young WF, Kaplan NM. Clinical presentation of diagnosis of pheochromocytoma. www.uptodate.com updated May 12, 2014.
11. Bravo EL, Gifford RW. Pheochromocytoma. Endocrinol Metab Clin North Am. 1993;22:329.
12. Waguespack SG, Rich T, Grubbs E, Yink AK, Perrier ND, Ayala-Ramirez M, et al. A current review of the etiology, diagnosis and treatment of pediatric pheochromocytoma and paraganglioma. J Clin Endocrinol Metab. 2010;95(5):2023–37.
13. Sheps SG, Jiang NS, Klee GG, van Heerden JA. Recent developments in the diagnosis and treatment of pheochromocytoma. Mayo Clin Proc. 1990;65(1):88–95.
14. Pomares FJ, Canas R, Rodriguez JM, et al. Differences between sporadic and multiple endocrine neoplasia type 2A phaeochromocytoma. Clin Endocrin (Oxf). 1998;48:195.
15. Domi R, Sula H. Pheochromocytoma, the challenge to anesthesiologists. J Endocrinol Metab. 2011;1(3):97–100.
16. Phitayakorn R, McHenry CR. Perioperative considerations in patients with adrenal tumors. J Surg Oncol. 2012;106:604–10.
17. Lentschener C, Gaujoux S, Tesniere A, Dousset B. Point of controversy: perioperative care of patients undergoing pheochromocytoma removal-time for a reappraisal? Eur J Endocrinol. 2011;165:365–73.
18. Pacak K. Approach to the Patient: Preoperative Management of the Pheochromocytoma Patient. J Clin Endocrinol Metab. 2007. 92 (11).
19. Turkistani A. Anesthetic management of pheochromocytoma: a case report. MEJ Anesth. 2009;20(1):111–4.
20. Sherif L, Hegde R, Shetty K, Gurumurthy T, Jain P. Anesthetic management of a rare case of extra adrenal pheochromocytoma—a case report. The Internet Journal of Anesthesiology. 2008. 21(1).

21. Lord MS, Augoustides JG. Perioperative management of pheochromocytoma: focus on magnesium, clevidipine, and vasopressin. J Cardiothorac Vasc Anesth. 2012;26(3):526–31.
22. Domi R, Laho H. Management of pheochromocytoma: old ideas and new drugs. Niger J Clin Pract. 2012;15(3):253–7.
23. Bruynzeel H, Feelders RA, Groenland HN, van der Meiracker AH, van Eijck CHJ, Lange JF, de Herder WW, Kazemier G. Risk factors for hemodynamic instability during surgery for pheochromocytoma. J Clin Endocrinol Metab. 2010;95(2):678–85.
24. Hamilton A, Sirrs S, Schmidt N, Onrot J. Anaesthesia for phaeochromocytoma in pregnancy. Can J Anaesth. 1997;44:654–7.
25. Santeiro ML, Stromquist C, Wyble L. Phenoxybenzamine placental transfer during the third trimester. Ann Pharmacother. 1996;30:1249.
26. James MFM. Adrenal Medulla. The anesthetic management of pheochromocytoma. In: Anaesthesia for patients with endocrine disease. Oxford: Oxford University Press; 2010; p. 149–68 (Chapter 8).
27. Hull CJ, Bachelor AM. Anesthetic management of patient with endocrine disease. In: Wylie and Churchill Davidson's. A practice of anesthesia. 7th ed. 2003; p. 811–27.
28. Takahashi K, Sai Y, Nosaka S. Anaesthetic management for caesarean section combined with removal of phaeochromocytoma. Eur J Anaesthesiol. 1998;15:364.
29. Anis Baraka (2011). Undiagnosed Pheochromocytoma Complicated with Perioperative Hemodynamic Crisis and Multiple Organ Failure, Pheochromocytoma—A New View of the Old Problem, Dr. Jose Fernando Martin (Ed.). ISBN: 978-953-307-822-9, InTech, doi:10.5772/25963. Available from: http://www.intechopen.com/books/pheochromocytoma-a-new-view-of-the-old-problem/undiagnosed-pheochromocytoma-complicated-with-perioperative-hemodynamic-crisis-and-multiple-organ-failure.

Part VI
The Abdomen

Section Editor: Michael T. Bailin

Michael T. Bailin
Department of Anesthesiology, Baystate Health,
Springfield, MA, USA

The Full Stomach

27

Scott Switzer and Derek Rosner

You are called urgently to the radiology suite to provide sedation for a 25-year old, otherwise healthy male undergoing MRI of the head. He is s/p MVA (motor vehicle accident) with an open femur fracture and has become agitated. The radiologist is uncomfortable providing conscious sedation.

Medications:	Methyphenidate LA, Dilaudid (hydromorphone) 2 mg (In ED)
Allergies:	None
PMHx:	ADHD
Physical Exam:	
Vital Signs:	HR 115 BP 140/90 RR 24 SpO_2 99% NC O_2@3 L/m
HEENT:	C-collar in place
	Full lumberjack beard
	Pupils miotic, equal, sluggish
	Uncooperative with airway exam
Otherwise unremarkable	
Labs: Unremarkable other than blood alcohol level of 0.25%	
NPO status unknown	
Other commonly used GERD, LES	

(1) **What constitutes a "Full Stomach"?**

In anesthesia, the term "full stomach" applies to patients that have recently ingested foods and/or have pharmacologic, metabolic, anatomic, or hormonal conditions, which impair gastric emptying. Full stomach patients are at a greater risk for pulmonary aspiration of gastric contents during all phases of an anesthetic.

S. Switzer (✉) · D. Rosner
Department of Anesthesiology, Baystate Medical Center, 759 Chestnut St., Springfield, MA 01107, USA
e-mail: scott.switzer@baystatehealth.org

D. Rosner
e-mail: intubateu@gmail.com

© Springer International Publishing AG 2017
L.S. Aglio and R.D. Urman (eds.), *Anesthesiology*,
DOI 10.1007/978-3-319-50141-3_27

The most important factors leading to complications from aspiration are the gastric volume and pH. Studies point to gastric volumes around 20 cc/kg (←check this number) and a pH <2.5 correlating to more severe complications of aspiration.

As an example, pregnant patients in the third trimester are considered "full stomach" even if they have obeyed fasting criteria.

(2) **What are the risk factors that increase the likelihood of gastric aspiration?**

Risk factors that increase the likelihood of gastric aspiration include anatomic, pharmacologic, metabolic, autonomic, and hormonal states that impair gastric emptying or impair protective airway reflexes. These include, but are not limited to:

Autonomic neuropathy
Augmented adrenergic state (stress, pain, etc.)
Alcohol intoxication
Opioid administration/sedation
Anticholinergic medications
Traumatic head injury
Encephalopathy
Nasogastric intubation (impaired gag reflex, altered LES tone)
Bowel obstruction/acute abdominal pathology
Obesity
Pregnancy
Hiatal hernia

A diabetic patient with profound autonomic neuropathy may have impaired gastric emptying. In addition, patients with large hiatal hernias, morbid obesity, and pregnancy may have a higher likelihood of gastric aspiration because of the cephalad displacement of the gastroesophageal junction and loss of lower esophageal sphincter (LES) tone [1].

(3) **How does obesity or GERD affect the risk for gastric aspiration? What if the GERD is well controlled?**

Morbidly obese patients with large truncal adiposity may have displacement of their gastroesophageal junction cephalad, altering LES pressure and increasing the risk for gastric aspiration. In addition, obese patients are at greater risk for developing type 2 diabetes-induced autonomic neuropathy, which could slow gastric emptying. Patients with GERD generally are NOT at greater risk for gastric aspiration, unless their GERD is secondary to a large hiatal hernia or another process which has altered LES tone. Patients with well-controlled GERD are generally considered low risk for gastric aspiration [1].

(4) **What pharmacologic measures can be employed (have been demonstrated) to minimize the risk of gastric aspiration?**

While there are no agents that have demonstrated a decrease in the risk of gastric aspiration, some pharmacologic interventions can be employed to potentially mitigate any sequelae. The only agents available that BOTH decrease gastric volume and increase gastric pH are proton pump inhibitors (PPI) and histamine-2 blockers, such as famotidine (H2-blocker) or esomeprazole (PPI). Other agents that can be considered in high risk patients include metoclopramide, a gastric pro-kinetic agent that works by blocking dopamine receptors. This agent both increases LES tone and promotes gastric motility. Sodium citrate is a non-particulate antacid which can be used to increase gastric pH.

(5) **What factors affect LES pressure?**

The LES is a 2–4 cm high pressure region at the gastroesophageal junction. Different from the remainder of esophagus, the LES maintains an increased resting tone secondary to cholinergic influences and calcium influxes. However, many ingestible, pharmacologic, and anatomic factors can alter this relationship. The following is a list of the most common factors:

<u>Foods:</u>

Chocolate
Ethanol
Peppermint
Caffeine

<u>Hormones:</u>

CCK
Progesterone
Secretin
Glucagon
Somatostain
VIP

<u>Autonomic nervous system:</u>

Beta-adrenergic agonists
Alpha-adrenergic antagonists
Anticholinergics

<u>Others:</u>

Theophylline
Smoking
Morphine, meperidine
Calcium-channel blockers
Diazepam
Dopamine

(6) **What factors are involved in the decision to place a nasogastric tube (NGT) prior to the induction of general anesthesia?**

In patients with a full stomach, it would be beneficial to decrease the volume of gastric contents prior to the administration of medications, which will ablate the protective airway reflexes. This is especially true in cases in which there is significant abdominal distention due to obstruction of the GI tract, leading to the accumulation of GI gas and liquid secretions. The goal of "decompressing the stomach" is a worthy one, but should be considered carefully.

NGT insertion is uncomfortable at best, and uncooperative patients may not tolerate the procedure without significant sedation, possibly jeopardizing the protective pharyngeal reflexes we wish to protect. The procedure can also cause bleeding, and trauma to the naso/oropharynx, making laryngoscopy more difficult. In addition, it should be noted that NGT suction will rarely yield a completely empty stomach.

The presence of a gastric tube in the esophagus and stomach can also compromise LES tone, and has been identified as a risk factor for aspiration. For this reason, many practitioners will remove the NGT prior to induction.

In this patient, several factors argue against NGT placement prior to the induction of general anesthesia. First, the history of head trauma raises the possibility of a fracture of the cribriform plate, leading to possible intracranial injury during placement. Secondly, given this patient's altered and deteriorating mental status NGT placement could provoke agitation, retching or emesis, and would most certainly lead to an aggravated sympathetic response. All of these are to be avoided in the brain injured patient. It is therefore reasonable to argue that NGT placement in this patient would be unwarranted and potentially dangerous.

(7) **What is a "protected airway"?**

The ideal "protected airway" is a conscious patient with intact airway reflexes. When these conditions are not present, a "protected airway", as described by anesthesia providers, is a cuffed endotracheal tube inflated in the trachea. An LMA would NOT be an example of a protected airway.

(8) **What is a "rapid sequence induction?"**

Rapid sequence induction in anesthesia refers to the process and sequence of drug delivery in an effort to secure a patient's airway expeditiously, minimizing the risk of gastric aspiration. In a rapid sequence induction, after application of ASA standard monitors and denitrogenation, an induction agent is introduced intravenously followed by a fast acting muscle relaxant, in rapid succession. In addition, cricoid pressure is applied before the patient is anesthetized in an effort to compress the esophagus against the posterior portion of the cartilaginous ring, minimizing the risk for gastric aspiration. Prior to direct laryngoscopy, NO positive pressure breaths are delivered. Once an endotracheal tube is confirmed to be in the appropriate location with bilateral breath sounds and the cuff is inflated, the airway is considered secure and cricoid pressure is relieved.

(9) **What is cricoid pressure? What is the utility of cricoid pressure during rapid sequence induction?**

Cricoid pressure, or Sellick's maneuver, refers to the application of downward (posterior) force, applied to the anterior aspect of the cricoid cartilage during rapid sequence induction, with the aim to prevent the reflux and aspiration of gastric contents. As the cricoid cartilage is the only continuous ring in the glottis, it is used to compress, and hopefully occlude the esophagus posteriorly against the anterior aspect of the vertebral bodies. Traditionally, 10–20 N of force are applied prior to induction, with an increase of 30–40 N after induction. Cricoid pressure is not released until the establishment of a protected airway is confirmed via auscultation of the lungs, and if possible, the detection of expired CO_2.

Despite the intuitive usefulness of this maneuver, clinical benefit has not been repeatedly demonstrated. Several studies have shown that practitioners, even when well trained, do not perform effective compression of the cricoid ring, either by failing to accurately locate the cricoid, by applying an incorrect amount of force to the cricoid, or by applying force in such a way as to displace the esophagus laterally, rather than posteriorly. Additionally, even correctly applied cricoid pressure has been shown to obscure the view of the glottis, or to interfere with the passage of the endotracheal tube during intubation. Other complications associated with the application of cricoid pressure include nausea, vomiting and aspiration in non-anesthetized patients, esophageal rupture, and exacerbation of unrecognized airway or cervical spine injuries.

Largely due to the unproven clinical benefit of cricoid pressure and the potential for delaying the expeditious establishment of a protected airway, there is considerable controversy surrounding the utility of cricoid pressure during RSI. Despite this, it is still considered by many to be standard of practice, and should not be abandoned without consideration of the clinical situation at hand.

(10) **What neuromuscular blocking drugs should be employed during a rapid sequence induction? How would you choose?**

Both classes of muscle relaxants (depolarizing and non-depolarizing) can be employed for a rapid sequence induction. Classically, succinylcholine, a depolarizing muscle relaxant, is employed to facilitate endotracheal tube placement in a rapid sequence induction. However, if contraindications to succinylcholine exist (history of malignant hyperthermia or an elevated potassium level, etc.), rocuronium, a non-depolarizing muscle relaxant, can be employed. The conventional dose of rocuronium for a standard anesthetic induction is 0.6–0.7 mg/kg. However, for a rapid sequence induction utilizing rocuronium, the dose is increased to 1.2 mg/kg to decrease to time to achieve adequate intubating conditions.

(11) **What are the pros and cons to MAC anesthesia for this patient?**

In this case, MAC anesthesia could be employed. The benefits of this technique include avoidance of airway instrumentation, given his potential cervical spinal injury, and avoidance of possible difficulties with both mask ventilation (note full lumberjack beard) and intubation (cervical spine collar in place). However, given the patient's intoxicated state, unknown NPO status, and recent agitation, providing safe and adequate sedation may be a challenge. In addition the patient's inaccessible position in the MRI scanner would lead most to establish a secure airway prior to beginning the study. If a MAC anesthetic is chosen, avoidance of agents that would abolish pharyngeal reflexes (in the event of aspiration) or cause respiratory depression (given the patient's airway state, potential intracranial hypertension, and distant location in the scanner) is appropriate. Acceptable agents for a MAC anesthetic might include the alpha-2 agonist dexmedetomidine and the NMDA-antagonist ketamine (assuming no intracranial hypertension exists).

(12) **What are the pros and cons to awake fiberoptic intubation for this patient?**

Advantages of an awake fiberoptic intubation in this patient include securing the airway in a fashion that allows the patient to spontaneously breathe and does not abolish pharyngeal reflexes in the event of emesis. However, difficulties in performing an awake fiberoptic intubation in this patient are numerous. Patient compliance may be an obstacle given the patient's intoxicated state. Fiberoptic placement orally may be impaired by the patient's "full lumberjack beard", cervical spinal collar and decreased mouth opening, given that he did not cooperate during the initial airway exam. A nasal approach could be employed to bypass the oropharyngeal challenges with appropriate vasoconstriction and nasopharyngeal anesthesia. Caution should be noted that given this patient is s/p MVA with distracting injuries and a head injury. A cribriform plate fracture cannot be ruled out until imaging has been completed.

(13) **What is the proper course of action if the patient vomits during induction with an unprotected airway?**

The patient should be immediately turned to the lateral, head down position to promote regurgitant gastric flow away from the glottis. Gentle oropharyngeal suction should then be performed to clear the upper airway. Given this patient's uncertain c-spine stability, care must be taken when performing this maneuver (logroll with at least three caretakers). This is now an emergent situation and immediately securing the airway is the priority. If not already done, succinylcholine should be administered to obtain optimal intubating conditions. A direct laryngoscopy with in-line stabilization of the neck is a reasonable course of action, as this is generally the most expeditious method of intubation. Having an available video laryngoscope may be useful; however, fiberoptic intubation at this point would generally not be optimal. This is due to the likely presence of gastric contents in the oropharynx and the time required to implement this technique. Given the patient's recent agitation, developing intracranial hypertension from head trauma is a possibility. Avoidance of hypercarbia (via hypoventilation) through speedy establishment of a definitive airway would be beneficial.

(14) **What is the role of fiberoptic bronchoscopy in the immediate post- aspiration period? Bronchoalveolar lavage?**

Once the airway is secured, the patient should be adequately anesthetized, neuromuscular paralysis should be obtained with a non-depolarizing agent, and hemodynamic stability should be ensured. Immediate bronchoscopic evaluation can be used to determine the extent of airway contamination by gastric contents, and to clear obstructions/secretions from the trachea and proximal smaller airways. While extensive and careful suction may aid in diminishing the pulmonary complications of gastric aspiration, using saline to perform bronchoalveolar lavage should be used with caution, as this can spread gastric contamination further into the distal airways, and potentially worsen pulmonary complications.

In this patient, attention should be paid to adequate ventilation during bronchoscopy to avoid hypercarbia in the setting of possible intracranial HTN.

(15) **What is Mendelson's syndrome?**

Described by Curtis Mendelson, a New York obstetrician in 1946, Mendelson's syndrome refers to the bronchopulmonary complications of aspiration of gastric contents following the induction of general anesthesia. Signs and symptoms typically manifest over a biphasic course, with an early phase at 1–2 h, and then again at 4–6 h due to neutrophil infiltration. Hypoxia, dyspnea, and cyanosis are the cardinal signs, but hemodynamic instability may accompany massive aspiration events which progress to ARDS and multisystem organ failure. Damage to the lungs (chemical pneumonitis) is mainly due to the low pH of gastric contents. Edema, atelectasis and pulmonary hemorrhage are common sequelae. Postobstructive pneumonia or secondary bacterial pneumonia can also develop in the aftermath of aspiration events.

(16) **What are the expected radiographic findings in the period following aspiration of gastric contents?**

Alveolar/lobar infiltrates in the dependent lung segments (especially the right lower and middle lobes in supine patients) may take up to 48 h to fully appear, and several weeks to completely resolve. Appearance of chest X-ray findings may therefore lag significantly behind the development of symptoms, and likewise, resolution of X-ray findings may lag behind improvements in clinical conditions. Significant volume loss on chest radiograph typically indicates bronchial obstruction with postobstructive collapse.

(17) How do you care for a patient with significant sequelae of gastric aspiration? What is the role of steroids or antibiotics?

Treatment following a significant aspiration event includes prevention of further aspiration by positioning the patient at 45° head up, protecting the airway, as needed, through endotracheal intubation and ventilating with a standard, lung-protective strategy. Supportive care includes goal-directed O_2 administration (SpO_2 is reasonable) and hemodynamic support with IV fluids and vasopressors as needed. Originally corticosteroids were routinely administered following gastric aspiration events. However, more recent work has called their routine use into question due to increased risk for gram negative pneumonias and increased ICU length of stay. Antibiotics are not indicated for pure chemical pneumonitis. However, high risk patients (those with gastroparesis, proton pump inhibitor or H2 antagonist use or periodontal disease) may warrant a course of antimicrobial prophylaxis with gram negative and anerobic coverage [2].

18 What ventilator settings would be appropriate for a patient with known aspiration of gastric contents?

Patients who have suffered from aspiration of gastric contents generally develop a chemical pneumonitis. The severity of this can range from a transient irritated cough and no additional oxygen requirements, to full blown ARDS and multisystem organ failure. Patients who require mechanical ventilation should receive supplemental oxygen as required for goal-directed titration. SpO_2 is a reasonable marker, but $ScvO_2$ or arterial PO_2 can also be used in severe cases. Standard lung-protective strategies can be employed for ventilator settings. This generally entails low tidal volume ventilation (4–6 ml/kg) with PEEP (5–8 cm H_2O) and intermittent recruitment maneuvers to prevent/treat atelectasis.

(19) What is the plan for postoperative care of this patient? Would extubation be appropriate?

Chemical pneumonitis associated with gastric aspiration can range from mild to severe, therefore the postoperative care of this patient will be dependent upon the clinical course over the next several hours and operative interventions by the surgical team. If lung compliance and oxygen saturation are adequate without significant supplemental oxygen, and ventilation is sufficient (may verify with arterial blood gas measurements), extubation and oxygen supplementation via nasal cannula or face mask oxygen is reasonable.

Extubation to noninvasive ventilation may not be a successful strategy, as any process that leads to the patient developing dyspnea at this early stage will likely continue to evolve over the next several hours resulting in reintubation. An additional reason to leave the patient intubated, regardless of pulmonary function would be if there are plans to return to the OR for other surgeries in the very near future. A discussion with the surgical services involved in the care of this patient would be appropriate.

References

1. Ng A, Smith G. Gastroesophageal reflux and aspiration of gastric contents in anesthetic practice. Anesth Analg. 2001;93:494–513.
2. Raghavendran K, Nemzek J, Napolitano LM, Knight PR. Aspiration-induced lung injury. Crit Care Med. 2011;39(4):818–26.

Anesthesia for Liver Transplantation

28

John Stenglein

Case Presentation You are called to the ICU to evaluate a 45 y/o male with history of untreated hepatitis C and newly diagnosed hemochromatosis. He has a long history of depression and alcohol abuse. More recently, his clinical course has been complicated by portal hypertension, recurrent ascites, and he now presents with worsening encephalopathy.

Meds	spironolactone, propranolol, lactulose, neomycin, multivitamin
Med Hx:	Depression, anxiety, alcohol abuse. Hepatitis C infection, cirrhosis, portal hypertension
Surg Hx:	TIPSS procedure following variceal bleeding 1 year ago
Physical Exam:	165 lbs, 5′ 10″; BP = 100/64; HR = 100; RR = 18; O_2 Sat = 96 (room air); unremarkable airway exam; Palpable liver edge below costal margin
Patient c/o SOB relieved with lying supine	

Section 1: Physiology

1. What is the anatomy of the liver?

As the largest internal organ and gland, the liver weighs about 3–4 lbs. It is composed of four unequal lobes. The right (largest) and left lobes are separated by the falciform ligament. The much smaller caudate and quadrate lobes are located on the visceral side of the organ, between the other two lobes.

The liver is further divided into a total of eight segments, all of which is covered by a thin layer of connective tissue known as Glisson's capsule.

2. What is the porta hepatis?

This refers to the central hilum where the common bile duct, portal vein, and hepatic artery enter the liver.

3. What is the blood supply to the liver?

The liver has a dual blood supply and receives approximately 25% of cardiac output. The common hepatic artery arises from the celiac trunk (off the aorta) and sends off the cystic artery before entering the liver. Although it only provides a quarter of the total blood flow, it provides half of the hepatic oxygen supply. The portal vein is formed from the confluence of the splenic and superior mesenteric veins and receives blood from the digestive tract, spleen, pancreas, and gall bladder. It supplies the majority of hepatic blood flow (75%), although less oxygen than its arterial counter part. There is a reciprocal flow relationship between the two systems, known as the hepatic arterial buffer response (HABR), which is mediated by adenosine and functions to maintain the adequacy of perfusion [1].

4. What are hepatic sinusoids?

Hepatic sinusoids refer to a type of open pore vessel or discontinuous capillary. This type of discontinuous endothelium allows for the passage of proteins, as large as albumin to pass freely. The sinusoids are separated from the hepatocytes by the space of Disse.

Sinusoids receive oxygen-rich blood from the hepatic artery and the nutrient-rich blood from the portal vein. They are also the home of Kuppfer cells, which filter and process microbes, toxins, and antigens.

From the sinusoids, blood flow empties into the central vein of each lobule, which is the basic structural unit of the

J. Stenglein (✉)
Department of Anesthesiology, Baystate Medical Center, Tufts University School of Medicine, 759 Chestnut St, Springfield, MA 01199, USA
e-mail: john.stenglein@baystatehealth.org

© Springer International Publishing AG 2017
L.S. Aglio and R.D. Urman (eds.), *Anesthesiology*,
DOI 10.1007/978-3-319-50141-3_28

liver. The central veins coalesce into hepatic veins, which leave the liver and drain blood to the IVC.

5. What is a liver acinus?

This refers to the basic functional unit of the liver. It is formed around a portal canal, which is comprised of an arteriole and bile ductile, as well as nerves and lymph tissue. Blood from the portal canal is directed toward a central venule via sinusoids. This flow is divided into three circulatory zones, based on proximity to the canal. Zone 1 receives the highest flow, whereas Zone 2 and Zone 3 receive successively less in terms of both oxygen and nutrients, making hepatocytes in the latter zones more vulnerable to ischemia from circulatory disruption.

6. What is the hepatic portal venous system?

The hepatic portal venous system channels drainage from the gastrointestinal tract into the liver. Blood drained from the distal esophagus to the proximal anal canal joins venous return from the spleen and pancreas to empty into the venous system destined for the liver. This allows many of the substances absorbed by the GI tract to undergo the first pass effect, allowing selective metabolism and detoxification, before reaching the general circulation.

7. What are the functions of the liver?

The various functions of the liver are carried out by hepatocytes. The liver is responsible for hundreds of separate functions, usually in combination with other systems and organs. Some of the main functions are listed below, arranged by endocrine, anabolic, and catabolic features:

<u>Endocrine</u>
Produces Insulin-like growth factor I (IGF-I)
Produces thrombopoietin
Produces angiotensinogen (⇧ results in diminishes negative feedback loop for renin.)
Hydroxylates vitamin D
Deiodinates thyroxine and triiodothyronine (converting T3 to T4)
Metabolizes and conjugates steroid hormones
Stores glycogen for later conversion to glucose.
<u>Anabolic</u>
Produces antithrombin III
Produces Alpha-1 antitrypsin
Produces Protein C and S
Produces Plasinomogen
Produces Factors I, II, V, VII, IX, X XI, XII, XIII prekallikrein. (does not make III, IV, VIII, vWF)
Produces C-reactive protein, haptoglobin, ceruloplasmin, transferrin,
Produces pseudocholinesterase
Produces alpha acid glycoprotein
Produces glutathione—cofactor for elimination of oxidants
Produces ketones
Synthesizes albumin (plasma oncotic pressure/drug binding)
Synthesizes saturated fatty acids
Synthesizes cholesterol
Synthesizes bile salts (lipid absorption, transport, secretion)
Performs gluconeogenesis (glycogen as initial source, then lactate, glycerol, alanine, and glutamate)
<u>Catabolic functions</u>
Breaks down amino acids to ammonia
Eliminates and metabolizes toxins absorbed from GI tract (alcohol, drugs, etc.)
Eliminates ammonia through urea production.
Supports Biotransformation reactions
(phase I—making drugs more polar by adding polar/removing nonpolar groups)
(phase II—adding hydrophilic molecules)
Metabolizes glucose, fructose, lactate, citrate, and acetate
Degrades hemoglobin, bilirubin, fibrin split products,
Clears activated coagulation factors.
Inactivates aldosterone, ADH, insulin, estrogen, and androgens.

<u>Pathophysiology</u>

(1) What is cirrhosis? How long does it take to develop?

Cirrhosis is the end result of a variety of chronic liver diseases, all leading to irreversible scarring of the liver. The resultant fibrosis (scarring) is an impedance to flow and requires higher pressures for entering blood. Flow ultimately favors the lower resistance provided by portosystemic shunts and begins to bypass the liver (and hepatic functions) entirely.

Fortunately, the liver is an organ with a tremendous reserve. Normal function may be maintained when as little as 20% of the liver remains, which is why many of the insidious hepatic diseases can take years to manifest signs or symptoms. It also provides the key to successful living-donor transplantation.

(2) What is the most common cause of cirrhosis in the United States? Worldwide?

Although it is the most common cause of cirrhosis in the US, alcoholism only develops in 10–20% of excessive drinkers [2]. The metabolism of EtOH, catalyzed by alcohol dehydrogenase, results in significant oxidative damage, which depletes antioxidants and induces liver injury.

In contrast, viral hepatitides (specifically types B and C) are the most common causes of cirrhosis worldwide.

(3) How are the causes of liver failure categorized?

The etiology of liver failure can be divided into noncholestatic and cholestatic causes of cirrhosis.

Causes of Noncholestatic cirrhosis include:

Hepatitis (viral, ETOH, drug-induced)
Hemochromatosis
Alpha 1 antitrypsin
Cystic fibrosis
Wilson Disease
Budd–Chiari
Amyloidosis
Amanita intoxication
Solvents (such as CCl_4)

Causes of Cholestatic cirrhosis (intrahepatic or extrahepatic) include:

Primary biliary cirrhosis
Primary sclerosis cholangitis
Biliary atresia (most common pediatric cause for transplant)

(4) What is the distinction between acute and chronic liver failure?

Acute liver failure (aka fulminant hepatic failure) refers to the new onset of encephalopathy and an elevated INR (≥ 1.5) in patients without previous liver disease, over a period of less than 26 weeks. More than half of the cases are attributed to drug-related toxicity (usually acetaminophen). Due to the rapid progression of the disease, signs of portal hypertension and cirrhosis are generally absent.

Only 40% of patients with acute liver failure will recover spontaneously [3].

(5) What is the mechanism by which acetaminophen toxicity results in hepatic failure? Can anything be done to alter the clinical course?

In adults, the primary metabolic pathway for acetaminophen is glucuronidation.

The main metabolite is relatively nontoxic and is excreted into bile. A small amount of the drug is metabolized via the CYP-450 pathway into NAPQI, which is a strong, highly hepatotoxic, oxidizing agent. Following a supratherapeutic ingestion, the levels of NAPQI produced by the CYP system overwhelm the ability for conjugation/inactivation by the available glutathione stores. The toxic metabolites accumulate and begin to destroy liver cells.

Oral activated charcoal readily binds acetaminophen and can be of significant benefit if administered within 1 h following ingestion.

N-acetylcysteine (NAC) given within 8 h of overdose can dramatically decrease the risks of toxicity, as it is a precursor of glutathione and increases the concentration of the latter for conjugation of NAPQI.

(6) What are the five major types of viral hepatitis? How are they transmitted? What percentage will become chronically infected?

Hep A—The most common viral hepatitis (50% of all cases) due to a high degree of contagiousness. Primary spread is due to fecal–oral transmission. Course is usually benign and self-limited. However, an estimated 100 patients die each year in the US from acute hepatic failure related to infection [4]. Inactivated HAV vaccine may provide protection for 10 years or longer.

Hep B—Five-percent of world's population is chronically infected [5]. Ninety percent recover from the acute infection, however, 1–5% of adults will remain in carrier state. Eighty to ninety percent of infected children will become carriers. Primary spread is from contact with infected body fluids. According to the CDC, three doses of the HBV vaccine provide greater than 90% protection to infants, children, and adults who are immunized prior to exposure and boosters are no longer recommended for patients with normal immunity who have completed the series. In women who are seropositive for both HBsAg and HBeAg vertical transmission is approximately 90% [6].

Approximately 25% of those who become chronically infected during childhood and 15% of those who become chronically infected after childhood die prematurely from cirrhosis or liver cancer and the majority remain asymptomatic until the onset of cirrhosis or end-stage liver disease [7].

Hep C—An estimated 1.8% of US population carries HCV, representing the estimated 75% of acute infections, which have become chronic. It is generally transmitted through contact with infected blood. Progression from infection to cirrhosis or hepatocellular cancer may take decades, similar to HBV. Newly approved medications can cure infection upwards of 90% of individuals, depending on the subtype [8].

Hep D—HDV can propagate only in the presence of the hepatitis B virus (HBV), and is spread in a similar manner [9]. Transmission of HDV can occur either via simultaneous infection with HBV or be superimposed on a chronic infection. In combination with HBV, hepatitis D has the highest fatality rate of all the hepatitis infections, at 20%.

Hep E—HEV is similar to hepatitis A in both transmission and clinical course. However, during pregnancy the disease is much more severe and can result in acute hepatic failure. During the third trimester, the mortality rate from acute infection approaches 20% [10].

(7) How does the presence of an acute hepatitis infection or (chronic) cirrhosis impact the risks of surgery?

Acute hepatitis is considered a significant risk for elective surgery, predisposing patients to significant morbidity and mortality. Similarly, cirrhosis is a major risk factor for nonhepatic procedures. As such, elective procedures should be avoided in the decompensated state, as evidenced by increased INR, encephalopathy, or infection.

(8) What is Budd–Chiari Syndrome?

It is a rare condition caused by thrombosis of the major hepatic veins, which generally presents with abdominal pain, jaundice, ascites, and hepatomegaly. In about half of cases, patients are found to be hypercoagulable, relating to pregnancy, polycythemia vera, oral contraceptive agents, lupus anticoagulant, among other causes. The majority of patients do not respond/are not candidates for medical therapy and will require some type of invasive intervention, such as the surgical shunting of blood around the clot. Unfortunately, many will become transplant candidates secondary to progression to acute hepatic failure.

(9) What is acute fatty liver of pregnancy?

It is a microvesicular fatty infiltration of hepatocytes, possibly related to an inherited enzyme deficiency in the mitochondrial beta-oxidation of fatty acids [11]. The incidence is generally estimated at 1 in 7000 to 1 in 20,000 deliveries.

Symptoms usually present in the third trimester with nausea, vomiting, jaundice, abdominal pain, and encephalopathy. Laboratory evidence may reveal elevated LFTs and a prolonged PT. Liver biopsy is diagnostic and treatment involves the prompt delivery of the fetus, regardless of gestational age. Most patients recover; however in one population-based study in the UK of 57 patients, one woman required a liver transplant and a second case proved fatal [12].

(10) What is hemochromatosis?

It is an autosomal recessive disorder (0.5% homozygous in US [13]) associated with increased intestinal absorption of iron. Iron overload results in excessive and injurious deposition in tissues, especially the liver, heart, pancreas, and pituitary. Pathogenesis is usually less severe in women due to menstruation. Hemochromatosis may lead to diabetes, CHF, and increased pigmentation of skin ("bronze diabetes"). Labs reveal increased serum iron and ferritin, as well as increased transferrin saturation. Diagnosis is confirmed by liver biopsy. Treatment is scheduled phlebotomy. Excessive EtOH intake and coexisting viral hepatic infection worsen disease progression, and a late diagnosis may leave few options other than a transplant.

(11) What is Wilson disease?

It is an autosomal recessive disorder associated with the accumulation of copper. It is universally fatal if untreated, and most will die of liver disease [14]. It results from the defective excretion of copper into bile. Symptoms include wide-ranging neurologic dysfunction and hepatic dysfunction, eventually leading to cirrhosis. Initial testing includes LFTs, CBC, and serum ceruloplasmin, as well as an ocular slit-lamp exam and a 24-hour urine test for copper excretion. A Kayser Fleischer ring, referring to a crescent of pigmentation at the periphery of the cornea, may be present on exam and is included in a scoring system for diagnosis. Treatment often involves copper chelation with penicillamine depending on the severity of disease. Liver transplant can be lifesaving for patients with Wilson disease presenting with acute hepatic failure or chronic liver disease unresponsive to treatment.

(12) What is alpha-1 antitrypsin (AAT) deficiency?

AAT is an inherited disorder that involves both the lungs and liver. In the US, individuals with severe deficiency are estimated to be between 80–100,000 [15]. AAT is a serine protease inhibitor of elastase, trypsin, chymotrypsin, and thrombin. In the lung, this deficiency predisposes to panacinar emphysema due to a loss of elasticity. Therapy frequently involves the transfusion of purified pooled human antiprotease.

Accumulation of abnormal alpha-1 AT in the liver causes liver disease and is associated with cirrhosis and/or the development of hepatocellular carcinoma. Transplantation is reserved for patients with end-stage liver failure. Fortunately, a normal phenotype donor liver will produce and secrete normal AAT following transplant and is curative.

(13) What is carbon tetrachloride (CCl_4)?

A chemical, banned for consumer use in 1970, whose metabolism results in a highly toxic metabolite capable of causing centrilobular necrosis. It was previously used in cleaning solvents, refrigerants, and fire extinguishers. Use has declined significantly since it was realized that CCl_4 is one of the most dangerous hepatotoxins, capable of producing acute liver failure.

(14) What is portal hypertension?

The clinical definition of portal hypertension is the elevation of hepatic venous pressure gradient to >5 mmHg. It occurs in the setting of portal venous congestion (resistance to flow) and leads to the development of low pressure collateral routes for venous blood leaving the stomach and small intestine to return to the central circulation. A gradient ≥ 10 mmHg (termed clinically significant portal hypertension) is predictive of the development of complications of cirrhosis, including death.

Portosystemic shunting, resulting from this pressure increase, allows toxins and waste to enter the central circulation without having to pass through hepatic filtration. The presence of these substances in the circulation contributes to the development of encephalopathy. It may also produce a conduit for bacteria absorbed from GI tract to bypass the Kuppfer cells in the sinusoids [16].

Because of the reciprocal relationship between hepatic arterial flow and that from the portal venous system, portal hypertension results in an increased dependence on hepatic arterial flow for perfusion.

(15) How is portal HTN diagnosed?

A diagnosis of portal hypertension can be made in a patient with a known risk factor who has clinical manifestations consistent with the diagnosis. Although the direct portal pressure measurement is possible, the assessment more often focuses on the hepatic venous pressure gradient (HVPG), which quantifies the gradient attributed to sinusoidal resistance to blood flow.

The free hepatic venous pressure (FHVP) is obtained first by advancing a catheter from the RIJ down to the hepatic vein and measuring the venous pressure, which provides a correlate of intra-abdominal pressure (⇑ by ascites). Subsequent inflation/wedging of the balloon occludes the hepatic vein and provides a value reflective of portal venous pressure downstream, termed the wedged hepatic venous pressure (WHVP). This is conceptually similar to the wedge pressure measurement in the pulmonary artery, creating a distal column of static fluid reflective of the downstream pressure.

The HVPG is calculated by subtracting the FHVP from the WHVP and approximates the gradient between the portal vein and the IVC. Normal range is 3–5 mm Hg.

(16) What are varices? When do they become problematic?

Varices refer to the dilated submucosal veins that form lower resistance passages from the portal venous system to the azygous and hemiazygous veins, effectively a pop-off valve for portal hypertension. A gradient above 12 mmHg is generally the threshold pressure for variceal rupture.

Gastric varices bleed less commonly than esophageal varices, though significant gastric bleeding can be more difficult to control.

Variceal bleeding is one of the hallmarks of decompensated cirrhosis and unfortunately causes about a third of the cirrhosis-related deaths. As such, patients will frequently require endoscopic surveillance and treatment, as 20–30% of patients will bleed within 2 years of diagnosis of elevated portal pressures. Of the patients who survive the initial event, 60% will rebleed within 1 year [17].

(17) How are acute variceal bleeds managed?

Bleeding can be managed with banding, endoscopic ligation or sclerotherapy. Acute bleeding should also be treated with volume resuscitation, correction of severe coagulopathies, and lowering of the portal pressure. Intubation is often indicated for airway protection. Medications to reduce portal pressure include vasopressin, somatostatin, and/or octreotide. Although β-blockers can reduce portal pressures, hypotension from volume loss may not allow for safe utilization.

Balloon tamponade can also be an effective option for emergent variceal bleeding, but is associated with significant complications, including esophageal rupture and aspiration. Historically, the Blakemore–Sengstaken tube was passed down into the esophagus and a gastric balloon was inflated in the stomach. Upward traction with a 1 kg weight was applied based on the theory that the balloon would compress the GE junction and reduce blood flow to the varices. Continued bleeding, despite the upward pressure, would necessitate the inflation of the esophageal balloon to directly tamponade the involved vessels.

(18) What is fetor hepaticus?

It is described as a sweet, malodorous, and fecal smell of the breath. Portosystemic shunting allows thiols to pass directly to the lungs, where they can be exhaled and appreciated on exam.

(19) What is the role of the healthy liver in sudden hemorrhage?

The liver normally functions as a reservoir for blood in the splanchnic system. In healthy individuals, it is capable of redistributing up to one liter of blood into the systemic circulation when faced with sudden intravascular loss. In the setting of compromised hepatic function and altered blood flow, an individual's ability to tolerate sudden massive hemorrhage would be diminished.

(20) How does portal hypertension cause a low platelet count?

Thrombocytopenia is a well-known feature of cirrhosis and likely multifactorial in its etiology. Normally, the spleen pools approximately one-third of the circulating platelets, in part due to the prolonged transit time (10 min) to pass through splenic tissue. In the setting of portal hypertension, increased pressures are transmitted back through the splenic vein and eventually lead to splenic enlargement. A larger spleen slows down transit even further and prolonged exposure to splenic tissue translates to an increased chance of platelet destruction by phagocytic cells [18]. Associated factors may include depression of bone marrow function from alcoholism, and decreased production of thrombopoetin, synthesized in the liver.

(21) What are other common extrahepatic hepatic features of hepatic failure encountered in liver transplant patients (by system)?

Endocrine

- Hypoglycemia
- Gynecomastia

Neurologic

- Encephalopathy
- Cerebral Edema—up to 75% incidence in patients with grade IV encephalopathy [19]. It may lead to increased ICP, ischemia, herniation, etc. It may result from the osmotic effect of accumulated glutamine causing astrocyte swelling, a loss of autoregulation, or both [20].

Pulmonary

- Hyperventilation secondary to ammonia or acidosis
- Diaphragmatic compression by ascites or pleural effusion causing atelectasis
- R to L intrapulmonary shunts (up to 40% of cardiac output), which may lead to hypoxemia.
- Intrapulmonary Vascular Dilation (Hepatopulmonary Syndrome)

Cardiovascular

- Cardiomyopathy (ETOH, hemochromatosis)
- Elevated Mixed Venous O_2
- High cardiac output (hyperdynamic) low SVR state
- fluid sequestration in splanchnic bed.
- AV shunting (widespread AV malformations), decreased viscosity secondary to anemia also favor high cardiac output, as well as decreased SVR.
- Negative ionotropic effect of increased bile salts.
- Cholemia will also blunt the response to norepinephrine, angiotensin II, and isoproterenol.
- Increased levels of endogenous vasodilators.
- Low effective circulating volume increases the renin–angiotensinogen cascade, leading to excessive sodium retention.

Renal

- Prerenal azotemia from intravascularly depleted state.
- Hyponatremia

Hematologic

- Decreased production of clotting factors and tendency toward coagulopathy
- Thrombocytopenia (hepatic thrombopoetin production)

(22) What is platypnea? What is orthodeoxia?

Platypnea is the opposite of orthopnea. It refers to shortness of breath in the upright position. Orthodeoxia refers to low oxygen saturation also in the upright position. This constellation of symptoms is generally associated with hepatopulmonary syndrome and serves as evidence of right-to-left shunting.

In general, this clinical sign requires both an anatomic and functional component, and is exceedingly rare [21]. The former may refer to an ASD, PFO, or fenestrated ASD aneurysm. Less well understood, the functional component (in this case cirrhosis) results in a positional modification of abnormal shunting, causing redirection of IVC flow through the atrial communication. This effectively worsens the R to L shunt with the upright position [22].

(23) What are the causes and consequences of low albumin? How long does it remain in the circulation?

In general, the liver maintains the pool of approximately 500 g of circulating albumin by allocating approximately 15% of daily protein production [23]. The half-life of albumin is about 20 days. Although the liver is responsible for the production of albumin, low levels may also be attributed to increased renal loss or increased breakdown.

As the main determinant of oncotic pressure (80% [24]), low albumin may influence the tendency of capillary beds to draw fluid into vessels, resulting in worsening edema and ascites. It is important to note that albumin also plays a crucial role in plasma protein binding, due to its strong negative charge. Some of the highly bound drugs include warfarin, furosemide, benzodiazepines, and NSAIDS. Low albumin levels may result in a higher free fraction (metabolically active) of such medications.

(24) What is ascites? What favors its production? How is it treated?

Ascites refers to the accumulation of fluid in the peritoneal cavity, which can lead to varying degrees of abdominal distention. It can be either transudative or exudative, depending on the etiology. It is often characterized as having a "shifting dullness" or "fluid wave" on exam. Diagnosis is generally confirmed using ultrasound.

Ascites is most commonly associated with portal HTN. Low albumin levels and a tendency to retain fluid, both common in cirrhotics, only worsen this tendency. It is usually treated with salt restriction, diuretics (aldosterone antagonists) or paracentesis. In refractory cases, it is possible to surgically shunt fluid from the peritoneum back into the venous circulation (Leveen shunt), however, refractory ascites is considered as an indication for liver transplantation.

(25) What is a LeVeen shunt?

This procedure refers to the creation of a peritoneovenous shunt to drain peritoneal fluid into either the IJ or SVC, through a connecting subcutaneous drain. It is occasionally used to ease refractory ascites. Complications include shunt failure, fluid overload, infection, low-grade DIC or infection.

(26) What is spontaneous bacterial peritonitis (SBP)?

This refers to a "spontaneous" infection within the abdominal cavity in the absence of an obvious infectious source. It is common in patients with portal hypertension and ascites, revealed in 10–27% of routine paracentesis [25]. Diagnosis is confirmed if either bacteria or large numbers of neutrophils (>250 cells per mm^3) are found in the analyzed fluid. Symptoms generally include fever, increased WBC, pain, and malaise, although some patients may be asymptomatic [26]. The etiology may be related to increased gut wall permeability or impaired hepatic ability to clear portal bacteremia. Patients at risk of SBP are frequently started on antibiotic prophylaxis.

(27) What is hepatorenal syndrome (HRS)?

HRS refers to the often insidious deterioration of renal function in patients with acute or chronic liver failure. It is a frequent complication of cirrhosis and is thought to result from a decline in renal perfusion due, in part, to splanchnic dilation. Decreased perfusion from increased vasoactive mediators effectively mimics prerenal physiology.

It is estimated that 18% of individuals with cirrhosis and ascites will develop HRS within 1 year of diagnosis, and 39% will develop HRS within 5 years [27]. It is a diagnosis of exclusion and often signifies that the patient only has weeks to live without either recovery of hepatic function or transplant [28].

It is considered a functional disorder in that the kidneys from patients with HRS can be successfully transplanted to nonafflicted individuals with resolution of renal function.

(28) What is hepatopulmonary syndrome (HPS)?

HPS is present in up to 20% of patients who present for liver transplantation, as transplantation is the only effective medical therapy [29]. Most patients will eventually complain of dyspnea, either at rest or with activity, though may also display evidence of platypnea and orthodeoxia. Although the etiology is not entirely understood, the diagnostic criteria for HPS include portal hypertension, PaO_2 less than 80 mm Hg on room air and evidence of intrapulmonary vascular dilation (IPVD).

Diagnosis of IPVD can utilize contrast-enhanced echocardiography, radiolabelled albumin scanning, or pulmonary angiography. Using agitated saline as contrast, the injectate would normally only opacify the right heart chambers before being filtered by the pulmonary capillaries. However, if the opacificaiton is seen in the left heart following venous injection, this suggests a right-to-left intracardiac shunt or an intrapulmary shunt. With an intracardiac shunt, the bubbles will be seen with 3 beats, while an intrapulmonary shunt, indicative of IVPD, will send bubbles between 3 and 6 beats post-injection.

Nuclear scanning, in IVPD, would demonstrate passage of larger, tagged albumin molecules that would normally be trapped in the pulmonary vascular bed in nondilated states.

(29) What is portopulmonary hypertension (PPHTN)?

PPHTN is defined as pulmonary hypertension in the presence of portal hypertension, in a patient without other predisposing factors. It was previously a contraindication to transplant. It is thought to result from an imbalance between vasodilatory and vasoconstricting molecules, with toxins bypassing normal hepatic metabolism through portosystemic shunts.

Serotonin, normally degraded by the liver, is one etiologic factor that may lead to pulmonary smooth muscle hyperplasia and hypertrophy when present in the circulation, even while the systemic vascular resistance remains low [30].

TIPSS

(1) What is a TIPS procedure?

Transjugular intrahepatic portosystemic shunting, or a TIPS (or TIPSS) procedure as it is more commonly referred, is a technique generally used to treat portal hypertension and the associated consequences.

It generally performed in interventional radiology procedure rooms and involves the creation of a stented (artificial) pathway through the flow-resistant liver, between the portal vein and one of the hepatic veins. The conduit is designed to reduce the pressure backup to the spleen, stomach, lower esophagus, and intestines, and lower the risk of variceal rupture.

The internal jugular vein is usually accessed to pass a guidewire and introducer sheath through the following structures:

IJ to SVC to IVC to hepatic vein, through liver parenchyma into portal vein

Once the anatomy and pressure is confirmed, the tract is dilated with an angioplasty balloon before placing the mesh endograft (stent).

(2) What are the benefits of TIPS? Is the procedure done instead of transplantation?

Although the procedure is generally used to temporize the manifestations of decompensated cirrhosis, it may be utilized as a bridge to transplant. Early placement of TIPS improved 1-year survival to 86% compared with 61% in a group randomized to similar therapy without early TIPS [31].

The inserted stent is contained entirely inside the liver and can be removed at the time of transplant. Studies have shown that variceal bleeding is reduced in up to 90% of TIPS patients, although there are conflicting views as to whether there is an overall survival benefit.

(3) What type of anesthesia is appropriate for TIPS?

As a minimally invasive procedure, TIPS can be performed with local anesthesia and minimal IV sedation. However, patients have often decompensated to the point that they are encephalopathic and at higher risk for regurgitation/aspiration, requiring a secured airway.

(4) What are the risks of the procedure?

The operative mortality ranges from 0–2% in skilled hands [32]. Because the rerouted blood flow effectively bypasses the liver (first pass clearance of the gut), patients who have already experienced encephalopathy are increasingly vulnerable to the additional toxins now capable of bypassing any remaining hepatic detoxification.

Lastly, the procedure requires a certain quantity of IV contrast dye for proper visualization, which is both nephrotoxic and a potential allergen.

Transplant

(1) What are the indications for liver transplant?

Cirrhosis alone is not an indication for transplant. The indications for transplant include acute liver failure, cirrhosis with complications (variceal bleed, ascites, encephalopathy, HRS), certain neoplasms (HCC), and liver-based metabolic conditions with systemic manifestations.

The decision to transplant requires a risk-benefit analysis. The requirement for post-op immunosuppression may post-grave risks for the individual based on the etiology of the original insult and/or the presence of latent infections. The transplanted organ infrequently cures the underlying disease.

The suitability of patients with HCC for transplant is based upon the Milan Criteria, which attempts to ensure that transplant candidacy is limited to patients with a reasonable prognosis [33]. This criteria essentially limits transplants to individuals with smaller (<5 cm), nonmetastatic lesions that do not involve major vessels.

Unfortunately, necessary immunosuppression is also associated with higher risk of tumor regrowth.

(2) What is meant by the term orthotopic transplantation?

"Orthotopic" refers to the "normal or usual position." In the case of an orthotopic liver transplant (OLT), the donor liver will occupy the space, previously home to the patient's diseased organ.

(3) How are donors matched with recipients?

The primary criteria used to match donor liver grafts with recipients are ABO blood type and graft size. ABO incompatible transplantation (ILT) is generally limited to emergent situations.

(4) How many liver transplant candidates successfully receive a new organ?

Only about two-third of patients on the liver waitlist survive until transplantation [34].

In 2014, 6729 liver transplants were performed in US. In 2011, the median time to transplant in the United States was 12.6 months.

(5) What are the contraindications to transplant (may be center specific) [35]

- Sepsis
- Advanced cardiopulmonary disease (making surgery too risky)
- Metastatic disease not meeting criteria for cure (Milan Criteria)
- Hemangiosarcoma
- Intrahepatic cholangiocarcinoma
- Lack of adequate social support.
- AIDS
- Continued substance abuse within the last 6 months.
- Psychological issues severe enough to impact compliance
- Sustained ICP (intracranial pressure) > 50 or CPP (cerebral perfusion pressure) < 40 mmHg.

Relative Contraindications

- Advanced Age
- HIV
- BMI $\geq$ 40 (some centers will perform gastric sleeve before or during transplant)

(6) What other health issues should also be considered before transplant?

In anticipation of the need for immunosuppression, patients should be screened for the possibility for latent infections, including tuberculosis. Patients from endemic areas should also be screened for coccidiomycosis and strongyloides.

Vaccinations for Hep A, Hep B, pneumococcus, influenza, diphtheria, pertussis, and tetanus should be obtained before transplant, to ensure an adequate immune response prior to suppression.

As part of a multidisciplinary evaluation, patients should also adhere to the recommended screening for colon cancer. Needed dental extractions should be also carried out prior to transplantation, as immunosuppression increases the risks of any localized infection.

(7) What are the two major sources for donor organs?

The vast majority (96%) of transplanted livers are obtained from deceased donors [36]. However, the possibility of living-donor transplantation exists because of the redundant capacity of the liver. The right hepatic lobe (60% of liver) can be harvested and given to an adult, while the smaller left hepatic lobe can be transplanted to a child or adult of similar size. Due to the ability of the liver to regenerate, both the donor and recipient should regain normal liver function, assuming successful recovery. The lobes that are removed do not regrow, rather an expansion of the remaining lobes ensures the restoration of function.

In 2014, only 280 living-donor grafts were transplanted, in part out of concern for the well-being of donors, as several donor-related deaths have been reported.

(8) How are the available organs allocated in the United States?

The United Network for Organ Sharing (UNOS) was established in 1984. It develops policies and collects data for all US organ transplants as the supply of available organs falls short of the demand and warrants rationing. The approach generally prioritizes the sickest patients, de-emphasizing time spent on the waiting list. In regard to liver transplantation specifically, patients are ranked by MELD score and stratified by blood type.

(9) What is the Child-Pugh Score?

The CP score was the original scoring system adopted by the UNOS for the allocation of transplantable livers. It was a scoring system designed to prognosticate for cirrhotic patients undergoing surgical treatment of portal HTN. Scoring was based on the severity of five clinical measures (total bilirubin, albumin, PT, ascites, and encephalopathy).

The subjective assessment of the ascites and encephalopathy was one of the cited criticisms for the Child-Pugh score and it was eventually replaced by the MELD score for organ allocation.

(10) What is the MELD Score? How is it determined? How often is it calculated?

The Model-for-End-Stage-Liver-Disease was originally designed as a prognostic tool for cirrhotic patients undergoing TIPS procedures. It was eventually shown to be a strong predictor of 3-month mortality risk for the various causes of cirrhosis. UNOS adopted it in 2002 to replace the Child-Pugh score. The sickest patients have MELD scores updated every 7 days.

The MELD score is based upon a patient's creatinine, bilirubin, and INR. The score ranges from 6 to 40. Candidates with MELD scores less than 15 have better survival without transplantation, and, as such, patients become candidates for transplant with scores ≥ 15. For reference, most liver transplant candidates have MELD scores less than 25, while only 2% of the transplant list has a MELD score greater than 25 [37].

(11) What are MELD exception points?

Certain conditions are associated with shortened survival, which would not be appreciated by the traditional MELD scoring system. Additional points can be conferred by some of the following diagnosis: HCC, hepatopulmonary syndrome, portopulmonary HTN, cystic fibrosis, hepatic artery thrombosis, etc.

If providers feel that the MELD score/exception points do not accurately portray an individual's morbidity and mortality risk, they may still be considered for transplant by petitioning for additional MELD points from the regional review board.

(12) What does it mean to be deemed Status 1?

These patients, generally suffering from acute liver failure, are predicted to have a life expectancy of less than 7 days. As such, they are given the highest priority by the United Network for Organ Sharing.

(13) What are the survival rates post-transplantation?

One-year survival approaches 90% [38]. Three-year posthepatic transplant survival is about 80% and drops to about 55% at 5 years [39].

(14) What is liver dialysis? What is the indication?

Liver dialysis is a relatively new detoxification technique based on principles similar to those of hemodialysis. It is utilized primarily as a bridge to liver transplantation or to allow for hepatic regeneration following an acute insult. The molecular adsorbents recirculation system (MARS) utilizes two dialysis circuits with the goal being to introduce, and subsequently clean, albumin after it has absorbed albumin-bound toxins from a patient's blood. Adsorbed compounds include ammonia, bile acids, bilirubin, and iron.

A meta-analysis of 483 patients failed to show a significant mortality benefit from artificial hepatic support systems as compared to standard medical therapy. A subanalysis did, however, show a reduction in mortality in acute-on-chronic failure states [40]. A second prospective randomized study of 70 patients demonstrated a significant improvement in the degree of encephalopathy [41].

Preop

(1) What patient complaints may suggest hepatic dysfunction?

Patients with hepatic dysfunction generally present with dark urine, fatigue, anorexia, and nausea. They may also complain of low-grade fevers.

(2) What are common physical exam findings in a patient with liver failure?

Scleral icterus, jaundice, ascites, splenomegaly, palmar erythema, gynecomastia, asterixis, testicular atrophy, spider angiomata, petechiae, and ecchymosis.

(3) What is the role of the preoperative evaluation?

Once the degree of hepatic dysfunction has been appreciated, one of the major objectives of the preoperative evaluation is to identify any issues that can be optimized prior to surgery, such as a coexisting coagulopathy. The patient may benefit from the administration of vitamin K or a platelet transfusion, prior to the procedure.

It is also necessary to determine if the patient is likely to survive the anesthetic and surgery, as poor cardiovascular health can actually be a contraindication to transplant. The scarcity of available organs mandates that livers go to the sickest patients, but they must also have a reasonable likelihood of survival.

(4) What is hepatic encephalopathy?

Encephalopathy refers to reversible mental status changes resulting from hepatic dysfunction. Such a state will likely require the use of a proxy to obtain consent for anesthesia. It is often triggered by some acute insult, such as a GI bleed or infection, in the context of chronic liver dysfunction. Symptoms may range from subtle cognitive dysfunction to coma. More than half of patients with cirrhosis will eventually become encephalopathic to some degree [42].

The cognitive dysfunction is attributed to the accumulation of neurotoxic substances previously metabolized by the healthy liver. Portosystemic shunting ensures that nitrogenous waste (NH_3) completely bypasses any remaining hepatic function. However, ammonia levels often do not correlate well with the severity of symptoms and are not required for diagnosis.

These circulating toxins contribute to cytotoxic brain edema [43], increased GABA activity, disruption of the blood brain barrier, and may even lead to coma. The West Haven Criteria grade encephalopathic symptoms on scale of I to IV, in order of severity.

(5) What are liver function tests? How will the values change with progression to cirrhosis?

Aminotransferase (AST/ALT) levels generally provide evidence of hepatocellular injury rather than the actual function of the liver. As such, there is a poor correlation between the level of aminotransferase elevation and the severity of disease, as a decreasing mass of hepatocytes will no longer "spill" signals of cellular injury into the bloodstream.

Cholestasis or biliary obstruction is better evidenced by bilirubin, alkaline phosphatase, gamma-glutamyl transpeptidase (GGT), and LDH. Alkaline phosphate lacks specificity for hepatobiliary disease, though elevations can be indicative.

LDH is also a rather nonspecific signal of hepatic injury, as it may be elevated by nonhepatic causes. As an isolated elevation, it would be consistent with hepatic injury.

(6) What are the cutoffs for mild/moderate/large/and extreme elevations in aminotransferases?

Mild	100-249 IU/L)
Moderate	250-999 IU/L)
Large	1000-1999 IU/L)
Extreme	>2000 IU/L)

Mild elevations usually suggest fatty liver, NASH (nonalcoholic steatohepatitis), drug toxicity, and chronic viral infection. Larger increases (3–22×) are seen in patients with acute hepatitis or the exacerbation of chronic states.

(7) How does the ratio of AST/ALT aid in diagnosis?

AST ALT > 4:1 is typical of Wilson disease
AST ALT ~ 2:1 may suggest alcoholic liver disease
AST ALT < 1:1 is consistent with NASH

(8) What is meant by synthetic liver function? What indicators are relevant?

In contrast to serum markers of hepatic injury, the liver's ability to synthesize proteins may provide a clearer picture of overall function. Synthetic function is generally assessed by measuring albumin levels and the prothrombin time.

Although albumin is the most abundant protein synthesized by the liver, the 3-week half-life ensures that levels will remain normal long after the onset of any type of hepatocellular injury or dysfunction. It is therefore not a sensitive marker for acute liver injury.

The half-life of coagulation factors, specifically factor VII, can be as short as 4-h. This allows for much more rapid detection of changing function. As such, the PT/INR is routinely used to evaluate and follow liver patients as a marker for hepatic dysfunction. Again due to the physiologic redundancy, factor VII levels have to drop by 70% before the PT will be prolonged.

(9) Would you give this patient preoperative sedation? Should any other medications be considered?

Sedatives may worsen the fragile cognitive state of many patients with ESLD and should be used with extreme caution or avoided entirely. Sedation may mask signs of anacute decline (i.e. increased ICP) and medications may also be difficult to metabolize, with prolonged effects.

Interestingly, flumazenil (in the absence of benzodiazepines) has been shown to improve the level of consciousness in certain patients with severe encephalopathy [44].

(10) What is the benefit of lactulose?

Lactulose is a disaccharide frequently used as an osmotic laxative. It also lowers the intestinal pH, which lessens the presence of ammonia-producing bacteria and may improve cognitive function in patients with hepatic encephalopathy [45].

(11) What tests should the preoperative evaluation include?

Labs: ABO-Rh blood typing, LFTs, coagulation profile, CBC with differential, alpha-fetoprotein, calcium, and Vitamin D levels,
Viral serologies (CMV, Epstein Barr, HIV, hep A/B/C, rapid plasma reagin (syphilis),
Urinalysis
Drug (tox) screen

(12) What is the purpose of the cardiopulmonary evaluation?

Not surprisingly, the morbidity and mortality from liver transplants are increased in patients with CAD [46]. The cardiopulmonary evaluation in transplant patients should include screening for CAD, cardiomyopathy, valvular disease, underlying lung disease, hepatopulmonary syndrome, and pulmonary hypertension.

The AHA/ACC suggests noninvasive stress testing in liver transplant candidates with no active cardiac conditions if they have three or more risk factors for CAD. More aggressively, the 2013 guidelines from the American Association for the Study of Liver disease and the American Society of Transplantation recommended noninvasive cardiac testing for all adults being evaluated for liver transplantation [47].

Some have even advocated for patients with more than two cardiovascular risk factors to undergo angiography to assess the severity of disease [48], with the potential for revascularization prior to transplant in patients with significant coronary stenosis.

Intraoperative Management

(1) How are you going to induce anesthesia?

A rapid sequence induction is often indicated because of the emergent nature of transplant surgery. Similarly, the presence of ascites may raise intragastric pressure, decrease FRC, and render the patient a higher risk of aspiration. Issues with ongoing nausea, variceal bleeding, intrapulmonary shunting, etc., also favor rapid securement of the airway. In contrast, a nonreassuring airway exam may still warrant an awake technique.

(2) What lines/devices are you going to need to do the case safely?

In addition to the standard ASA monitors, the need for invasive monitoring and vascular access will be based severity of liver disease and type of procedure. In general, an arterial catheter will be required. Large-bore intravenous access is also obtained as surgical bleeding may be significantly increased based on associated coagulopathies. The need for massive transfusion of blood products should be anticipated and may warrant a preoperative conversation with the blood bank.

A rapid infusion system capable of high transfusion flow rates (>500 mL/min) is typically utilized. Systems, such as the Level-One or Belmont, incorporate a reservoir, pump, filters, and a heat exchanger. They are also designed to detect and avoid the presence of blood clots or air embolism, hypothermia, and/or line occlusion.

(3) What other monitors might you utilize?

Aside from standard monitors, anesthesiologists are increasingly relying on ultrasound images to monitor volume status, need for inotropic support, presence of emboli, and ventricular function. In a survey of anesthesiologists at liver transplant centers, more than 86% of survey respondents (n = 217) reported using transesophageal echocardiography in some or all transplant cases [49].

Approximately half of the liver transplant programs also use ICP monitoring, as a significantly elevated ICP can both worsen prognosis and be a contraindication to transplant [50]. Patients at risk for elevated ICP should have efforts made to minimize agitation/stimulation. Elevation of the head, mannitol, hyperventilation, hypertonic saline, and even barbiturates can be used in an attempt to reduce ICP below 20-25 and maintain CPP above 50–60 mmHg.

(4) How are you going to maintain anesthetic depth?

All volatile anesthetics produce a dose-dependent decrease in hepatic blood flow. However, inhalational anesthesia is still the mainstream for liver transplantation because volatile anesthetics have little overall influence on liver function and the depth of anesthesia is easily assessed. Sevoflurane and isoflurane have been shown to have less of a negative effect on portal blood flow, hepatic arterial flow, and total hepatic blood flow than halothane and enflurane and traditionally isoflurane has been favored due to the belief that it favors splanchnic blood flow.

Sevoflurane and isoflurane also maintain HABR more effectively than some of the other volatile anesthetics [51]. In either case, periods of severe hypotension during the surgery may require temporary discontinuation of the agent. Midazolam, with minimal hemodynamic effects, can be used for amnesia during these periods.

On the contrary, propofol has been shown to increase flow in both the hepatic arterial and portal venous circulation [52]. Perhaps due to the influence of rapid blood loss on the pharmacology of propofol or the lack of clearance during the anhepatic phase, it is not routinely utilized.

(5) What muscle relaxant are you going to use?

Although pseudocholinesterase may be reduced in the setting of hepatic dysfunction, this should not be a contraindication to the administration of succinylcholine.

Vecuronium undergoes hepatic elimination and will display prolonged neuromuscular blockade in patients with cirrhosis [53]. Rocuronium also undergoes hepatic metabolism and elimination and effects can be prolonged in a setting of hepatic dysfunction. Both may still be utilized with careful monitoring.

Cisatracurium is an attractive choice for neuromuscular blockade in ESLD patients because of its organ-independent elimination and lack of histamine release.

(6) How does liver disease affect drug metabolism and pharmacokinetics?

Reduction of protein synthesis may result in alterations in drug binding. This may result in increased free fractions of medications, potentially leading to increased volume of distribution outside of the vascular bed.

An altered volume of distribution, particularly with ascites, should also be considered, as well as the possibility of reduced drug metabolism secondary to hepatocyte dysfunction.

ESLD may potentiate the effects of morphine, meperidine, alfentanil, vecuronium, rocuronium, mivacurium, benzodiazepines, and dexmedetomidine, among others.

Despite being principally metabolized by the liver, fentanyl elimination is not significantly altered in liver disease [54].

(7) What is the role for inducing hypotension in liver transplantation?

Controlled hypotension is a technique that has been utilized for decades to reduce bleeding and the need for blood transfusion. Controlled hypotension is defined as a reduction of the systolic blood pressure to 80–90 mm Hg, a reduction of mean arterial pressure (MAP) to 50–65 mm Hg, or a 30% reduction of baseline MAP [55]. This approach has to be weighed against the risks of end-organ ischemia.

(8) What is venovenous bypass (VVB)?

Less involved than cardiac bypass, venovenous bypass for OLT consists only of a centrifugal pump and heparin bonded tubing. The procedure involves the cannulation of the IVC through the femoral vein and possibly also cannulation of the portal vein with diversion of blood flow back to the heart, usually via the axillary or internal jugular vein. It was a more popular technique in the 1980s and 1990s, particularly in the setting of major hemodynamic instability after test clamping of the IVC. It was advocated in patients with >30% drop in mean arterial pressure and >50% decrease in cardiac index during a 5-min test-clamping period [56].

The perceived benefits were the ability to maintain preload, improve renal perfusion, lessen intestinal venous congestion, and delay the development of metabolic acidosis. However, the risks of air embolism, thromboembolism and inadvertent decannulation had the potential to result in significant morbidity and mortality. The overall incidence of complications due to the use of VVB was reported to be between 10 and 30% [57].

Meanwhile, as the majority of patients undergoing OLT have liver cirrhosis with well-developed portal venous collaterals, the effect of portal clamping on hemodynamic status is negligible and the use of VVB is not uniformly used at all centers.

(9) What are the surgical stages of liver transplantation?

A. Preanhepatic (dissection phase). A wide subcostal incision is made. The liver is mobilized, remaining attached only via the IVC, portal vein, hepatic artery, and common bile duct.

B. Anhepatic phase—The anhepatic phase begins with placement of a clamp on the suprahepatic and infrahepatic IVC. Additionally the hepatic artery, portal vein, and CBD are clamped prior to removing the native liver. The donor liver is then anastomosed to the supra and infrahepatic IVC and portal vein.

C. Postanhepatic (neohepatic) phase. The new graft is flushed to remove air, debris, and preservatives. Venous clamps are removed and the hepatic artery is anastomosed. The common bile duct of the donor liver is then connected to the recipient via a choledochocholedochostomy.

(10) What are the anesthetic challenges of each stage?

Preanhepatic phase—With abdominal incision and drainage of ascites, hypovolemia can occur. This should be anticipated and colloids can be used to maintain preload. Typically, half the total blood loss occurs during this phase.

Anhepatic Phase—Cross-clamping of the IVC and portal vein decreases venous return by as much as 50%. With the decreased CO, hypotension is common. Distal venous pressure increase from the clamps can also interfere with both renal and intestinal perfusion. Placement of the donor liver may require retraction near the diaphragm, which may impede ventilation and oxygenation.

As the liver is no longer metabolizing citrate, transfusions can lead to ionized hypocalcemia and myocardial depression. Progressive acidosis secondary to intestinal and peripheral venous stasis should also be anticipated.

Fibrinolysis may also begin during this stage because of an absence of liver-produced plasminogen activator inhibitor, which results in the unopposed action of tissue plasminogen activator.

Neohepatic Phase—Reperfusion is associated with abrupt increase in potassium and hydrogen ion concentrations, which can be life threatening. Approximately one in three patients will exhibit signs of postreperfusion syndrome, which is defined by systemic hypotension and pulmonary hypertension. It is thought to result from a combination of acidosis, hyperkalemia, emboli, vasoactive substances, and even hypothermia.

Fibrinolysis is most severe after reperfusion and is caused by abrupt increase in tissue plasminogen activator from graft endothelial cell release. Increasingly, tissue thromboelastography (TEG) is being used to guide transfusions.

(11) What is ischemia-reperfusion injury?

This refers to injury sustained to the donor organ from both hypoxia and the production of reactive oxygen species, including superoxide, hydrogen peroxide, and hydroxyl radicals, which can lead to some degree of cellular necrosis or apoptosis. Similarly, the activation of Kuppfer cells and release of inflammatory cytokines by the donor liver, can add to the cellular damage.

Postoperative Management

(1) What are initial signs of graft function?

It is possible to observe signs of graft function in the operating room and early postoperative period. These include decreased calcium requirements, spontaneous increase in ionized calcium as citrate is metabolized, improvement in acidosis, increased urine output, a rise in core temperature, and bile output from the graft.

(2) How soon should LFTs begin to normalize?

During the first few postoperative days, transaminase levels will spike because of graft ischemia, procurement injury, organ preservation, and reperfusion injury. After this period, aminotransferase and bilirubin levels that do not trend downward suggest the possibility of hepatic artery thrombosis, which should lead to prompt ultrasonic evaluation.

(3) What are the major types of immunosuppression?

Immunosuppressive medications have revolutionized transplant medicine. The various types of immunosuppressants include:

Glucocorticoids, calcineurin inhibitors, macrolide antibiotics, inhibitors of purine and pyrimidine synthesis, and antibody therapy.

They can be further classified by induction versus maintenance, biologic (antilymphocyte antibodies/anticytokine receptor antibodies) versus pharmacologic, or by mechanism of action.

(4) How would you control the patient's post-op discomfort? Would you use an epidural for post-op pain control?

Epidural analgesia is contraindicated because of coagulopathy, which usually preexists, or develops during the perioperative period. Postoperative pain control is generally achieved with opioids, including patient-controlled analgesia.

References

1. Lautt WW. The 1995 Ciba-Geiby award lecture. Intrinsic regulation of hepatic blood flow. Can J Physiol Pharmacol. 1996;74:223.
2. Bardag-Gorce F, French BA, et al. The importance of cycling of blood alcohol levels in the pathogenesis of experimental alcoholic liver disease in rats. Gastroenterology. 2002;123:325.
3. Lee WM, Larson AM, Stravits RT. AASLD position paper: the management of acute liver failure: update 2011. American Association for the Study of Liver Diseases. Available at: http://www.aasld.org/practiceguidelines/Documents/Acuteliverfailure update2011.pdf (2011). Accessed 3 Aug 2015.
4. CDC. Prevention of hepatitis A through active and passive immunization. MMWR 1999; 48(No. RR-12):4.
5. World Health Organization. Hepatitis B. World Health Organization. Available at: http://www.who.int/csr/disease/hepatitis/whocdscsrlyo20022/en/index1.html (2015). Accessed 3 Aug 2015.
6. American College of Obstetricians and Gynecologists. ACOG Practice Bulletin No. 86: Viral hepatitis in pregnancy. Obstet Gynecol. 2007;110(4):941–56. PMID: 17906043.
7. Centers for Disease Control and Prevention. Hepatitis B FAQs for Health Professionals. Available at: http://www.cdc.gov/hepatitis/hbv/hbvfaq.htm#overview (2015). Accessed 3 Aug 2015.
8. U.S. Food and Drug Administration. Faster, Easier Cures for Hepatits C. Available at: http://www.fda.gov/ForConsumers/ConsumerUpdates/ucm405642.htm (2015). Accessed 3 Aug 2015.
9. Makino S, Chang MF, Shieh CK, et al. Molecular cloning and sequencing of a human hepatitis delta (delta) virus RNA. Nature. 1987;329(6137):343–6.
10. World Health Organization. Global Alert and Response (GAR); Hepatitis E. Available at: http://www.who.int/csr/disease/hepatitis/whocdscsredc200112/en/index1.html (2015). Accessed 11 July 2015.
11. Treem WR, Rinaldo P, et al. Acute fatty liver of pregnancy and long-chain 3-hydrocyacyl-coenzyme A dehydrogenase deficiency. Hepatology. 1994;19(2):339.
12. Knight M, Nelson-Piercy C, et al. A prospective national study of acute fatty liver of pregnancy in the UK. Gut. 2008;57(7):951.
13. Edwards CQ, Kushner JP. Screening for hemochromatosis. N Engl J Med. 1993;328(22):1616.
14. EASL Clinical Practice Guidelines: Wilson's disease. European Association for Study of Liver. J Hepatol. 2012;56(3):671–85.
15. Campos MA, Wanner A, et al. Trends in the diagnosis of symptomatic patients with alpha1-antitrypsin deficiency between 1968 and 2003. Chest. 2005;128(3):1179.
16. Kumar A, Sharma P. Hepatic venous pressure gradient measurement: time to learn. Indian J Gastroenterol. 2008;27(2):74–80.

17. Bosch J, Garcia-Pagan JC. Prevention of variceal rebleeding. Lancet. 2003;361:952–4.
18. Handin R, Lux S, Stossel T. Blood: principles and practice of hematology, Vol. 1. Lippincott Williams & Wilkins, 2003. P1021.
19. Lee VM. Acute liver failure. N Engl J Med. 1993;329(25):1892.
20. Biel A, Larsen FS. Pathophysiology of cerebral edema in fulminant hepatic failure. J Hepatol. 1999;31:771–6.
21. Cheng TO. Platypnea-orthodeoxia syndrome: etiology, differential diagnosis, and management. Cathet Cardiovasc Interv. 1999;47:64–6.
22. Cheng TO. Mechanisms of Platypnea-Orthodeoxia: what causes water to flow uphill. Circulation. 2002;105:e47.
23. Friedman LS, Martin P, et al. Liver function tests and the objective evaluation of the patient with liver disease. In: Zakim D, Boyer T, editors. Hepatology: a textbook of liver disease. 3rd ed. Philadelphia: WB saunders; 1996. p. 791.
24. Nicholson JP, Wolmarans MR, et al. The role of albumin in critical illness. Br J Anaesth. 2000;85(4):599–610.
25. Runyon BA. Spontaneous bacterial peritonitis: an explosion of information. Hepatology. 1988;1(8):171–5.
26. Koulaouzidis A, Bhat S. Spontaneous bacterial peritonitis. World J Gastroenterol. 2009;15(9):1042–9.
27. Gines A, Escorsell A, et al. Incidence, predictive factors, and prognosis of the hepatorenal syndrome in cirrhosis with ascites. Gastroenterology. 1993;105(1):229–36.
28. Alessandria C, Ozdogan O. MELD score and clinical type predict prognosis in hepatorenal syndrome: relevance to liver transplantation. Hepatology. 2005;41(6):1282.
29. Hendrickse A, Azam F, et al. Hepatopulmonary syndrome and portopulmonary hypertension. Curr Treat Options Cardiovasc Med. 2007;9(2):127–36.
30. Egermayer, et al. Role of serotonin in the pathogenesis of acute and chronic pulmonary hypertension. Thorax. 1999;54:161–8.
31. Garcia-Pagan JC, et al. Early use of TIPS in patients with cirrhosis and variceal bleeding. N Engl J Med. 2010;362(25):2370.
32. Freedman AM, Sanyal AJ, et al. Complications of transjugular intrahepatic portosystemic shunt: a comprehensive review. Radiographics. 1993;13(6):1185.
33. Mazzaferro V, Gegalia E, et al. Liver transplantation for the treatment of small hepatocellular carcinomas in patients with cirrhosis. N Engl J Med. 1996;334(11):693.
34. OPTN/SRTR 2011 Annual Report of the U.S. Organ Procurement and Transplantation Network and the Scientific Registry of Transplant Recipients: Transplant Data 1998–2011. Released December 19, 2012, http://optn.transplant.hrsa.gov/data/annual report.asp (2012). Accessed 28 Dec 2012.
35. Martin P, DiMartini A, et al. Evaluation for liver transplantation in adults: 2013 practice guidelines by the American Association for the Study of Liver Diseases and The American Society of Transplantation. Hepatology. 2014;59(3):1144.
36. http://optn.transplant.hrsa.gov/converge/latestData/rptData.asp. Retrieved on 7/13/2015.
37. Trotter JF, Osgood MJ. MELD scores of liver transplant recipients according to size of waiting list: impact of organ allocation and patient outcomes. JAMA. 2004;291(15):1871–4.
38. Lidofsky SD. Liver transplantation for fulminant hepatic failure. Gastroenterol Clin North Am. 1993;22(2):257.
39. Health Resources and Services Administration, U.S. Department of Health and Human Services. Organ procurement & transplantation network. Available at http://optn.transplant.hrsa.gov/latestData/rptStrat.asp (2015). Accessed 3 Aug 2015.
40. Kjaergard LL, Liu J, et al. Artificial and bioartificial support systems for acute and acute-on-chronic liver failure: a systematic review. JAMA. 2003;289(2):217.
41. Hassanein T, Tofteng F, et al. Efficacy of albumin dialysis (MARS) in patients with cirrhosis and advanced grades of encephalopathy: a prospective, controlled, randomized multicenter trial. Hepatology. 2004;38(LB04):726A.
42. Jalan R, Hayes PC. Hepatic encephalopathy and ascites. Lancet. 1997;350:1309.
43. Cordoba J, Blei AT. Brain edema and hepatic encephalopathy. Semin Liver Dis. 1996;16(3):271.
44. Pomier-Layragues G, Giguere JF, et al. Flumazenil in cirrhotic patients in hepatic coma: a randomized double-blind placebo-controlled crossover trial. Hepatology. 1999;29:347–55.
45. Prasad S, Dhiman RK. lactulose improves cognitive functions and health-related quality of life in patients with cirrhosis who have minimal hepatic encephalopathy. Hepatology. 2007;45(3):549–59.
46. Plotkin JS, Scott VL, et al. Morbidity and mortality in patients with CAD undergoing orthotopic liver transplant. Liver Transpl Surg. 1996;2(6):426.
47. Raval Z, Harinstein ME. Cardiovascular risk assessment of the liver transplant candidate. J Am Coll Cardiol. 2011;58(3):223.
48. Martin P, DiMartini A, et al. Evaluation for liver transplantation in Adults: 2013 practice guidelines by the American Association for the Study of Liver Diseases and the American Society of Transplantation. Hepatology. 2014;59(3):1144.
49. Wax DB, Torres A, et al. Transesophageal echocardiography utilization in high-volume liver transplantation centers in the united states. J Cardiothorac Vasc Anesth. 2008;22(6):811–3.
50. Vaquero J, Fontana RJ, et al. Complications and use of intracranial pressure monitoring in patients with acute liver failure and severe encephalopathy. Liver Tranpl. 2005;11(12):1581–9.
51. Matsumoto N, Kotumi M, et al. Hepatolobectomy-induced depression of hepatic circulation and metabolism in the dog is counteracted by isoflurane, but not by halothane. Act Anaesthesiol Scand. 1999;43:850–4.
52. Carmichael FJ, Crawford MW, et al. Effect of propofol infusion on splanchnic hemodynamics and liver oxygen consumption in the rat. Anesthesiology. 1993;79:1051–60.
53. Bencini AF, Scaf AH, et al. Hepatobiliary disposition of vecuronium bromide in man. Br J Anaesth. 1986;58:988–95.
54. Haberer JP, Schoeffler P, et al. Fentanyl pharmacokinetics in anaesthetized patients with cirrhosis. Br J Anaesth. 1982;54:1267–70.
55. Degoute CS. Controlled hypotension: a guide to drug choice. Drugs. 2007;67(7):1053–76.
56. Vertoli P, el Hage C, et al. Does adult liver transplantation without venovenous bypass result in renal failure. Anesth Analg. 1992;75:489–94.
57. Chari RS, Gan TJ, et al. Venovenous bypass in adult orthotopic liver transplantation: routine or selective use? J Am Coll Surg. 1998;186:683–90.

Anesthesia for Open Repair of Abdominal Aortic Aneurysm

29

Stefan Alexandrov Ianchulev

Case Presentation

A 77-year-old female patient has been scheduled for open surgic, repair of an infrarenal aortic aneurysm.

Relevant history: Exercise tolerance <4 METs due to arthritis and peripheral vascular disease. She has controlled hypertension, coronary artery disease with CABG × 3 fifteen years ago. She has vein grafts to the right and circumflex coronary arteries, with an internal mammary graft to the left anterior descending coronary artery. Four years ago the patient had an acute myocardial infarction. At that time both left carotid artery and aortic valvular stenosis were noted. She underwent left CEA and AVR later that year.

Additional history includes moderate renal artery stenosis and breast cancer, s/p lumpectomy.
PSH: Left hip replacement, CEA, CABG × 3, AVR
Meds: Amlodipine, atorvastatin, bumetanide, metoprolol, aspirin
Allergies: simvastatin (muscle aches), cefazolin (anaphylaxis)
Exam:
Height: 165 cm, Weight: 93 kg, BMI: 35.
BP 140/88 h 64, Mallampati: 2, TMD: 2FB; AAOx3
Tests:
Labs: Na 141, K 4.3, Cl 101, HCO3 30, BUN 23, Cr 0.94, Hb 11.5, Hct 35, PT 10.9, PTT 36.2, INR 1.0, GFR 54
ECG: SR, HR 66, First degree AVB, with LBBB.
Echo: EF 50%, moderate mitral regurgitation, Moderate hypokinesis of the anterior, posterior and inferior LV walls. Elevated pulmonary artery pressure estimated at 50 mmHg, Prosthetic aortic valve with *P*max = 2.8 m/s.

1. What is abdominal aortic aneurysm (AAA)?

AAA represents a dilatation of the abdominal aorta which can extend above the renal arteries. If the aneurysm extends above the diaphragm, it is classified as a thoracoabdominal aortic aneurysm (TAAA). Adventitial degradation is a central feature of the disease. Factors promoting development of the disease are shear stress, inflammation and hypercoagulability, potentiated by oxidized LDLs. The aorta and peripheral vessels affected by the atherosclerotic process become susceptible to aneurysm development and dissection. Dissection may lead to intramural hematoma formation. True aneurysm affects all layers of the aortic wall, and pseudoaneurysm is an intimal expansion through a damaged muscularis layer. The natural history of the disease is a continuous progression of atherosclerosis [1].

2. What are major risk factors for developing an AAA?

Smoking, hypertension, familial predisposition, advancing age (greater than 40), low HDL, high LDL, increased fibrinogen, and atherosclerosis. Low platelet count may result from a consumptive process in patients with aneurysms. Currently, it is recommended to screen males older than 65 who have smoked.

3. What is the incidence and prevalence of AAA?

There are more than 45,000 patients with abdominal aortic aneurysm undergoing surgical repair each year. A population-based study from Norway in the late 1990s found a prevalence of 8.9 and 2.2% in males and females respectively. In the US, approximately 1% of males between 55 and 65 years of age have a clinically significant aneurysm and the prevalence increases by 2–4% for each decade of life thereafter. Women are affected four times less frequently than males and about a decade later in life [2].

S.A. Ianchulev (✉)
Department of Anesthesiology, Tufts Medical Center, 800 Washington St., Boston, MA 02111, USA
e-mail: sianchulev@tuftsmedicalcenter.org

© Springer International Publishing AG 2017
L.S. Aglio and R.D. Urman (eds.), *Anesthesiology*,
DOI 10.1007/978-3-319-50141-3_29

4. How does AAA present?

AAA are most often found incidentally, and if electively repaired, the risk of all-cause mortality is less than 8%. Acute dissection will present with abdominal, back or groin pains, pulsatile mass and possible hemodynamic compromise. A patient with these findings must be immediately evaluated to prevent further dissection or rupture.

5. What is the risk of rupture of an AAA?

Risk of rupture depends on the diameter of the internal lumen and increases with growth of the aneurysm. An important dimension to keep in mind is a diameter of 4.5 cm. A study following patients with AAA showed that on average the size increased by 0.3 cm/year and the cumulative 6 year risk of rupture was less than 2% when the size was less than 4.5 cm. Risk of rupture increased to above 20% in AAA greater than 5 cm in diameter. Rupture carries high mortality; approximately 23–69%, compared to 1.4–6.5% if not ruptured [3].

6. What are recommendations for AAA screening?

One time ultrasound screening is recommended in patients ages 65–75 with known risk factors and followed by active monitoring of a detectable aneurysm. No benefit has been found in screening of women or men over 75 with negative previous screening. Life style modification and medical therapy may slow growth and delay the need for repair. When the internal diameter of the aneurysm reaches 5.5 cm the risk of rupture is equal to the operative mortality risk and thus aneurysm sizes greater than 6.0 cm or lumen size twice the normal aortic diameter should be repaired [4].

7. What are the current recommendations for AAA repair?

Class	Location of AAA	Size	Procedure	Level of evidence
I.	Infrarenal/juxtarenal	≥5.5 cm	Repair	Level B
I.1.	Infrarenal/juxtarenal	4.0–5.4 cm	Monitored q 6–12 months	Level A
II.1.	Infrarenal/juxtarenal	5.0–5.4 cm	May have repair	Level evidence B
II.2.	Suprarenal of thoracoabdominal or type IV aneurysm	5.5–6.0 cm	Repair is probably indicated	Level of evidence B
II.3.	AAA	<4.0 cm	Monitoring by US q 2–3 years is reasonable	Evidence level B
III.	Asymptomatic infrarenal/juxtarenal	<5.0 cm in men and 4.5 cm in women	Intervention not recommended	Level of evidence A

(continued)

Recommendation for interventions in AAA [5]

8. How do you approach an elective AAA patient in preparation for surgery?

When a patient presents for elective aortic aneurysm repair, the surgeon will recommend one of two approaches to manage the AAA; open repair versus endovascular aortic repair (EVAR). The 2005 ACC/AHA Guidelines recommend open surgical repair for patients with low-to-moderate risk of surgical complications and endovascular repair for high surgical risk individuals [5].

9. How do you classify abdominal aortic aneurysms; does classification affect anesthesia management?

Classification of AAA is based on the relationship of the aneurysm to the renal arteries, with suprarenal, juxtarenal and infrarenal AAA as typical labels. An infrarenal AAA will have at least 10 mm of a normal aortic segment adjacent to the most cephalad end of the aneurysm [4]. A suprarenal AAA may involve the celiac arteries. Thus it is important to understand the implications of vessel involvement and possible additional surgical interventions. This information plays a significant role in deciding open surgical repair versus EVAR, and profoundly influences intraoperative anesthetic management.

Additionally, aneurysms may be classified as fusiform, involving all layers of the aortic wall, saccular or pseudoaneurysms when they are more focal and localized and do not involve all mural layers, and inflammatory, which are prone to significant intraoperative bleeding.

10. Which patients should undergo open repair of AAA?

Patients who are deemed low or average risk of perioperative surgical complications may undergo open repair. Octogenarians have an operative mortality rate less than 10% and may be appropriate open repair candidates. Some studies have shown that preoperative management of coronary artery disease (diagnostic tests followed by an intervention) has helped reduce the rate of perioperative major adverse cardiac event (MACE) to about 2%. Other studies were not so optimistic [2]. An association between presence of renal plus cardiac disease and mortality has been established. Patients with advanced cardiac and renal disease may benefit from EVAR.

11. Which patients are more suitable for EVAR?

Patients who represent high risk of postoperative surgical complications and patients with favorable anatomical and clinical attributes may be suitable for EVAR.

Anatomic Factors influencing decision for EVAR versus open repair.

(a) Vascular access—iliac arteries
(b) Aneurysm morphology (tortuosity, thrombus)
(c) Aneurysm neck length and morphology (calcification, thrombus, length, angle)
(d) Involvement of renal and celiac arteries
(e) Thrombus presence

12. What scoring system is used to guide surgical decision making?

A scoring system has been set up based on the aortic angle and tortuosity, and the presence of intraluminal thrombus. The scores are 1 through 3 points with higher total number of points signifying poorer EVAR outcomes [4].

Aortic angle and tortuosity scoring

Grade	Tortuosity index	Aortic angle	Amount of thrombus
0	≤1.05	160°–180°	No visible thrombus
1	≥1.05 ≤ 1.15	140°–159°	<25% of cross-sectional area
2	>1.15 ≤ 1.20	120°–139°	25–50% of cross-sectional area
3	>1.20	<120°	>50% of cross-sectional area

Clinical factors:

(a) Various scoring systems have been used to define benefit of open versus EVAR approach—APCHE, POSSM, ASA, SVS/AAVS.
(b) Age, cardiac, pulmonary, and renal status of the patient.
(c) EVAR still considered intermediate to high cardiac risk procedure with 3–7% mortality.
(d) Preexisting renal insufficiency associated with poor EVAR outcomes.
(e) Diabetes mellitus is associated with significantly higher device related complications and early mortality rates. However, the insulin controlled DM II patients had lower incidence of endoleaks than the non-insulin controlled DM II and nondiabetic patients.
(f) Patient preferences should be considered. The EVAR—1 trial showed better outcomes in the first 4 years, but increased risk of endoleaks and re-interventions thereafter. Patient preference for EVAR is above 80%. (SIR Guideline 56, 57–58) [4].
(g) Patients with high risk factors for either approach require a multidisciplinary evaluation and decision.

13. What short- and long-term outcome differences exist between approaches?

The short-term outcomes of EVAR have been found to be superior to open repair with regard to 30-day mortality, hospital length of stay, and number of blood transfusions. However, these advantages disappeared in the long term where the mortality from either procedure was equal at 6 years. Other differences between groups related to dye exposure and fluoroscopy, occurrence of endoleaks and the need for re-intervention which were higher in the EVAR group. Thus cost savings from the short-term EVAR advantages were lost. Current literature does not support EVAR for small AAA [6]. Ruptured AAA can successfully be managed by EVAR [7].

Obese and frail patients can benefit significantly from EVAR with regard to short-term outcomes. Continuous improvement of endograft technology and design with availability of branched and fenestrated grafts, as well as total percutaneous access has helped shift the risk–benefit balance toward EVARs [6].

14. What are key dangers of open surgical repair?

In the open group, organ ischemia and humoral changes due to cross-clamping have been identified as major reasons for perioperative mortality and morbidity. The open approach has also been associated with higher blood product and fluid utilization, protracted ICU stay and early morbidity, including acute kidney injury and pneumonia.

15. What additional considerations apply for a ruptured AAA?

Stable patients with a suspected ruptured AAA, should undergo a CT angiography to determine AAA morphology. Unstable patients should be taken immediately to the operating room. A hybrid operating room allows more flexibility for on-the-table decision to maximize control of dissection and bleeding. Sometimes a supraceliac balloon can be inserted to stabilize hemodynamics initially and give the anesthesiology team time to catch up with fluids and blood products.

16. What is the significance of abdominal compartment syndrome (ACS) in the context of ruptured AAA?

Patients with significant fluid or blood product resuscitation, and those with coagulopathy are more prone to developing this condition. A high degree of vigilance is needed for early recognition before it impacts other organs. ACS may cause liver or renal failure, interrupt venous return, induce coagulopathy and may quickly become lethal.

17. What is the relevance of pre-existing cardiac disease for the patient undergoing AAA repair?

Open repair is considered a high-risk vascular procedure with regard to cardiac morbidity and mortality. The pooled prevalence of myocardial infarction and death in the perioperative period in vascular surgery patients is 4.9% and 2.4% respectively. In the long term they approach 8.9 and 11.2%. A detailed understanding of the cardiac status, in terms of ischemic potential and ventricular function is important.

18. What symptoms or signs indicate further preoperative cardiac evaluation is necessary in patients with AAA?

Unstable angina, uncontrolled heart rhythm and chronic heart failure symptoms should prompt immediate evaluation and optimization of therapy prior to surgery. This follows the latest recommendations from the American Heart Association and American College of Cardiology for perioperative evaluation of the cardiac patient presenting for noncardiac surgery. This guideline-based approach should not simply target clearance for the surgical procedure but give the patient and caregivers the ability to make informed decisions, help optimize the current therapy and provide recommendations for the perioperative management of the cardiac problems. Emergency procedures should focus on resuscitation of the patient and stratification of cardiac risk should occur in the postoperative phase.

19. When is preoperative myocardial revascularization helpful?

There is a significant prevalence of coronary artery disease and carotid artery disease in patients with AAA. The Coronary Artery Revascularization Prophylaxis (CARP) trial did not find improvement of short-term outcome or long-term survival despite aggressive revascularization prophylaxis. Patients with the absence of multiple preoperative cardiac risk variables experienced the best long-term survival after vascular surgery [8]. Similar results were established by the Dutch Echocardiographic Cardiac Risk Evaluation Applying Stress Echo (DECREASE) in high-risk patients. This is also reflected in the current AHA/ACC recommendations for CABG, recommending only those patients who experience unstable angina symptoms benefit from revascularization despite the higher incidence of periprocedural complications in those patients. Patients who underwent prophylactic revascularization did exhibit 5.5% mortality from the CABG itself thus reducing the actuarial benefit from the procedure.

20. Does this patient require further cardiac workup?

This patient has an extensive cardiac history with significant changes in myocardial performance. Transthoracic (TTE) or transesophageal (TEE) echocardiography can be helpful in defining current (post revascularization and AVR) myocardial function and will diagnose left ventricular aneurysm or thrombus. TTE is better in the diagnosis of left ventricular apical thrombus. Additional testing is not necessary as the patient is an unlikely candidate for further cardiac optimization. Since there has not been a change in activity level and no new onset of shortness of breath, the value of additional tests, considering their invasiveness and inherent risks may be counterproductive.

21. When is percutaneous coronary intervention (PCI) indicated prior to AAA repair?

Prophylactic PCI may be reserved for those patients with unstable angina or evidence of myocardial ischemia. Significant atherosclerotic disease poses a periprocedural risk to patients undergoing PCI related to vascular access. More recently, alternative sites for PCI access have been utilized, including the radial and brachial arteries.

22. Would you perform other noninvasive diagnostic testing and when?

Noninvasive diagnostic tests should only be performed in patients deemed to be an intermediate risk and followed by an intervention if indicated. Tests are currently not recommended for those patients where further diagnosis will not lead to an intervention. Perioperative medical management and optimization is indicated.

23. What is the significance of poorly controlled preoperative hypertension?

The preoperative visit should include vital sign testing, and unexplained hypertension in a patient with AAA should prompt investigation to rule out renal artery stenosis (RAS). RAS can contribute to poorly controlled hypertension via the renin–angiotensin–aldosterone mechanism. Uncontrolled or long-standing hypertension may mask hypovolemia and significant left ventricular hypertrophy may be present. These patients are often very susceptible to minor changes in the intravascular volume. Induction of general anesthesia in hypovolemic patients can cause significant hypotension with poor response to therapy. Evidence suggests that blood pressure less than 20% of normal can have adverse effects including renal and myocardial hypoperfusion [9].

24. What is the function of BNP ("B-type" or brain natriuretic peptide) and when should it be a preoperative lab test?

When evaluating a patient with intermediate risk factors, one should consider the brain natriuretic peptide (BNP) as a test for well-managed cardiac disease. The prognostic value of BNP has been shown in an analysis by Young et al. with an odds ratio of 15.0 to predict postoperative major adverse cardiac events (MACE). The authors point out that the BNP has a high rule-out and low rule-in value for MACE. As such, this test should be added to the battery of tests these patients undergo [10].

25. What is the role of measuring hematocrit and creatinine to predict outcome?

Preoperative hematocrit (Hct) has been related to surgical outcome. Patients with low preoperative Hct (<28) have a higher risk of postoperative acute coronary events and incidence of transfusion. Transfusion itself carries risk of transfusion related problems including transfusion related acute lung injury, immunocompromise, and hemolytic reactions, among others. A recent article in the British Journal of Anesthesia related preoperative anemia to poor outcomes and increased health care resources [11]. Current recommendations are to consider treating elective surgery patients with a multimodal approach of erythropoietin, iron and vitamin B12 preoperatively. Some medical centers have established "anemia clinics" as part of their perioperative surgical home initiatives.

Preoperative evaluation of creatinine (Cr) and glomerular filtration rate (GFR) can provide estimates of kidney function, which relates to perioperative morbidity and mortality. Patients with worse renal function may fare poorly and experience higher incidence of in hospital complications [12]. Preoperative Cr greater than 2 mg/dL and GFR less than 60 ml/min are independent predictors of mortality in both the short and long term [13, 14]. Perioperative beta-blockers and statin therapy in renally impaired patients have been proven to be beneficial [1].

26. What cardiac workup will you do in this patient? What if coronary graft failure is suspected?

Patients with significant vascular disease have a higher incidence of atherosclerosis with up to 50% manifesting significant carotid artery disease. One should include assessment of new ECG findings with regard to rate, rhythm and conduction abnormalities. Evidence of unstable angina or recent acute coronary syndrome will need further evaluation and a decision to order additional tests and or procedures. Stress echocardiography or cardiac catheterization may further clarify the condition. The patient described here has a significant cardiac surgery history and advanced age. If atherosclerotic changes in the grafts are causing preoperative ischemia or new failure symptoms, treatment options include PCI with or without stenting. This patient carries a high risk of an adverse perioperative event if cardiac surgery was performed prior to AAA repair. Cardiac catheterization may be the safest option to improve graft blood flow. Guidelines for Surgery after percutaneous coronary intervention are shown in Fig. 29.1.

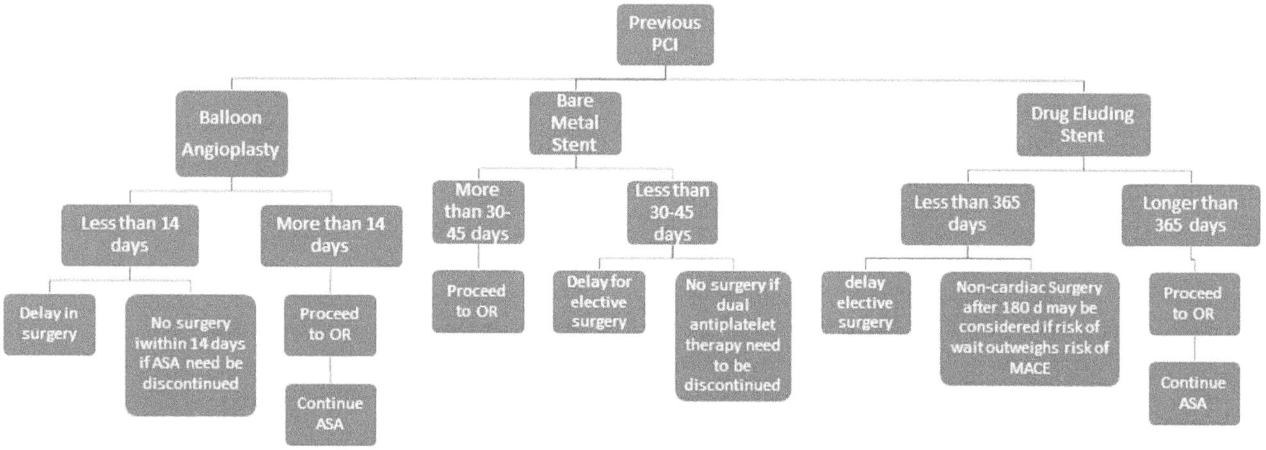

Fig. 29.1 Guidelines for surgery after percutaneous coronary intervention (based on the 2014 Guidelines from American Heart Association) [19]

27. What preoperative interventions are indicated regarding (a) cardiac rhythm disturbances, (b) medication management (beta-blockers, clonidine, ACE inhibitors, and statins)?

(a) Uncontrolled cardiac dysrhythmia and high grade AV block, such as second degree Mobitz II, needs to be evaluated, and if indicated, an implantable cardiac rhythm management device inserted.
(b) Beta-blockers are indicated in patients who can tolerate them and have significant impact on reduction of perioperative ischemia. However, their role has been questioned in otherwise stable patients. The POISE study evaluated the all-cause mortality and concluded that while the rate of postoperative myocardial infarction was lower, the rate of death or stroke in the extended release metoprolol group was significantly higher in a 30-day postoperative period. New initiation of beta-blockers may not be warranted in stable patients. Clonidine has not been shown to affect the incidence of perioperative MI in the POISE II study and was associated with increased incidence of hypotension and nonfatal cardiac arrest [15]. ACE inhibitors have been found to have beneficial effects on acute vascular events in atherosclerotic disease, but their impact on blood pressure with induction of anesthesia and refractoriness to treatment make them less desirable on the day of surgery. Statins are consistently shown to improve outcomes after vascular surgical interventions. More recent trials have confirmed the benefits of statins on improved renal outcomes, lower resource utilization and overall hospital costs [6].

28. How would you evaluate respiratory status in patients undergoing major vascular surgery? What recommendation should be made regarding smoking cessation?

Patients undergoing open AAA repair may experience numerous possible pulmonary complications. Most intra-abdominal surgery predisposes to atelectasis, pneumonia, weakened cough, reduced vital capacity, worsening of COPD, and can lead to respiratory failure. Careful review of current pulmonary status should involve smoking (past and current), asthma control, timing of medications, previous lung-related hospitalizations and intubations, as well as the presence of chronic bronchitis. Smoking cessation just prior to the surgical procedure is not recommended. Increased airway irritability can lead to worsening of pulmonary status in the perioperative period. There are benefits to smoking cessation longer than a few days prior to procedure as the intra-arterial carbon monoxide content significantly diminishes and oxygenation improves.

Arterial blood gas measurement may be recommended in heavy smokers and patients with advanced COPD to assess the severity of CO_2 retention. Values greater than 45 mmHg arterial CO_2 are associated with higher postoperative morbidity. Patients with significant COPD may benefit from bronchodilators. Perioperative beta-blocker therapy should be carefully instituted if needed with selective beta-blockers (bisoprolol, metoprolol, esmolol). Glucocorticoid therapy may be beneficial in managing COPD exacerbation.

Patients with significant limitations of their respiratory status may benefit from epidural analgesia in the immediate postoperative period. Incentive spirometry and continuous positive airway pressure are the only modalities where benefit has been proven [1].

29. How would you address coagulation in this patient?

Vascular patients are predisposed to hypercoagulable states. This may compromise graft patency in vascular surgery patients postoperatively. It is important to assess coagulation status with a careful history and physical examination preoperatively. When regional analgesia is planned for postoperative pain control, careful review and planning of perioperative anticoagulation must be performed. Intraoperative coagulopathy may be induced by heparinization, as a surgical complication, or by use of other anticoagulation or antiplatelet therapy. Vascular surgery affects fibrinolysis, antithrombin III, fibrinogen levels, and proteins C and S. The need for perioperative heparinization should be discussed with the surgeon and included in the planning for epidural analgesia management.

30. If the patient had diabetes what would you recommend?

Diabetes is a common disease with significant impact on organs and systems. Current recommendations suggest tight perioperative blood glucose management with values between 90 and 150 mg/dL. Recommendations of the American College of Endocrinology limit maximum blood glucose during the hospitalization to 180 mg/dL. In the ICU blood glucose may be even tighter controlled with ranges between 90 and 110 mg/dL. The problem of acute hypoglycemia should be taken seriously as neurologic injury can be severe and insidious.

31. What intraoperative monitors would you choose? Discuss arterial, venous, and pulmonary catheters.

Open AAA repair is a major intraabdominal or retroperitoneal surgery with significant fluid shifts and cross-clamp ischemic time. Appropriate monitoring in addition to standard ASA recommendations include an arterial line and a central venous catheter. Vascular surgical patients can have significant atherosclerotic disease and may exhibit significant discrepancy between the measured blood pressure in both arms. The arterial line should be placed in the arm with higher blood pressure.

At least a triple lumen 7Fr. catheter is recommended for central venous pressure monitoring and administration of vasoactive or inotropic agents. It has been shown that the values of central venous and pulmonary artery pressure do not correlate with measured circulating blood volume. The usefulness of a pulmonary artery catheter is debatable due to associated morbidity and mortality while requiring significant expertise in its interpretation. Much of its utility has been replaced by transesophageal echocardiography (TEE). TEE has become an indispensable tool in the management of the cardiac patient for noncardiac surgery.

32. What additional monitoring may be helpful?

Continuous cardiac output monitors like continuous pulse volume recording from the arterial line are useful in managing fluid status of the patient. Currently stroke volume variation (SVV) is not recommended to follow for volume optimization. However, stroke volume and stroke volume index are useful in guiding therapy. Additional monitors to consider are cerebral oximetry, motor and somatosensory evoked potentials. The cerebral oximeter may give information on the balance of oxygen delivery and demand of the prefrontal areas of the cerebrum. Use of this technology has been associated with decreased hospital stay and cost. Monitoring SSEPs and MEPs may have value in discovering spinal cord ischemia. They require more technical personnel, anesthetic planning, and necessitate additional knowledge.

33. How is the AAA approached surgically?

Open AAA repair can be accomplished either through the retroperitoneal or midline approach. The retroperitoneal approach has better exposure and induces less bowel trauma and fluid shifts.

34. What are the goals of hemodynamic management in the patient undergoing open AAA repair?

Current literature suggest that "less is more" regarding fluid management during open AAA repair. The goal is to maintain euvolemia and cardiac performance avoiding liberal fluid administration. Excess fluid administration will cause edema, hemodilution and can lead to postoperative issues including bacterial transudation through the bowel walls secondary to bowel edema. Postoperatively, fluid mobilization within the first three days, will pose significant burden on the cardiovascular system, and may result in longer ventilator support, and pulmonary edema. Enhanced recovery after surgery (ERAS) protocols address many the aforementioned issues, including preoperative, intraoperative and postoperative elements. Literature suggests that standardization may improve outcomes.

35. What kind of venous access should this patient have?

Given the potential of significant blood loss and fluid shifts in open repair, large bore intravenous catheters are recommended. Two peripheral large bore (for example two 14 g IVs) and a central line should be sufficient. If peripheral access is inadequate, a large bore central line, 8 or 9 French, should be considered.

36. What intravenous fluids will you use?

Euvolemia is a beneficial goal for patients with significant fluid shifts during the procedure. The ASA Choosing Wisely initiative favors reducing colloid use. Crystalloids will extravasate to the extravascular space due to disruption of the glycocalyx membrane of the vasculature from humoral factors or direct vessel injury. Colloids remain in the vascular space longer, but are associated with renal damage and coagulopathy. More recently, hypertonic saline has gained attention but can be associated with significant hyperosmolarity and hypernatremia impacting renal performance. Patients receiving hypertonic saline had significantly less fluid administered during the procedure. Strandvik et al. found that despite the decrease of ICP and effective blood pressure restoration in ICU patients, it did not affect outcome [16].

37. What type of anesthetic technique will you use for open surgery of AAA?

General and combined general and epidural techniques can be employed. While the inhalational technique can allow for ischemic preconditioning, an epidural can be beneficial in reducing the sympathetic outflow, inducing bradycardia and mitigating hypertension. A disadvantage to the epidural technique is vasodilation necessitating more IV fluids. Many providers elect to place the epidural preoperatively and start dosing it after the major blood loss and reperfusion periods have occurred.

38. What antibiotics are appropriate for this patient?

Patients presenting for intraabdominal procedures should receive prophylactic antibiotics prior to incision. Cefazolin will be inappropriate in this patient due to her cefazolin

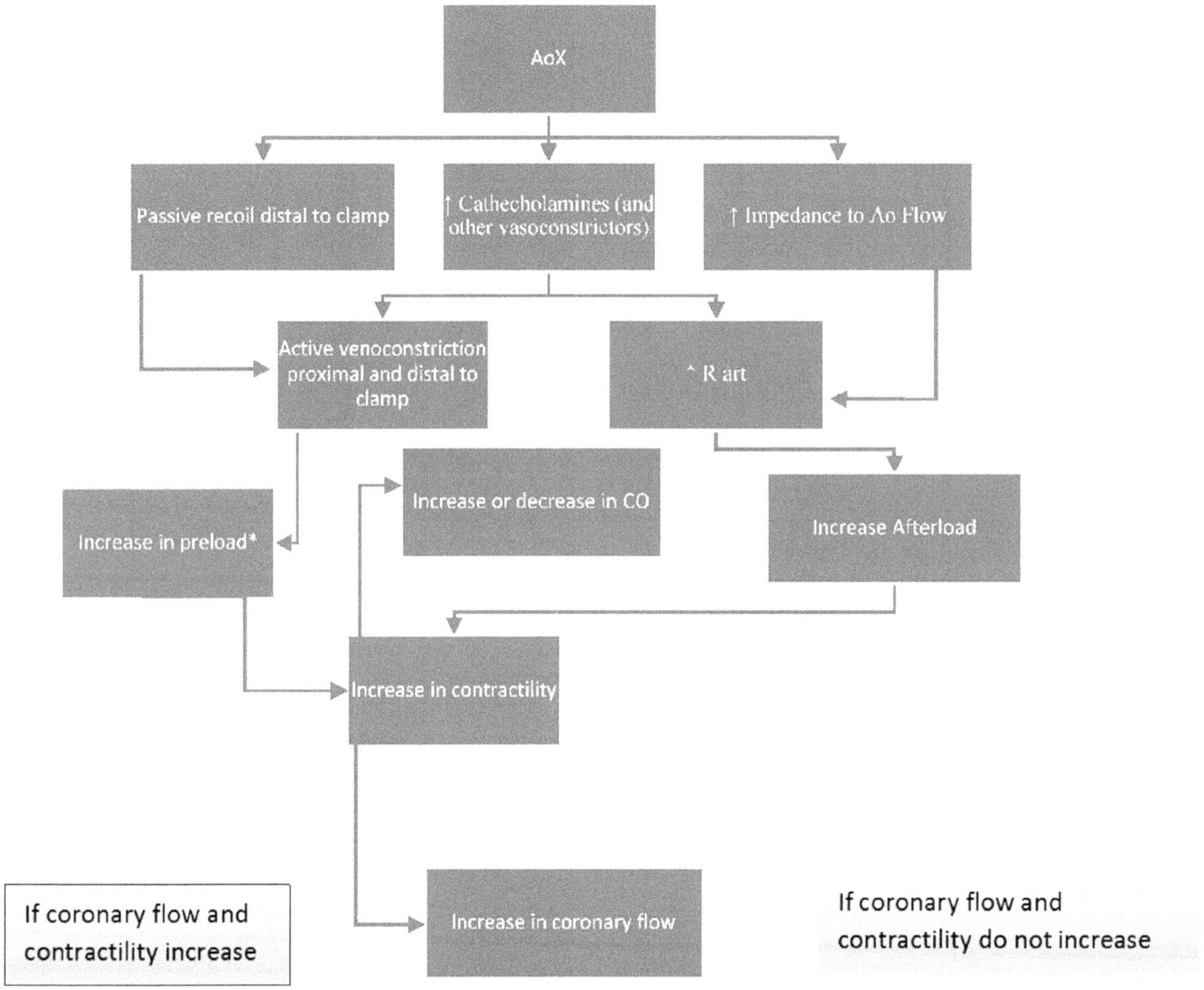

Fig. 29.2 Systemic hemodynamic response to aortic cross-clamping. Preload (*asterisk*) does not necessarily increase with infrarenal clamping. Depending on splanchnic vascular tone, blood volume can be shifted into the splanchnic circulation, and preload will not increase. *Ao* aortic; *AoX* aortic cross-clamping; *R art* arterial resistance. (Adapted from Gelman S: The pathophysiology of aortic cross-clamping. Anesthesiology 82: 1026–1060, 1995, with permission of Wolters Kluwer)

Table 29.1 Percent change in cardiovascular variables on initiation of aortic occlusion

		Percent change occlusion	
Cardiovascular variable	Supraceliac	Suprarenal–infraceliac	Infrarenal
MAP	54	5[a]	2[a]
PCWP	38	10[a]	0[a]
LVEDA	28	2[a]	9[a]
LVESA	69	10[a]	11[a]
EF	−38	−10[a]	−3[a]
Patients with WMA	92	33	0

Adapted from Roizen MF, Beaupre PN, Alpert RA et al.: Monitoring with two-dimensional transesophageal echocardiography. Comparison of myocardial function in patents undergoing supraceliac, suprarenal–infraceliac, or infrarenal aortic occlusion. J Vasc Surg 1:300–305, 1984, with permission of Elsevier

[a]Statistically different from the group undergoing supraceliac aortic occlusion

anaphylaxis (β-Lactam antibiotic), and thus vancomycin or clindamycin are appropriate choices. This procedure should not involve bowel damage and thus coverage with metronidazole or aminoglycoside is unnecessary [17].

39. Describe the impact of aortic cross-clamping during surgery and how to manage it.

An aortic cross-clamp is needed for control of the aorta above the aneurysm. Increasingly proximal occlusion induces more profound physiological effects. Aortic occlusion impacts hemodynamics (Fig. 29.2), cardiac performance (Table 29.1), and release of humoral factors (prostaglandins, catecholamines, vasoconstrictors, activation of renin-angiotensin-aldosterone system).

The initial occlusion increases the peripheral resistance and leads to a decrease in venous return and cardiac output. Redistribution of blood ensues with shift toward the splanchnic circulation and muscles in cases of an infrarenal cross-clamp. Venoconstriction occurs as a result of the catecholamine surge. This leads to an increase in intracranial and lung blood volumes. Suprarenal occlusion is less well tolerated since there is less ability for circulatory redistribution. The load on the heart increases and is much more likely to cause left ventricular segmental wall motion abnormalities. Patients with compromised coronary perfusion may experience ischemia and not be able to maintain cardiac output.

The impact on muscles and organs distal to the cross-clamp is significant. Their perfusion relies on pressure dependent collaterals. An increase in blood pressure augments distal perfusion and can attenuate the ischemia. The hypertensive response to aortic cross-clamp may be attenuated with afterload reduction agents like clevidipine or nicardipine as well as preload reduction agents like nitroglycerin. Inducing mild hypotension prior to cross-clamp allows for better tolerance of the afterload increase. Ischemic preconditioning has been associated with up to 23% decrease in myocardial and renal injury in human studies [18].

40. Can renal protection be instituted during aortic cross-clamping, and is it effective?

No current renal protective strategy has been proven to be more effective or superior to another. Evidence shows that appropriate hydration is associated with better outcomes. Some practitioners have employed bicarbonate infusion without success, and this can be associated with higher sodium load. The use of mannitol prior to clamp application and after clamp removal increases the urine output through osmotic diuresis, but this has not been proven to have a renal protective effect. The free radical scavenging ability of mannitol may be protective in ischemia reperfusion situations, although evidence is still inconclusive. Overall, the relationship of urine output to postoperative incidence of AKI has not been established. Fenoldopam has not proven to be of value. Renal dose dopamine exerts its action through increase in the cardiac output and perfusion. Loop diuretics may be beneficial by decreasing ATP utilization in normovolemic patients. Administering diuretics to hypovolemic patients may be harmful. In cases of prolonged clamp duration, selective hypothermia with direct infusion of cold Ringer's Lactate may be beneficial [18].

41. What mesenteric and hepatic protection strategies are appropriate in high aortic cross-clamping?

Aortic cross-clamp above the celiac arteries carries a high risk of bowel and liver ischemia and release of interleukins and tumor necrosis factor. This has been associated with bacterial translocation and worsened postoperative course and outcomes. The best solution is to keep the ischemic time as short as possible or to bypass the clamp with a graft. Some authors recommend high doses of methylprednisolone at the beginning of anesthesia, allowing two hours for the pharmacologic effect, but this has been associated with renal dysfunction in the postoperative period. A bicarbonate infusion may be considered for prolonged hepatic ischemic time.

42. What is the impact of aortic cross-clamp on coagulation?

There are two general ways open repair of AAA affects coagulation. Blood loss and associated fluid administration with hemodilution of factors and platelets may induce coagulopathy, and this is more significant in anemic patients. Second, the clamp itself can stimulate the release of plasminogen activator. Thromboelastography has revealed increased clotting factor activity during clamping and decreased speed of clot solidification after unclamping of the aorta.

43. How do you manage unclamping?

Aortic cross-clamp has rendered a significant part of the body ischemic and reliant on collaterals. Depending on the level of cross-clamp application this effect can be significant. Release of an infrarenal cross-clamp is better tolerated than a supraceliac occlusion given equal ischemic time. Aortobifemoral grafts allow for sequential reperfusion and diminished acid load. Reperfusion is associated with systemic flooding of humoral factors and lactic acid, all contributing to significant hypotension and vasodilatation. Profound acidosis in the cardiac patient can impact myocardial performance.

Prophylactic sodium bicarbonate administration is not recommended as the intracellular milieu may not be affected and the CO_2 byproduct of its metabolism may worsen respiratory status. However, if reperfusion significantly impacts myocardial performance, its use may be justified.

Preparation for unclamping is an important process where volume status should be optimized. Electrolyte abnormalities should be corrected. In the case of supraceliac cross-clamp and multiple blood transfusions, circulating citrate may not be metabolized by the liver, and ionized hypocalcemia and coagulation abnormalities may persist. Calcium administration and replacement may be prudent.

44. How do you manage significant blood loss?

Significant blood loss is possible during open repair of AAA. Current recommendations are to replace plasma and platelets after eight units of blood have been administered or after six units have been given and more is anticipated. Recent research in trauma and major transfusion has shown that 1:1:1 ratio of PRBC, FFP, and platelets yields best results. Recombinant factor availability has allowed for targeted replacement of those blood components that have been depleted. The role of factor eight concentrates and fibrinogen concentrates is still under evaluation. In emergent procedures where coagulopathy has become difficult to manage, factor VIIa may be considered. Utilization of cell saver and rapid infusion devices are commonplace and should be considered.

45. What kind of spinal cord monitoring or protection should be utilized in open AAA repairs?

Spinal cord ischemia occurs in 1–11% of cases. Much of it is related to perfusion of the anterior spinal cord by the single anterior radicular artery of Adamkiewicz. It has a variable origin between T8 and L1/L2. It is unknown whether the aortic cross-clamp and graft will affect spinal cord perfusion as collateralization is often poor. The perfusion of the anterior spinal cord may be monitored intraoperatively with SSEPs and MEPs. If suspicion of inducing spinal artery ischemia is high, this may necessitate the insertion of a spinal drain, particularly in cases with supraceliac cross-clamping. Insertion of a silastic spinal drain catheter at spinal level L3-4, requires understanding CSF production and tolerable drainage. Some current spinal drain catheters, which have larger bores, have built in valves allowing for draining only when the intracranial pressure (ICP) exceeds 5–10 mmHg. One should never drain more than 10–12 cc of CSF in an hour as the ensuing low intracranial pressure poses a risk of rupturing of bridging intracranial veins and inducing subarachnoid bleeding. The outcome of such an event carries high mortality and morbidity. Another maneuver to preserve spinal cord perfusion is to increase perfusion pressure by augmenting mean arterial pressure.

46. How do you manage temperature during the procedure?

Thermoregulation is impaired under general anesthesia. Redistribution of heat during the initial 2 h can lead to significant hypothermia. Fluid administration, exposure and ambient temperature can exacerbate the loss of body temperature. Hypothermia impacts various processes including drug metabolism, coagulation, and may result in increased blood loss. As an accepted quality measure as well as good practice, efforts should be made to keep the patient normothermic. There may be a beneficial effect of mild local hypothermia during the aortic cross-clamp period to improve ischemia tolerance, but the detrimental effects of generalized hypothermia are well documented. The use of a warming device on the lower body during cross-clamping of the aorta is not recommended as it may aggravate ischemia secondary to increased metabolic demand.

47. What postoperative pain management strategies should be considered?

Open AAA repair carries significant pain potential and a functional thoracic epidural catheter is beneficial. If there are contraindications to an epidural catheter insertion, a tranversus abdominal plane (TAP) block and intravenous opioids should be considered. The postoperative pain management strategy should begin in the preoperative period and planned during the preoperative visit. The impact of an epidural catheter with combined opioid and local anesthetic infusion in the postoperative period has several benefits including better quality postoperative respiratory function. In patients at higher risk for postoperative ileus (transperitoneal surgical approach), using a local anesthetic infusion (omitting opioids) has been shown to be beneficial. Generally, multimodal pain control, consisting of nonsteroidal medication like acetaminophen, epidural infusion of local anesthetic and judicious use of opioids should be considered.

References

1. Miller RD, Eriksson LI, Fleisher L, Wiener-Kronish JP, Young WL. Miller's anesthesia. 7th ed. Philadelphia: Churchill Livingstone; 2009.
2. Aggarwal S, et al. Abdominal aortic aneurysm: a comprehensive review. Exp Clin Cardiol. 2011;16(1):11–5.
3. Baril DT, Kahn RA, Ellozy SH, Carroccio A, Marin ML. Endovascular abdominal aortic aneurysm repair: emerging developments and anesthetic considerations. J Cardiothorac Vasc Anesth. 2007;21(5):730–42.

4. Walker TG, Kalva SP, Yeddula K, Wicky S, Kundu S, Drescher P, d'Othee BJ, Rose SC, Cardella JF; Society of Interventional Radiology Standards of Practice Committee; Interventional Radiological Society of Europe; Canadian Interventional Radiology Association. Clinical practice guidelines for endovascular abdominal aortic aneurysm repair: written by the Standards of Practice Committee for the Society of Interventional Radiology and endorsed by the Cardiovascular and Interventional Radiological Society of Europe and the Canadian Interventional Radiology Association. J Vasc Interv Radiol. 2010. 21(11):1632–55. doi:10.1016/j.jvir.2010.07.008.
5. Hirsch AT, Haskal ZJ, Hertzer NR, Bakal CW, Creager MA, Halperin JL, Hiratzka LF, Murphy WR, Olin JW, Puschett JB, Rosenfield KA, Sacks D, Stanley JC, Taylor LM Jr, White CJ, White J, White RA, Antman EM, Smith SC Jr, Adams CD, Anderson JL, Faxon DP, Fuster V, Gibbons RJ, Hunt SA, Jacobs AK, Nishimura R, Ornato JP, Page RL, Riegel B; American Association for Vascular Surgery; Society for Vascular Surgery; Society for Cardiovascular Angiography and Interventions; Society for Vascular Medicine and Biology; Society of Interventional Radiology; ACC/AHA Task Force on Practice Guidelines Writing Committee to Develop Guidelines for the Management of Patients With Peripheral Arterial Disease; American Association of Cardiovascular and Pulmonary Rehabilitation; National Heart, Lung, and Blood Institute; Society for Vascular Nursing; TransAtlantic Inter-Society Consensus; Vascular Disease Foundation. ACC/AHA 2005 Practice Guidelines for the management of patients with peripheral arterial disease (lower extremity, renal, mesenteric, and abdominal aortic): a collaborative report from the American Association for Vascular Surgery/Society for Vascular Surgery, Society for Cardiovascular Angiography and Interventions, Society for Vascular Medicine and Biology, Society of Interventional Radiology, and the ACC/AHA Task Force on Practice Guidelines (Writing Committee to Develop Guidelines for the Management of Patients With Peripheral Arterial Disease): endorsed by the American Association of Cardiovascular and Pulmonary Rehabilitation; National Heart, Lung, and Blood Institute; Society for Vascular Nursing; TransAtlantic Inter-Society Consensus; and Vascular Disease Foundation. Circulation. 2006 Mar 21;113(11):e463–654.
6. Subramian B, Singh N, Roscher C, Augustides JGT. Innovations in treating aortic disease: the abdominal aorta. J Cardiothorac Vasc Anesth. 2012;26(5):959–65. doi:10.1053/j.jvca.2010.10.003.
7. Veith FJ, Cayne NS, Berland TL, Mayer D, Lachat M. EVAR for Ruptured Abdominal Aortic Aneurysms: tips for improving survival rates among patients who undergo endovascular repair of rAAAs. Endovascular Today. 2011. Available at http://evtoday.com/2011/03/evar-for-ruptured-abdominal-aortic-aneurysms/.
8. McFalls EO, Ward HB, Moritz TE, et al. Coronaryartery revascularization before elective major vascular surgery. N Engl J Med. 2004;351:2795–804.
9. Walsh M, et al. Relationship between intraoperative mean arterial pressure and clinical outcomes after noncardiac surgery: toward an empirical definition of hypotension. Anesthesiology. 2013;119 (3):507–15.
10. Young,YR, et al. Predictive value of plasma brain natriuretic peptide for postoperative cardiac complications–a systemic review and meta-analysis. J Crit Care. 2014. 29(4):696 e691–10.
11. Baron DM, Hochrieser H, Posch M, Metnitz B, Rhodes A, Moreno RP, PearseRM, and Metnitz P for the European Surgical Outcomes Study (EuSOS) group for the Trials Groups of the European Society of Intensive Care Medicine and the European Society of Anaesthesiology. Preoperative anaemia is associated with poor clinical outcome in non-cardiac surgery patients. British Journal of Anaesthesia. 2014; 113 (3): 416–23, doi:10.1093/bja/aeu098.
12. Pasqualini L, Schillaci G, Pirro M, et al. Renal dysfunction predicts long-term mortality in patients with lower extremity arterial disease. J Intern Med. 2007;262:668–77.
13. Lee TH, Marcantonio ER, Mangione CM, et al. Derivation and prospective validation of a simple index for prediction of cardiac risk of major noncardiac surgery. Circulation. 1999;100:1043–9.
14. Welten GM, Chonchol M, Hoeks SE, et al. Statin therapy is associated with improved outcomes in vascular surgery patients with renal impairment. Am Heart J. 2007;154:954–61.
15. Devereaux PJ, et al. Clonidine in patients undergoing noncardiac surgery. N Engl J Med. 2014;370(16):1504–13.
16. Strandvik GF. Hypertonic saline in critical care: a review of the literature and guidelines for use in hypotensive states and raised intracranial pressure. Anaesthesia. 2009;64:990–1003. doi:10.1111/j.1365-2044.2009.05986.x.
17. American Society of Health–System Pharmacists. Clinical Practice Guidelines forAntimicrobial Prophylaxis in Surgery. In *ASHP Therapeutic Guidelines*. Retrieved from http://www.ashp.org/surgical-guidelines.
18. Barash PG. Clinical anesthesia. 6th ed. Philadelphia: Wolters Kluwer/Lippincott Williams & Wilkins; 2009.
19. Fleisher LA, Fleischmann KE, Auerbach AD, et al. ACC/AHA guideline on perioperative cardiovascular evaluation and management of patients undergoing noncardiac surgery: executive summary: a report of the american college of cardiology/american heart association task force on practice guidelines. J Am Coll Cardiol. 2014;64(22):2373–405. doi:10.1016/j.jacc.2014.07.945.

Further Reading

20. POISE Study Group, Devereaux PJ, Yang H, Yusuf S, Guyatt G, Leslie K, Villar JC, Xavier D, Chrolavicius S, Greenspan L, Pogue J, Pais P, Liu L, Xu S, Málaga G, Avezum A, Chan M, Montori VM, Jacka M, Choi P. Effects of extended-release metoprolol succinate in patients undergoing non-cardiac surgery (POISE trial): a randomised controlled trial. Lancet. 2008 May 31;371(9627):1839–47. doi:10.1016/S0140-6736(08)60601-7. Epub 2008 May 12.

30 Anesthesia for Endovascular Aortic Aneurysm Repair (EVAR)

Stefan Anexandrov Ianchulev

Case presentation:

A 70-year-old male patient has been scheduled for endovascular repair of an infra-renal aortic aneurysm.

Major Medical History: Cardiovascular system: Exercise tolerance <4 METs, HTN, CAD with moderately decreased ejection fraction, stable angina, PVD, carotid artery stenosis, left CEA 2009. Renal artery stenosis, hip osteoarthritis, severe COPD, on steroids and recent exacerbation requiring hospitalization, presents for 5.5 cm infrarenal AAA repair.

Physical Exam:	165 cm, 95 kg; BMI 34.5
Heart sounds:	Normal; Lungs without rhonchi or wheezes
BP 140/88; HR 64; Mallampati class: 2	
AAOx3	
PSH:	Left CEA
Meds:	Norvasc, Lipitor, Toprol, ASA, Folic Acid, Fish Oil, taper schedule steroids, MVI
Medical Consultation concludes:	No further risk stratification needed for cardiac workup; acceptable risk
Allergies:	Simvastatin, Augmentin, Bactrim, IV Dye (Iodine), Codeine, Procainamide, Keflex

Laboratory test results:

- Labs: Na 141, K 4.3, Cl 101, HCO3 30, BUN 23, Cr 1.4, Hb 11.5, Hct 31, PT 10.9, PTT 36.2, INR 1.2, GFR 54
- ECG: NSR, IAV block; LBBB
- CXR: signs of hyperinflation, lower standing diaphragm.

1. How would you approach this patient based on the history, physical exam, and previous tests?

This patient presents with the concomitant diagnoses of CAD, peripheral vascular disease, COPD, obesity, and chronic kidney insufficiency. Additional tests like dipyridamole stress test and dobutamine stress echo have low sensitivity (20–30%), but high specificity (95–100%). Subjecting this patient to stress testing may prompt further investigation if positive and should lead to a final intervention with regard to the CAD. If this final intervention is not desirable or too high of a risk due to patient's general condition, then these tests should be avoided. Each test the patient is subjected to in the process of preparation for surgery has its own risk, which is additive to the inherent risk of the planned surgical procedure. Risk stratification can occur postoperatively. However, optimal medication coverage should be instituted prior to surgery. The beneficial effects of statins and beta blockers in this patient population have been established. It is important to consider the type of anesthesia in this patient. General anesthesia (GA) has been associated with higher cardiovascular morbidity compared to regional anesthesia (RA) [1].

2. Is the LBBB block of significance in this patient?

Isolated long-standing LBBB does not mandate further testing or treatment in this setting. If pulmonary artery catheterization is planned, precautionary measures to treat complete heart block should be in place. Catheter induced right bundle block is usually transient, but longer duration may result in prolonged asystole requiring CPR. The availability of resuscitative medications and external pacing capability is advised. It may be difficult or impossible to detect ST depression or elevation in a patient with LBBB.

3. What are your considerations regarding the renal status of this patient?

An elevated creatinine and BUN in the setting of significant cardiovascular disease signify chronic renal

S.A. Ianchulev (✉)
Department of Anesthesiology, Tufts Medical Center, 800 Washington St, PO Box 29802111 Boston, MA, USA
e-mail: sianchulev@tuftsmedicalcenter.org

© Springer International Publishing AG 2017
L.S. Aglio and R.D. Urman (eds.), *Anesthesiology*,
DOI 10.1007/978-3-319-50141-3_30

impairment. It would be prudent to obtain the glomerular filtration rate (GFR) to assign the chronic kidney disease (CKD) stage. More advanced stages correlate with higher morbidity and mortality in the perioperative setting. The CKD stage is defined based on the glomerular filtration rate, age, gender, and race according to the formula: $186 \times (\text{Creat}/88.4) - 1.154 \times (\text{Age}) - 0.203 \times (0.742$ if female) $\times$ (1.210 if black).

Chronic kidney disease poses significant risk for renal dysfunction in cases where intravenous dye is used. A stage change in the renal insufficiency has been reported to occur between 18% and 29% of cases [2]. The presence of CKD should prompt further discussion with the patient and evaluation of recent changes in BUN, Cr, and GFR. A plan for preprocedural hydration should be considered.

4. Is COPD common in patients with AAA? How should the COPD be addressed in this patient?

Many elderly patients have COPD, particularly those with significant smoking history. It is important to evaluate the patient for evidence of exacerbation and optimal therapy. Significant reversibility on PFTs may signify the need for further therapy optimization. Significant pulmonary disease renders patients at much higher risk for mortality and significant morbidity due to diminished pulmonary reserve.

Associated bronchitis and sputum production should be assessed. History of intubation for COPD exacerbation may impact the type of anesthesia administered. An in-depth discussion of general versus regional or even local anesthesia should be performed. The patient's preferences need to be respected but possibilities of prolonged intubation and related complications should be addressed. Home oxygen requirement, acute changes in symptoms, or baseline function should prompt the evaluation of arterial blood gases for baseline CO_2 retention. Higher bicarbonate on the electrolyte panel may signify metabolic compensation for respiratory acidosis due to CO_2 retention. Oral steroid use should be noted and replacement may be required.

5. What additional risks occur with increasing severity of the COPD? What is the implication of COPD on the anesthesia decision?

COPD is another risk factor for prolonged postoperative ventilation and associated complications. Given the low invasiveness of the procedure, regional anesthesia should be considered. Loco-regional anesthesia has been associated with better perioperative pulmonary outcomes and shorter LOS. Edwards in 2011 showed a preponderance of pneumonia and failure to wean from the ventilator in the general anesthesia versus the regional anesthesia group [1]. Given a recent exacerbation of COPD in this patient, loco-regional anesthesia should be the preferred choice.

5. How does obesity impact outcome in AAA repair?

Obesity has been associated with worse outcomes in both open and endovascular abdominal aortic aneurysm repair as determined from the NSQIP study in 2007 by Giles [3]. Obesity is often associated with obstructive sleep apnea, hyperlipidemia, and type II diabetes. These associated comorbidities present additional risk for the surgical patient.

7. How do you approach a patient with limited exercise capacity?

Patients who cannot walk up one flight of stairs or walk on ground level at 3 km/hour based on a 5 m walk test in 6 s, have increased incidence of adverse events [4]. The walk test has been established as an independent predictor of increased postoperative morbidity and mortality. The patients in the Afilalo study had more than 2 times adverse outcomes over those who were able to do walk the distance in less than 6 s.

8. What are the implications of fluoroscopy?

Patients with renal impairment carry additional risk based on dye exposure and load during the procedure. Patients who have intravenous dye allergy are most commonly allergic to the iodine in iodine containing dyes. This scenario is best managed by avoiding iodine and substituting with nonionic dyes. In EVAR imaging iodine dye is used. Pretreatment with corticosteroids and H1/H2 blockers is advised. N-acetyl cysteine may have a role in renal protection. Adequate hydration should be performed before the procedure, but caution should be taken not to put this patient in acute congestive heart failure. Alternatively, intraoperative imaging may be performed with carbon dioxide as the contrast agent in patients at very high risk for renal impairment, weighed against the risk of significant gas embolism.

9. What factors determine suitability for EVAR?

(I) Aneurysm-related anatomic factors:

(a) Vascular access to the iliac arteries, and their size and tortuosity may necessitate an alternative approach with a higher incision and side graft access instead of percutaneous access. A minimum intraluminal diameter of 7 mm is needed for successful percutaneous access.
(b) Aneurysm morphology (tortuosity, thrombus) may affect suitability for graft fit. An angiogram must be performed

to locate the more important arterial branches supplying the kidneys, intestines, and possibly the anterior radicular artery.

(c) Aneurysm neck length and morphology (calcification, thrombus, length, angle) must be known. A minimum of 10 mm neck is required for a proper sit of the proximal graft end. Overall size matters as well, as very large aneurysms have the propensity for early graft failure (Type I and Type II).

(d) Thrombus in the aneurysm poses risk of dislodgement and distal embolization.

(II) Involvement of renal and celiac arteries

Advances in graft development allows for implantation of grafts which may cover the ostium of large arterial branches. Secondary stenting through fenestrations in the graft during the procedure allows for reestablishing perfusion in those branches. There are patient-specific fenestrated grafts with orifices for the renal, celiac, and superior mesenteric arteries. Additional vascular access through the brachial or axillary arteries may be required. This should be discussed with the surgeon pre-operatively.

10. How is surgical outcome related to the anatomic factors of planning EVAR over open surgery?

A scoring system (see Tables 30.1, 30.2, 30.3 and 30.4) has been set up based on the aortic angle and tortuosity, and the presence of intraluminal thrombus. The scores are one through three points with higher total number of points signifying poorer EVAR outcomes [2].

11. What clinical factors impact surgical decision-making for endovascular (EVAR) versus open repair (OR) of AAA?

(a) Various scoring systems have been used to define benefit of OR versus EVAR approach—APCHE, POSSM, ASA, SVS/AAVS.

(b) Age, cardiac, pulmonary, and renal status of the patient.

(c) EVAR is still considered intermediate to high cardiac risk procedure with 3–7% mortality.

(d) Preexisting renal insufficiency is associated with poor EVAR outcomes.

(e) Diabetes Mellitus is associated with significantly higher device related complications and early mortality rates. However, the insulin controlled DM II patients had lower incidence of endoleaks than the noninsulin controlled DM II and nondiabetic patients.

(f) Albumin less than 3.6 g/dl is a patient-related risk factor associated with higher morbidity and mortality.

(g) Smoking is a contributing factor to postoperative pulmonary complications. It has been found that those patients who stopped smoking between 1 and 8 weeks before surgery had higher complication rate compared to those who either continued smoking or stopped longer than 8 weeks.

(h) Patient preferences should be considered: EVAR—1 trial showed better outcomes in the first 4 years, but increased risk of endoleaks and re-interventions thereafter. Current study showed patient preference for EVAR to be above 80% (SIR Guideline 56, 57–58).

(i) Patients with major risk factors for either approach require a multidisciplinary evaluation and decision.

12. How does preoperative evaluation of the patient with AAA for EVAR differ from open repair?

There is no difference between the preoperative evaluations of these patients. The EVAR procedure evokes more concerns with regard to renal status of the patient. While the procedure itself may be less invasive, the patients presenting for EVAR are generally sicker. They may be at much higher risk if general anesthesia is performed. Based on their physical status, these patients may be counseled for regional or even local anesthesia. It is even more important to understand how the surgical procedure will be carried out and when bailout to an open approach is indicated [5]. Some centers recommend that multidisciplinary teams should be involved when an OR is considered. The recommendations of the American College of Cardiology and the American Heart Association are a useful tool in the guidance of preoperative cardiac tests.

Patients presenting for EVAR are at risk of complications associated with aneurysmal rupture or iliac arterial damage

Table 30.1 Aortic angle and tortuosity scoring [2]

Aortic angle and tortuosity scoring		
Grade	Index	Aortic angle
0	≤1.05	160°–180°
1	>1.05 ≤ 1.15	140°–159°
2	>1.15 ≤ 1.20	120°–139°
3	>1.2	<120°

Table 30.2 Thrombus scoring [2]

Thrombus scoring	
Grade	Amount of thrombus
0	No visible thrombus
1	<25% of cross-sectional area
2	25–50% of the cross-sectional area
3	>50% of cross-sectional area

Table 30.3 Aortic neck length scoring [2]

Aortic neck length scoring	
Grade	Aortic neck length (mm)
0	>25
1	>15 but <25
2	>10 but <15
3	<10

Table 30.4 Proximal aortic diameter scoring [2]

Proximal aortic diameter scoring	
Grade	Aortic neck diameter (mm)
0	<24
1	≥24 <26
2	≥26 <28
3	>28

requiring the ability to administer large volume of fluids or blood products.

Generally, all vascular patients should be on aspirin and statins if not contraindicated.

13. What is your rationale for inserting venous and arterial catheters? How will you manage volume?

This patient should have two large bore peripheral intravenous catheters. A radial arterial line should be inserted preferably on the right side in case a brachial artery approach from the left is needed during the procedure for additional surgical access. The need for a central line should be based on expected hemodynamic instability or need for vasoactive medications. Poor peripheral access should also prompt central venous access.

Measuring CVP is unreliable as predictor of intravascular volume. Insertion of a central line for this purpose is unnecessary. The use of a pulmonary artery catheter (PAC) is associated with significant morbidity and mortality as well as a lack of reliability to adequately represent left sided filling pressures volume status. Assessing volume status of the patient is best done with transesophageal echocardiography (TEE). Utilizing TEE may require deeper sedation or general anesthesia.

Hydration of the patient should be performed intravenously before the procedure and a fluid deficit should be corrected. The help of various less invasive devices and algorithms are available to aid in this process. These include measurement of pulse pressure variation and stroke volume variations. These methods have not been validated in spontaneously breathing patients or in patients with significant dysrhythmia. There are inherent problems in the assumptions made for these devices, so caution is advised when this benefit is sought. Either 0.9% normal saline or isotonic bicarbonate solution may be used for perioperative hydration especially for patients with elevated creatinine. Intraoperative measurements of hematocrit, electrolytes and arterial blood gas are recommended.

14. What EVAR grafts are in current use?

Common grafts used for endovascular repair of AAA are mentioned in Table 30.5 (It is not the scope of this chapter to review specific graft related selection criteria, but we felt it is of importance to understand some of the grafts' characteristics). Other grafts are in the process of development and trials.

15. Will you chose general versus regional or MAC anesthesia?

The complexity of the surgical intervention and physiologic perturbation, coupled with advances in operating room

Table 30.5 Common grafts used for endovascular repair of AAA*

Graft	Manufacturer	Properties
Zenith Flex AAA	Cook, Bloomington, IN	Bifurcated three piece modular graft made of polyester fabric and is self-expanding. Proximal size is 22–36 mm with 8–24 mm iliac limbs
Powerlink AAA	Endologix, Irvine, CA	A unibody self-expanding graft made of polytetrafluoroethylene. Proximal component is 25 or 28 mm diameter and the iliac graft size is 16 mm. It is available with and without suprarenal fixation
Excluder AAA endoprosthesis	Gore and Associates, Flagstaff, AR	A two piece modular self-expanding graft. Various sizes are available to fit in the iliac arteries as well as to allow anchorage below the renal arteries
AneuRx endoprosthesis	Medtronic, Minneapolis, MN	A two piece modular device
Talent endoprosthesis	Medtronic, Minneapolis, MN	A modular device which employs suprarenal attachment struts

*Other grafts are in process of development and trials

technology, make it necessary for an anesthesiologist to manage the patient in a hybrid interventional radiology suite operating room.

The establishment of National Surgical Quality Improvement Program (NSQIP) allowed for retrospective analysis of various standard parameters. With regard to type of anesthetic, in a study by Edwards and colleagues based on NSQIP, general anesthesia was associated with greater pulmonary morbidity and length of stay in the hospital compared with spinal and local/MAC management in EVAR patients [1]. This study suggests that the use of less invasive anesthesia technique may be beneficial in limiting perioperative morbidity and decrease cost associated with EVAR in high risk patients. The EUROSTAR study also commented on the benefits of local/MAC and regional anesthesia being the greatest in the high risk group. The EUROSTAR study showed among more than 5500 patients that regional and local anesthesia with MAC have advantages over GA groups.

In the patient above, epidural or spinal anesthesia is recommended if the anatomy of the AAA allows for easy surgical approach and uncomplicated graft deployment. Local anesthesia with sedation can be utilized after discussion with the patient. With greater complexity epidural anesthesia with intravenous sedation will ensure longer lasting anesthesia. Local anesthesia and regional anesthesia have the benefit of reduced ICU admissions, hospital length of stay, and early complications. These patients also experienced mortality benefit in the long term. Additionally the fluids and vasopressor administered were less. Postoperative cardiac and pulmonary complications were also fewer.

The afterload reduction may be beneficial in the patient with compromised ejection fraction. This has to be weighed against the need of preload maintenance and fluid administration. A gentle onset of the epidural is recommended.

16. What factors do you take into account when planning regional anesthesia when a patient will be anticoagulated for EVAR?

The risk of epidural hematoma is low if the insertion is clean and the administration of intravenous heparin is at least 1 h after insertion. Removal of the epidural catheter should be performed 2–4 h after the last heparin administration and documentation of normal coagulation factors. It is recommended that the platelet count be monitored in patients receiving heparin longer than 4 days. For low molecular weight heparin administration, the recommendations are to avoid neuraxial manipulation for 10–12 h after the last dose in the DVT prophylaxis regimen. If the dosing is at DVT treatment level, at least 24 h should pass prior to neuraxial anesthesia administration.

Anticoagulants like clopidogrel, dabigatran, prasugrel, and several others necessitate careful review of dosing and communication with the medical and surgical teams. Typically use of the agents will require discontinuation of 5–10 days prior to institution of neuraxial anesthesia [6].

17. How would you manage intraoperative hemodynamics?

Preserving homeostasis and perfusion to vital organs is crucial in these patients. Hydration and maintenance of intraoperative mean arterial pressure while avoiding or minimizing vasopressors in the setting of unrecognized hypovolemia is of high importance.

18. What fluids will you use, and why do you choose one type over another?

Current studies have shown significant impact of perioperative fluid management on outcomes [5]. Optimum fluid management, as described in the literature as goal-directed therapy (GDT), is advised in patients with compromised renal function undergoing significant contrast exposure and fluoroscopy. However, none of the recommended strategies have reached Level 1 recommendation [7]. The utility of urine output under general anesthesia has not been validated, nor has pressure contour analysis of arterial pressure in spontaneously breathing awake patients.

While the intravascular volume is important to maintain, the type of fluid used has not made a clear outcome difference in many studies. The eternal question of colloid versus crystalloid still has not been answered. There is, however, evidence that larger Dalton size colloids may contribute to postoperative renal injury as well as a negative impact on coagulation. Use of balanced crystalloid solution for this patient exposed to a significant dye load would generally be considered standard of care.

Avoiding hypovolemia is the best renal protection according to evidence based research. Medications such as loop diuretics, mannitol, renal dose dopamine, or fenoldopam have not been associated with superior outcomes. Mannitol has the purported benefit of free radical scavenging. An osmotic diuresis may allow for faster dye clearance and so minimize its impact.

Avoiding vasopressors if possible is important, particularly so under general anesthesia where the splanchnic blood flow is diminished. Judicious use when needed is acceptable to counteract anesthesia induced vasodilatation. In a patient with compromised myocardial performance, a pure alpha agonist may cause further decrease in cardiac output and compromise organ perfusion further.

19. What are your concerns with regard to blood loss?

Simple EVAR for a well-defined infrarenal AAA can be accomplished with minimal blood loss. However, complex AAA repair carries potential for significant blood loss from the access sites. In these patients, frequent point of care monitoring of Hgb/Hct and ABGs is appropriate. While RBC transfusion has been associated with adverse outcomes and higher morbidity, oxygen carrying capacity must be maintained.

20. How will you manage intraoperative blood pressure in this patient for EVAR?

Blood pressure management is an important part of intraoperative management. Earlier grafts were very prone to dislodgement due to lack of anchoring attachments and the need for balloon expansion. High blood pressure and tachycardia could dislodge the graft during initial deployment. To avoid this, induced hypotension and brief asystole induced with adenosine were recommended. The need for balloon expansion of the graft could pose a significant afterload increase and have significant impact on myocardial performance and blood pressure. Later trifurcated balloons were developed which had less impact on afterload. The modern age has brought self-expanding grafts which avoid those hemodynamic perturbations. The current state of the art recommends mild hypotension, keeping systolic blood pressure below 100 mmHg during graft deployment. Prolonged hypotension and advanced age have been associated with increased incidence of delirium and longer hospital stay.

21. How will you manage heparin anticoagulation?

Five thousand units of intravenous heparin are usually administered initially. A target ACT of 2–2.5 times normal is typical for EVAR. As the length of procedure increases, ACT may guide additional heparin administration.

22. Knowing the concern for urinary catheter associated infections, would you insert a Foley catheter in a patient for EVAR?

Placement of an indwelling urinary catheter is recommended as copious urine may be produced, and the significant dye load can compromise kidney function. Appropriate hydration and careful assessment of fluid input and output is mandatory. An initially uncomplicated procedure may turn into a difficult time consuming technical challenge, or require open conversion which currently occurs with a 2% frequency.

23. Would you elect to perform an EVAR in a ruptured AAA?

There is an increasing tendency to treat ruptured AAA with endovascular stents and other minimally invasive techniques. Success with this approach has been largely reported by some groups. Others report less successful management with EVAR. Advantages of less invasiveness, less manipulation and damage to periaortic structures and bowels, decreased bleeding and minimized hypothermia, and associated issues has made many surgeons attempt EVAR for rupture. As experience increases, so does the success rate. Some authors have recommend a standard protocol and approach to the patient with ruptured AAA. They advise the performance of the procedure in only very well-equipped imaging centers, minimized fluid administration and tolerance to transient hypotension. However, this has not been widely accepted due to lack of conclusive evidence and fear that he attempt of endovascular treatment may delay treatment and even increase risk [8]. Local anesthesia is preferred in these cases. The use of supraceliac balloon aortic occlusion can mitigate against circulatory collapse but makes the insertion of the stent more challenging. Caution is advised in such cases to make an early diagnosis of abdominal compartment syndrome in ruptured AAA. If this occurs, laparotomy and hematoma evacuation will improve oliguria and high ventilator pressures. Monitoring of bladder pressures is recommended for these patients. It appears that the greatest benefit of EVAR is in the patients who are hemodynamically unstable or in hemorrhagic shock. An average of 49% of all ruptured AAA were treated endovascularly. In those centers who were successful the most important issues were proper aortic balloon control, early recognition of abdominal compartment syndrome and the establishment of a structured system and protocol for management of the patient with the ruptured AAA. From an anesthetic point of view, a large bore IV should be placed and sufficient blood cross-matched. Neuraxial anesthesia is not considered appropriate. Van Beek concluded in his meta-analysis of short-term survival that endovascular repair of ruptured AAA is not inferior to OR [9].

24. What factors limit the success of local anesthesia and sedation in ruptured AAA treated by EVAR?

(a) Pain from expanding hematoma
(b) Increased intra-abdominal pressure and respiratory insufficiency
(c) Ischemic pain in the limbs and buttocks
(d) Metabolic acidosis with insufficient respiratory compensation and hypotension leading to confusion and agitation

25. What are the types of Endoleaks? (see Table 30.6)
26. Is there a role for CSF drainage or evoked potential monitoring in the endovascular repair of AAA?

Normally AAA, particularly below the renal arteries do not require CSF drainage. If the level of the proximal graft insertion is set at a higher level, the chances of occluding the anterior radicular artery increase. The artery of Adamkiewicz originates between T5 and L5 and most commonly between T9 and T12 directly from the aorta. Collaterals to the spinal cord can originate from the inferior mesenteric artery, internal iliac, and middle sacral arteries. The inferior mesenteric artery is occluded in infrarenal AAA. Some surgeons advocate the use of aortic balloon occlusion for 10–15 min to check for neurological deficit in awake patients or use SSEPs/MEPs in patients under general anesthesia prior to stent deployment. A spinal catheter to drain CSF can be inserted postoperatively. Neurological deficits should initially be treated with an increase in mean blood pressure to improve the spinal cord perfusion pressure (perfusion pressure = MAP-ICP or CVP whichever is higher). If this does not yield the expected result, CSF drainage is indicated. There are significant risks associated with CSF drains. The incidence of epidural hematoma is not to be underestimated particularly when the patients undergo anticoagulation. Active monitoring for symptoms associated with it should be instituted with all patients. Another risk is the accidental drainage of large amount of CSF. Draining more than 10–12 ml of CSF per hour is contraindicated. Loss of significant CSF amount can lead to tenting of the

Table 30.6 Types of endoleaks

Enodleaks types	Description	Repair
Type I	Inadequate seal between the aortic wall and the proximal or distal end of the graft. High potential for rupture	Immediate
Type II	Retrograde filling of the aneurysmal sac occurs due to intercostal, lumbar, testicular, or inferior mesenteric branches. Most would thrombose over time	Delayed. When this leak type leads to continuous aneurysmal expansion the leak should be addressed
Type III	Structural failure of the graft with blood flow in the sac	Immediate repair
Type IV	Leaks associated with the porosity of the material. It can be primary (at time of deployment) or secondary (late occurrence after initial seal has been established)	Delayed
Type V	Persistent pressurization of the aneurysmal sac without identifiable cause	Delayed

dura and tear of some of the bridging veins resulting in SAH with grave consequences.

27. What type of pain management do these patients require postoperatively?

Patients presenting for EVAR have minimal pain when access has been percutaneous. However, retroperitoneal or lower abdominal access to the iliac vessels can be significantly more painful. While local anesthesia is sufficient in the first case, the latter is better served with epidural analgesia or intravenous PCA. Elderly patients can be very sensitive to the actions of opioids and therefore careful planning is needed. The benefit of epidural placement in these patients is early extubation and better pain control with less opioids.

28. Where should your patient recover?

Vascular patients often require intensive care management and frequent observations. The ICU setting is best for these purposes. However, EVAR performed under local anesthesia and MAC may be recovered in a step down unit or PACU overnight prior to sending to the general hospital floor. Many hospitals do not have a stepdown vascular unit, and these patients will go to the ICU. Monitoring these patients greatly depends on the invasiveness of the procedure. Open repair, regardless of the approach, will require ICU management for the immediate postoperative period. EVAR patients have less fluid administered during the procedure and generally less vasoactive medications, so their postoperative course is generally less complicated form the hemodynamic point of view.

29. What is postimplantation syndrome?

This is a post EVAR condition characterized by fever, elevated C-reactive protein and leukocytosis in the absence of infection. Etiology of the postimplantation syndrome may be related to reaction to the graft material, endothelial modification or thrombotic material isolation. In general this process is self-limiting. It may last between 2 to 10 days and will respond well to nonsteroidal medications.

30. What are the long-term results of EVAR?

The 30 day short-term mortality is drastically decreased in EVAR patients compared to OR. The hospital stay is reduced, but the there is no benefit in long term survival. At 2 years the cumulative survival rates were around 90% in both groups [10]. The EVAR-1 study enrolled more than 1000 patients with the primary endpoint of all-cause mortality in patients older than 60 years of age and AAA larger than 5.5 cm. The results showed significantly improved 30 day mortality of 1.7% versus 4.7% in the OR group. However, -secondary interventions in the initial 30 days were more in the EVAR group. No significant difference in the endpoint of the study was found but aneurysm-related mortality was lower in the EVAR group. However, rates of all other complications and reinterventions were lower in the OR group compared to EVAR.

Another trial, EVAR-2 compared the all-cause mortality in EVAR patients versus medically managed patients unfit for surgery with the same selection requirement as the EVAR-1. Operative mortality in the EVAR group in this study was higher than the EVAR-1. The overall mortality in this group was 64% without difference in the EVAR or medical managed groups. However, additional monitoring and interventions in the EVAR group ware associated with significant cost [11]. EVARs should be monitored lifelong and usually occurs with yearly CT angiography and radiographic films. Currently a sac pressure monitoring device can be inserted during the initial surgery for remote pressure monitoring. The device consists of a piezoelectric membrane which charges a capacitor (Remon device). The membrane is activated with ultrasound waves. Once charged the device can measure ambient pressures and transmit them via ultrasound to the probe. Studies with the device have shown that patients who have evidence by CT angiogram of decreased sac size, also exhibit decreased sac pressures. Another device with radiofrequency transmission is the EndoSure. Pressure measured by it correlated well with the catheter measured pressure in the sac [12].

References

1. Edwards MS, et al. Results of endovascular aortic aneurysm repair with general, regional, and local/monitored anesthesia care in the American college of surgeons national surgical quality improvement program database. J Vasc Surg. 54(5):1273–82.
2. Walker TG, et al. Clinical practice guidelines for endovascular abdominal aortic aneurysm repair: written by the standards of practice committee for the society of interventional radiology and endorsed by the cardiovascular and interventional radiological society of Europe and the Canadian interventional radiology association. J Vasc Interv Radiol. 2010;21(11):1632–55.
3. Giles KA, et al. The impact of body mass index on perioperative outcomes of open and endovascular abdominal aortic aneurysm repair from the national surgical quality improvement program 2005–2007. J Vasc Surg. (official publication, the Society for Vascular Surgery [and] International Society for Cardiovascular Surgery, North American) 2010;52(6):1471–77.
4. Afilalo J, et al. Gait speed as an incremental predictor of mortality and major morbidity in elderly patients undergoing cardiac surgery. J Am Coll Cardiol. 2010;56(20):1668–76.

5. Subramian B, Singh N, Roscher C, Augustides JGT. Innovations in treating aortic disease: the abdominal aorta. J Cardiothorac Vasc Anesth. 2012;26(5):959–65. doi:10.1053/j.jvca.2010.10.003.
6. Narouze S, et al. Interventional spine and pain procedures in patients on antiplatelet and anticoagulant medications: guidelines from the American society of regional anesthesia and pain medicine, the European society of regional anaesthesia and pain therapy, the American academy of pain medicine, the international neuromodulation society, the North American neuromodulation society, and the world institute of Pain. Reg Anesth Pain Med. 2015;40(3):182–212.
7. Saratzis AN, et al. Acute kidney injury after endovascular repair of abdominal aortic aneurysm. J Endovasc Ther. 2013;20(3):315–30.
8. Livesay JJ, Talledo OG. Endovascular aneurysm repair is not the treatment of choice in most patients with ruptured abdominal aortic aneurysm. Tex Heart Inst J. 2013;40(5):556–9.
9. van Beek SC, et al. Editor's choice—endovascular aneurysm repair versus open repair for patients with a ruptured abdominal aortic aneurysm: a systematic review and meta-analysis of short-term survival (1532-2165 (Electronic)).
10. De Bruin JL, et al. Long-term outcome of open or endovascular repair of abdominal aortic aneurysm. N Engl J Med. 2010;362 (20):1881–9.
11. Brown LC, et al. The UK EndoVascular Aneurysm Repair (EVAR) trials: randomised trials of EVAR versus standard therapy (2046-4924 (Electronic)).
12. Baril DT, et al. Endovascular abdominal aortic aneurysm repair: emerging developments and anesthetic considerations. J Cardiothorac Vasc Anesth. 2007;21(5):730–42.

Morbid Obesity

31

John Stenglein

CASE

A 43-year-old woman is sent for preoperative evaluation prior to laparoscopic gastric banding. She stands 5 ft 5 in. tall and weighs 440 lbs. BMI = 73

She does not exercise due to longstanding pain in her knees, "I'm bone on bone," she exclaims. She does report worsening SOB with her regular activities.

Medications	Lisinopril 20 mg oral daily
	Simvastatin 20 mg oral daily
	Metformin 500 mg BID
	Orlistat 120 mg, prior to meals.
Allergies	NKA
Past Medical History	
She has a history of hypertension, hypercholesterolemia, diabetes mellitus, and OSA. She states that her nightly CPAP is set to 12 cm H_2O. She lost 100 lb while taking Fen–Phen about 20 years ago, but gained it back.	
Physical Exam	
VS:	154/75, 105 Pulse, 22 RR, 94% O_2 Sat. on room air.
Hyperpigmentation is noted on the skin folds of her posterior neck.	
EKG:	
NSR with RVH	
Abnormal Labs	
HCT 51%	
Polysomnogram	
AHI = 32	

1. How is obesity defined? What is the incidence of obesity and morbid obesity?

J. Stenglein (✉)
Department of Anesthesiology, Baystate Medical Center, Tufts University School of Medicine, 759 Chestnut Street, Springfield, MA 01199, USA
e-mail: john.stenglein@baystatehealth.org

© Springer International Publishing AG 2017
L.S. Aglio and R.D. Urman (eds.), *Anesthesiology*,
DOI 10.1007/978-3-319-50141-3_31

Obesity refers to an abnormally high percentage of body fat. The degree of obesity is generally estimated by the Body Mass index (BMI). More than 1/3 of US adults are considered obese, with a BMI $\geq$ 30 [1].

Approximately 4% of US adults are categorized as morbidly obese with a BMI $\geq$ 40 [2].

2. How is BMI calculated? What are the adult classifications?

BMI = weight (kg)/Height (m^2)

<18.5	Underweight	
18.5–24.9	Normal	
25.0–29.9	Overweight	
30.0–34.9	Obesity	(class 1)
35.0–39.9	Obesity	(class 2)
$\geq$40	Morbid obesity	(class 3)
$\geq$50	Super morbid obesity	

3. What are the limitations of BMI? Why is it utilized?

The calculated BMI does not take into account the nature of the patient's frame or degree of muscularity. Therefore, the calculation generally overestimates obesity in patients with more lean body mass and underestimates it in those with less lean body mass.

While BMI-defined obesity showed high specificity (95% for men and 99% for women), it demonstrated poor sensitivity (36% for men and 49% for women) [3].

The utility of BMI is its convenience as a screening tool, not for diagnosis. It is strictly a height and weight-based calculation, and as such does not require calipers, submersion tubs, radiation-based scans, or impedance measurements.

4. What are the different physiologic types of fat distribution?

Obesity can be described as peripheral or central. Central or android obesity is generally associated with increased oxygen consumption and higher rates of heart disease. Higher levels of proinflammatory cytokines, also seen in central obesity, are thought to contribute to increased levels of insulin resistance [4]. Gynecoid or peripheral obesity relates to patients with adipose tissue primarily deposited in the hips, buttocks, and thighs. It has been shown to be less metabolically active and not as strongly associated with cardiovascular disease.

5. What is metabolic syndrome? What is the incidence? What are the clinical implications?

Metabolic syndrome is a constellation of conditions associated with higher rates of heart disease and diabetes. It applies to individuals in whom at least three out of the following five diagnoses have been made: central obesity, hypertension, hypertriglyceridemia, low HDL, and elevated fasting glucose [5].

The incidence of metabolic syndrome in the US is approximately 40% by age 60 [6]. Patients at risk for metabolic syndrome should be screened appropriately for the comorbid conditions associated with the diagnosis, as this may impact anesthetic management and risk stratification.

6. When is bariatric surgery recommended?

Bariatric surgery is generally reserved for patients with a BMI of at least 40 kg/m^2. However, an individual with a BMI above 30 kg/m^2 may also be a candidate if any associated conditions are expected to improve with significant weight loss. Prior to surgery, patients are routinely involved in a multidisciplinary evaluation to select individuals in whom the likelihood of success justifies the risks of the procedure.

7. What other diseases are commonly associated with obesity?

Obesity may be related to hypothyroidism, Cushing syndrome, insulinoma, hypogonadism, and hypothalamic disorders, to name a few. Related syndromes may also include Prader–Willi, leptin-deficiency, and Bardet–Biedl. Prior to surgery, a workup should exclude many of the various medical causes that may render a patient prone to excessive weight gain.

8. What diseases commonly result from obesity?

Obesity increases the risk of CAD, CVA, HTN, and NIDDM. It is also associated with liver disease, gallbladder disease, OSA, polycythemia, osteoarthritis, and infertility. It may also raise the risks of developing endometrial, breast and colon cancers as well as being an independent risk factor for DVT [7].

9. What are some of the major physiologic changes commonly associated with obesity classified by organ system?

<u>Pulmonary</u>

Pulmonary volume, etc.	Abbreviation	Effect
Functional residual capacity	FRC	↓
Vital capacity	VC	↓ (50% in Obese vs. 20% in "controls" under GA)
Inspiratory capacity	IC	↓
Expiratory reserve volume	ERV	↓
Total lung capacity	TLC	↓
Residual volume	RV	No Δ
Closing capacity	CC	No Δ (FRC may lower volumes below CC)
Dead space		No Δ
Respiratory muscle efficiency		↓
Chest wall compliance		↓

Decreased respiratory muscle efficiency
Decreased chest wall compliance

<u>Cardiovascular</u>
Increased metabolic demands (**CO up 20–30 cc/kg of excess fat**)
Increased blood volume (**polycythemia secondary to chronic Hypoxia**)
Increased stroke volume (**Ventricular dilation—eccentric LVH, decreased compliance L/min/kg of adipose tissue**)
<u>GI</u>
Increased gastric volume (more strongly associated with binge eating, rather than obesity).
Increased abdominal pressure.
Increased incidence of GERD and hiatal hernia.

Endocrine
High sympathetic tone may predispose to insulin resistance
Higher glucose levels may predispose to wound infections.
High RAAS levels may impair natriuresis and increase BP (renin–angiotensin–aldosterone system)
Hematology
Increased levels of clotting factors may predispose to DVT.

10. What is Roux-en-Y gastric bypass? How much weight loss is commonly expected with the procedure?

This procedure involves the creation of an anastomosis of the proximal gastric pouch to a segment of the proximal jejunum, bypassing most of the stomach and the duodenum. Patients lose an average of 50–60% of excess body weight within 1–2 years.

11. What other surgical procedures are available to facilitate weight loss?

Procedures can be classified as either restrictive, malabsorptive, or both. The simplest restrictive procedure entails the laparoscopic placement of an inflatable gastric band around the upper portion of stomach. This serves to create a small pouch, which fills quickly upon eating to promote a feeling of fullness. This lower risk surgery offers the benefits of being reversible and having less chance of malabsorption.

A sleeve gastrectomy is also performed laparoscopically and promotes weight loss through the removal of approximately 80% of the stomach. This reduces the amount of food that can be consumed (restrictive) and may also decrease both absorptive and endocrinologic functions of the stomach.

Obstructive Sleep Apnea (OSA)

1. What is OSA? Why is it important to determine if a patient is at risk for OSA?

Obstructive sleep apnea (OSA) is defined as the cessation of airflow during sleep, for at least 10 s, despite continuing ventilatory effort. To diagnose OSA, these events must occur five or more times per hour and result in a decreased SpO_2 of at least 4%.

In addition to the physiologic consequences of chronic hypoxemia and hypercarbia, patients with OSA are at higher risk for postoperative respiratory complications. This may potentially alter the anesthetic plan and postoperative disposition [8].

2. When should you suspect occult OSA?

OSA is generally associated with central obesity, increased neck circumference, and/or micrognathia. It should also be considered in the differential diagnosis for patients presenting with RVH, LVH, polycythemia, or pulmonary hypertension. Although obesity is the biggest risk factor for OSA, it is possible to have one without the other. Only about 70% of patients with OSA are obese, so screening should not be limited solely to overweight patients.

3. What is the incidence of OSA?

It has been estimated that 4% of men and 2% of women have symptoms consistent with OSA. Furthermore, 82% of these men and 92% of these women, with moderate or severe sleep apnea, have not been diagnosed [9].

4. How should you screen for suspected OSA? What is the STOP-BANG questionnaire?

The STOP questionnaire, first published in Anesthesiology in 2008, was validated in surgical patients at preoperative clinics as a screening tool for OSA. Later, the inclusion of the four additional questions increased the sensitivity to predict moderate and severe sleep-disordered breathing, as compared to the original questionnaire.

The STOP-BANG questions are answered "yes" or "no."

1. Snoring—Do you snore loudly (louder than talking or loud enough to be heard through closed doors)?
2. Tired—Do you often feel tired, fatigued, or sleepy during the daytime?
3. Observed—Has anyone observed you stop breathing during your sleep?
4. Blood pressure—Do you have or are you being treated for high blood pressure?
5. BMI—Is your BMI greater than 35 kg/m^2
6. Age—Are you over 50 years old?
7. Neck circumference—For males, is your shirt collar 17 in./43 cm or larger?

   For females, is your shirt collar 16 in./41 cm or larger?

8. Gender—Are you male?

High risk of OSA: answering yes to three or more items
Low risk of OSA: answering yes to less than three items

The sensitivities of the STOP-BANG screening tool for an AHI (apnea hypopnea index) of >5, >15, and >30 were 86.1, 92.8, and 95.6%, respectively, with negative predictive values of 84.5 and 93.4% for moderate and severe OSA [10].

5. How is OSA diagnosed? What are the gradations?

OSA is diagnosed with a polysomnogram or "sleep study." This test detects and records the EEG, EKG, electrooculogram, pulse oximetry, capnography, airflow, esophageal pressure, blood pressure, pharyngeal and extremity electromyography, and room noise.

It is designed to detect episodes of both apnea and hypopnea. Apnea is defined as airflow cessation lasting at least 10 s, while hypopnea is a 50% reduction in flow for a similar period. Either must be sufficient to cause a 4% drop in oxygenation in order to be considered an "event."

The severity of sleep apnea, reported as the apnea–hypopnea index, is based on the number of "events" per hour of sleep.

5–15 events = mild
16–30 events = moderate.
≥ 30 events = severe

The consensus is that moderate or severe disease should be treated with CPAP [11].

6. What is the significance of an AHI (apnea hypopnea index) score of 32 in this patient?

An AHA score 32 suggests severe OSA, which may have implications for premedication, choice of analgesics, as well as postoperative disposition and monitoring.

7. What are the different types of sleep apnea?

Sleep apnea can be categorized as central, obstructive, or mixed. Central sleep apnea refers to a lack of respiratory effort in the presence of signals normally sufficient to trigger inhalation. Chemoreceptor detection of rising carbon dioxide and decreasing pH or oxygen levels fail to initiate a breath at the normal physiologic thresholds. In OSA, the respiratory drive is still intact, although airflow is compromised by the interference of dynamic anatomical obstruction.

8. What are the systemic effects of OSA?

Prolonged OSA may increase the reliance on hypoxia to drive ventilation, rather than initially being stimulated by increasing levels of CO_2. The sensitivity to both triggers may actually be blunted, resulting in chronic hypoxemia and hypercarbia. Unlike the more obvious complaint of hypersomnolence, the silent effects of chronic hypoxemia may result in high sympathetic tone, contributing to systemic and pulmonary hypertension, secondary polycythemia (HCT 51%); right-sided heart failure, left-sided heart failure, and premature death.

9. What is the pathophysiology behind cor pulmonale?

Diffuse hypoxic pulmonary vasoconstriction may lead to a generalized increase in pulmonary vascular resistance (PVR) during the low oxygen states associated with obstructive sleep apnea. High sympathetic tone, triggered by the hypoxemia and hypercarbia associated with apnea, will add to the already increasing vascular resistance. Furthermore, extreme thoracic pressures generated from breathing against an obstruction, may lead to irreversible pulmonary arteriolar remodeling. To a certain point, the right heart will compensate for the afterload increase in the pulmonary arterial circulation. However, with continued progression, right heart failure may eventually ensue.

10. What is Pickwickian Syndrome? (Obesity-Hypoventilation Syndrome)

In 1837, Charles Dickens published his first novel, The Posthumous Papers of the Pickwick Club. Joe, one of the characters in the novel, was described as a relentless eater who suffered from excessive daytime somnolence. In the 1950s, this character description of Joe was linked to a growing appreciation for sleep-disordered breathing, coining the term "Pickwickian Syndrome." Today, obesity-hypoventilation syndrome is considered a type of sleep-disordered breathing, which is an umbrella term for the many sleep-related breathing disorders.

Obesity-hypoventilation syndrome is diagnosed in individuals with a BMI > 30 kg/m^2, an awake arterial carbon dioxide $\geq$ 45 mmHg, and no alternative explanation for hypoventilation. Most patients with this diagnosis have concurrent OSA.

11. Would you consider ambulatory surgery in a morbidly obese individual? What role would OSA play in your decision?

Although obesity alone does not necessarily influence perioperative complications or unplanned admission, the associated comorbidities, including OSA, may place a patient at higher risk for ambulatory surgery. It is generally accepted that patients with BMI > 40 kg/m^2, and optimized comorbid conditions, can still safely undergo ambulatory surgery. However, a BMI > 50 kg/m^2 may be less suitable, regardless of other conditions [12].

A review of the published literature demonstrated that inadequately treated OSA patients carry higher risk for complications following ambulatory surgery. If optimized, patients may still be considered if they are able to use a positive airway pressure (PAP) device after the procedure. Those who are unable or unwilling to use a PAP device after discharge should be carefully considered for surgery with postoperative monitoring. A presumed diagnosis of OSA, based on screening tools such as the STOP-BANG questionnaire, may restrict ambulatory care to procedures and individuals in whom postoperative pain relief can be provided predominantly with non-opioid-based analgesics [13].

Preoperative considerations

1. Would you order additional tests for this patient?

Given the patient's history of metabolic syndrome, inability to exercise, worsening shortness of breath, and previous exposure to Fen–Phen, a chemical stress echo would be reasonable to obtain, if no recent similar study had been performed. Angina or dyspnea on exertion (DOE) may not be apparent in obese populations secondary to limited mobility.

According to the 2014 AHA-ACC Guidelines for non-cardiac surgery, it would be reasonable for patients with "dyspnea of unknown origin" to undergo preoperative evaluation of LV function. Also, "*for patients with elevated risk and poor (<4 METS) or unknown functional capacity, it may be reasonable to perform exercise testing with cardiac imaging to assess for myocardial ischemia if it will change management.*"

Echocardiographic evidence of right heart dysfunction or pulmonary hypertension may favor more invasive intraoperative monitoring. More informed risk stratification may also help guide the preoperative conversation about the risks and benefits of surgery.

2. Does the patient's CPAP setting (12 cmH_2O) cause any concern? What might provide some reassurance for induction?

A CPAP setting of >10 cmH_2O, may imply difficult mask ventilation, as significant pressure is required to maintain airway patency [14]. Review of previous surgical and anesthetic records, in the context of patient's weight at the time, would be the most reliable predictor of difficulty at induction. In similar circumstances, this may allow one to proceed with the presumption that an individual is able to be mask ventilated or safely intubated, based on past experience.

In the absence of this assurance, neck circumference has been shown to be the single biggest predictor of problematic intubation in obese individuals. At 40 cm, only about 5% of patients will present with difficulty, while at 60 cm, the incidence approaches 35% [15].

3. Would you give any preoperative sedation?

Obese patients have increased sensitivity to central nervous system depressants. They may be more susceptible to decreased tone in the posterior airway, as redundant adipose tissue in the pharynx may collapse with sedation. This may complicate both preoxygenation before, and mask ventilation after, induction. Unless this particular patient was exceedingly anxious, the risks of using an anxiolytic may favor avoiding any preoperative sedation.

4. Would you premedicate with an H-2 antagonist, a prokinetic agent, and/or a nonparticulate antacid prior to induction?

After routine fasting and in the absence of other gastroenterological pathology, obese, non-diabetic surgical patient, are not more predisposed to high-volume, low-pH gastric contents than their lean counterparts [16].

However, it is generally accepted that the risks of an aspiration event may be increased by the presence of a hiatal hernia and/or GERD, which are both more common in obese individuals [17]. An increase greater than 3.5 kg/m^2 in BMI is associated with a 2.7-fold increase in risk for developing new reflux symptoms [18]. Also, intragastric pressure may be higher in patients with abdominal obesity, predisposing to hiatal herniation and/or reflux symptoms, relating to an increased incidence of transient lower esophageal sphincter relaxation [19].

The anesthesiologist should consider steps to minimize the risks of an aspiration event, particularly if an unfavorable airway exam is a contraindication to an RSI. Premedication may lessen the risks of an awake intubation.

5. What are your preoperative concerns in a patient who has previously undergone some type of weight loss procedure?

Any alteration of the normal anatomy may negatively impact gastric transit time, resulting in prolonged retention of stomach contents. Second, patients who have had surgical alteration of their stomach or intestines are at heightened risk of malabsorption. Vitamin deficiencies or generalized malnutrition may reduce resilience to the surgical and physiological insults associated with subsequent procedures.

Change in the position or function of the gastroesophageal junction or pylorus, may reduce the propersity of the normal anatomy to prevent reflux of digestive contents into either the stomach or esophagus.

6. Would you insert an elective nasogastric tube in a vomiting, pre-op patient prior to an emergent laparoscopy, 6 weeks after having undergone a gastric bypass?

Insertion of naso- or orogastric tubes may put a fresh, anastomotic suture line at risk for perforation. Such action should only be undertaken after thorough consideration of the risks and benefits and conversation with the surgeon.

Intraoperative Considerations

1. Why is preoxygenation so vital in obese patients? How can you increase the effectiveness of apneic deoxygenation?

Oxygen consumption increases with enlarged body mass, and this will result in a shorter time to apneic deoxygenation. Rather than several maximum vital capacity breaths, it has been shown that breathing pure oxygen for at least 3 min, with a good seal, will lengthen the period before the patient begins to desaturate [20]. Preoxygenation in a head-up position (25°) has also been shown to prolong this period [21]. Lastly, the use of CPAP 10 cm H_2O during preoxygenation will minimize atelectasis and ensure maximal preinduction oxygen loading [22].

2. What airway challenges may be associated with morbid obesity?

The initial airway assessment may be complicated by the obscuration of landmarks by excessive adiposity. It may be difficult to accurately assess thyromental distance, hyomental distance, and sternomental distance, due to an inability to palpate the structures themselves. Moreover, the chin may be in close proximity to chest, potentially restricting mouth opening. Additionally, the laryngoscope handle may contact the chest and make blade insertion difficult.

Once the blade is inserted, the deposition of adipose in the visible structures may decrease the pharyngeal area, change the shape of the airway, and add difficulty to both ventilation and intubation. An inverse relationship generally exists between the degree of obesity and the pharyngeal area. Furthermore, adipose tissue may impact the position of the hyoid bone, causing the epiglottis to override the entrance to the glottis.

The detection of breath sounds may also present a challenge, increasing reliance on end-tidal carbon dioxide to ensure ventilation. The only means of truly ensuring tube placement above the carina may be bronchoscopy. These same factors complicating induction will also impact the risks and approach to both emergence and extubation.

3. Describe the characteristics and utility of successful "ramp" positioning.

The purpose of ramping is to horizontally align the patient's external auditory meatus with the sternal notch. Ideally, this will also align the oral, pharyngeal, and laryngeal axis to favor visualization of the glottic opening and passage of an endotracheal tube, similar to the "sniffing position" in non-obese patients.

4. How are you going to induce anesthesia? Is there an indication for awake intubation?

Due to the patient's habitus, she is unlikely to tolerate apnea for very long. Based on her degree of obesity and high CPAP requirement, she is also more likely to be a difficult mask. Her potential for increased gastric pressure, due to overlying tissue, would also favor rapid intubation and securement of her airway through either a rapid sequence or a modified rapid sequence induction.

However, a non-reassuring airway exam should be prioritized over a heightened risk of aspiration or increased oxygen demand. If the loss of the airway is a legitimate concern, an awake intubating technique would be favored. Steps can then be taken to minimize the potential consequences of an aspiration.

5. What is your plan for analgesia?

Multimodal analgesia is likely to reduce postoperative hypoventilation, as compared to a purely opioid-based technique. Drugs and classes to consider would include NSAIDS, alpha-2 agonists, and NMDA antagonists, such as ketamine. Although potentially more challenging in obese patients, regional anesthesia may result in a lower incidence of respiratory depression for amenable procedures, by providing targeted analgesia.

6. What are your concerns surrounding patient positioning?

When caring for morbidly obese individuals, one must be aware of the increased pressure on contact points—from stirrups, the lateral position, or on any dependent structure. With this in mind, an effort should be made to minimize the duration of procedures and also to frequently examine and/or reposition anything deemed to be at risk for injury.

As an extreme example, there are case reports of postoperative rhabdomyolysis in obese individuals, resulting from operative pressure on gluteal muscles. This has been known to cause renal failure and death [23, 24]. Aside from focal contact points, the Trendelenburg position may worsen already diminished thoracic compliance. The anesthesiologist may be forced to set limits on position based on the patient's physiologic tolerance.

It is necessary to consider the weight limit for most operating room tables is dependent upon the position of the bed itself. The maximum allowable weight when reversed or articulated may be significantly less than the cited value for the supine position in "normal" orientation.

7. Would you have any reservations about doing a prone procedure on a morbidly obese patient?

Although prone positioning is not contraindicated in morbidly obese (MO) patients, it should be approached with caution. Studies have shown a significant decrease in stroke volume with repositioning, which may be related to increasing intrathoracic pressure. Increased compression of abdominal contents may directly impact the IVC and similarly decrease venous return. In contrast, SVR and PVR generally increase, which should be anticipated and considered in the context of the patient's cardiac function.

Morbid obesity is associated with an increase in hypertension, diabetes, vascular disease; all of which have been linked to a higher incidence of postoperative visual loss with prone procedures.

It may be beneficial to allow a patient to assess his or her own position prior to induction. Awake intubation followed by awake prone positioning has been advocated as a technique to allow morbidly obese patients to position themselves in such a manner to minimize ocular pressure and other contact points, while assessing for any cardiopulmonary compromise before going to sleep [25]. Efforts to minimize direct pressure on the abdomen may minimize the physiologic insult of the prone position.

Intraoperative airway or cardiovascular emergency may require immediate supination of the patient. Emergent "flipping" of larger patients poses increased risks to both patient and staff, particularly since waiting for additional help may worsen outcome.

8. What other challenges should be anticipated when caring for MO patients?

Obtaining both initial and adequate vascular access may present a formidable challenge. Use of ultrasound, either peripherally or centrally, should be considered early to facilitate adequate venous access for a safe anesthetic in the context of the procedure and patient history.

The presence of conical-shaped arms may complicate hemodynamic monitoring. The alternative placement of the noninvasive cuff on the forearm or placing an arterial catheter (via ultrasound) may be required to ensure appropriate intraoperative monitoring. It should be noted that forearm cuff measurements generally overestimate true systolic and diastolic values.

9. What EKG changes have been associated with obesity?

Restricted diaphragmatic expansion, due to increased abdominal fat, may lead to leftward shift in P-wave, QRS, and T-wave axes [26]. Similarly, adipose deposits in the chest wall may diminish QRS voltage. LVH and T-wave flattening are also seen with increasing frequency in this population.

Pharmacology

1. What is Fen–Phen? What are your concerns? How does the pharmacological mechanism of Orlistat differ?

Fen–Phen (fenfluramine–phentermine) was a weight loss medication whose peak popularity occurred in the 1990s. It was found to increase metabolism and decrease appetite. Fenfluramine was an SSRI, while phentermine functioned as both an SNRI and a dopamine releasing agent. Due to the increased incidence of valvular heart disease and pulmonary hypertension in consumers, it was taken off the market in 1997. The manufacturer has since paid out billions of dollars in settlements.

Given the patient's history, it would be reasonable to recommend a preoperative cardiac echocardiogram to assess valvular function, pulmonary arterial pressure, and function of the right heart, based on this exposure.

Orlistat, a FDA-approved lipase inhibitor, interferes with the breakdown of ingested triglycerides. Instead of being absorbed, undigested fats are excreted in the feces.

2. How will the patient's obesity affect your choice of medications?

Lipid-soluble drugs will have a higher volume of distribution in obese patients. This will decrease peak concentrations, diminish the amount of drug available at the target receptor, and prolong the elimination half-life. Water-soluble drugs have a more limited volume of distribution and should generally be based on ideal body weight, rather than the total weight of the patient.

3. What is ideal body weight (IBW)? How is it calculated?

IBW is statistically based on actuarial tables to be associated with the lowest mortality for a specific height and gender. It is often utilized in the insurance industry. Broca's index is one of several mathematical equations used to estimate ideal body weight. That value is often used to predict pharmacokinetics for obese patients.

IBW (kg) = height (cm) $- x$
$X = 100$ for adult males
$X = 105$ for adult females.

4. What common anesthetic medications are dosed on ideal body weight (IBW) versus total body weight (TBW)?

Lipophilic drugs are generally dosed on TBW, as they will have an increased volume of distribution, as compared to lipophobic compounds. Common examples of lipophilic drugs include propofol, midazolam, fentanyl, sufentanil, dexmedetomidine, and succinylcholine.

Although propofol is highly lipophilic, it is recommended that induction be based on lean body mass (LBM), while infusions be calculated based on TBW, as the volume of distribution is somewhat time-dependent. LBM is usually approximated as 120% of IBW. Similarly, the rapid metabolism of remifentanil, by plasma esterases, favors dosing based on IBW, despite being highly lipophilic.

Lipophobic drugs are generally dosed by IBW. This list includes alfentanil, ketamine, vecuronium, rocuronium, and morphine.

It is generally recommended that maximum local anesthetic doses for infiltration be based upon ideal body weight. However, in the context of obesity, local anesthetic doses may actually be reduced by 25% for spinals and epidurals, as engorged epidural veins and fat may impinge on the volume of the epidural space and result in higher than anticipated levels.

5. Which inhaled anesthetics may be better suited for MO patients?

The low blood–gas solubility coefficient of desflurane makes it a popular choice for the maintenance of anesthesia in the obese population. Lower solubility minimizes the accumulation of desflurane in adipose tissues and favors faster recovery. However, due to the pungent nature of the gas, it may not be appropriate for all patients.

Nitrous oxide also has low blood–gas solubility coefficient. However, due to the potential concern for intestinal inflation or a time-dependent risk of postoperative nausea and vomiting, it may be best reserved for emergence, facilitating an early decrease in the concentration of the volatile agent.

Postoperative Management

1. What is the benefit to recovery in the semi-fowler's position?

The semi-Fowler's position refers to a supine patient with the head of bed raised to an angle between 30 and 45°. It has been shown to increase the FRC, pulmonary compliance, and oxygenation in postoperative patients by displacing or unloading the intraabdominal contents from the diaphragm.

2. How should postoperative pain be controlled?

Although multimodal analgesia should be continued in the postoperative period, patient-controlled analgesia (PCA) has been shown to be safe for morbidly obese patients following gastric bypass surgery, with appropriate monitoring and the avoidance of a basal rate infusion [27].

References

1. Ogden C, Carroll M, Kit B, et al. Prevalence of childhood and adult obesity in the United States, 2011-2012. JAMA. 2014;311 (8):806–14. doi:10.1001/jama.2014.732.
2. Levy J. US obesity rate inches up to 27.7% in 2014. Gallup-Healthways Well-Being Index, Gallup, Inc. 21 June 2015. Web. http://www.gallup.com/poll/181271/obesity-rate-inches-2014.aspx.
3. Romero-Corral A, Somers VK, et al. Accuracy of body mass index to diagnose obesity in the US adult population. Int J Obes (Lond). 2008;32(6):959–66.
4. Alam K, Lewis JW, Stephens JM, et al. Obesity, metabolic syndrome and sleep apnoea. All proinflammatory states. Obes Rev. 2007;8:119–27.
5. Alberti KG, Zimmet P, Shaw J. The metabolic syndrome—a new worldwide definition. Lancet. 2005;366:1059.
6. Liberopoulos EN, Mikhailidis DP, Elisaf MS. Diagnosis and management of the metabolic syndrome in obesity. Obes Rev. 2005;6:283–96.
7. Holst AG, Jensen G, et al. Risk factors for venous thromboembolism. Circulation. 2010;121:1896–903.
8. Cullen DJ. Obstructive sleep apnea and postoperative analgesia—a potentially dangerous combination. J Clin Anesth. 2001;13(2):83–5.
9. Chung F, Elsaid H. Screening for obstructive sleep apnea before surgery: why is it important? Curr Opin Anaesthesiol. 2009;22 (3):405–11.
10. Ong TH, Raudha S, et al. Simplifying STOP-BANG: use of a simple questionnaire to screen for OSA in an Asian population. Sleep Breath. 2010;14:371–6 Epub 2010 Apr 26.
11. Eckman DM. Anesthesia for bariatric surgery. In: Miller RD, et al., editors. Miller's anesthesia. 8th ed. Philadelphia: Churchill Livingstone. p. 2204.
12. Joshi GP, Ahmad S, Riad W, Eckert S, Chung F. Selection of patients with obesity undergoing ambulatory surgery: a systematic review of the literature. Anesth Analg. 2013;117(5):1082–91.
13. American Society of Anesthesiologists Task Force on Perioperative. Management of patients with obstructive sleep apnea. Practice guidelines for the perioperative management of patients with obstructive sleep apnea. Anesthesiology. 2014;120(2):268–86.
14. Eckman DM. Anesthesia for bariatric surgery. In: Miller RD, et al., editors. Miller's anesthesia, 8th ed. Philadelphia: Churchill Livingstone. p. 2209.
15. Brodsky JB, Lemmens HJ, et al. Morbid obesity and tracheal intutbation. Anesth Analg. 2002;94:732.
16. Harter RL, Kelly WB, Kramer MG, et al. A comparison of the volume and pH of gastric contents of obese and lean surgical patients. Anesth Analg. 1998;86:147.
17. Menon S, Trudgill N. Risk factors in the aetiology of hiatus hernia: a meta-analysis. Eur J Gastroenterol Hepatol. 2011;23(2):133–8.
18. Nilsson M, Johnsen R, Ye W, et al. Obesity and estrogen as risk factors for gastroesophageal reflux symptoms. JAMA. 2003; 290:66.

19. Ogunnaike BO, Whitten CW. Evaluation of the obese patient. In: Longnecker, et al., editors. Anesthesia, 1st edn. New York: McGraw Hill Professional. p. 381.
20. Drummond GB, Park GR. Arterial oxygen saturation before intubation of the trachea; an assessment of oxygenation techniques. Br J Anaesth. 1984;56:987–92.
21. Dixon BJ, Dixon JB, et al. Preoxygenation is more effective in the 25 degrees head-up position for the morbidly obese patient. Obes Surg. 2003;13:4–9.
22. Coussa M, Proietti S, et al. Prevention of atelectasis formation during the induction of GA in morbidly obese patients. Anesth Analg. 2004;98:1491–5.
23. Bostanjian D, Anthone GJ, Hamouti N, et al. Rhabdomyolysis of gluteal muscles leading to renal failure: a potentially fatal complication of surgery in the morbidly obese. Obes Surg. 2003;13:302–5.
24. Collier B, Goreja MA, Duke BE III. Postoperative Rhabdomyolysis with bariatric surgery. Obes Surg. 2003;13:941–3.
25. Douglass J, Fraser J, Andrzejowski J. Awake intubation and awake prone positioning of a morbidly obese patient for lumbar spine surgery. Anaesthesia. 2014 Feb;69(2):166–9.
26. Alpert MA, Boyd TE, et al. Effect of weight loss on the ECG of normotensive morbidly obese patients. CHEST. 2001;119(2).
27. Choi YK, Brolin RE, et al. Efficacy and safety of patient-controlled analgesia for morbidly obese patients following gastric bypass surgery. Obes Surg. 2000 Apr;10(2):154–9.

Laparoscopy

32

Carmelita W. Pisano

Case:

A 68-year-old female presents with a long-standing history of menorrhagia and is scheduled to undergo a laparoscopic total hysterectomy

Past Medical History:	
Cardiac:	Hypertension
Pulmonary:	Obstructive Sleep apnea (OSA)
	Chronic Obstructive Pulmonary
	Disease, Stage II
GI:	Gastroespohageal Reflux Disease
	(GERD)
Endocrine:	Diabetes Mellitus Type II (DMII)
Medications:	Atenolol 25 mg orally twice daily
	Hydrochlorothiazide 25 mg orally daily
	Lisinopril 40 mg orally daily
	Nexium 40 mg orally daily
	Spiriva 2 puffs twice daily
	Albuterol 2 puffs prn
Allergies:	NKDA
Social Hx:	Ex smoker: 30 pack-years; quit 5 years ago
Physical Exam:	
Vital Signs:	BP: 125/75 HR: 51
	SaO2: 97% on Room Air
	Weight: 305 lbs Height: 68 in. BMI: 46.4
Lungs:	Clear to auscultation bilaterally
METS:	4–5

(continued)

Labs:	Chemistry: 140| 102|18/ 150 Why hyponatremic, and bicarb a touch low?
	4.2| 24 | 0.9\ These abnl labs may make people 'overthink'.
CBC:	8\7.9/250
	/28\
ECG:	NSR @ 58 bpm
PFTs:	FEV_1: 60%
	FEV_1/FVC: 0.6

1. Define laparoscopy.
   Laparoscopy is defined as a minimally invasive procedure where a laparoscope is used to enter the peritoneum. Once the peritoneal cavity is entered, insufflating gas creates a pneumoperitoneum. Laparoscopy may be used to examine abdominal or pelvic (pelviscopy) organs, diagnose conditions, and/or perform surgery [1].
2. Name some surgical procedures currently performed laparoscopically.
   Laparoscopic procedures can be performed on all abdominal organs and includes gastrectomy, anti-reflux and bariatric procedures, cholecystectomy, hepatic and pancreatic resections, bowel and rectal surgery, adrenalectomy, and splenectomy [2]. Urological procedures performed laparoscopically include prostatectomy and nephrectomy. Laparoscopic gynecological surgeries include hysterectomy, ovarian, and tubal procedures [3].
3. What are the advantages of laparoscopic surgery? Which specific patient populations benefit most from laparoscopic procedures?
   Advantages of laparoscopic surgery are several-fold. Recovery time is shortened. This is mostly due to minimal bowel manipulation during laparoscopy, reducing the incidence of postoperative ileus. Because of the smaller incisions associated with laparoscopic

C.W. Pisano (✉)
Department of Anesthesiology, Perioperative and Pain Medicine, Brigham and Women's Hospital, 75 Francis Street, Boston, MA 02115, USA
e-mail: cpisano@partners.org

© Springer International Publishing AG 2017
L.S. Aglio and R.D. Urman (eds.), *Anesthesiology*,
DOI 10.1007/978-3-319-50141-3_32

procedures, resultant scars are more cosmetic and there is less postoperative pain [4]. Decreased intraoperative blood loss and less frequent surgical wound infections are also seen [5]. For particular patient populations, i.e., morbidly obese patients and patients with significant cardiopulmonary comorbidities, the benefits of a minimally invasive procedure are truly apparent with respect to less postoperative pulmonary complications.

4. What are the disadvantages of laparoscopic surgery?
   In addition to the steep learning curve for surgeons learning laparoscopic techniques, other disadvantages of laparoscopic surgery include poor depth perception and loss of dexterity due to limited range of motion using laparoscopic instruments [6].
5. What are some absolute and relative contraindications to laparoscopic surgery?
   Most contraindications to laparoscopic surgery are relative and these risks must be compared to the benefits of a less invasive procedure. Relative contraindications include patients with pre-existing increased intracranial pressure (and/or space occupying lesion), severe hypovolemia and known right-to-left intracardiac shunts, for example, a patent foramen ovale [7].
6. What are optimal surgical conditions for laparoscopic surgery?
   Optimal surgical conditions include gastrointestinal decompression via a bowel prep and or naso/orogastric tube placement. This permits easier and safer formation of the pneumoperitoneum for surgical exposure decreasing the chance of injury to organs when the instruments are inserted. Neuromuscular blockade relaxes abdominal wall muscles facilitating formation of the pneumoperitoneum [1, 8].
7. What is the gas of choice used to create the pneumoperitoneum during laparoscopy and why?
   The gas of choice used to create the pneumoperitoneum is carbon dioxide (CO_2). This is due to its easy accessibility, low cost, and fairly inert and non-combustible properties. Carbon dioxide (CO_2) is highly soluble and rapidly buffered in blood and eliminated by the lungs [9].
8. What are the disadvantages to using carbon dioxide (CO_2)?
   A disadvantage to using CO_2 as an exogenous gas for insufflation is that it is irritating to the peritoneum. Use of carbon dioxide may also lead to hypercarbia and respiratory acidosis and also cause metabolic, hormonal, and immunological adverse effects [10]. Although the incidence is low due to the high solubility of CO_2 in blood, the formation of a gas (CO_2) embolism could be catastrophic.

Preoperative concerns:

1. What concerns do you have about this patient's history and physical with regards to laparoscopic surgery?
   Her baseline pulmonary history (COPD) and obstructive sleep apnea (OSA) can predispose her to postoperative pulmonary complications. Morbid obesity may make the procedure more technically challenging for the surgeon to perform, and other obstacles, such as difficult airway, difficulty with ventilation in head-down position and positioning injuries may materialize. This patient is also anemic, which is likely due to her presenting symptom of menorrhagia, and may lead to a lower threshold for blood transfusion.
2. How does this patient's medical history predispose her to postoperative pulmonary complications? What are the GOLD criteria? How are they best used?
   This patient has Stage II COPD. The GOLD criteria are used to classify patients with COPD based on the severity of their degree of obstruction (Table 1). The degree of obstruction is determined by pulmonary function tests, specifically FEV_1 and FEV_1/FVC [11]:

In order to better predict who may develop postoperative pulmonary complications, the GOLD criteria must be used in conjunction with other factors such as level of activity, smoking history, etc. The hypercarbia that develops during laparoscopy due to the use of CO_2 could be difficult to manage in patients with moderate to severe COPD resulting in hypercarbic respiratory failure postoperatively. Based on this patient's age, history of moderate COPD and OSA, and surgical site, she would be expected to have an increase in postoperative pulmonary complications, such as hypoxemia, atelectasis, hypercapnia, pneumonia, and ventilatory failure [12]:

- Age: The risk of postoperative pulmonary complications increases as a patient ages (>65) regardless of their baseline pulmonary status.
- COPD: See above table. Patients with mild COPD along with other significant comorbidities, and patients with moderate to severe COPD have a significant increased risk of postoperative pulmonary complications. Considering the patient's overall medical condition at the time of surgery, the relative risk of pulmonary complications is 2.7–4.7 [13].
- OSA: Though not currently routinely screened preoperatively in all patients, new data suggests an association between OSA and postoperative pulmonary complications [12].

- Surgical site: For incisions closer to the diaphragm, the risk of postoperative pulmonary complications increases.

Intraoperative concerns:

1. What are the three main causes of the physiological changes seen with laparoscopic surgery?
   Whether separate or in combination, the occurrence of the following are the main causes of the physiological changes seen during laparoscopic surgery:
   (a) Pneumoperitoneum: A pneumoperitoneum is essential for performing laparoscopic surgery. Creating, maintaining and dealing with the consequences of increased intra-abdominal pressure can lead to many problems intraoperatively [14].
   (b) Carbon dioxide: Although CO_2 for insufflation is the preferred gas based on its inert and non-combustible properties, absorption of this gas into the blood stream can cause pathophysiological effects on multiple organ systems.
   (c) Patient position: Trendelenburg and reverse Trendelenburg both have profound effects on a patient's hemodynamics.
2. What effect does laparoscopy have on the arterial to end-tidal CO_2 gradient (P_aCO_2-$P_{ET}CO_2$)?
   In ASA I & II patients, the reliability of $P_{ET}CO_2$ for monitoring P_aCO_2 is generally not affected by the use of CO_2 as an insufflation gas during laparoscopy. This may not be the case for ASA III & IV patients, however. For these patients, the increase in alveolar dead space and/or increased ventilation/perfusion mismatch that occurs with laparoscopic insufflation may increase the normal alveolar–arterial (A-a) gradient (normally 3–5 mmHg) where even with a normal $P_{ET}CO_2$, the P_aCO_2 may be significantly elevated [15].
3. Does this patient need an arterial line? Why or why not?
   Based on this patient's history of Stage II COPD and OSA and the fact that $P_{ET}CO_2$ may not accurately reflect P_aCO_2, an arterial line may be beneficial. This will allow direct monitoring of P_aCO_2 which will aid in the management of the hypercarbia which occurs with laparoscopy.
4. What are the typical causes of hypercarbia seen during laparoscopic surgery?
   The hypercarbia observed during laparoscopy could be a result of diffusion of CO_2 from the peritoneal cavity; hypoventilation; increase in the production of CO_2 (i.e., lactate and ketoacids); increased dead space (i.e., pulmonary embolism, severe COPD) [16].
5. What effect does CO_2 absorption have on the cardiovascular system?
   Hypercarbia has direct and indirect stimulating effects on the cardiovascular system. When CO_2 is absorbed across the peritoneum, it is normally excreted through the lungs. This is due to its high solubility and diffusibility. If the patient is hypoventilated or has significant pulmonary disease where managing ventilation may be challenging, hypercarbia may occur and could cause acidosis [17]. Mild hypercarbia can stimulate the sympathetic system resulting in tachycardia and increased myocardial contractility. Moderate to severe hypercarbia causes myocardial depression as well as direct vasodilatation due to the resultant acidosis [18]. Severe hypercarbia can also cause cardiac arrhythmias especially in the setting of hypoxia.
6. How does increased intra-abdominal pressure affect the cardiovascular system?
   Normal intra-abdominal pressure is 0–5 mmHg and with insufflation it increases to 10–15 mmHg. Pressures exceeding 15 mmHg can cause abdominal compartment syndrome and compromise organ function. Creation of the pneumoperitoneum causes an increase in systemic vascular resistance (SVR) (due to compression of the abdominal organs and blood vessels) and to a lesser extent, a decrease in cardiac output (CO), which results in an overall increase in mean arterial blood pressure (MAP). The degree of overall increase in MAP is proportional to the increase in intra-abdominal pressure. In addition to the mechanical compression of the pneumoperitoneum, the increase in MAP is also a result of the release of catecholamines, vasopressin and the activation of the renin–angiotensin system. With intra-abdominal pressures exceeding 20 mmHg, a decrease in heart rate, blood pressure, and cardiac output may occur due to decreased preload. The observed decreases in cardiac output are related to decreased venous return from compression of the inferior vena cava. In order to minimize these effects, insufflation should occur slowly and at the lowest pressure to achieve adequate surgical conditions (<15 mmHg). Vasodilatory agents, opioids, etc., may be used to treat increases in SVR, while preloading with intravenous fluids prior to insufflation may prevent the decreases in venous return and cardiac output [1].
7. What cardiac arrhythmias can be seen with peritoneal distention?
   Rapid insufflation with high flow rates can result in cardiac dysrhythmias including severe bradycardia, nodal rhythms as well as asystole. This is likely due to the rapid stretch of the peritoneal cavity with insufflation, which can result in significant vagal stimulation [19].

Table 1 The GOLD criteria are used to classify patients with COPD

GOLD COPD staging			
Stage I	Mild COPD	$FEV_1/FVC < 0.70$	$FEV_1 \geq 80\%$ normal
Stage II	Moderate COPD	$FEV_1/FVC < 0.70$	FEV_1 50–79% normal
Stage III	Severe COPD	$FEV_1/FVC < 0.70$	FEV_1 30–49% normal
Stage IV	Very severe COPD	$FEV_1/FVC < 0.70$	$FEV_1 < 30\%$ normal, or $< 50\%$ normal with chronic respiratory failure present

8. How does the Trendelenburg position affect the cardiovascular system?
   Head-down tilt or Trendelenburg position results in increased venous return (preload) and cardiac output. This is easily tolerated in healthy patients, however, in patients with poor left ventricular function, an increase in central volume and pressure may be deleterious [20].
10. How does increased intra-abdominal pressure (pneumoperitoneum) affect the respiratory system?
   The pneumoperitoneum is the primary factor that influences pulmonary function during laparoscopic surgery. These influences include elevation of the diaphragm, increase in intrathoracic pressure and therefore, a decrease in lung compliance, an increase in airway pressure, and a reduction in the functional residual capacity. Most healthy, ASA I and ASA II patients tolerate these pulmonary changes without issue. However, in ASA III and ASA IV patients, specifically patients with pre-existing pulmonary disease, these effects can have severe consequences [21].
11. What effect does CO_2 absorption have on the respiratory system?
   Hypercarbia seen during laparoscopic surgery as a result of CO_2 absorption into the blood can stimulate the respiratory center. Carbon dioxide levels above 100–150 mmHg will result in respiratory depression [21]. During laparoscopic surgery, attention must be paid to effective ventilation strategies to ensure adequate elimination of carbon dioxide. Hypercarbia can produce bronchodilation and severe hypercarbia with resulting acidosis may cause pulmonary vasoconstriction [19].
12. How does the Trendelenburg position affect the respiratory system?
   On its own, the Trendelenburg position does not induce any significant pulmonary changes. However, in the setting of a pneumoperitoneum, the Trendelenburg position can exaggSerate the effects of the pneumoperitoneum by reducing lung compliance, increasing the airway pressure and reducing the functional residual capacity [21].
13. How does the pneumoperitoneum affect the renal system?
   The pneumoperitoneum affects the renal system through its mechanical compressive effects. This compressive effect accounts for about 50% of the decrease in glomerular filtration rate that is observed during laparoscopic surgery. Renal plasma flow and urine output are also decreased. These effects may remain despite adequate hydration; therefore, it is thought that the oliguria observed during laparoscopic surgery is due to neurohumoral alterations secondary to hypercarbia, as well as due to the compressive effects of the pneumoperitoneum [22]. With intra-abdominal pressures below 15 mmHg, the oliguria is reversible [23].
14. How does hypercarbia affect the central nervous system?
   Hypercarbia during laparoscopic surgery can have direct effects on the central nervous system. Cerebral blood flow varies proportionately with $PaCO_2$. Cerebral blood flow increases 1–2 mL/100 g/min for each 1 mmHg increase in $PaCO_2$. Therefore, intracranial pressure may be increased with CO_2 insufflation and resultant hypercarbia. Mild hypercarbia directly causes cortical depression and increases the seizure threshold, however, increased levels of CO_2 directly stimulates the subcortical hypothalamic centers and may result in increased cortical excitability and seizure activity. At extreme levels of hypercarbia, general anesthesia is induced due to cortical and subcortical depression, which is most likely due to reduced intracellular pH causing intracellular perturbations [14, 24].
15. Should nitrous oxide be used during laparoscopic surgery? Why or why not?
   There is controversy on whether or not nitrous oxide should be used during laparoscopic surgery. The two main issues are the potential of nitrous oxide to cause bowel distention and postoperative nausea and vomiting. The argument for increased bowel distention revolves around the fact that nitrous oxide is about 30 times more soluble than nitrogen, which means in a closed air-containing space (i.e., bowel), nitrous oxide will enter faster than nitrogen can be eliminated, thereby increasing the size of the closed air-containing space. However, studies have shown no significant effect on surgical conditions when nitrous oxide was used during laparoscopy. In addition, several studies found no increase in the incidence of postoperative nausea and vomiting when nitrous oxide was used during laparoscopic surgery [25, 26].

16. Is local or regional anesthesia a reasonable choice for laparoscopic surgery? Why or why not?
Although general anesthesia is the anesthetic technique of choice for laparoscopic surgery, local and regional anesthetic are optional and feasible techniques. Local anesthesia involves infiltration of local anesthetics into the surgical incisions (by surgeon) to minimize surgical incision pain, however, the abdominal cavity is not anesthetized, which may result in discomfort for the awake patient. Intravenous sedative and narcotics may be given for patient comfort. Regional neuraxial anesthesia entails injecting a local anesthetic near the spinal cord (spinal or epidural). The block would need to reach the T4 level for laparoscopic surgery [27]. The advantages of local or regional anesthesia for laparoscopic surgery are the avoidance of general anesthesia and its associated risks (e.g., airway trauma, sore throat, postoperative nausea, and vomiting) and need for less opioid use [28]. Disadvantages of local anesthesia include increased patient anxiety and pain (specifically shoulder pain as a result of CO_2 insufflation), which may require administration of sedatives and/or opioids, which may lead to respiratory depression [28]. Disadvantages of regional anesthesia used for laparoscopic surgery include requirement of a high level (T4) block, which could potentially lead to cardiac depression, bradycardia, hypotension due to the sympathectomy, and shoulder pain, among others [29].
17. What are the potential intraoperative complications that may occur during laparoscopy?
Several potential intraoperative complications may occur during laparoscopic surgery:
Complications with access into the peritoneal cavity. Access to the peritoneal cavity can be obtained by several methods. The closed method involves blindly passing the Veress needle into the abdominal cavity via a small incision at the umbilicus [30]. The pneumoperitoneum is established once the Veress needle is verified to be in the correct position. The open method involves the surgeon making an incision at the umbilicus through the skin, abdominal fascia and peritoneum under direct vision, followed by insertion of a Hassan trocar and establishment of the pneumoperitoneum [30]. Both methods of access could potentially cause complications. The rate of complication associated with the placement of the Veress needle or a trocar was approximately 0.3% [30]. These complications include injuries to major retroperitoneal blood vessels and/or bowel, solid organ injury, abdominal wall hematoma, wound infection, avulsion of adhesion, and fascial dehiscence and herniation [30, 31]. Although major vascular and bowel injuries with trocar insertion are rare, studies have shown that use of the open method may decrease the incidence of these more serious complications [30].
Complications related to the formation of the pneumoperitoneum. Complications related to the creation of the pneumoperitoneum by insufflating a gas include subcutaneous emphysema, mediastinal emphysema, and pneumothorax, which are due to the improper placement of the Veress needle or trocar [31]. Other complications related to the insufflation of CO_2 include cardiac dysrythymias, carbon dioxide retention and respiratory acidosis, postoperative pain related to retained intra-abdominal gas and venous CO_2 gas embolism [31]. The pneumoperitoneum may also lead to several hemodynamic changes, including stimulation of the neurohumoral vasoactive system with resultant release of catecholamines and increased heart rate, mean arterial pressure and systemic and pulmonary vascular resistance and decreases in venous return, preload and cardiac output [31]. In ASA I and ASA II patients these physiological changes are tolerated well when the intra-abdominal pressure is kept at or below 15 mmHg.
Other complications. Other complications include those that could occur as a result of the Trendelenburg position, such as venous congestion of the head and neck, increased intracranial and intraocular pressure, corneal and conjunctival edema, endobronchial intubation, and hypoxemia [14].
18. How may a pneumothorax manifest? How would you detect/diagnose a pneumothorax?
Pneumothorax is a known complication of laparoscopic abdominal surgeries. It is characterized by the abnormal collection of air or gas in the pleural space. During laparoscopic procedures, the CO_2 is under pressure in the abdomen and can track along anatomical paths, such as the esophageal hiatus, and enter the pleural space and cause separation between the lung and the chest wall [32]. Associated risk factors for the development of a pneumothorax during laparoscopic surgery include surgery times exceeding 200 min, positive end-tidal $CO_2 > 50$ mmHg, advanced patient age and operator inexperience [32, 33]. A pneumothorax can be detected intraoperatively by decreased total lung compliance, increased airway pressure and increased P_aCO_2 and $P_{ET}CO_2$. Significant hemodynamic changes, such as jugular venous distention, hypotension, absent breath sounds, bulging diaphragm, and expanding subcutaneous emphysema may be observed, especially with a tension pneumothorax [32]. Changes in the electrocardiographic (ECG) pattern may be a sensitive marker of a pneumothorax. Here, the amplitude of the QRS complex in the anterior precordial leads is reduced [34]. A pneumothorax may also be detected postoperatively with the patient exhibiting signs of restlessness and respiratory

distress. To confirm both an intraoperative and a postoperative pneumothorax, a chest radiograph should be obtained, unless there is suspicion of a tension pneumothorax, where needle decompression may be warranted before obtaining imaging. Also, ultrasonography has been shown to aid in the diagnosis of a pneumothorax and can also help determine the treatment [35].

19. How is a pneumothorax treated?
    A laparoscopic gas-induced pneumothorax usually resolves spontaneously, as CO_2 quickly diffuses out of the chest. Administering 100% oxygen for both an intraoperative or postoperative pneumothorax, in addition to adding PEEP and increasing the minute ventilation intraoperatively is appropriate. Serial X-ray films and/or arterial blood gases should be obtained to monitor resolution of the pneumothorax. Insertion of a chest tube is usually unnecessary with a laparoscopic gas-induced pneumothorax [32, 35].
20. What could result from an endobronchial intubation?
    Endobronchial intubation during laparoscopic surgery may present as hypoxemia and increased airway pressures [36]. Several factors during laparoscopic surgery may contribute to the high risk of endobronchial intubation. Though patient position (Trendelenburg) may be a factor, it appears that the pneumoperitoneum from abdominal insufflation is the main contributing factor to endotracheal tube migration during laparoscopic surgery [37].
21. What are the differences between air and CO_2 (gas) embolism?
    A gas (or air) embolism occurs when a blood vessel is open and a pressure gradient exists that leads to gas entering the blood vessel. Gas embolism may occur as a result from injury of blood vessels during the blind insertion of the Veress needle with insufflation of CO_2 directly into the vessel during laparoscopic surgery [14]. Distinguishing a gas embolism from an air embolism is important since the latter may have catastrophic consequences. The main differences include composition of the embolism and its solubility in blood and the effect of using nitrous oxide in its presence [38]. The composition of an air embolism is 79% nitrogen and 21% oxygen, where the CO_2 (gas) embolism) is 100% CO_2 [14, 38]. This is an important distinction when it comes to the size of the embolism, where one could see cardiovascular collapse with an air embolism but not with an equally sized CO_2 embolism because of the high solubility of CO_2 in blood. Air embolism occurs when air is entrained into an open blood vessel, usually above the heart.
22. What are the possible signs of a significant CO_2 embolism? How may you diagnose a CO_2 embolism?
    The clinical presentation of carbon dioxide embolism ranges from asymptomatic to cardiovascular collapse and death [39]. The presentation depends on the rate and volume of CO_2 entrapment and the patient's condition. Due to its high blood solubility, CO_2 embolism usually causes less detrimental effects than those produced by air. The bronchoconstriction or changes in pulmonary compliance that are caused by air embolism are not usually seen with CO_2 embolism [39]. At its worst, carbon dioxide embolism may present as a "gas lock" effect, which can cause right and left heart failure due to right ventricular obstruction, paradoxical embolism with or without a patent foramen ovale, dysrthythmia or asystole, pulmonary hypertension, systemic hypotension and cardiovascular collapse [39]. A "mill-wheel" murmur can be auscultated if the embolism is large enough. Without an increase in minute ventilation, the end-tidal CO_2 would decrease, though the arterial partial pressure of CO_2 would be increased [39]. The most sensitive method of diagnosing a CO_2 embolism is transesophageal echocardiography, with the transgastric inferior vena cava view being the ideal window for monitoring the appearance of carbon dioxide bubbles. However, transesophageal Doppler has recently been shown to be nearly as sensitive as transesophageal echocardiograpy and less expensive [39].
23. How would you treat a CO_2 embolism?
    Immediate cessation of insufflation, release of the pneumoperitoneum, discontinuation of nitrous oxide, and increase in the FiO2 to 100 percent should occur if CO_2 embolism is suspected [40]. The patient should also be hyperventilated and placed in steep head-down and left lateral decubitus position (Durant's maneuver) to decrease the amount of gas that advances through the right side of the heart to cause obstruction of the right ventricular outflow tract [40]. In cases with profound hemodynamic compromise, a central venous or pulmonary artery catheter may be introduced for aspiration of the gas.

Postop:

1. What postoperative issues can be associated with laparoscopic surgery?

In addition to shoulder pain due to the retention of intra-abdominal gas, the effects of the pneumoperitoneum on respiratory function may continue into the postoperative period, requiring supplemental oxygen, non-invasive or high oxygen flow delivery systems [14]. Patients may also experience oliguria. The incidence of postoperative nausea and vomiting following laparoscopic surgery can be as high as 42% [41]. This is likely due to the rapid stretch of the peritoneum during abdominal insufflation, which may activate neurogenic pathways involved in inducing nausea and vomiting [42].

References

1. Wetter P, Kavic M, et al. Prevention and management of laparoscopic surgical complications, 3rd edn. Society of Laparoscopic Surgeons; 2012.
2. Cunninham A. Anesthestic implications of laparoscopic surgery. Yale J Biol Med. 1998;71:551–78.
3. Kono R, Nagase S, et al. Indications for laparoscopic surgery of ovarian tumors. Tohoku J Exp Med. 1996;178(3):225–31.
4. Amornyotin S (2013) Anesthetic management for laparoscopic cholecystectomy, endoscopy. In: Amornyotin S, editor. ISBN 978-953-51-1071-2, InTech. doi:10.5772/52742.
5. Leonard IE, Cunningham AJ. Anesthetic consideration for laparoscopic cholecystectomy. Best Pract Res Clin Anesthesiol. 2002;16(1):1–20.
6. Westebring-van der Putten EP, Goossens RHM, et al. Haptics in minimally invasive surgery—a review. Minim Invasive Ther. 2008;17(1):3–16.
7. Hayden P. Anaesthesia for laparoscopic surgery. Continuing Educ Anaesth Crit Care Pain. 2011;11(5):177–80.
8. Martini CH, Boon M, et al. Evaluation of surgical conditions during laparoscopic surgery in patients with moderate vs deep neuromuscular block. Br J Anesth. 2014;112(3):498–505.
9. Srivastava A, Niranjan A. Secrets of safe laparoscopic surgery: anaesthetic and surgical considerations. J Minim Access Surg. 2010 Oct–Dec;6(4):91–4.
10. Neuhaus SJ, Gupta A, et al. Helium and other alternative insufflation gases for laparoscopy. Surg Endo. 2001 June;15 (6):553–60.
11. Vestbo J, et al. Global strategy for the diagnosis, management and prevention of chronic obstructive pulmonary disease: GOLD executive summary. Am J Respir Crit Care Med. 2013;187:347–65.
12. Smetan GW. Postoperative pulmonary complications: an update on risk assessment and reduction. Clevel Clin J Med. 2009;76 (4):60–5.
13. Licker M, Schweizer A, et al. Perioperative medical management of patients with COPD. Int J Chron Obstruct Pulmona Dis. 2007;2 (4):493–515.
14. Yao FF, Fontes ML, et al. Anesthesiology: problem-oriented patient management, 7th edn. Lippincott Williams & Wilkins; 2012. pp. 671–704.
15. Kodali BS. Capnography and laparoscopy. In: Capnography: a comprehensive educational website, 8th edn.
16. Bibhukalyani D. Acid-base disorders. Indian J Anaesth. 2003;47 (5):373–9.
17. Nguyen NT, Wolfe BM. The physiological effects of pneumoperitoneum in the morbidly obese. Ann Surg. 2005;241(2):219–26.
18. Veekash G, Wei LX, et al. Carbon dioxide pneumoperitoneum, physiological changes and anesthetic concerns. Ambul Surg. 2010 July;16(2):41–6.
19. Rist M, Hemmerling TM, et al. Influence of pneumoperitoneum and patient position on preload and splanchnic blood volume in laparoscopic surgery of the lower abdomen. J Clin Anesth. 2001;13:244–9.
20. Hirvonen EA, Nuutinen LS, et al. Hemodynamic changes due to Trendelenburg positioning and pneumoperitoneum during laparoscopic hysterectomy. Acta Anaesth Scan. 1995;39(7):949–55.
21. Min KS, Kyu WS, et al. The effect of pneumoperitoneum and trendelenburg position on respiratory mechanics during pelviscopy surgery. Kor J Anesth. 2010;59(5):329–34.
22. London ET, Hung SH, et al. Effect of intravascular volume expansion on renal function during prolonged CO_2 pneumoperitoneum. Ann Surg. 2000;231(2):195–201.
23. Al-Kandari A, Gill IS. Difficult conditions in laparoscopic urologic surgery. Berlin: Springer; 2011.3.
24. Zucker KA. Surgical laparoscopy. Lippincott, Williams & Wilkins; 2001.17.
25. Taylor E, Feinstein R, et al. Anesthesia for laparoscopic cholecystectomy. Is nitrous oxide contraindicated? Anesthsiology. 1992;76:541–3.
26. Singh P, Gupta M, et al. Nitrous oxide during anesthesia for laparoscopic donor nephrectomy: Does it matter? Indian J Urol. 2008 Jan–Mar;24(1):126–7.
27. Tzovaras G, Fafoulakis F, et al. Spinal vs general anesthesia for laparoscopic cholecystectomy. Arch Surg. 2008;143(5):497–501.
28. Sinha R, Gurwara AK, et al. Laparoscopic surgery using spinal anesthesia. JSLS. 2008 Apr–Jun;12(2):133–8.
29. Perrin M, Fletcher A. Laparoscopic abdominal surgery. BJA: CEACCP. 2004;4(4):107–10.
30. Perugini RA, Callery MP. Complications of laparoscopic surgery. In: Holzheimer RG, Mannick JA, editors. Surgical treatment: evidence-based and problem-oriented. Munich: Zuckschwerdt; 2001.
31. Pryor A, Mann WJ, et al. Complications of laparoscopic surgery. In: Marks, J, Falcone, T, editors. UpToDate. 2015 June.
32. Machairiotis N, Kougioumtzi I, et al. Laparoscopy induced pneumothorax. J Thorac Dis. 2014;6(Suppl 4):S404–6.
33. Bala V, Kaur MD, et al. Pneumothorax during laparoscopic cholecystectomy: a rare but fatal complication. Saudi J Anaesth. 2011 Apr–Jun;5(2):238–9.
34. Ludemann R, Krysztopik R, et al. Pneumothorax during laparoscopy. Surg Endosc. 2003 Dec;17(12):1985–9.
35. Jang DM, Seo HS, et al. Rapid identification of spontaneously resolving capnothorax using bedside M-mode ultrasonography during laparoscopic surgery: the "lung point" sing (two cases report). Kor J Anesth. 2013;65(6):578–82.
36. Mackenzie M, MacLeod K. Repeated inadvertent endobronchial intubation during laparoscopy. Br J Anaesth. 2003;91:297–8.
37. Gupta N, Girdhar KK, et al. Tube migration during laparoscopic gynecological surgery. J Anaesth Clin Pharmacol. 2010 Oct–Dec;26(4):537–8.
38. Groenman FA, Peters LW, et al. Embolism of air and gas in hysteroscopic procedures: pathophysiology and implication for daily practice. J Minim Invasive Gynecol. 2008 Mar–Apr;15 (2):241–7.
39. Park EY, Kwon JY, et al. Carbon dioxide embolism during laparoscopic surgery. Yonsi Med J. 2012;53(3):459–66.
40. Zirky AA, DeSousa K, et al. Carbon dioxide embolism during laparoscopic sleeve gastrectomy. J Anaeth Clin Pharmacol. 2011 Apr–Jun;27(2):262–5.
41. Iitomi T, Toriumi S, et al. Incidence of nausea and vomiting after cholecystectomy performed via laparotomy or laparoscopy. Masui. 1995;44:1627–31.
42. East JM, Mitchell DIG. Postoperative nausea and vomiting in laparoscopic versus open cholecystectomy at two major hospitals in Jamaica. West Indian Med J. 2009;58(2):130–7.

Carcinoid Disease

33

Tara C. Carey

CASE:

A 47-year-old man presents for exploratory laparotomy and small bowel resection.

HPI:	The patient has been having ongoing abdominal cramping in the setting of known metastatic carcinoid disease. The patient was diagnosed with a small bowel carcinoid 6 years prior and had hepatic metastasis at the time of diagnosis. He has persistent diarrhea and daily flushing episodes. He is undergoing resection for disease control and for symptomatic relief
MEDS: –Amlodipine 10 mg qd –Pantoprazole 40 mg qd –Oxycontin 80 mg PO TID –Oxycodone 5 mg PO q4 hr prn breakthrough pain (avg 20 mg/day) –Octreotide LAR 40 mg SQ monthly	
PMHx: –Metastatic carcinoid with multiple small bowel tumors and hepatic metastases –Hypertension –Chronic low back pain	
EXAM:	Ht: 69″, Wt: 75 kg, HR: 80 bpm, BP: 114/74, T 36.5 C
HEENT:	No telangiectasia. Pupils equal, round, and reactive to light.
CV:	RRR, no murmurs, rubs, or gallops. No evidence of jugular venous distension.
Resp:	Clear to auscultation, no wheezing, no crackles.
Abdomen:	Well-healed surgical scars. No hepatomegaly.
Extremities:	No peripheral edema.

T.C. Carey (✉)
Department of Anesthesiology, Perioperative, and Pain Medicine, Harvard Medical School, Brigham and Women's Hospital, 75 Francis Street, CWN L1, Boston, MA 02115, USA
e-mail: tccarey@partners.org

© Springer International Publishing AG 2017
L.S. Aglio and R.D. Urman (eds.), *Anesthesiology*,
DOI 10.1007/978-3-319-50141-3_33

1. What are carcinoid tumors?

Carcinoid tumors are rare, slow-growing neuroendocrine tumors that are derived from the enterochromaffin cells, or Kulchitsky cells, of the neuroendocrine system [1]. Carcinoid tumors are now referred to as well-differentiated neuroendocrine tumors [2]. The incidence is estimated to be ~ 2–4 per 100,000 people per year [3, 4]. Carcinoid tumors are associated with multiple endocrine neoplasia (MEN) type 1 syndrome [5, 6].

Carcinoid tumors most commonly present in the gastrointestinal tract (65%), less often in the tracheobronchial tree or lungs (25%), and rarely other areas of the body (i.e., ovaries, pancreas) (10%). In the gastrointestinal (GI) tract, carcinoid tumors most commonly arise in the small bowel (40%) and appendix (19%) [2].

These tumors release a variety of vasoactive substances including serotonin, dopamine, norepinephrine, histamine, bradykinins, tachykinins, and prostaglandins that lead to the symptoms of carcinoid syndrome [4–6].

2. What is carcinoid syndrome?

Carcinoid syndrome is caused by tumor release of vasoactive substances into the systemic circulation leading to the development of a variety of symptoms, including cutaneous flushing, diarrhea, bronchospasm, abdominal cramping, and right-sided heart failure. Flushing and diarrhea are the most commonly experienced symptoms [6, 7], with 90% of patients experiencing flushing and 70% with diarrhea, where those with wheezing (20%) and bronchospasm (10%) are far less common [7]. The flushing of carcinoid syndrome primarily involves the face, neck, and chest and may be associated with a burning sensation.

Carcinoid syndrome is only experienced by ~10% of patients with carcinoid tumors [3, 8, 9]. This is because carcinoid syndrome is most commonly seen in patients with primary tumors of the gastrointestinal system that have metastasized to the liver. Prior to hepatic metastases, the hormones and peptides released by the primary tumor of the GI system are inactivated by hepatic metabolism via the portal circulation. Once the primary tumor has metastasized to the liver, these chemical substances bypass hepatic metabolism and are released directly into the systemic circulation and cause the symptoms of carcinoid syndrome.

Carcinoid syndrome may develop in the absence of hepatic metastases when the primary tumor releases vasoactive substances directly into the systemic circulation. This is true for primary carcinoid tumors located outside of the gastrointestinal tract, as is the case with bronchial, ovarian, and pancreatic tumors [5].

3. What are your preoperative considerations in a patient with suspected carcinoid disease?

A thorough preoperative history and physical exam are necessary to identify patients with carcinoid syndrome, as they may be at higher risk of developing intraoperative carcinoid crisis. This includes assessing for history of flushing, diarrhea, wheezing, shortness of breath, and bronchospasm. It is imperative to evaluate for symptoms associated with carcinoid heart disease and right-sided heart failure (i.e., jugular venous distension, hepatomegaly, peripheral edema, fatigue, etc.), as this significantly increases the patient's risk of morbidity and mortality associated with the procedure [10]. It is important to ascertain how long a patient has been symptomatic, as 50% of patients with carcinoid syndrome will develop carcinoid heart disease [11], and this usually occurs within 24–28 months after onset of carcinoid syndrome [12]. Lastly, one should evaluate whether the patient is treated with octreotide and their current dose. Patients receiving octreotide at baseline may require higher doses to treat symptoms if they develop in the perioperative period [3].

Physical exam should include assessment for wheezing, presence of telangiectasias, signs of right-sided heart failure, presence of murmur, and evaluation of volume status given the risk of volume depletion in the setting of frequent diarrhea.

4. What preoperative laboratory or imaging studies are useful in assessing for the presence of carcinoid disease?

Laboratory evaluation to aid in the diagnosis of a carcinoid tumor includes serum measurement of chromogranin A and 24-h urine measurement of 5-hydroxyindole-3-acetic acid (5-HIAA). Chromogranin A is a glycoprotein secreted by carcinoid tumors and is elevated in 56–100% of people with carcinoid tumors [13]. Because this level correlates with bulk of disease, it can be followed serially to evaluate for disease progression or response to treatment [13]. 5-HIAA is a metabolite of serotonin and is frequently elevated in patients with carcinoid disease, especially in patients with hepatic metastases, and may therefore be normal in patients who have gastrointestinal carcinoid without metastatic disease. Elevated concentration of 5-HIAA is positively correlated with disease progression and worsened prognosis [12]. High levels of 5-HIAA preoperatively has also been demonstrated to be a risk factor for increased perioperative complications and death [10].

An octreotide scan, or somatostatin receptor scintigraphy, is the most sensitive imaging modality for identifying the presence of carcinoid tumors and metastatic disease [14]. Radiolabeled octreotide is injected into the body and binds to the somatostatin receptors of carcinoid tumors, which can then be viewed on imaging. Conventional MRI and CT scan should also be reviewed to evaluate for the presence of metastatic disease.

5. (A) How common is carcinoid heart disease in patients with carcinoid tumors and what are the implications of carcinoid heart disease?

Carcinoid heart disease (CHD) occurs in more than 50% of patients with known carcinoid syndrome [11] and may be the presenting symptom of carcinoid syndrome in up to 20% of patients [15]. CHD is associated with an increase in morbidity and mortality in patients with carcinoid disease [15–18]. Patients with CHD have a 31% 3-year survival rate compared to 60% in patients without CHD [12]. Given the increased morbidity and mortality associated with CHD, these patients are at increased risk of perioperative complications, and it is critical to identify these patients in the preoperative setting.

(B) Describe the pathophysiology of carcinoid heart disease and what valvular abnormalities are most commonly seen.

CHD is classically characterized by plaque-like deposits of fibrous tissue on the endocardial surfaces of valve leaflets, chordae tendineae, papillary muscles, and cardiac chambers [16]. High concentrations of serotonin, along with other vasoactive substances, released by carcinoid tumors into the vena cava and, subsequently, the right heart, are implicated in triggering the pathological formation of these plaque-like deposits [15, 16]. These mediators then pass through the pulmonary circulation and are degraded before they are able to trigger the same pathological response in the left heart [15, 16]. As a result, the valves of the right heart are affected in >90% of patients with CHD, with only 10% of patients having evidence of left heart involvement [15, 16]. Left heart involvement is more commonly seen in patients with a patent foramen ovale, allowing flow of these mediators into the left heart prior to their degradation by the pulmonary circulation [15, 16]. The most common valvular abnormalities seen in CHD are tricuspid insufficiency and pulmonary stenosis.

(C) What should your preoperative assessment include to evaluate for the presence of CHD?

Clinically, patients may initially have subtle, nonspecific symptoms of fatigue or dyspnea on exertion. As the valvular disease progresses, more classic signs and symptoms of right-sided heart failure may be evident. A focused physical exam should be performed to evaluate for the presence of murmur, elevated jugular venous pressure, peripheral edema, hepatosplenomegaly, and ascites [15]. Having frequent episodes of daily flushing (>3 episodes/day) has been shown to be an independent risk factor for development and progression of CHD [18].

(D) What additional laboratory or imaging studies are useful in evaluating for the presence and/or severity of CHD?

Laboratory evaluation of patients with carcinoid tumors can help to identify patients who are more likely to have CHD. Higher levels of 5-hydroxyindole-3-acetic acid (5-HIAA) in the urine have been correlated with increased risk of developing CHD and progression of CHD on echocardiography [15, 16, 18]. N-terminal pro-brain natriuretic peptide (NT-proBNP), a natriuretic peptide released by the atria and ventricles in response to increased wall stress secondary to volume and/or pressure overload, has been shown to have a high sensitivity (87%) and specificity (80%) in predicting CHD, even in patients without carcinoid syndrome. An NT-proBNP >260 pg/mL can be used to rule out significant carcinoid heart disease [15–17].

Patients who have carcinoid syndrome, especially with frequent flushing episodes, symptoms or exam findings concerning for CHD, high levels of 5-HIAA or NT-proBNP, should be further evaluated with transthoracic echocardiography to better evaluate for and/or characterize the severity of the patient's CHD.

6. What additional laboratory or diagnostic studies would you want preoperatively?

As outlined above, serum chromogranin A, 24-h urine collection of 5-HIAA, and, in some cases, NT-proBNP are useful in characterizing the burden of disease in patients with carcinoid. In addition to these studies, a chemistry panel should be obtained to evaluate for the presence of volume depletion, electrolyte abnormality, and hyperchloremic metabolic acidosis in the setting of diarrhea. Imaging studies, including octreoscan, should be reviewed to evaluate for the presence of liver metastases and burden of disease. If you suspect carcinoid heart disease, obtaining an electrocardiogram and transthoracic echocardiogram is prudent to better characterize cardiac function.

7. In addition to standard ASA monitors, what access and intraoperative monitoring do you think is necessary to manage this patient?

One should obtain large bore intravenous access given the potential need for fluid resuscitation in the event of carcinoid crisis. This is even more critical if there is a high risk of blood loss with the planned surgical procedure. Preinduction intra-arterial monitoring is necessary, given the need for continual hemodynamic monitoring during induction of anesthesia and the remainder of the procedure. Central venous access may also be necessary, especially when vasopressor support is likely, as may be the case in patients with carcinoid heart disease or other significant medical comorbidities.

8. What is carcinoid crisis?

Carcinoid crisis is a more severe, and potentially life-threatening, manifestation of the signs of carcinoid syndrome, where release of vasoactive substances from the carcinoid tumor or metastases leads to the development of severe flushing, bronchospasm, tachycardia, and/or hemodynamic instability to the point of complete vascular collapse [1].

9. When is carcinoid crisis more likely to develop?

Carcinoid crisis can be triggered by induction of anesthesia, direct tumor manipulation, embolization procedures, chemotherapy with resultant tumor lysis, physical exam, stress, anxiety, pain, light plane of anesthesia, hypertension, hypotension, hypercapnia, hypothermia, and use of medications that may trigger carcinoid crisis (sympathomimetics and histamine releasing drugs) [11, 19]. While these perioperative events are considered to be periods where patients are at increased risk of developing carcinoid crisis, it is critical to remain ever vigilant as crisis has been shown to occur spontaneously in the patient with carcinoid disease [19].

10. Which patients are at risk for developing carcinoid crisis?

Patients with known carcinoid syndrome, hepatic metastases, or primary carcinoid tumors outside of the GI tract are thought to be at higher risk of developing carcinoid crisis. Multiple studies and published guidelines suggest that only patients with symptomatic carcinoid, or carcinoid syndrome, are at risk of developing carcinoid crisis. Some even suggest that patients without preoperative symptoms do not require prophylactic treatment [7, 20, 21]. In a retrospective study by Massimino et al., they found that carcinoid crisis was just as likely to occur in patients without carcinoid syndrome as those with carcinoid syndrome, and the only predictor of intraoperative carcinoid crisis was the presence of hepatic metastasis [20]. Massimino et al. [20] discuss that even in the absence of hepatic metastases on preoperative imaging, any patient with carcinoid disease should be presumed to be at risk for carcinoid crisis given that a significant percentage of patients have hepatic metastases that are not apparent on preoperative imaging, but are instead identified intraoperatively.

11. What steps can be taken to minimize the development of carcinoid crisis?

Avoiding intraoperative carcinoid crisis begins with a thorough preoperative evaluation, as outlined above, to better characterize the patient's burden of disease, presence of metastases, and presence of carcinoid heart disease. Management of these patients frequently requires multidisciplinary communication with the surgical team, oncologist, endocrinologist, and, if applicable, cardiologist, to ensure the patient is optimized for surgery.

Adequate preoperative anxiolysis can be achieved with benzodiazepines or a nonhistamine releasing opioid, to avoid stress induced catecholamine release. Medications targeted toward blocking the production or effects of vasoactive substances released by the tumor can be administered preoperatively. These medications include H1 and H2 blockers. Some reports recommend administration of corticosteroids or serotonin blockers, like cyproheptadine [5], but the effectiveness of these agents is debated [22]. Octreotide is the mainstay of pre, intra, and postoperative treatment of carcinoid disease and carcinoid crisis.

Intraoperatively, a slow, controlled induction is essential to minimize sympathetic stimulation and avoid carcinoid crisis. In cases where the patient is at risk for aspiration, the need for rapid sequence intubation must be weighed against the potential for less hemodynamic control and risk of carcinoid crisis. In these situations, remifentanil can be an ideal agent to use for blunting the sympathetic response to laryngoscopy as it is a potent analgesic that is rapidly titratable [23].

Given that carcinoid crisis can also develop in response to light anesthesia and tumor manipulation, it is imperative to ensure that the patient is adequately anesthetized, especially during more stimulating parts of the procedure. Close intraoperative communication with the surgical team is essential in the care of these patients. If symptoms develop during tumor manipulation, the surgeon should stop surgical stimulation until adequate hemodynamic control is achieved.

12. What is octreotide?

Octreotide is a somatostatin analogue that binds to the somatostatin receptor and prevents release of vasoactive substances by carcinoid tumors. Octreotide has proven to be invaluable in the treatment of carcinoid syndrome and in the prevention and treatment of carcinoid crisis [5, 9].

13. How and why is octreotide used in the perioperative period in patients with carcinoid disease? What is the dose?

Patients with carcinoid syndrome are frequently on octreotide for management of their disease in the preoperative setting. If not already on octreotide prior to surgery, these patients may require preoperative treatment in the weeks leading up to surgery. Interdisciplinary planning with the surgeon, endocrinologist, and oncologist is necessary to help determine whether or not the patient would benefit from preoperative treatment with octreotide.

There is not a clear consensus on which patients should receive a prophylactic bolus dose of octreotide. Where some guidelines recommend the use of prophylactic octreotide only in patients with preoperative symptoms, other institutions routinely administer prophylactic octreotide to any patient with carcinoid disease, even if they are asymptomatic preoperatively [20]. As outlined above, patients with carcinoid heart disease, patients with highly elevated levels of 5-HIAA, hepatic metastases, and carcinoid syndrome have all been associated with more advanced disease, and therefore may all benefit from prophylactic treatment with octreotide. Until there is a more reliable predictor for development of carcinoid crisis, the patient specific and surgical specific risk factors must be assessed in order to decide whether or not prophylactic treatment is warranted.

The recommended prophylactic dose of octreotide required to prevent carcinoid crisis is widely variable, and ranges from a bolus of 50–500 mcg IV preoperatively, with or without the use of an intraoperative infusion of 50–150 mcg IV/h [3, 11, 20]. Infusions up to 500 mcg/h have been reported [11]. Patients who have been on chronic octreotide therapy for symptom management have been shown to require higher doses of octreotide to treat carcinoid crisis [3]. It is, therefore, important to clarify whether a patient was taking octreotide preoperatively and to quantify their dose.

Octreotide should be readily available for any patient with known or presumed carcinoid disease, even without carcinoid syndrome, as these patients are at risk of developing intraoperative carcinoid crisis [19, 20]. In the event of carcinoid crisis, an octreotide bolus of 100–500 mcg every 5–10 min should be administered until physiological derangements resolve.

14. Is octreotide always effective?

While octreotide is considered the mainstay in treatment of carcinoid crisis and associated with decrease in frequency of intraoperative complications [5], it is not 100% effective in reversing the signs of carcinoid crisis [9, 20]. The anesthesiologist and surgeon should work together to minimize triggers for development of carcinoid crisis and be prepared with additional treatment modalities including fluid resuscitation and vasopressors.

15. What adverse side effects, if any, are associated with octreotide treatment?

Common adverse effects of treatment with octreotide are relatively minor compared to the life-threatening symptoms associated with carcinoid crisis. They include headache, nausea, vomiting, abdominal cramping, cholestasis, and insulin suppression with resultant hyperglycemia [3]. Patients who are receiving octreotide should have their glucose monitored in the perioperative setting to avoid complications associated with hyperglycemia.

16. What are your goals for induction?

As stated above, patients with carcinoid disease are at risk of developing carcinoid crisis during induction of general anesthesia. A slow, controlled induction with continual hemodynamic monitoring is essential in patients at risk of carcinoid crisis. It is imperative to ensure a deep plane of anesthesia prior to laryngoscopy.

17. Is neuraxial anesthesia appropriate in patients with carcinoid?

Neuraxial anesthesia was previously thought to be relatively contraindicated in patients with carcinoid syndrome secondary to reports of profound hypotension after epidural or spinal placement [24, 25]. More recent data suggest that neuraxial anesthesia may be safely tolerated by patients with carcinoid disease, with case reports of both spinal and epidural anesthesia being well tolerated in patients with known carcinoid syndrome [13, 22, 26]. Neuraxial anesthesia has the advantage of decreasing sympathetic response to surgical stimulation, and pain in the postoperative setting, thereby decreasing the risk of carcinoid crisis. If neuraxial anesthesia is performed, close hemodynamic monitoring is essential as patients may have a profound hypotensive response requiring intervention. In patients with epidural anesthesia, local anesthetics should be administered in a graded fashion to avoid profound hypotension. In patients where spinal anesthesia is to be performed, preoperative optimization with adequate hydration may allow for increased hemodynamic stability. Combination of a moderate dose of local anesthetic with opioids, allows for reduced local anesthetic dose, and may minimize sympathectomy and prevent blocking of the cardiac accelerator fibers [22].

18. What medications should be used or available when providing an anesthetic for a patient with a known carcinoid tumor?

Octreotide is invaluable in the prevention and treatment of carcinoid crisis, and should be available during any case where a patient has known carcinoid disease. Antihistamines can be used to prevent flushing and bronchospasm associated with histamine release. Antiserotonergic agents, such as cyproheptadine, ondansetron, along with corticosteroids to reduce bradykinin production can also be used, though the data on the effectiveness of these agents is inconconclusive [9]. Hypertension should be treated with beta-blockers or by deepening the plane of anesthesia with propofol, volatile agents, or remifentanil [23].

19. What medications should be avoided in patients with carcinoid disease and why?

Medications that stimulate histamine release should be avoided as they may potentiate an exaggerated release of histamine from the tumor. These medications include benzylquinolone, nondepolarizing, neuromuscular blockers (atracurium and, historically, mivacurium), succinylcholine, morphine, and meperidine. Ketamine should be avoided as it causes increase in sympathetic nervous system stimulation. Catecholamine releasing drugs such as ephedrine, norepinephrine, epinephrine should be avoided as they can actually worsen the hypotension secondary to carcinoid crises. In the case of bronchospasm, ipratropium and corticosteroids are preferred to beta-agonists, like albuterol, as they may potentiate mediator release [5].

20. What vasopressor would you use in patients with carcinoid disease and why?

Direct acting peripheral vasoconstrictors, such as phenylephrine, or vasopressin, are preferred in patients with carcinoid disease, as they do not induce catecholamine release [8, 20].

21. Describe the management of carcinoid crisis.

If the patient begins to exhibit signs of carcinoid crisis, i.e., flushing, bronchospasm, or hemodynamic instability, swift management is essential to avoid catastrophic consequences. The surgical team should immediately be notified to cease surgical manipulation until the patient is hemodynamically stable. Octreotide should be administered in incremental doses of 100–500 mcg IV every 5–10 min until the crisis resolves. Fluids should be liberally administered to aid in resuscitation. If the patient has ongoing hypotension, phenylephrine and vasopressin are the vasopressors of choice. While epinephrine and ephedrine should be avoided as they have the potential to worsen hypotension via potentiation of mediator release, there are case reports of successful use of epinephrine and ephedrine in patients with carcinoid crisis. These agents are best reserved for cases of refractory hypotension and cardiovascular collapse unresponsive to the above measures. As stated above, in the case of bronchospasm, ipratropium is preferred to beta-agonists or epinephrine.

22. What are the postoperative considerations for patients with carcinoid syndrome?

Patients are still at risk of developing carcinoid crisis in the postoperative setting. Patients may require advanced level monitoring in the intensive or intermediate care unit to allow for close monitoring of the patient's cardio-respiratory status and to ensure adequate analgesia. Patients may require ongoing treatment with octreotide infusion, for up to 48 h, until they can be transitioned to their home regimen.

References

1. Oberg K. Neuroendocrine gastrointestinal and lung tumors (carcinoid tumors), carcinoid syndrome, and related disorders. In: Melmed S, Polonsky KS, Larsen PR, Kronenberg HM, editors. Williams textbook of endocrinology. 12th ed. Philadelphia: Elsevier Saunders; 2011.
2. Turner JR. The gastrointestinal tract. In: Kumar V, Abbas AK, Aster JC, editors. Robbins and cotran pathologic basis of disease. 9th ed. Philadelphia: Elsevier Saunders; 2015.
3. Seymour N, Sawh SC. Mega-dose intravenous octreotide for the treatment of carcinoid crisis: a systematic review. Can J Anaesth. 2013;60(5):492–9. doi:10.1007/s12630-012-9879-1.
4. Choi CK. Anesthetic considerations and management of a patient with unsuspected carcinoid crisis during hepatic tumor resection. Middle East J Anaesthesiol. 2014;22(5):515–8.
5. Grant F. Anesthetic considerations in the multiple endocrine neoplasia syndromes. Curr Opin Anaesthesiol. 2005;18(3):345–52.
6. Wijeysundera D, Sweitzer B. Preoperative evaluation. In: Miller R, editor. Miller's Anesthesia. 8th ed. Philadelphia: Elsevier Saunders; 2015.
7. Patel C, Mathur M, Escarcega RO, Bove AA. Carcinoid heart disease: current understanding and future directions. Am Heart J. 2014;167(6):789–95. doi:10.1016/j.ahj.2014.03.018.
8. Powell B, Mukhtar AA, Mills GH. Carcinoid: the disease and its implications for anaesthesia. Contin Educ Anaesth Crit Care Pain. 2011;11:9–13. doi:10.1093/bjaceaccp/mkq045.
9. Mancuso K, Kaye AD, Boudreaux JP, Fox CJ, Lang P, Kalarickal PL, Gomez S, Primeaux PJ. Carcinoid syndrome and perioperative anesthetic considerations. J Clin Anesth. 2011;23 (4):329–41. doi:10.1016/j.jclinane.2010.12.009.
10. Kinney MAO, Warner ME, Nagorney DM, Rubin J, Schroeder DR, Maxson PM, Warner MA. Perianaesthetic risks and outcomes of abdominal surgery for metastatic carcinoid tumours. Br J Anaesth. 2001;87:447–52. doi:10.1093/bja/87.3.447.
11. Gupta P, Kaur R, Chaudhary L, Jain A. Management of bronchial carcinoid: An anaesthetic challenge. Indian J Anaesth. 2014;58 (2):202–5. doi:10.4103/0019-5049.130830.
12. Fox DJ, Khattar RS. Carcinoid heart disease: presentation diagnosis and management. Heart. 2004;90(10):1224–8. doi:10.1136/hrt.2004.040329.
13. Woo KM, Imasogie NN, Bruni I, Singh SI. Anaesthetic management of a pregnant woman with carcinoid disease. Int J Obstet Anesth. 2009;18(3):272–5. doi:10.1016/j.ijoa.2009.01.009.
14. Oberg K, Kvols L, Caplin M, Delle Fave G, de Herder W, Rindi G, Ruszniewski P, Woltering EA, Wiedenmann B. Consensus report on the use of somatostatin for the management of neuroendocrine tumors of the gastroenteropancreatic system. Ann Oncol. 2004;15 (6):966–73. doi:10.1093/annonc/mdh216.
15. Gustafsson BI, Hauso O, Drozdov I, Kidd M, Modlin IM. Carcinoid heart disease. Int J Cardiol. 2008;129(3):318–24. doi:10.1016/j.ijcard.2008.02.019.
16. Grozinsky-Glasberg S, Grossman AB, Gross DJ. Carcinoid heart disease: from pathophysiology to treatment—'something in the way it moves'. Neuroendocrinology. 2015;101(4):263–73. doi:10.1159/000381930.
17. Ramage JK, Ahmed A, Ardill J, Bax N, Breen DJ, Caplin ME, Corrie P, Davar J, Davies AH, Lewington V, Meyer T, Newell-Price J, Poston G, Reed N, Rockall A, Steward W, Thakker RV, Toubanakis C, Valle J, Verbeke C, Grossman AB. Guidelines for the management of gastroenteropancreatic neuroendocrine (including carcinoid) tumours (NETs). Gut. 2012;61 (1):6–32. doi:10.1136/gutjnl-2011-300831.
18. Bhattacharyya S, Toumpanakis C, Chilkunda D, Caplin ME, Davar J. Risk factors for the development and progression of carcinoid heart disease. Am J Cardiol. 2011;107(8):1221–6. doi:10.1016/j.amjcard.2010.12.025.
19. Guo LJ, Tang CW. Somatostatin analogues do not prevent carcinoid crisis. Asian Pac J Cancer Prev. 2014;15(16):6679–83.
20. Massimino K, Harrskog O, Pommier S, Pommier R. Octreotide LAR and bolus octreotide are insufficient for preventing intraoperative complications in carcinoid patients. J Surg Oncol. 2013;107:842–6. doi:10.1002/jso.23323.
21. Boudreaux JP, Klimstra DS, Hassan MM, Woltering EA, Jensen RT, Goldsmith SJ, Nutting C, Bushnell DL, Caplin ME, Yao JC. North American neuroendocrine tumor society (NANETS) the NANETS consensus guideline for the diagnosis and management of neuroendocrine tumors: well-differentiated neuroendocrine tumors of the Jejunum, Ileum, Appendix, and Cecum. Pancreas 2010;39(6):753–66. doi:10.1097/MPA.0b013e3181ebb2a5.
22. Orbach-Zinger S, Lombroso R, Eidelman LA. Uneventful spinal anesthesia for a patient with carcinoid syndrome managed with

long-acting octreotide. Can J Anaesth. 2002;49(7):678–81. doi 10.1007/BF03017444.
23. Farling PA, Durairaju AK. Remifentanil and anaesthesia for carcinoid syndrome. Br J Anaesth. 2004;92:893–5. doi:10.1093/bja/aeh135.
24. Mason RA, Steane PA. Carcinoid syndrome: its relevance to the anaesthetist. Anaesthesia. 1976;31:228–42.
25. Vaughan DJA, Brunner MD. Anesthesia for patients with carcinoid syndrome. Int Anesthesiol Clin. 1997;35:129–42.
26. Monteith K, Roaseg OP. Epidural anaesthesia for transurethral resection of the prostate in a patient with carcinoid syndrome. Can J Anaesth. 1990;37(3):349–52. doi:10.1007/BF03005589.

Kidney Transplantation

34

Jonathan Ross

Case

A 52 year old male with hypertension, GERD, Type 2 diabetes, and currently on hemodialysis three times weekly is scheduled for a living, related donor kidney transplant from his sister, who is ABO compatible. The patient had dialysis on the evening before presenting to the hospital for surgery. This morning, laboratory studies show a WBC of 7.2, HCT of 31, RBC of 9.8, Na 132, K 5.6, Glucose 141, Cr 8.1, and BUN 77. On exam, you note that the patient is 5′10″ tall, and weighs 88 kg. He appears well and is afebrile. Vital signs include BP 91/44, HR 98, RR 16, SpO2 96% on room air. His lungs are clear, and heart rate and rhythm are regular. In anticipation of the surgery, he has not had any intake of food or drink today.

What screening is undertaken prior to becoming a candidate for kidney transplant?
Prior to being placed on the list for a transplant, or being eligible for donation of a live organ, all patients undergo a series of evaluations. Prescreening of transplant candidates should involve a comprehensive overview of all organ systems to ensure the overall health of the candidate. Routine CBC, electrolyte, renal, coagulation, and liver bloodwork should be performed on a regular basis as long as the patient is on the candidate list. As well, urinalysis (if the candidate is not anuric), a cardiac workup, and a chest radiograph or CT scan should be performed during the evaluation process [1, 2].

The immune compatibility of the recipient must be assessed and matched with potential donor organs. The individual HLA markers are encoded on the 6th chromosome, and thus can be obtained easily by genetic testing. The closer the HLA match between donor and recipient, the lesser the chance of immune-mediated rejection of the organ.

What immediate preoperative considerations are necessary prior to transplant?
When an organ is eventually assigned to a patient, recipients can fall into two categories—the 'emergency' transplant (i.e., very short notice due to the use of a cadaveric donor organ), and the 'scheduled' transplant (a living related or nonrelated donor organ) [3]. Given the fact that all patients will start from a condition that is essentially an end-stage renal disease (ESRD), it is important in both of these categories to optimize electrolytes and volume status. Immediate preoperative laboratory studies, including a CBC, electrolytes, and coagulation panel are therefore important, with corrections made as needed prior to moving to the operating theater. An unscheduled dialysis session may be warranted if electrolytes are significantly imbalanced, with care given to minimize ultrafiltration in order to preserve intravascular volume [4, 5].

In patients who are diabetic, normalization of blood glucose is essential to minimize infection risk, promote appropriate wound healing, and successful vascular anastomosis [6]. An insulin infusion (with dextrose drip as indicated) has entered the literature as the most rapid and accurate method of titrating blood glucose, however a sliding scale insulin treatment continues to be used in many facilities as well [7, 8].

What comorbidities are common in patients with ESRD?
Once renal output (measured as glomerular filtration rate, GFR) drops below 15 ml/min/1.73 m^2, patients are typically started on dialysis and considered to have ESRD. Virtually every organ system is affected in patients with renal disease, for a variety of reasons. The cardiovascular and hematologic systems are the most consequential for the surgical patient.

J. Ross (✉)
Department of Anesthesia, Baystate Medical Center, 759 Chestnut Street, Springfield, MA 01199, USA
e-mail: jonathan.ross@bhs.org

© Springer International Publishing AG 2017
L.S. Aglio and R.D. Urman (eds.), *Anesthesiology*,
DOI 10.1007/978-3-319-50141-3_34

What cardiovascular comorbidities are seen in these patients?

The volume and pressure increases seen in progressive renal disease typically cause permanent arterial injury, leading to hypertension (from uncontrollable volume overload), as well as worsening vascular response to fluid shifts [9, 10]. Patients also tend to have disregulation of the renin-angiotensin system, since juxtaglomerular cells in the healthy kidney are the principal controlling factor in renin release. There is no clear-cut data for changes in renin production in patients with ESRD; some patients seem to have reduced angiotensin II levels, and some patients have increases in levels of this vasoactive hormone [11].

What Hematologic issues are seen in ESRD patients?

Besides volume overload, the blood also develops increased levels of metabolic waste products, which can result in a metabolic acidosis, hyponatremia, hyperkalemia, hypermagnesemia, and hyperchloremia. Since the changes are usually slow and insidious, the heart can compensate (to some extent) for the higher potassium level, however, if symptoms of hyperkalemia are evident, treatment with calcium is warranted, followed by medications to decrease the serum potassium level (see below) [12]. Hypermagnesemia can cause muscle relaxation and weakness, amongst other more serious cardiac conduction side effects if levels increase [13].

Patients with poor renal function also tend to have decreased erythropoietin levels, which results in reduced production of red blood cells. There is therefore a tendency toward anemia (normochromic and normocytic). In addition to this baseline anemia, the dialysis machine causes significant physical damage to RBCs. Patients frequently receive injections of synthetic epo- or darbepoetin to partially compensate for the underlying issue [14]. Despite the injections, the observed hematocrit remains lower than a nonrenal failure patient. To avoid a relative insufficiency in tissue oxygenation, circulation becomes somewhat hyperdynamic. Patients may also develop an increased 2,3 DPG level in order to shift the oxyhemoglobin dissociation curve to the right, promoting increased tissue oxygenation [15].

This patient has an elevated potassium level, despite having had dialysis the day before. Is this a contraindication to proceeding? How does an elevated potassium level affect the heart?

Potassium and sodium are principal components of the action potential, which is the electrochemical signal propagation seen in the heart and nervous system. Inappropriately high levels of potassium reduce the excitability of the heart, decreasing both pacemaking and overall conduction of electrical signals. As the potassium levels rise, the SA node signal is suppressed, the HIS-bundle conduction becomes inefficient, and the patient enters various stages of heart block, bradycardia, and eventually cardiac arrest [16].

Patients with chronic renal disease tend to have an elevated serum potassium level due to the inability of the damaged kidney to effectively eliminate the superfluous fraction of this electrolyte. Fortunately, the slow and chronic buildup of potassium seen in these patients allows for some cardiac compensation to occur, and the typical signs of hyperkalemia-related EKG changes (i.e., cardiac conduction changes) occur at a higher than expected serum potassium level. In this particular case, as long as the EKG does not show changes of hyperkalemia (peaked T-waves, p-wave flattening, AV-block, etc.), it is reasonable to proceed with the surgery [17].

If the potassium level was 6.6 mEq/L instead of 5.6, how would this affect the decision to proceed with the surgery?

Although patients with renal failure can have chronically elevated potassium levels, serum levels above 6.0 mEq/L ARE typically a contraindication to surgical procedures, since even small increases in serum potassium from that point can lead to serious conduction abnormalities in an unpredictable manner. The potassium should be decreased prior to coming to the OR. This can be accomplished via an additional round of dialysis, and can transiently be achieved through the use of potassium-reducing medications. An infusion of insulin and glucose will assist in reducing potassium levels, as will albuterol, or bicarbonate. These medications function by driving potassium into the intracellular compartment, decreasing the circulating level.

Is an arterial line necessary for this case? What about other monitors?

An arterial line is typically not required for kidney transplantation. The use of an arterial line is designed to assist with blood pressure monitoring in surgeries where there is either a high probability of serious hemodynamic fluctuations, a significant number of blood samples required for laboratory or point-of-care analysis, a patient with significant comorbidities (such as advanced aortic stenosis), a patient whose body habitus makes standard blood pressure cuffs unreliable, or cases where vasoactive drugs are used to achieve specific blood pressures at specific times (e.g., an aneurysm clipping). Standard ASA monitors are an appropriate choice if none of these factors are expected.

What type of venous access will be needed for this case?

A typical renal transplant is not a procedure with a high blood loss potential, and should be manageable with one or two 18G IVs [18]. Neither central access nor CVP monitoring is typically needed, unless indicated by a comorbid condition, or lack of alternative vascular access options.

What are the choices for anesthesia type in this case?

Kidney transplant is a procedure usually performed under a general anesthetic. There is literature supporting a neuraxial technique, including the use of spinal anesthesia, epidural alone, and CSE [19, 20]. Issues requiring consideration in selecting a regional anesthetic technique include the surgical use of heparin (or other anticoagulants) in order to reduce the risk of graft thrombosis, and the increased bleeding tendency of patients on long-term dialysis.

What kinds of changes to drug metabolism are expected in patients about to receive a renal transplant?

There are several marked changes in physiology in the pretransplant patient that can result in altered metabolism of common medications. Decreases in serum albumin levels results in a higher plasma level of protein-bound drugs. Oddly, the amount of propofol (a highly protein-bound drug) needed for induction or maintenance of anesthesia increases in these patients [21, 22]. This is a result of the hypervolemia and hyperdynamic circulation (a result of anemia, see above) in these patients (Table 34.1).

Is there any controversy regarding the use of sevoflurane in ESRD or in patients undergoing a renal transplant?

Historically, the use of sevoflurane has been associated with the potential for production of renal toxic compounds, including inorganic fluoride ions [24], and the production of 'compound A' (a fluorinated ether) when interacting with CO_2 absorbers containing a strong base, such as NaOH [25, 26]. In reality, studies have not demonstrated development of nephrotoxicity from fluoride ions at the levels produced by sevoflurane, either in humans or animal models [27]. Animal studies in rats have, however, demonstrated the potential for temporary renal toxicity from the combination of sevoflurane, low fresh gas flow rates, and strong-base CO_2 absorbers. Since, in humans, the enzyme pathway utilized for transforming the rebreathed compound A into a nephrotoxic material is 10–30 fold less active than in rats, no studies have demonstrated a transient renal dysfunction stemming from sevoflurane use in humans [28, 29]. The FDA does suggest that the use of fresh gas flow over 2L/min when using sevoflurane for greater than 1 h, however, no other country has a similar restriction in place.

What is the difference in transplanting kidneys from living related, living nonrelated, and cadaveric sources?

There are several advantages of a living donor (related or nonrelated) transplant over a cadaveric donor. The advantages include:

- A shorter wait for transplantation. The supply of deceased donor organs is limited, and can have a significant waiting time for a patient awaiting transplantation. For some patients with end-stage renal disease, their overall health can decline rapidly while waiting for a transplant. A living donor, as a volunteer, can effectively eliminate the wait time for the intended recipient, and also, by removing that recipient from the waiting list, shortens the list for all recipients [2].
- Faster recovery time for the recipient. Although modern stasis methods help with preservation of tissue, an organ from a living donor has a higher chance of functioning immediately after implantation, decreasing the overall hospital length of stay [3].
- Improved long-term outcome. There is a higher overall graft survival rate from a living donor organ rather than a cadaveric kidney. For the first two years after transplant,

Table 34.1 Changes to Drug Pharmacokinetics in ESRD

Agent	Pharmacokinetics [23]
Propofol	Increased amounts needed
Etomidate	Not affected
Ketamine	Not affected
Morphine	Metabolites can accumulate, causing increased CNS/respiratory depression
Fentanyl, Remifentanil, Sufentanil	Essentially unaffected
Succinylcholine	Unaffected, but patients may have elevated baseline potassium
Nondepolarizing relaxants	Decreased amounts needed (delayed clearance) except with atracurium/cisatracurium
Neostigmine	Prolonged effect
Glycopyrrolate, Atropine	Prolonged effect
Midazolam	Unaffected

there is typically excellent function from any graft. After that time, the failure rate of cadaveric kidneys is higher than in living donors. Although the exact reason for this is unknown, it may be related to inflammatory cytokine circulation at the time of brain death, prior to explantation of the organ [30].

The overall outcome between living related versus living-unrelated kidney transplants is similar in terms of renal function decline over time and graft survival length [31, 32]. The major concern with an unrelated donor is in the frequency of rejection (see below), however, modern immunosuppression methods are quite effective in 'hiding' the HLA incompatibilities of nonrelated donors from the cellular response system.

What kinds of graft (transplanted organ) rejections can occur?

In a kidney transplant, the principal types of rejections include:

- *Hyperacute*: rejection immediately, within minutes to hours of transplantation. This type of rejection is due to preexisting antibodies against major antigens on the new tissue. This is similar to an ABO mismatch in blood transfusions. The body will generate a systemic inflammatory immune response to any foreign tissue that triggers a hyperacute reaction [33]. This is an uncommon type of rejection, since antibody screening with the preoperative blood samples can test for a positive crossmatch of T-cells or B-cells. However, there are examples of HLA compatible kidneys undergoing this type of reaction as well, so it is still an important contributor to failed transplantations. It is believed that a prior blood transfusion, pregnancy, or previous transplant is the original cause for the creation of the responsible circulating cytotoxic IgG HLA antibodies. Besides an inflammatory response, these antibodies can also agglutinate red blood cells and cause widespread clumping of blood cells inside the new kidney arteries, starving the kidney of oxygen, and leading to tissue death [33, 34].
- *Acute*: One week to several months following transfusion. This type of graft rejection is related to the attack of protective cells (cellular immunity) rather than the formation of antibodies (humoral immunity). Cytotoxic T-cells, killer cells, and other cytokine-mediated immune cells migrate into the foreign tissue and cause apoptosis, resulting in tissue death. This type of reaction can be mitigated with proper immunosuppressive treatment, and is believed to occur in 15–20% of all kidney transplants. Multiple (treated) episodes of acute rejection can lead to chronic rejection [35, 36].
- *Chronic*: More than one year after graft placement. Almost all transplant patients eventually develop some form of chronic rejection. This type of rejection involves the fibrosis (scarring) of the structural and functional components of the donor kidney from cell death and restructuring.

What is done to decrease the chances of immune-mediated rejection of the organ?

Although plasmapheresis is occasionally utilized in patients receiving living kidneys from non-HLA matching donors, the principal method of decreasing rejection of the transplanted kidney is the use of immunosuppressants. A combination of monoclonal antibodies, steroids, calcineurin inhibitors, and TOR inhibitors are used to decrease the immune response over time [37, 38]. There are three phases of the immunosuppressive regimen:

- *Induction therapy*, which involves the greatest level of immunosuppression. It is started before or during the transplant. This phase is the most significant to the anesthesiologist, since some of these medications will be required during the procedure, most commonly, steroids and campath (see below).
- *Maintenance therapy*, designed to prevent acute rejection over the first several months
- *Long-term immunosuppression*, which is individually titrated for optimal effect.

The surgeon asks for an infusion of Campath during the case. What is Campath?

Alemtuzumab (Campath) is a monoclonal antibody that was originally used in treatment of B-cell and T-Cell lymphoma [39]. It binds to the surface of lymphocytes and targets them for destruction. This function has been adapted for use in organ transplantation, since it effectively makes this medication an excellent immunosuppressant.

What are some of the principal surgical complications of kidney transplant?

There are a number of surgical morbidities that are seen in patients who undergo renal implantation [40–42]. Since the kidney is a bridge between the circulatory and the urinary system, functional problems can occur with either of these components.

From a vascular point of view, the most immediately obvious would be an anastomotic failure of the renal vessels to the new kidney. Since each renal artery receives approximately 12–15% of the cardiac output, potentially hundreds of milliliters of blood loss per minute can occur in the event of vessel rupture. Fortunately, this is an uncommon occurrence in kidney transplant procedures. More commonly seen is renal artery thrombosis, which occurs from a low-flow state in the renal artery, stemming either from an inappropriately tight anastomosis causing obstruction, vascular 'kinking,' or significant hypotension. Arterial kinking presents as acute cessation of urine flow. If this complication is recognized quickly (by Doppler ultrasound), it is possible to salvage the organ. Doppler ultrasound is also utilized to diagnose complications in the venous connections of the kidney. An acute venous thrombosis can result in edema of the kidney, and also cause loss of the organ [43].

- Other complications include errors in connecting the urinary system, which can result in backflow of urine and hydronephrosis (if too tight), or urine leaking (often from necrosis of the tip of the ureter). Ultrasound would demonstrate a perinephric fluid collection, and the patient often presents with fever and decreased urine output.

The patient had dialysis the morning of the surgery. Are there any concerns with the timing of dialysis?
Although dialysis removes many waste products from the body and typically provides the benefit of normalizing electrolytes, the ultrafiltration component can result in major body fluid shifts, and hypovolemia is a significant possibility. Fluid boluses and increased rates of continuous infusions may be warranted [44].

The blood vessels are anastomosed, and the organ 'pinks up' as blood starts to flow through it. You notice an increase in etCO$_2$ and peaked T-waves. What is the cause?
The longer the 'down time' of an organ as it sits outside of the body, the more waste metabolites will build up. Cadaveric kidneys are typically placed in cold storage in a solution that contains high potassium (to prevent intracellular diffusion of potassium), and can remain viable for up to 40 h [45]. The goal for living donors is to have ischemic times less of than 30 min (when on ice), and no more than 3–5 min when warm [46, 47]. Without perfusion, toxic metabolites build up in the preserved organ quickly. Cooling shows the overall metabolism of the kidney and decreases waste product production. However, it does not stop cellular functioning altogether. Without oxygen, energy consumption within the cells is necessarily anaerobic, and if available fuel sources are exhausted, some cells will undergo apoptosis and rupture, releasing more toxic products. When perfusion is restored, the built up toxic metabolites are 'washed' into circulation. These waste products include potassium (which can cause the peaked T-waves seen in this question), and carbon dioxide, which is buffered by the bicarbonate system in the blood and breathed out of the lungs, increasing the etCO$_2$. Both of these effects are transient, and only seen very soon after connecting the transplanted organ to vascular support, unless the organ ischemia continues.

What are the fluid goals for the case?
The primary concern for the new kidney is to avoid ischemia and acute tubular necrosis (ATN) [48]. This is principally achieved by keeping a positive fluid balance. Presuming that the patient does not have severe CHF or some other significant contraindication to high fluid balance, fluids are typically given to maintain a CVP between 10 and 15 mmHg, and PA pressure of 18–20 mm, in an effort to optimize renal blood flow. Since neither a CVP nor a PA catheter is commonly placed during a kidney transplant, and given that (until the graft is in place) the patient is anuric, other estimates of fluid balance must typically be used. Often patients will be 'tanked up' with crystalloid to the point where they can maintain a systolic blood pressure between 130 and 150 mmHg while under anesthesia. This usually requires fluid administration in the 10–20 ml/kg/h range [44, 49].

What types of fluids are used to achieve this?
Typically, a form of crystalloid is utilized as the principal fluid. Although there is literature on the use of hexastarches and other artificial colloids, either normal saline or a combination of half-normal saline with bicarbonate (for isotonicity) is most often seen in transplant regimens. Traditionally, potassium-including solutions are not administered during these procedures, due to the fear of worsening the hyperkalemia seen in patients with inadequate graft perfusion. Since relying entirely on normal saline can lead to a hyperchloremic metabolic acidosis, the use of half-normal saline (with bicarb) interspersed with normal saline has come into favor. Several liters are expected to be infused during the case, in order to maximize the vascular fluid space. A blood volume >70 ml/kg is positively associated with faster return to function of the transplanted kidney [50].

Is there any contraindication to the use of diuretics during transplantation?
Loop diuretics are commonly used to increase urine flow through the transplanted kidney. Mannitol, as an osmotic agent, improves renal blood flow (by increasing blood volume), and is associated with better outcomes in terms of initiating renal function from the transplanted organ. The only potential issue with diuretics would be in a patient who, due to severe comorbid disease, could not achieve an appropriate blood volume via crystalloid transfusion, and entered a hypovolemic state. This is unlikely when dealing with the urine volumes produced by a newly transplanted

kidney, but can be seen in some cases where renal function is immediately established [51, 52].

Is there any contraindication to the use of pressors during transplantation?

Traditionally, use of any vasoactive with alpha-constrictor properties has been discouraged. As with any transplanted system, there is hesitation on the part of surgeons when considering the use of these vascular constricting mediations for fear of decreasing flow to the organ in question. Despite this intrinsic fear, the literature suggests that there may not be as significant of an impact in the use of low-dose phenylephrine or ephedrine in kidney transplantation as previously believed, and this question is still an ongoing investigation [53, 54].

The surgeon asks for a low-dose dopamine infusion. Is there any merit to requesting low-dose dopamine?

Low-dose dopamine (0.5–2.5 mcg/kg/min) is believed to preferentially activate the dopamine (D1) receptors in renal vascular beds, theoretically increasing blood flow to the region, and thereby improving graft survival rates. However, the merit of this practice has come into question, as multiple studies have shown that there is no correlation between low-dose dopamine and graft survival rates, possibly due to the fact that a transplanted kidney does not respond to dopamine in the same way as an endogenous kidney. There is also a question of decreased long-term survival and other negative side effects, which appear to correlate with patients receiving low-dose dopamine infusions during their transplant and subsequent hospital stay [55].

Should the post-transplant patient recover in the PACU or the ICU?

The typical renal transplant should be extubatable following the procedure and would not be a candidate for ICU level of care unless they demonstrate signs of sepsis, fluid overload, or other acute cardiopulmonary events. PACU staff should be available to observe for signs of hyperacute graft rejection or renal circulatory problems (pain out of proportion for surgery and anuria), which can require immediate surgical re-exploration.

The patient has severe hypertension in the PACU, with a blood pressure of 230/115. What is a Goldblatt kidney?

Goldblatt kidney, or nephrogenic hypertension, is a condition where the kidney is actively undergoing ischemia, which it interprets as insufficient pressure (or flow), and releases renin in order to increase blood pressure (and thus, presumably, blood flow) [56]. The result is increased systemic hypertension mediated via the renin-angiotensin system. Although the pressure can be temporarily lowered with vasodilators, the required treatment is relief of the renal artery stricture. In a post-transplant patient, the most likely cause is at the site of renal artery anastomosis, which may be overly tightly sewn, clotted, or kinked. A surgical reexploration is warranted.

What are the options for postoperative pain relief?

Due to the size of the organ being implanted, kidney transplantation is almost always performed as an open procedure. As such, the incision will require significant postoperative pain management. Since the location is retroperitoneal, and should not involve visceral manipulation or peritoneal incision, the most significant pain source is the incision itself. The most common pain management technique is the use of PCA analgesia with morphine or dilaudid. Studies do show that epidural analgesia is superior for pain management, but it continues to be a less commonly utilized modality of management for these procedures. [44, 57, 58, 59]. NSAID use has been shown to be detrimental to patients with renal disease, and is not typically utilized in renal transplant pain management [60, 61]. Tylenol metabolism is altered in patients with renal transplantation and its use may also be best avoided or reduced [62].

References

1. Kittleson MM. Preoperative cardiac evaluation of kidney transplant recipients: does testing matter? Am J Transplant (official journal of the American Society of Transplantation and the American Society of Transplant Surgeons). 2011;11(12):2553–4.
2. Brennan TV, Fuller TF, Vincenti F, Chan S, Chang CK, Bostrom A, et al. Living donor kidney transplant recipients and clinical trials: participation profiles and impact on post-transplant care. Am J Transplant (official journal of the American Society of Transplantation and the American Society of Transplant Surgeons). 2006;6(10):2429–35.
3. Torkaman M, Khalili-Matin-Zadeh Z, Azizabadi-Farahani M, Moghani-Lankarani M, Assari S, Pourfarziani V, et al. Outcome of living kidney transplant: pediatric in comparison to adults. Transpl Proc. 2007;39(4):1088–90.
4. Wolfe RA, Ashby VB, Milford EL, Ojo AO, Ettenger RE, Agodoa LY, et al. Comparison of mortality in all patients on dialysis, patients on dialysis awaiting transplantation, and recipients of a first cadaveric transplant. New Engl J Med. 1999;341(23):1725–30.
5. Rostaing L, Maggioni S, Hecht C, Hermelin M, Faudel E, Kamar N, et al. Efficacy and safety of tandem hemodialysis and immunoadsorption to desensitize kidney transplant candidates. Exp Clin Transplant (official journal of the Middle East Society for Organ Transplantation). 2015;13(Suppl 1):165–9.
6. Reese PP, Israni AK. Best option for transplant candidates with type 1 diabetes and a live kidney donor: a bird in the hand is worth two in the bush. Clin J Am Soc Nephrol CJASN. 2009;4(4):700–2.
7. Dukes JL, Seelam S, Lentine KL, Schnitzler MA, Neri L. Health-related quality of life in kidney transplant patients with diabetes. Clin Transplant. 2013;27(5):E554–62.

8. Fourtounas C. Transplant options for patients with type 2 diabetes and chronic kidney disease. World J Transplant. 2014;4(2):102–10.
9. Malyszko J, Bachorzewska-Gajewska H, Tomaszuk-Kazberuk A, Matuszkiewicz-Rowinska J, Durlik M, Dobrzycki S. Cardiovascular disease and kidney transplantation evaluation of potential transplant recipient. Pol Arch Med Wewn. 2014;124(11):608–16.
10. Keddis MT, Bhutani G, El-Zoghby ZM. Cardiovascular disease burden and risk factors before and after kidney transplant. Cardiovasc Hematol Disord: Drug Targets. 2014;14(3):185–94.
11. Hestin D, Mertes PM, Hubert J, Claudon M, Mejat E, Renoult E, et al. Relationship between blood pressure and renin, angiotensin II and atrial natriuretic factor after renal transplantation. Clin Nephrol. 1997;48(2):98–103.
12. Nasir K, Ahmad A. Treatment of hyperkalemia in patients with chronic kidney disease: a comparison of calcium polystyrene sulphonate and sodium polystyrene sulphonate. J Ayub Medical Coll Abbottabad JAMC. 2014;26(4):455–8.
13. Gill K, Fink JC, Gilbertson DT, Monda KL, Muntner P, Lafayette RA, et al. Red blood cell transfusion, hyperkalemia, and heart failure in advanced chronic kidney disease. Pharmacoepidemiol Drug Saf. 2015;24(6):654–62.
14. Belonje AM, de Boer RA, Voors AA. Recombinant human Epo treatment: beneficial in chronic kidney disease, chronic heart failure, or both? Editorial to: "correction of anemia with erythropoietin in chronic kidney disease (stage 3 or 4): effects on cardiac performance by Pappas et al." Cardiovasc Drugs Ther/Sponsored International Society of Cardiovascular Pharmacotherapy. 2008;22(1):1–2.
15. Mucke D, Strauss D, Eschke P, Gross J, Grossmann P, Daniel A. Adenine nucleotide- and 2,3-diphosphoglycerate metabolism in human erythrocytes in chronic kidney insufficiency. Z fur Urol und Nephrol. 1977;70(1):39–49.
16. Welch A, Maroz N, Wingo CS. Hyperkalemia: getting to the heart of the matter. Nephrol Dial Transplant (Official Publication of the European Dialysis and Transplant Association—European Renal Association). 2013;28(1):15–6.
17. Bugge JF. Hyperkalemia, heart failure and reduced renal function. Tidsskrift for den Norske laegeforening: tidsskrift for praktisk medicin, ny raekke. 2010;130(13):1354–5.
18. de Weerd AE, van Agteren M, Leebeek FW, Ijzermans JN, Weimar W, Betjes MG. ABO-incompatible kidney transplant recipients have a higher bleeding risk after antigen-specific immunoadsorption. Transplant Int (Official Journal of the European Society for Organ Transplantation). 2015;28(1):25–33.
19. Hadimioglu N, Ertug Z, Bigat Z, Yilmaz M, Yegin A. A randomized study comparing combined spinal epidural or general anesthesia for renal transplant surgery. Transpl Proc. 2005;37(5):2020–2.
20. Lopez-Herrera-Rodriguez D, Guerrero-Dominguez R, Acosta Martinez J, Sanchez Carrillo F. [Epidural analgesia for renal transplant surgery]. Rev Esp Anestesiol Reanim. 2015;62(1):54–5.
21. Nathan N, Debord J, Narcisse F, Dupuis JL, Lagarde M, Benevent D, et al. Pharmacokinetics of propofol and its conjugates after continuous infusion in normal and in renal failure patients: a preliminary study. Acta Anaesthesiol Belg. 1993;44(3):77–85.
22. Osborne R, Joel S, Grebenik K, Trew D, Slevin M. The pharmacokinetics of morphine and morphine glucuronides in kidney failure. Clin Pharmacol Ther. 1993;54(2):158–67.
23. Elston AC, Bayliss MK, Park GR. Effect of renal failure on drug metabolism by the liver. Br J Anaesth. 1993;71(2):282–90.
24. Bito H, Atsumi K, Katoh T, Ohmura M. Effects of sevoflurane anesthesia on plasma inorganic fluoride concentrations during and after cardiac surgery. J Anesth. 1999;13(3):156–60.
25. Iyer RA, Anders MW. Cysteine conjugate beta-lyase-dependent biotransformation of the cysteine S-conjugates of the sevoflurane degradation product compound A in human, nonhuman primate, and rat kidney cytosol and mitochondria. Anesthesiology. 1996;85(6):1454–61.
26. Versichelen LF, Bouche MP, Rolly G, Van Bocxlaer JF, Struys MM, De Leenheer AP, et al. Only carbon dioxide absorbents free of both NaOH and KOH do not generate compound A during in vitro closed-system sevoflurane: evaluation of five absorbents. Anesthesiology. 2001;95(3):750–5.
27. Driessen B, Zarucco L, Steffey EP, McCullough C, Del Piero F, Melton L, et al. Serum fluoride concentrations, biochemical and histopathological changes associated with prolonged sevoflurane anaesthesia in horses. J Vet Med A Physiol Pathol Clin Med. 2002;49(7):337–47.
28. Funk W, Gruber M, Jakob W, Hobbhahn J. Compound A does not accumulate during closed circuit sevoflurane anaesthesia with the Physioflex. Br J Anaesth. 1999;83(4):571–5.
29. Kharasch ED, Schroeder JL, Sheffels P, Liggitt HD. Influence of sevoflurane on the metabolism and renal effects of compound A in rats. Anesthesiology. 2005;103(6):1183–8.
30. Yabu JM, Fontaine MJ. ABO-incompatible living donor kidney transplantation without post-transplant therapeutic plasma exchange. J Clin Apheresis. 2015.
31. Ahmadi F, Ali-Madadi A, Lessan-Pezeshki M, Khatami M, Mahdavi-Mazdeh M, Razeghi E, et al. Pre-transplant calcium-phosphate-parathormone homeostasis as a risk factor for early graft dysfunction. Saudi J Kidney Diseas Transplant (An Official Publication of the Saudi Center for Organ Transplantation Saudi Arabia). 2008;19(1):54–8.
32. Ahmad N, Ahmed K, Khan MS, Calder F, Mamode N, Taylor J, et al. Living-unrelated donor renal transplantation: an alternative to living-related donor transplantation? Ann R Coll Surg Engl. 2008;90(3):247–50.
33. Boehmig HJ, Giles GR, Amemiya H, Wilson CB, Coburg AJ, Genton E, et al. Hyperacute rejection of renal homografts: with particular reference to coaglation changes, humoral antibodies, and formed blood elements. Transpl Proc. 1971;3(2):1105–17.
34. Chung BH, Joo YY, Lee J, Kim HD, Kim JI, Moon IS, et al. Impact of ABO incompatibility on the development of acute antibody-mediated rejection in kidney transplant recipients presensitized to HLA. PLoS ONE. 2015;10(4):e0123638.
35. Brocker V, Mengel M. Histopathological diagnosis of acute and chronic rejection in pediatric kidney transplantation. Pediatr Nephrol. 2014;29(10):1939–49.
36. Wu WK, Famure O, Li Y, Kim SJ. Delayed graft function and the risk of acute rejection in the modern era of kidney transplantation. Kidney Int. 2015.
37. Lim WH, Eris J, Kanellis J, Pussell B, Wiid Z, Witcombe D, et al. A systematic review of conversion from calcineurin inhibitor to mammalian target of rapamycin inhibitors for maintenance immunosuppression in kidney transplant recipients. Am J Transplant (Official Journal of the American Society of Transplantation and the American Society of Transplant Surgeons). 2014;14(9):2106–19.
38. Ledesma-Gumba MA, Danguilan RA, Casasola CC, Ona ET. Efficacy of risk stratification in tailoring immunosuppression regimens in kidney transplant patients at the national kidney and transplant institute. Transpl Proc. 2008;40(7):2195–7.
39. Csapo Z, Benavides-Viveros C, Podder H, Pollard V, Kahan BD. Campath-1H as rescue therapy for the treatment of acute rejection in kidney transplant patients. Transpl Proc. 2005;37(5):2032–6.
40. Di Carlo HN, Darras FS. Urologic considerations and complications in kidney transplant recipients. Adv Chronic Kidney Disease. 2015;22(4):306–11.

41. Jensen KK, Roder O, Bistrup C. Surgical complications and graft survival in pediatric kidney transplant recipients treated with a steroid-free protocol: experiences from a Danish university hospital. Transpl Proc. 2013;45(9):3258–61.
42. Jiang M, Gandikota N, Ames SA, Heiba S. Identification of urologic complications after kidney transplant. Am J Kidney Disease (official journal of the National Kidney Foundation). 2011;58(1):150–3.
43. Plainfosse MC, Calonge VM, Beyloune-Mainardi C, Glotz D, Duboust A. Vascular complications in the adult kidney transplant recipient. J Clin Ultrasound JCU. 1992;20(8):517–27.
44. Sprung J, Kapural L, Bourke DL, O'Hara JF Jr. Anesthesia for kidney transplant surgery. Anesthesiol Clin N Am. 2000;18 (4):919–51.
45. Goh CC, Ladouceur M, Peters L, Desmond C, Tchervenkov J, Baran D. Lengthy cold ischemia time is a modifiable risk factor associated with low glomerular filtration rates in expanded criteria donor kidney transplant recipients. Transpl Proc. 2009;41 (8):3290–2.
46. Gandolfo MT, Rabb H. Impact of ischemia times on kidney transplant outcomes. Transplantation. 2007;83(3):254.
47. Kouwenhoven EA, de Bruin RW, Heemann U, Marquet RL. JN IJ. Does cold ischemia induce chronic kidney transplant dysfunction? Transpl Proc. 1999;31(1–2):988–9.
48. Tripathi M, Das CJ, Agarwal KK, Khangembam BC, Dhull VS. Spontaneously resolving lower polar ATN in a transplant kidney with dual vascular supply demonstrated on 99mTc EC renography. Clin Nucl Med. 2013;38(5):390–1.
49. Carlier M, Squifflet JP, Pirson Y, Gribomont B, Alexandre GP. Maximal hydration during anesthesia increases pulmonary arterial pressures and improves early function of human renal transplants. Transplantation. 1982;34(4):201–4.
50. O'Malley CM, Frumento RJ, Hardy MA, Benvenisty AI, Brentjens TE, Mercer JS, et al. A randomized, double-blind comparison of lactated Ringer's solution and 0.9% NaCl during renal transplantation. Anesth Analg. 2005;100(5):1518–24, table of contents.
51. Lauzurica R, Teixido J, Serra A, Torguet P, Bonet J, Bonal J, et al. Hydration and mannitol reduce the need for dialysis in cadaveric kidney transplant recipients treated with CyA. Transpl Proc. 1992;24(1):46–7.
52. Smith DE, Gambertoglio JG, Vincenti F, Benet LZ. Furosemide kinetics and dynamics after kidney transplant. Clin Pharmacol Ther. 1981;30(1):105–13.
53. Alcaraz A, Luque P, Mendes DR, Calatrava P, Heredia EN, Jimenez W, et al. Experimental kidney transplantation in pigs from non-heart-beating donors: evaluation of vasoactive substances and renal artery flow. Transpl Proc. 2001;33(6):2971–2.
54. Day KM, Beckman RM, Machan JT, Morrissey PE. Efficacy and safety of phenylephrine in the management of low systolic blood pressure after renal transplantation. J Am Coll Surg. 2014;218 (6):1207–13.
55. Fontana I, Germi MR, Beatini M, Fontana S, Bertocchi M, Porcile E, et al. Dopamine "renal dose" versus fenoldopam mesylate to prevent ischemia-reperfusion injury in renal transplantation. Transpl Proc. 2005;37(6):2474–5.
56. Hurley JK, Lewy PR. Goldblatt hypertension in a solitary kidney. The J Pediatr. 1977;91(4):609–11.
57. Hadimioglu N, Ulugol H, Akbas H, Coskunfirat N, Ertug Z, Dinckan A. Combination of epidural anesthesia and general anesthesia attenuates stress response to renal transplantation surgery. Transpl Proc. 2012;44(10):2949–54.
58. Shah VR, Butala BP, Parikh GP, Vora KS, Parikh BK, Modi MP, et al. Combined epidural and general anesthesia for paediatric renal transplantation-a single center experience. Transpl Proc. 2008;40 (10):3451–4.
59. Hammouda GE, Yahya R, Atallah MM. Plasma bupivacaine concentrations following epidural administration in kidney transplant recipients. Reg Anesth. 1996;21(4):308–11.
60. Woywodt A, Schwarz A, Mengel M, Haller H, Zeidler H, Kohler L. Nephrotoxicity of selective COX-2 inhibitors. J Rheumatol. 2001;28(9):2133–5.
61. Gooch K, Culleton BF, Manns BJ, Zhang J, Alfonso H, Tonelli M, et al. NSAID use and progression of chronic kidney disease. Am J Med. 2007;120(3):280 e1–7.
62. Martin U, Temple RM, Venkat-Raman G, Prescott LF. Paracetamol disposition in renal allograft recipients. Eur J Clin Pharmacol. 2002;57(12):853–6.

Part VII

Eye, Ear, and Throat Surgery

Section Editor: Dennis J. McNicholl

Dennis J. McNicholl
Department of Anesthesiology, Perioperative and Pain Medicine,
Brigham and Women's Hospital, Boston, MA, USA

Open Eye Injury

35

Alvaro Andres Macias

CASE:

77-year-old male presents to the emergency department with a ruptured right eye after falling at home. He remembers hitting the side of his face on the edge of a chair but denies loss of consciousness.

Medications:	Simvastatin 20 mg PO daily
	Amlodipine/valsartan 1 tablet (10 mg/160 mg) PO daily
	Warfarin 5 mg PO daily
	Aspirin 81 mg PO daily
	Metoprolol 25 mg PO BID
	Fluticasone propionate 88 μg inhaler
	Apraclonidine hydrochloride 0.5% left eye 1–2 gtts BID
Allergies:	NKDA
Past medical history:	
Cardiac:	Hypertension
	Hypercholesterolemia
	Atrial fibrillation
	CHF with a dilated LV, s/p AICD placement 2 years ago
Pulmonary:	Former smoker (1 ppd × 10 years, quit 15 years ago)
	Mild COPD
ENT:	Glaucoma in left eye

(continued)

Physical exam:				
Vital signs:	BP 130/98	HR 85	RR 16	SpO2: 98% on room air
General:	AAO × 3, c/o pain on right side of face			
HEENT:	Right eye: open wound with partial loss of ocular contents. Visual acuity cannot be evaluated at the moment			
	Bruising around right orbit, 2 cm laceration under right eye, covered with dried blood			
Cardiac:	Irregularly irregular heart sounds, no murmurs			
Lungs:	Clear to auscultation and percussion, no wheezing			
NPO status:	Had lunch 2 h prior to arrival in emergency department			
Labs:	Hematocrit: 40%			
	Glucose: 156 mg/dL			
	Potassium: 4.0 mg/dL			
	INR: 2.5			

Introduction

Anesthetic management of patients presenting for urgent or emergent eye surgery after penetrating eye injury can be challenging. There is a risk of extrusion of ocular contents if intraocular pressure becomes elevated at any point during anesthesia induction, maintenance or extubation. Patient movement during the surgical procedure must be avoided at all times for the same reason. Additional concerns include risk of aspiration in patients with a full stomach, and the possibility of associated traumatic injuries (e.g., orbital or cranial trauma).

According to 2002 statistics, there were about 262,000 product-related eye injuries managed in U.S. hospital emergency departments. The highest number of injuries was related to household (124,998), workplace (96,938), and sports (35,633) [1]. A foreign body in the eye is the most

A.A. Macias (✉)
Department of Anesthesiology, Perioperative and Pain Medicine, Brigham and Women's Hospital/Massachusetts Eye and Ear, 75 Francis St, Department of Anesthesiology, CWN L1, Boston, MA 02115, USA
e-mail: amacias@partners.org

© Springer International Publishing AG 2017
L.S. Aglio and R.D. Urman (eds.), *Anesthesiology*,
DOI 10.1007/978-3-319-50141-3_35

common type of eye trauma, accounting for 35% of all eye injuries. Open wounds and contusions each account for about 25% of injuries, while the rest are burns. Nearly 35% of eye injuries occur in patients ≤17 years old. Although eye injury is not a significant cause of total blindness, it is the most common cause of monocular blindness [2].

Surgery has been shown to preserve vision in up to 75% of patients. The outcome is primarily related to the degree of injury to the posterior segment of the globe [3]. A 2009 report showed that 40% of 109 eyes with penetrating injuries or ruptured globes had a good outcome with surgical intervention, achieving a final visual acuity score of 6/12 (20/40) or better on the Snellen scale [4].

1. **What is the normal intraocular pressure at rest, and how does it change with blinking or squinting?**

The normal intraocular pressure (IOP) is 10–20 mmHg. The IOP changes depending on the production of aqueous humor and external pressures applied to the eye. Regular blinking can increase the IOP by 5–10 mmHg and forceful blinking can increase the IOP up to 90 mmHg [5].

2. **What physiologic or pathophysiologic factors can change the IOP?**

IOP has a diurnal variation and is more commonly elevated in the mornings [6]. It also changes with posture; it increases by 2–4 mmHg when lying supine. The Valsalva maneuver can also have a significant effect increasing the IOP up to 75–100 mmHg. Any extraocular pressure brings the IOP higher initially (e.g., digital compression, orbital mass, etc.) but then the IOP goes lower as the outflow of aqueous humor increases. Penetrating trauma has a dual effect; initially it causes the IOP to increase with the extrinsic force on the globe, but then the IOP usually decreases as there is loss of some intraocular contents to the exterior.

3. **How is IOP affected by glaucoma?**

Glaucoma is an optic neuropathy that is the result of a combination of multiple factors, one of them being an increase in IOP. However, some patients may develop "low pressure glaucoma" (aka normal-tension glaucoma) wherein the IOP measurement is normal, yet patients still manifest damage to the optic nerve and gradual loss of sight. For this reason, some have asserted that the definition of normal range of IOP being 10–22 mmHg is rather subjective [7].

4. **What are the most common causes of ocular trauma?**

- A foreign body in the eye is the most common type of eye trauma, accounting for 35% of all eye injuries [2].
- Open wounds and contusions each account for about 25% of injuries, while the rest are burns.
- Nearly, 35% of eye injuries occur in patients ≤17 years old.

5. **Should a patient with an open eye injury be brought emergently to the operating room?**

The recommendation is to repair and/or close the eye within 24 h after the trauma has occurred to decrease the chance of intraocular infection and other significant ocular complications. A full ophthalmologic examination is required to assess the magnitude of the damage to the eyeball and its contents [8]. However, factors such as the type of trauma (penetrating or blunt) and the age of the patient have an effect on the type of surgical repair and time window required for treatment. Signs of motility restriction from entrapment of tissues can lead to ischemia and fibrosis, so it should be repaired within the next 48 h, ideally 24 h. A primary repair is intended to reestablish integrity of the globe, to permit resolution of ocular hypotony, and to protect the eye globe against infection. Foreign bodies should be left in place until surgical removal can be performed. The rationale for this is that the foreign body may have a tamponade effect that would decrease extrusion of vitreous humor. If there is any prolapsed uveal tissue this should be surgically replaced back into the eye except if it is necrotic or contaminated. Any prolapsed vitreous should be identified and removed. Involvement of the lens is an important risk factor for endophthalmitis. If the lens capsule is breached, a primary lensectomy is required [9]. In cases of perforating lesions, it is rarely necessary to close the exit wound because these are often self-sealing and do not typically represent a portal for infection. The manipulation of the globe required to gain access to the exit wound may actually increase the risk of hemorrhage or prolapse of uveal tissue leading to more complications.

6. **What are the concerns in patients with ocular trauma requiring anesthesia?**

   - The mechanism of eye trauma, and the possibility of associated traumatic injuries or increased intracranial pressure (e.g., orbital and/or skull fractures, subdural hematoma, or intracranial trauma).

- Level of consciousness (especially in cases of head trauma).
- Findings of the eye exam performed by the ophthalmologist, including the size of any ocular perforation. Larger defects have a greater chance of extrusion of ocular contents.
- History of prior anesthetics, with particular attention to any history of a difficult airway or nausea and vomiting.
- Timing of last oral intake of fluids and/or solids.
- Standard issues noted in any preanesthetic consultation (e.g., allergies, medications, and past medical history).
- Toxicology screen (if relevant to presentation).

7. **What is the most common type of anesthesia used for open globe procedures and why?**

General anesthesia is the most common type of anesthesia used. The main goal is to provide the patient with profound analgesia, and to prevent coughing, retching, or vomiting, as well as forceful blinking or crying, in order to avoid harmful increases in intraocular pressure (IOP) [2]. In pediatric patients, general anesthesia is the ideal technique. Regional anesthesia is not recommended in pediatric patients that are awake.

8. **Can regional anesthesia be used for ruptured eye surgery?**

Although controversial, there are case reports of using regional anesthesia for ruptured eye surgery. It can be used in very specific cases such as in patients with a potentially difficult airway, or in situations where the likelihood of salvaging vision is low, making concerns regarding increases in IOP less paramount. There are case reports describing successful use of regional ophthalmic blocks after selected types of traumatic eye injury (e.g., for intraocular foreign body removal or repair of dehiscence of a previous surgical wound) [10]. If the wound is in the anterior segment of the eye and relatively small, a regional block is more likely to succeed.

The use of local anesthesia for these cases is not indicated. These patients have other comorbidities and risk factors that preclude them from being good candidates for this type of anesthesia. Pain control and immobility is the key for surgical repair. These procedures tend to be lengthy and keeping a patient immobile for more than 2 h can be a challenge. As previously mentioned, the frequent presence of a full stomach makes these patients poor candidates for sedation.

9. **What kind of precautions should be taken in patients on anticoagulants and/or antiplatelet agents where regional anesthesia is considered?**

For cataract surgery patients at a high risk of clotting and embolic complications due to cardiac or vascular pathology, administration of therapeutic doses of aspirin and warfarin are continued throughout the perioperative period. One large retrospective study noted no higher incidence of sight-threatening bleeding complications after regional anesthesia (e.g., eye block) in patients taking aspirin, warfarin (INR as high as 4.6), or clopidogrel up until the time of cataract surgery, compared with those who discontinued the therapy [11].

However, limited data is available regarding the risk of bleeding during cataract surgery in patients receiving dual antiplatelet therapy (e.g., aspirin plus clopidogrel) [12]. Dual antiplatelet therapy is often used after placement of a drug-eluting stent, and fatal stent clotting may develop if antiplatelet medications are prematurely stopped. In these cases, we suggest delaying eye surgery, if possible, until after the minimum period recommended for daily administration of dual antiplatelet therapy or perform these cases under topical anesthesia.

Regarding the newer anticoagulants, there is not enough evidence to make any kind of recommendations at the moment.

10. **Are there any preoperative laboratory studies needed in preparation for urgent or emergent eye surgery?**

By way of comparison, routine preoperative testing is not required before elective cataract surgery as it does not improve outcomes or decrease the number of complications [13]. Preoperative testing before emergent or urgent eye surgery is based on the patient's past medical history and current comorbidities. For patients on warfarin an INR is recommended. However, the cutoff for ophthalmic regional anesthesia is controversial. For the newest anticoagulants, there is not enough experience to date to offer firm recommendations regarding safety of regional anesthesia or surgery. However, as previously mentioned, regional anesthesia is rarely the preferred technique in patients with ocular trauma.

11. **What are the recommendations for managing pacemakers and AICDs during elective and emergent eye surgery?**

Currently, the recommendation is to leave the AICD active with a magnet available in the room. The use of electrocautery during eye surgery is extremely low. A survey conducted by the Ophthalmic Anesthesia Society showed that 83% of members left the AICDs active when only bipolar electrocautery was used with no reports of AICD malfunction or discharge [14]. It is always important to mention to the surgeon that an active AICD can fire if a triggering arrhythmia occurs, and that this may cause patient movement. There is typically a delay of between 4 and 15 s from the time of arrhythmia detection and patient movement from the discharge of the device.

12. **What is the oculocardiac reflex (OCR) and its most common manifestations?**

Aschner and Dagnini first reported the OCR in 1908 [15]. Afterwards, some isolated reports appeared in the literature. In 1956, Sorenson and Gilmore reported a case of cardiac arrest in a patient who had one of his ocular rectus muscles retracted [16]. In 1958, Kirsch reported a case of fatal cardiac arrest after manipulation of the extraocular muscles [17]. The incidence is variable, but the number of cases of cardiac arrest during eye surgery is reported as high as 1 in 3500 anesthetics [17].

How is it defined?

- C. Yi and D. Jee defined OCR as >10% decrease in HR or occurrence of any arrhythmia induced by traction during single muscle surgery of recession–resection type performed on one extraocular muscle (EOM) [18].

How does it present?

- Most commonly there is decrease in pulse rate associated with traction applied to extraocular muscles and/or compression of the eyeball, pinching of the conjunctiva with forceps, intraorbital injection of local anesthetics, and postoperative pressure on the bandage.
- It generally presents with bradycardia, junctional rhythm, asystole, and very rarely death.

Who is at higher risk?

- It is more common in children (90% under 15) and young adults and more common during general versus regional anesthesia. Interestingly enough, there is some evidence showing that a BIS <50 lowers the incidence [18].

What factors can accentuate the presentation of the OCR?

- Hypoxia and hypercarbia may contribute to the severity of the OCR by rapidly converting bradycardia to cardiac arrest, or may increase the sensitivity of the patient to the reflex.

Name the structures involved in the OCR:

- Long ciliary nerve and short ciliary nerve
- Ciliary ganglion
- Geniculate ganglion
- Fifth cranial nerve
  1. main sensory nucleus of the trigeminal nerve
  2. short internuncial fibers in the reticular formation
  3. motor nucleus of the vagus nerve.
- Vagus Nerve

Is it possible to effectively prevent the occurrence of the OCR?

- Neither IM nor IV atropine is entirely effective in abolishing or preventing the occurrence of the oculocardiac reflex.
- A study by Bosomworth and associates used IV atropine prophylactically in 17 patients after induction of anesthesia and just prior to operation [19]. The atropine dose selected was one-half that (0.1–0.4 mg) used for premedication. They showed that during the first half an hour of operation, only one patient in the atropine group developed a change of cardiac rhythm (bradycardia) during eye muscle traction. When the duration of surgery extended beyond 30 min, 4/17 patients developed arrhythmias.

What is the treatment?

- Removal of the inciting stimulus is always indicated. Once the reflex does occur, IV atropine is the most favored therapeutic agent; usually 0.2–1 mg IV is adequate. It is important to remember that since vagal tone appears to vary with age, even large doses of atropine may fail to accelerate the slowed heart in infants and geriatric patients.

13. **What kind of anxiolytics can be used?**

Benzodiazepines are usually used, as they do not increase IOP [20]. In patients whose respiratory drive is compromised, sleep apnea patients or in patients with associated intoxication (alcohol, opiates), benzodiazepines should be avoided altogether or used with caution as they can induce respiratory depression leading to CO_2 retention and secondary increase in IOP.

Dexmedetomidine in doses of 0.6 μg/kg IV over 10 min prior to induction has shown to prevent significant increases of IOP when succinylcholine is used [21].

14. **What is the optimal strategy for aspiration prophylaxis when an RSI is used for open globe procedures?**

Metoclopramide can be used to increase peristalsis and enhance gastric emptying although its use as part of RSI is controversial. It is also important to remember the potential side effects of this medication including dyskinesia and extrapyramidal symptoms [5].

Sodium citrate may be the most effective prophylaxis against chemical pneumonitis as it immediately decreases gastric acidity. Caution must be taken due to its sour taste triggering nausea and vomiting. These are untoward side effects that will elevate IOP [22].

Avoid emptying the stomach with an orogastric or nasogastric tube as it may cause more injury locally (especially nasopharyngeal a nasogastric tube). Attempting to place any kind of tube may lead to coughing, gagging or similar responses that will increase the IOP and potentially lead to extrusion of the ocular contents.

15. **What should be your plan for induction of anesthesia? What type of muscle relaxant should you use? Why?**

Rapid-sequence induction (RSI) technique with succinylcholine is the most commonly and preferred technique used as many of these patients present with a full stomach.

Succinylcholine 1.5 mg/kg offers the best intubating conditions, and has the shortest duration of action, but increases the IOP temporarily. It is clear that an adequate dose of the selected anesthetic induction agent (e.g., propofol 1.5–2.5 mg/kg) [23] should be used to minimize the chances of clinically significant increases in IOP. *There are no published reports of extrusion of ocular contents after administration of succinylcholine in this manner* [24, 25].

If RSI is indicated but the use of succinylcholine is contraindicated (e.g., hyperkalemia, malignant hyperthermia risk, neuromuscular disorder or prolonged immobility) a non-depolarizing muscle relaxant such as rocuronium is recommended. A standard intubating dose of rocuronium is 0.6 mg/kg; however, for RSI using rocuronium a dose of 1.2 mg/kg is used. This higher dose has the advantage of relatively rapid onset of action (and may offer the same excellent intubation conditions as a dose of 1.5 mg/kg of succinylcholine) without causing a significant increase in IOP. One potential disadvantage is that the onset of action is 90–140 s [26]. which, when compared to succinylcholine, means there is a slight increase in the amount of time that the airway is unprotected and therefore putting the patient at risk o aspiration. Another potential disadvantage of using higher dose rocuronium is the prolonged duration of action and time to return of adequate muscle function for reversal agents to be given. Sugammadex is a medication which has the ability to encapsulate and inactivate rocuronium and vecuronium, thereby addressing the issue of their duration of action.

16. **What induction agent could be used in this case?**

With the exception of ketamine, virtually all induction agents (including inhaled anesthetics, hypnotics, and opioids) lower ICP [5] and would therefore be suitable choices for induction of anesthesia for open globe procedures.

Ketamine is generally avoided because it may cause nystagmus and blepharospasm [5]. Additionally, there is controversy regarding whether ketamine increases IOP.

A reasonable induction sequence is an anesthetic induction agent (e.g., propofol 1.5–2.5 mg/kg IV), preceded by an opioid (e.g., fentanyl 1–2 μg/kg or remifentanil 1–1.5 μg/kg IV) and a muscle relaxant (see muscle relaxant section). Also, 1.0–1.5 mg/kg lidocaine may be administered 2 min before induction to attenuate the increase of IOP caused by laryngoscopy [27]. Doses of the anesthetic induction agent, opioid, and lidocaine are commonly reduced in elderly patients (e.g., propofol may be reduced to as little as 0.5–1.5 mg/kg).

Etomidate is less often used in this setting because it may induce myoclonus (i.e., skeletal muscle movement) severe enough to increase IOP and may increase secretions, even though it otherwise induces a significant reduction in IOP [28]. If etomidate is selected for induction of anesthesia, myoclonus may be decreased or eliminated by administration of a benzodiazepine (e.g., midazolam 1–2 mg), opioid (e.g., fentanyl 1–2 μg/kg), and muscle relaxant [29].

17. **How would you maintain anesthesia in this patient?**

A deep plane of anesthesia is maintained during ophthalmologic surgery, in order to prevent movement or coughing. This can be accomplished with either a potent inhaled anesthetic or a total intravenous anesthetic technique and the use of muscle relaxants.

Inhaled anesthetics beneficially decrease the production and increase the outflow of aqueous humor, decrease extraocular tension, and lower arterial blood pressure, thereby lowering IOP. In this regard, a total intravenous anesthetic (TIVA) technique is at least as effective in accomplishing a reduction in IOP as an inhalational anesthetic technique [23]. Hybrid techniques (e.g., remifentanil infusion 0.5–2 μg/kg plus an inhaled anesthetic) have also been used with good success.

When the patient is deemed to be at extremely high risk for postoperative nausea and vomiting, TIVA with propofol may be selected, in conjunction with multimodal antiemetic therapy.

18. **How would you extubate this patient?**

Extubation of the trachea should be accomplished before there is a tendency to cough. The administration of intravenous lidocaine, 1–2 mg/kg IV, before extubation of the trachea may be helpful in attenuating coughing, but may prolong awakening due to the sedative side effects of intravenous local anesthesia. A smooth extubation is always recommended. However, a deep extubation is not recommended in cases of full stomach, difficult airway, or in patients with associated injuries that may affect the airway.

19. **How would you manage pain after surgery?**

Pain after eye trauma can be managed with a multimodal approach. Usually opioids, NSAIDS and acetaminophen can be used. Depending on how much damage the eye has suffered and on the kind of surgery performed, an eye block can be done by the surgeon at the end of the case while the patient is still under general anesthesia. It is important to understand that performing a regional technique while the patient is still anesthetized poses an extra challenge for the surgeon or the anesthesiologist performing the block, as feedback from the patient is lost.

20. **What kind of antibiotic regimen is adequate coverage for open globe procedures?**

Over time, prophylactic antibiotic regimens have been refined to manage potential infections, and these have improved the probability of functional success with surgical intervention [30].

Recommended antibiotic regimens are as follows [31]:

- Intravitreal vancomycin: 1 mg/0.1 mL in 1 cc syringe.
- Intravitreal ceftazidime: 2.25 mg/0.1 mL in 1 cc syringe.
- PCN Allergy: Intravitreal gentamicin: 100 μg/0.1 mL in 1 cc syringe or amikacin 200–400 μg/0.1 mL in 1 cc syringe.
- Suspect Bacillus cereus: Intravitreal clindamycin: 0.5 mg/0.1 mL (optional). All *B. cereus* is sensitive to Vancomycin.
- Suspect fungus: Intravitreal Amphotericin B: 5–10 μg/0.1 mL.

21. **In terms of regaining useful sight, what is the outcome data for these patients who have sustained an open globe injury?**

The patient's level of light perception in the affected eye immediately after the injury can be used as a general predictor of outcome. In cases where patients were lacking any light perception in the traumatized eye, the U.S. Eye Injury Register reported that 16% improved and 2% even achieved 20/40 or better visual acuity. Among patients who still had light perception after their injury, 69% improved with surgery with 19% achieving normal visual acuity [29].

22. **Are there specific considerations in pediatric patients presenting with penetrating ocular trauma?**

It is recommended that attempts to gain intravenous access prior to inducing anesthesia should be avoided, as this will agitate the pediatric patient and could lead to significant increases in IOP. Ideally, these patients should be induced via mask using an inhalational agent. IV placement should follow after induction. NPO guidelines should be followed in patients who are not fasted if the surgical team agrees with the waiting time needed [29].

References

1. Product Summary Report-Eye Injuries Only, 2. U.S. Consumer Product Safety Commission, Directorate for Epidemiology. Nat Elec Injur Surv Syst (NEISS). 2003; 1.
2. Macias AA, Bayes J, McGoldrick KE (2015, 01 15). Anesthesia for emergent eye surgery. *UpToDate*. Retrieved 04 25, 2015, from http://www.uptodate.com/contents/anesthesia-for-emergent-eye-surgery?source=search_result&search=anesthesia+eye&selectedTitle=1%7E150.
3. Rahman I, Maino A, Devadson D, Leatherbarrow B. Open globe injuries: factors predictive of poor outcome. Eye. 2006;20:1336–41.
4. Andreoli CM, Gardiner MF. Open globe injuries: emergent evaluation and initial. UptoDate; 2009. Retrieved 24 Feb 2016 from http://www.uptodate.com/contents/open-globe-injuries-emergent-evaluation-and-initial-management.
5. Barash P, Cullen BF, Stoelting RK, Cahalan M, Stock C, Ortega R. Clinical anesthesia. 7th ed. Philadelphia: Lippincott Williams and Wilkins; 2013.
6. Coleman DJ, Trokel S. Direct-recorded intraocular pressure variations in a human subject. Arch Ophthalmol. 1969;82:637–40.
7. Chauhan BC, Drance SM. The influence of intraocular pressure on visual field damage in patients with normal tension and high tension glaucoma. Arch Ophthalmol. 1990;31:1145.
8. Agrawal R, Shah M, Mireskandari K, Yong GK. Controversies in ocular trauma classification and management: review. Int Ophthalmol. 2013;33:435–45.
9. Thompson WS, Rubsamen PE, Flynn HW Jr, Schiffman J, Cousins SW. Endophthalmitis after penetrating trauma. Risk factors and visual acuity outcomes. Ophthalmology. 1995;100:1696–701.
10. Scott IU, McCabe CM, Flynn HW, Lemus DR, Schiffman JC, Reynolds DS, Pereira MB, Belfort A, Gayer S. Local anesthesia with intravenous sedation for surgical repair of selected open globe injuries. Am J Ophthalmol. 2002;134:707–11.
11. Jamula E, Anderson J, Douketis JD. Safety of continuing warfarin therapy during cataract surgery: a systematic review and meta-analysis. Thromb Res. 2009;124:292–9.
12. Grzybowski A, Ascaso FJ, Kupidura-Majewsk K, Packer M. Continuation of anticoagulant and antiplatelet therapy during

phacoemulsification cataract surgery. Curr Opin Ophthalmol. 2015;26:28–33.
13. Chen CL, Lin GA, Bardach NS, Clay TH, Boscardin WJ, Gelb AW, Maze M, Gropper MA, Dudley RA. Preoperative medical testing in Medicare patients undergoing cataract surgery. N Engl J Med. 2015;1530–8.
14. Bayes J. Management of implanted cardiac defibrillators during eye surgery. Anesth Analg. 2008;372:671.
15. Naccarati S. The oculocardiac reflex (Dagnini-Aschner phenomenon)-its use in medicine and psychology. Arch Neur Psych. 1921;5(1):40–57. doi:10.1001/archneurpsyc.1921.02180250043004.
16. Sorenson EJ, Gilmore JE. Cardiac arrest during strabismus surgery; a preliminary report. Am J Ophthalmol. 1956;41:748–52.
17. Kirsch R. The prevention of cardiac arrest in ocular surgery. South Med J. 1958;51:1448–53.
18. Yi C, Jee D. Influence of the anaesthetic depth on the inhibition of the oculocardiac reflex during sevoflurane anaesthesia for paediatric strabismus surgery. Br J Anaesth. 2008;101:234–8.
19. Bosomworth PP, Ziegler CH, Jacoby J. The oculo-cardiac reflex in eye muscle surgery. Anesthesiology. 1958;19:7–10.
20. Carter K, Faberowski LK, Sherwood MB, Berman LS, McGorray S. A randomized trial of the effect of midazolam on intraocular pressure. J Glaucoma. 1999;8:204–7.
21. Jaakola ML, Ali-Melkkilä T, Kanto J, Kallio A, Scheinin H, Scheinin M. Dexmedetomidine reduces intraocular pressure, intubation responses and anaesthetic requirements in patients undergoing ophthalmic surgery. Br J Anaesth. 1992;68:570–5.
22. American Society of Anesthesiologists Committee. Practice guidelines for preoperative fasting and the use of pharmacologic agents to reduce the risk of pulmonary aspiration: application to healthy patients undergoing elective procedures: an updated report by the American Society of Anesthesiologists Committee on Standards and Practice Parameters. Anesthesiology. 2011;114 (3):495–511.
23. Schäfer R, Klett J, Auffarth G, Polarz H, Völcker HE, Martin E, Böttiger BW. Intraocular pressure more reduced during anesthesia with propofol than with sevoflurane: both combined with remifentanil. Acta Anaesthesiol Scand. 2002;46:703–6.
24. Vinik H. Intraocular pressure changes during rapid sequence induction and intubation: a comparison of rocuronium, atracurium, and succinylcholine. J Clin Anesth. 1999;11:95–100.
25. Libonati MM, Leahy JJ, Ellison N. The use of succinylcholine in open eye surgery. Anesthesiology. 1985;62(5):637–40.
26. Chiu CL, Jaais F, Wang CY. Effect of rocuronium compared with succinylcholine on intraocular pressure during rapid sequence induction of anaesthesia. Br J Anaesth. 1999;82:757–60.
27. Drenger B, Pe'er J, BenEzra D, Katzenelson R, Davidson JT (1985). The effect of intravenous lidocaine on the increase in intraocular pressure induced by tracheal intubation. *Anesth Analg* 64, 1211–13.
28. Jm Berry, Merin RG. Etomidate myoclonus and the open globe. Anesth Analg. 1989;69:256–9.
29. Sinha AC, Baumann B. Anesthesia for ocular trauma. Trends Anesth Crit Care. 2010;21:184–8.
30. Pieramici DJ, MacCumber MW, Humayun MU, Marsh MJ, de Juan E Jr. Open-globe injury. Update on types of injuries and visual results. Ophthalmology. 1996;103:1798–803.
31. Ahmed Y, Schimel AM, Pathengay A, Colyer MH, Flynn HW Jr. Endophthalmitis follow open-globe injuries. Eye. 2012;26(2): 212–7.

Anesthesia for Tympanomastoidectomy

36

Martha R. Cordoba Amorocho

24-year-old female with hearing loss due to cholesteatoma presents for right tympanomastoidectomy.

Medications:	inhaler 2 puffs q4h PRN (last used 3 months ago)
	lorazepam 2mg PO q6h PRN anxiety
Allergies:	NKDA
Past Medical History:	Asthma and panic attacks
Past Surgical History:	Appendectomy 3 yrs ago, with PONV
Ob/Gyn:	Last menstrual period 2 weeks ago
Physical examination:	VS: 5'5", 156 lbs
	HR 82, BP 120/64, RR 10, O_2 sat 99% on room air
	HEENT: normocephalic, PERRLA, oropharynx WNL
	CV: Regular rate and rhythm, no murmurs
	Pulm: CTA B/L
	Airway assessment:: Mallampati I
	normal mouth opening
	adequate neck range of motion
	Otherwise unremarkable

1. **What are the important considerations for this patient's preoperative assessment?**

The preoperative evaluation of patients undergoing tympanomastoidectomy does not differ much from other day surgery ENT cases. These are usually elective surgeries, with limited blood loss and fluid shifts. Acute mastoiditis unresponsive to intravenous antibiotics is an exception that may require urgent or emergent surgery, given the potential for complications such as facial palsy, sepsis, or intracranial infection [1].

It is important to evaluate the patient's risk for PONV and tailor the anesthetic plan accordingly. As the patient's head will be rotated during the procedure, it is important to establish a tolerable range of neck motion with the patient in the awake state, so as to avoid potential neck injuries resulting from patient positioning after the patient is under general anesthesia.

As best as can be predicted from the preoperative evaluation, some assessment should be made regarding the patient's ability to safely tolerate mild/moderate decreases in blood pressure (in cases where deliberate hypotension is being considered) or the effects of epinephrine contained in the local anesthetics.

Common symptoms of ear disorders include hearing loss, vertigo, and nausea. Due to these symptoms, patients may be uncomfortable before the surgery. If the patient uses a hearing aid, efforts should be made to allow for its use for as long as possible before induction, and to replace the device (s), if possible, during emergence to facilitate communication and minimize anxiety [2].

2. **The patient has been reading about risks of general anesthesia, and she is strongly interested in having her surgery done under sedation. What do you say to her?**

The majority of tympanomastoidectomies are performed under general anesthesia because of the discomfort of the procedure as well as the risk of a poor outcome if the patient were to move during the case. However, these procedures can also be performed under MAC and local anesthesia, and be well-tolerated by the patient with minimum discomfort [3]. For improved success, it is necessary that the hospital, anesthesiologists and surgeons have sufficient experience performing these surgeries under sedation.

M.R. Cordoba Amorocho (✉)
Department of Anesthesiology, Perioperative and Pain Medicine, Brigham and Women's Hospital, 75, Francis Street, CWN-L1, Boston, MA 02115, USA
e-mail: Mcordoba-amorocho@partners.org

© Springer International Publishing AG 2017
L.S. Aglio and R.D. Urman (eds.), *Anesthesiology*,
DOI 10.1007/978-3-319-50141-3_36

Adequate sedation and analgesia can be accomplished with different medications. Dexmedetomidine seems to be comparable to midazolam-fentanyl for sedation and analgesia in tympanoplasty [4]. Propofol can also be used for sedation in these cases [5].

It is crucial to select patients carefully for MAC. Ideally they should not be obese, not be at increased risk for aspiration, not have history of claustrophobia or panic attacks and have a reassuring airway. Patients should be made aware of what to expect during the procedure, such as operating room noise, and what would be expected from them, such as stillness and tolerance of relatively awake state. For the patient in this case example, her history of panic attacks makes the option of MAC less appealing for all involved.

3. **Why is local anesthetic infiltration by the surgeon important for the anesthesiologist?**

Injection of lidocaine with epinephrine is performed by the surgeon at the beginning of the case. Local anesthetic injection can rarely cause transient facial nerve palsy [6]. This paralysis can be distressing for the patient under sedation, or if still present while recovering after general anesthesia.

Systemic absorption of epinephrine can produce hemodynamic instability with hypertension or cardiac arrhythmias. Anesthesiologists typically try to allow blood pressure and heart rate to return to normal levels without treatment, but a severe or acute episode may require direct vasodilator agents or alpha-antagonist as the preferred treatments.

4. **What are some specific intraoperative considerations for tympanomastoidectomy?**

Some issues are particularly relevant while caring for a patient undergoing middle ear surgery. These include attention to patient positioning, use of a surgical microscope requiring a bloodless surgical field, use or avoidance of nitrous oxide, implications of facial nerve monitoring and preservation, need for smooth emergence, and PONV prevention and treatment.

5. **What precautions should be taken regarding patient positioning for these cases?**

During surgery, the head of the surgical bed and the patient's airway is usually turned 90 or 180° away from the anesthesiologist. Proper preparation is required in order to keep the patient safe while the table is rotated and afterwards. It is critical to adequately secure the ETT or LMA, to position the monitor cables in a way that avoid tangles and disconnections, and to have make sure the anesthesia circuit tubing and intravenous lines of sufficient length.

Also, for this surgery, the patient's head and neck will be extended and rotated away from the surgical side, with the operative ear up. Excessive pressure in the dependent ear and eye should be avoided, as well as any extreme positions that could produce cervical nerve injury. The patients should be safely secured to the table to prevent falls, as the surgical beds are often tilted dramatically during these cases.

6. **Why does the use of a surgical microscope matter for this procedure, and how does this affect your anesthetic technique?**

The surgeon operates with a microscope and while these procedures have very minimal blood loss, any bleeding appears magnified and obstructs visualization of the surgical field. Controlled hypotension is frequently used to achieve a bloodless operative field, which is needed for a successful tympanomastoidectomy. This can be achieved either using inhalational anesthetics or total intravenous anesthesia technique (TIVA).

It seems reasonable to aim for a mild to moderate (15–20%) reduction in blood pressure, avoiding any profound hypotension (MAP <60–65). Hypotension carries the risk of increased morbidity and mortality due to ischemic organ failure. A cardiovascular evaluation should consider the ability of the patient to tolerate mild hypotension, and preclude the use of controlled hypotension in certain patients who have significant carotid stenosis or coronary artery disease.

Several different agents have been used successfully to provide controlled hypotension for middle ear surgery, including clonidine [7], esmolol [8], nitroprusside [9], magnesium sulfate [10] and remifentanil. Remifentanil infusion, added to propofol or an inhaled anesthesia, is currently preferred in clinical practice, as it provides good surgical conditions without the side effects of cardiovascular hypotensive agents [11]. Remifentanil also decreases patient movement during surgery and results in a more rapid emergence at the end of the case. Dexmedetomidine could be helpful; however research regarding its use for tympanomastoidectomy is still limited [12, 13].

Regarding the choice of the inhaled agent used for maintenance of the anesthesia, sevoflurane [14], isoflurane, and desflurane [15], all enable acceptable surgical conditions and hypotension for middle ear surgeries.

7. **Are there any issues with the use of nitrous oxide during these cases?**

The middle ear cavity is filled with air and is non-distensible. Nitrous oxide is more soluble than nitrogen in blood, as a result, when nitrous oxide is used, it can move more quickly into the middle ear than nitrogen can be displaced, potentially producing a pressure increase in the middle ear. The opposite happens once nitrous oxide is discontinued, with negative pressure in the middle ear as nitrous oxide diffuses into the blood. These mechanical effects can cause tympanic membrane rupture and interfere with maintenance of the position of graft material and/or of ossicular reconstruction prostheses.

Additionally, there are concerns about the potential for nitrous oxide causing an increase in the patient's risk of developing PONV. Barometric changes in the middle ear produced by nitrous oxide may even be the cause for an increase in PONV in these surgeries [16].

The lack of any clear benefit derived from the use of nitrous oxide, combined with the above mentioned drawbacks, suggest avoiding it during tympanomastoidectomy; but if used, it should be discontinued at least 30 min before the tympanoplasty or ossiculoplasty in order to allow re-equilibration of the middle ear cavity.

8. **How does facial nerve monitoring affect your anesthesia plan?**

Injury to the facial nerve is a concern during tympanomastoidectomy. Hence, facial nerve electromyography monitoring (FNM) is used during these procedures. FNM electrodes are placed into the ipsilateral orbicularis oris and orbicularis oculi muscles, with ground electrodes placed in the neck or chest.

Muscle relaxant agents are contraindicated during the maintenance of the anesthetic, as injury to the facial nerve can occur anywhere along its course and if the patient is paralyzed this injury may go unrecognized. However succinylcholine can be used to facilitate intubation during induction. Some practitioners prefer to intubate without any muscle relaxant at all; using only propofol and remifentanil. If a muscle relaxant is used during intubation, return of neuromuscular function should be verified [17] (to rule out pseudocholinesterase deficiency) before surgery can proceed. As the patient is not paralyzed, the surgeon should communicate clearly before any painful stimulation.

Remifentanil can be added to an inhaled anesthetic or TIVA with propofol to decrease the chance of patient movement. If remifentanil is used vigilance is required, as always during anesthesia. While mild controlled hypotension is adequate, profound bradycardia or severe hypotension can occur when adding remifentanil, as tympanomastoidectomy is not a very painful procedure. If bradycardia occurs, glycopyrrolate, atropine, ephedrine, or epinephrine can be given, as needed, but sometimes it may be necessary to simply discontinue the use of remifentanil.

9. **What do you plan to use to secure the airway for this patient; an ETT or a LMA?**

Most of the considerations, whether to use a LMA or not for tympanomastoidectomy, are similar to any other surgical procedure. The LMA has been determined to be a safe alternative to the ETT, with no evidence of increased airway complications [18, 19]. Also, the choice of airway device does not seem to influence middle ear pressure with or without nitrous oxide use [20].

Some anesthesiologists prefer an LMA, as it can be reliably placed without the use of muscle relaxants, and can be removed at the end of the case with less stimulation, facilitating a smooth emergence. However, considering the fact that the airway will likely be away from the anesthesiologist during the case, many prefer to use an ETT.

10. **What is your plan for emergence of anesthesia?**

Maintaining a steady pressure in the middle ear and avoiding postoperative bleeding are crucial for surgical success during tympanomastoidectomy. Hence, it is important to prevent coughing and bucking during emergence, if possible. However, there are no guaranteed techniques to achieve these results.

The anesthesia provider can choose to remove the ETT when the patient is awake, or while the patient is still deeply anesthetized.

Awake extubation is generally believed to be a safe technique, as it occurs after the return of the protective airway reflexes. However, it can be accompanied by a significant incidence of coughing, bucking, and even laryngospasm. Alternatively, anesthesiologists prefer to use a LMA for these cases, as removing it once the patient is awake at the end of the case, is usually smoother than removing an ETT.

Close communication with the surgeon is necessary for a smooth awake extubation. The surgeon should be able to anticipate the end time for the procedure; this allows the anesthesiologist to titrate the medications adequately. The surgeon should be gentle while cleaning the surgical area after the procedure and while applying the mastoid dressing, in order to decrease the chance of stimulating a patient who may be "light" but not ready for extubation.

The advantage of deep extubation is the belief that it can produce a smoother emergence than awake extubation. However, deep extubation leaves the airway unprotected. If deep extubation is performed, careful consideration should be given to patient selection. Patients at risk for aspiration, airway obstruction (e.g., OSA), postoperative respiratory depression or patients with difficult airway (known or suspected) should likely be excluded.

If a deep extubation is attempted, it is reasonable and safe to do so in the operating room, and wait for the patient to emerge from anesthesia in the room, while continuing standard monitoring. The anesthesia provider should be ready to manage any possible post-extubation airway complication, such as laryngospasm.

11. **How significant is the role of PONV and how would you manage it?**

The incidence of PONV following otologic surgery is high, between 50–80% [21]. This can be a result of the anesthesia itself and probably also from direct manipulation of the middle ear structures, and indirect disturbance of the inner ear structures.

Treating and preventing PONV is crucial for improving the patient's experience, as nausea and vomiting can be more distressing than pain. Also, any retching and vomiting can cause changes in the pressure gradient of the middle ear and interfere with healing of the surgical site. Persistent vertigo, nausea, and vomiting may require hospital admission and even prolonged hospitalization.

The likelihood of PONV in a given patient will further increase if other risks factors are identified. These additional risks factors are female gender (from puberty), nonsmoking status, history of PONV or motion sickness, childhood (after infancy or younger adulthood), duration of surgery (each 3-minute increase in duration increases PONV risk by approximately 60%), and administration of nitrous oxide, volatile anesthetics or postoperative opioids [22].

As the incidence of PONV for these procedures is high, it seems reasonable to routinely offer prophylaxis to all patients, unless specific contraindications exist. Different antiemetic medications are available, whose selection will depend on the time of their administration, their potential side effects and contraindications.

Serotonin receptors antagonists, such as ondansetron, are customarily given at the end of the surgery, and the possible side effects are increase in liver enzymes, QT prolongation, constipation, and headache. Dexamethasone is administered shortly after the induction of anesthesia. Droperidol is given at the end of the surgery; however has an FDA issued black box warning of possible death and life-threatening QT prolongation or torsades de pointes. Transdermal scopolamine is applied at least 4 h before the end of the surgery. Promethazine and prochlorperazine are administered at the end of surgery. Scopolamine, promethazine, and prochlorperazine can cause sedation, dry mouth, and dizziness. The antihistamines diphenhydramine, and hydroxyzine may also be effective and are used as rescue medications, however they may also cause sedation [23].

Transdermal scopolamine [24, 25], midazolam [26], dexamethasone [27, 28], prochlorperazine [29], and ondansetron [30], as single-dose medications, have been proven to decrease the incidence of PONV after middle ear surgery.

Multimodal antiemetic therapy, as opposed to single-agent therapy, has been shown to work better. The granisetron-dexamethasone [31] and dexamethasone-midazolam [32] combinations have shown to be effective for these procedures.

A technique that includes use of propofol should be considered on patients at high risk of PONV undergoing middle ear surgery. Patients receiving propofol, compared with isoflurane, had significantly less nausea and vomiting [33]. This continues to be of benefit even while remifentanil is added. TIVA with propofol and remifentanil was characterized by lower incidence and severity of PONV when compared with sevoflurane and remifentanil [34]. Even when cost is a concern, a mixed technique combining inhaled anesthesia with a propofol infusion deserves consideration, as recovery during the first 24 h after surgery seems to be associated with a lower incidence of PONV [35].

A peripheral nerve block of the great auricular nerve (GAN) performed by the surgeon after induction of general anesthesia decreased the incidence of PONV, compared with the use of intravenous morphine [36]. The surgeon should consider using local anesthesia, not just for cases performed under MAC, but also for surgeries done under general anesthesia.

References

1. Levine AI, Govindaraj S, DeMaria JS, Gooden C, Chandrasekhar S. Otologic surgery anesthesiology and otolaryngology. New York: Springer; 2012 (pp. 173–182).
2. Liang S, Irwin MG. Review of anesthesia for middle ear surgery. Anesthesiol Clin. 2010;28(3):519–28.
3. Sarmento KMDA Jr, Tomita S. Retroauricular tympanoplasty and tympanomastoidectomy under local anesthesia and sedation. Acta Otolaryngol. 2009;129(7):726–8.
4. Parikh DA, Kolli SN, Karnik HS, Lele SS, Tendolkar BA. A prospective randomized double-blind study comparing dexmedetomidine vs. combination of midazolam-fentanyl for tympanoplasty surgery under monitored anesthesia care. J Anaesthesiol Clin Pharmacol. 2013;29(2):173–8.
5. Thota RS, Ambardekar M, Likhate P. Conscious sedation for middle ear surgeries: a comparison between fentanyl-propofol and fentanyl-midazolam infusion. Saudi J Anaesthesia. 2015;9(2):117–21.
6. Caner G, Olgun L, Gültekin G, Aydar L. Local anesthesia for middle ear surgery. Otolaryngol-Head Neck Sur. 2005;133(2):295–7.
7. Marchal JM, Gómez-Luque A, Martos-Crespo F, Sanchez De La Cuesta F, Martínez-López MC, Delgado-Martinez AD. Clonidine decreases intraoperative bleeding in middle ear microsurgery. Acta Anaesthesiol Scand. 2001;45(5):627–33.

8. Celebi N, Artukoglu F, Dal D, Saricaoglu F, Celiker V, Aypar U. Effect of hypotensive anesthesia on cognitive functions. A comparison of esmolol and remifentanil during tympanoplasty. Saudi Med J. 2007;28(9):1357–61.
9. Degoute CS, Ray MJ, Manchon M, Dubreuil C, Banssillon V. Remifentanil and controlled hypotension; comparison with nitroprusside or esmolol during tympanoplasty. Can J Anaesth. 2001;48(1):20–7.
10. Ryu JH, Sohn IS, Do SH. Controlled hypotension for middle ear surgery: a comparison between remifentanil and magnesium sulphate. Br J Anaesth. 2009;103(4):490–5.
11. Degoute CS, Ray MJ, Gueugniaud PY, Dubreuil C. Remifentanil induces consistent and sustained controlled hypotension in children during middle ear surgery. Can J Anaesth. 2003;50(3):270–6.
12. Ayoglu H, Yapakci O, Ugur MB, Uzun L, Altunkaya H, Ozer Y, Ozkocak I. Effectiveness of dexmedetomidine in reducing bleeding during septoplasty and tympanoplasty operations. J Clin Anesth. 2008;20(6):437–41.
13. Richa F, Yazigi A, Sleilaty G, Yazbeck P. Comparison between dexmedetomidine and remifentanil for controlled hypotension during tympanoplasty. Eur J Anaesthesiol. 2008;25(05):369–74.
14. Jellish WS, Owen K, Edelstein S, Fluder E, Leonetti JP. Standard anesthetic technique for middle ear surgical procedures: a comparison of desflurane and sevoflurane. Otolaryngol-Head Neck Sur. 2005;133(2):269–74.
15. Kaygusuz K, Yildirim A, Kol IO, Gursoy S, Mimaroglu C. Hypotensive anaesthesia with remifentanil combined with desflurane or isoflurane in tympanoplasty or endoscopic sinus surgery: a randomised, controlled trial. J Laryngol Otol. 2008;122(07):691–5.
16. Nader ND, Simpson G, Reedy RL. Middle ear pressure changes after nitrous oxide anesthesia and its effect on postoperative nausea and vomiting. Laryngoscope. 2004;114(5):883–6.
17. Cai YR, Xu J, Chen LH, Chi FL. Electromyographic monitoring of facial nerve under different levels of neuromuscular blockade during middle ear microsurgery. Chin Med J. 2009;122(3):311–4.
18. Taheri A, Hajimohamadi F, Soltanghoraee H, Moin A. Complications of using laryngeal mask airway during anaesthesia in patients undergoing major ear surgery. Acta Otorhinolaryngol Ital. 2009;29(3):151–5.
19. Ayala MA, Sanderson A, Marks R, Hoffer M, Balough B. Laryngeal mask airway use in otologic surgery. Otol Neurotol. 2009;30(5):599–601.
20. Hohlrieder M, Keller C, Brimacombe J, Eschertzhuber S, Luckner G, Abraham I, von Goedecke A. Middle ear pressure changes during anesthesia with or without nitrous oxide are similar among airway devices. Anesth Analg. 2006;102(1):319–21.
21. Fujii Y. Clinical strategies for preventing postoperative nausea and vomiting after middle ear surgery in adult patients. Current Drug Safety. 2008;3(3):230–9.
22. Gan TJ. Risk factors for postoperative nausea and vomiting. Anesth Analg. 2006;102(6):1884–98.
23. Gan TJ, Meyer T, Apfel CC, Chung F, Davis PJ, Eubanks S, Watcha M. Consensus guidelines for managing postoperative nausea and vomiting. Anesth Analg. 2003;97(1):62–71.
24. Honkavaara P, Saarnivaara L, Klemola UM. Prevention of nausea and vomiting with transdermal hyoscine in adults after middle ear surgery during general anaesthesia. Br J Anaesth. 1994;73(6):763–6.
25. Reinhart DJ, Klein KW, Schroff E. Transdermal scopolamine for the reduction of postoperative nausea in outpatient ear surgery: a double-blind, randomized study. Anesth Analg. 1994;79(2):281–4.
26. Jung JS, Park JS, Kim SO, Lim DG, Park SS, Kwak KH, et al. Prophylactic antiemetic effect of midazolam after middle ear surgery. Otolaryngol-Head Neck Sur. 2007;137(5):753–6.
27. Ahn JH, Kim MR, Kim KH. Effect of iv dexamethasone on postoperative dizziness, nausea and pain during canal wall-up mastoidectomy. Acta Otolaryngol. 2005;125(11):1176–9.
28. Liu YH, Li MJ, Wang PC, Ho ST, Chang CF, Ho CM, Wang JJ. Use of dexamethasone on the prophylaxis of nausea and vomiting after tympanomastoid surgery. Laryngoscope. 2001;111(7):1271–4.
29. Van Den Berg AA. A comparison of ondansetron and prochlorperazine for the prevention of nausea and vomiting after tympanoplasty. Can J Anaesth. 1996;43(9):939–45.
30. Ku PK, Tong MC, Lo P, van Hasselt CA. Efficacy of ondansetron for prevention of postoperative nausea and vomiting after outpatient ear surgery under local anesthesia. Otol Neurotol. 2000;21(1):24–7.
31. Gombar S, Kaur J, Kumar Gombar K, Dass A, Singh A. Superior anti-emetic efficacy of granisetron–dexamethasone combination in children undergoing middle ear surgery. Acta Anaesthesiol Scand. 2007;51(5):621–4.
32. Yeo J, Jung J, Ryu T, Jeon YH, Kim S, Baek W. Antiemetic efficacy of dexamethasone combined with midazolam after middle ear surgery. Otolaryngol-Head Neck Sur. 2009;141(6):684–8.
33. Jellish WS, Leonetti JP, Murdoch JR, Fowles S. Propofol-based anesthesia as compared with standard anesthetic techniques for middle ear surgery. Otolaryngol-Head Neck Sur. 1995;112(2):262–7.
34. Jellish WS, Leonetti JP, Fahey K, Fury P. Comparison of 3 different anesthetic techniques on 24-hour recovery after otologic surgical procedures. Otolaryngol-Head Neck Sur. 1999;120(3):406–11.
35. Lee DW, Lee HG, Jeong CY, Jeong SW, Lee SH. Postoperative nausea and vomiting after mastoidectomy with tympanoplasty: a comparison between TIVA with propofol-remifentanil and balanced anesthesia with sevoflurane-remifentanil. Korean J Anesthesiol. 2011;61(5):399–404.
36. Suresh S, Barcelona SL, Young NM, Seligman I, Heffner CL, Coté CJ. Postoperative pain relief in children undergoing tympanomastoid surgery: is a regional block better than opioids? Anesth Analg. 2002;94(4):859–62.

The Difficult Airway

37

Dennis J. McNicholl

Case Presentation

Obese 30-year-old female involved in a MVA including head/facial injuries and open fracture involving the lower extremity presents to the emergency department. Patient is in a cervical collar.

PMHx:	Obesity	
	Asthma	
Medications:	Oral contraceptives	
Allergies:	None known	
PSHx:	C/S × 2	
	Sinus surgery	
Physical Exam:	Height 5′6″ (167 cm)	Weight: 210 lbs (95.5 kg) (BMI 34)
VS: HR 106	BP 108/59 RR 22	SpO_2 96% on NRB

General: alert, oriented to person, place, and time. No memory of accident, in C-collar
Neuro: Nonfocal, able to move all extremities, 5/5 except for LLE (3/5), sensation intact
HEENT: PERRLA, LEFT facial laceration
CV: tachycardic, no murmur, capillary refill <3 s
Pulm: Breath sounds equal B/L, no wheezing
Abdomen: obese, nontender, nondistended
Extremities: LEFT open tib-fib fx
NPO Status: last meal 3 h prior to accident

QUESTIONS:
You receive a STAT page from the Emergency Department requesting airway management assistance for this patient involved in an MVA who is en route to your facility. On your way to the Emergency Department, what concerns do you have about managing this patient's airway?

There are many "unknowns" at this stage, so several scenarios may be running through your head in anticipation of the patient's arrival. What is their level of consciousness? Is the patient already intubated, or will they even need intubation in the immediate term before any evaluation or imaging is done in the emergency department? What was the mechanism of injury and how much energy transfer was involved in the accident? How likely is a neck injury? Have attempts already been made to intubate by pre-hospital personnel? Could there be blood in the airway? Is the patient hemodynamically stable or getting worse as time passes? All of these are good considerations to focus your attention and prepare for what might need to be done. More will be revealed when the patient arrives and additional history is gathered.

Upon arrival, the patient is on a backboard in a cervical collar. She is alert and oriented to name and date but has no recollection of what happened in the accident. What are some of the next priorities in managing the airway?

Perhaps the first order of business is to identify whether or not intubation is needed at this time. Assessment of vital signs (and their trend), mental status (and its trend), mechanism of injury, need for surgery (immediate or delayed), and any plans for imaging in the ED before deciding on surgery will all impact the decision about when or whether to intubate. With all these seemingly simultaneous decisions to make, it is worth bearing in mind the patient's multiple

D.J. McNicholl (✉)
Department of Anesthesiology, Perioperative and Pain Medicine, Brigham and Women's Hospital, 75 Francis St., Boston, MA 02115, USA
e-mail: dmcnicholl@partners.org

© Springer International Publishing AG 2017
L.S. Aglio and R.D. Urman (eds.), *Anesthesiology*,
DOI 10.1007/978-3-319-50141-3_37

risks for nonoptimal status (due to trauma, cervical collar, full stomach, etc.) and to plan accordingly.

Urgency for securing the airway would include respiratory distress, worsening mental status, hemodynamic instability portending shock, or aspiration.

How would you evaluate this patient's airway?

This patient presents in an awake state, which is a major advantage as it allows a more thorough airway evaluation in terms of history and physical examination. Indeed, the ASA Guidelines recommend that, whenever feasible, before the initiation of anesthetic care and airway management, an *airway history and physical examination* should be conducted [1].

The *airway history* in meant to detect medical, surgical, and anesthetic factors that may indicate the presence of a difficult airway. Examination of previous anesthetic records, if available in a timely manner, may yield useful information about airway management. The older the anesthetic record is, the more diminished its utility is likely to be. However, even without the actual records, some more information may be gleaned from related history questions—was the patient told of any anesthetic/airway issues after a prior surgery, was it a surgery that required intubation or not, have they gained or lost a substantial amount of weight since the last surgery, etc.

The *airway physical examination* should similarly be conducted whenever feasible. The purpose is to detect physical characteristics that may indicate the presence of a difficult airway. It is also recommended that multiple airway features should be assessed.

Is there anything in this patient's medical history that may be of concern with respect to managing the airway?

The patient's history with a focus on the airway can be revealing and should be ascertained. The past surgical history for this patient includes sinus surgery. If practical and feasible, more information about this should be sought, such as if there were any difficulties with the intubation for that procedure, or how recently it was performed (concern for friable tissue or inflammation should a nasal approach to intubation or use of a nasal trumpet be considered as she presents now), and the original indication for the surgery (e.g., polyps, tumor removal, epistaxis).

Another diagnosis this patient carries is asthma, and in characterizing this condition it would be useful to know if she has ever been intubated for this condition (not only could it provide information about the intubation, but would also likely be indicative of severe baseline airway disease). Other pertinent history is the frequency of inhaler use and whether oral steroids have been required to control symptoms.

One important history question is whether or not the patient snores. Compared to other history questions, this one is somewhat different in that the patient typically cannot rely on themselves for an accurate answer (though there are some patients who will admit to being woken up by the sound of their own snoring). Even when a patient does admit to snoring or being told that they snore, this information only occasionally will be recorded in the medical record, thus it may be "under the radar" of most practitioners. The practitioner for whom it probably matters the most is the anesthesiologist, as snoring is a risk factor for difficult mask ventilation.

In conducting a thorough airway history, it is important to keep in mind that even patients with no past surgical history can have revealing information about intubation if they have had nonsurgical conditions that require intubation (e.g., asthma, COPD exacerbation, sepsis, etc.)

Given this patient's presentation, what do you expect to find on physical examination that would likely be important for managing the airway?

This patient is awake and can participate in an airway exam at least to some degree. With the presence of the cervical collar, any exam will naturally be more limited. A basic evaluation under other circumstances would naturally include the range of motion of the neck, but this would clearly be ill-advised in a case such as this one. Cervical collars also restrict mouth opening (another basic part of the airway exam under normal circumstances).

The ASA Guidelines recommend that multiple airway features be assessed. It lists 11 features in all, though it also states this is not an exhaustive list, nor is it mandatory to evaluate all of them (again, the caveat of using judgment with respect to the clinical context about whether to evaluate certain aspects of the airway).

Of all the components of the airway physical exam only four, in fact, actually require patient cooperation:

- Visibility of the uvula (Mallampati class 3 or 4)
- Interincisor distance (less than 3 cm)
- Range of motion of the head and neck (cannot extend neck or touch chin to chest)
- Relationship of the maxillary and mandibular incisors during voluntary protrusion of the mandible (cannot bring mandibular incisors anterior to maxillary incisors)

The other seven components of the airway exam do not require patient cooperation and can be assessed externally by visual observation or with the gentle use of a tongue depressor. These assessments can provide significant and often critical information about the likelihood of encountering difficulty with intubation. These features include the following:

- Length of upper incisors (relatively long)
- Relationship of maxillary and mandibular incisors during normal jaw closure (prominent "overbite")

- Shape of the palate (highly arched or narrow. This may be assessed with gentle application of a tongue depressor)
- Compliance of the submandibular space (stiff, indurated, occupied by mass, or nonresilient)
- Thyromental distance (less than three "ordinary finger breadths" which is typically ~6 cm)
- Length of neck (short)
- Thickness of neck (thick)

One physical feature that is not on this list but may be of clinical significance during intubation is that of the tongue size relative to the size of the oral cavity. This feature is somewhat related to the compliance of the submandibular space, in that this is the compartment into which the tongue would normally be displaced during direct laryngoscopy. Toward this point, the combination of a large tongue size and decreased submandibular compliance would compound the difficulty encountered compared to that for either feature alone.

Additionally, this patient has an elevated BMI, which raises concerns for both difficult mask ventilation (DMV) and difficult intubation (DI).

Would you consider delaying the management of this patient's airway to try to obtain prior medical records?

Overall, obtaining additional history is important and may lead to a change in approach to managing the airway. If the patient's history reveals something concerning or serious, prior records should be obtained if they will be available in a timely manner and if it is practical to do so. In some cases, additional consultation (e.g., from an otorhinolaryngologist) may be in order to safely manage a difficult airway.

Obtaining prior records may be as fast and simple as looking up an anesthesia record in your own hospital's electronic medical record system, or may be as prohibitively cumbersome as filing a request at another institution.

The decision of whether or not to delay intubation for the sake of obtaining prior records depends on how important the information might be in managing the patient's airway at that moment in time, and keeping in mind the amount of time that may actually be available to obtain that information. In urgent/emergent situations such as in this case, the patient's clinical status will guide the necessity of trying to garner additional history or obtain prior records.

Should trauma imaging studies (e.g., CT scans, X-rays, FAST exam) be done before or after securing the airway? Would CT imaging of the head and neck help you decide what approach to take in securing the airway?

The timing of when trauma imaging should take place is typically the purview of the emergency medicine physician or trauma team. While additional imaging may be useful to know, even "normal" results of a cervical CT scan cannot rule out some injuries (e.g., spinal cord contusion, ligamentous instability), thus the change in management from an airway management perspective would likely be minimal. It would be prudent to assume the c-spine is unstable at this stage of the clinical course.

What potential problems do you foresee in managing this patient's airway?

The ASA Difficult Airway Algorithm is designed to aid in identifying potential airway problems and planning the approach *in advance*; it is not intended to be invoked at the onset of an airway crisis.

After the patient's history has been taken and airway physical examination has been completed, enough information should be available to assess the likelihood and clinical impact of the six basic airway management problems (as stated in the ASA Difficult Airway Algorithm) relative to the current clinical scenario. These problems are as follows:

- Difficulty with patient cooperation or consent
- Difficult mask ventilation
- Difficult supraglottic airway placement
- Difficult laryngoscopy
- Difficult intubation
- Difficult surgical airway access

It is noteworthy to observe from this list that ability to ventilate comes before ability to intubate. While so much focus is placed on the anesthesiologist's ability to intubate, mask ventilation is the real lifesaving skill set when caring for a patient who is known or suspected to be a difficult intubation. In the case presented here, the luxury of evaluating the patient's airway in the same manner as for an elective case is not available. This places more emphasis on correctly evaluating this patient's risk factors for difficult mask ventilation.

How will you formulate your plan for managing this patient's airway?

The ASA Difficult Airway Algorithm delineates four basic choices with respect to managing the airway:

- Awake intubation versus intubation after general anesthesia
- Noninvasive versus invasive initial approach to intubation
- Video-assisted laryngoscopy as an initial approach to intubation
- Preservation versus ablation of spontaneous ventilation

A similar decision-tree approach to airway management is the Airway Approach Algorithm (AAA) [2]. This algorithm has been described as a method to be used *before* applying the ASA Difficult Airway Algorithm.

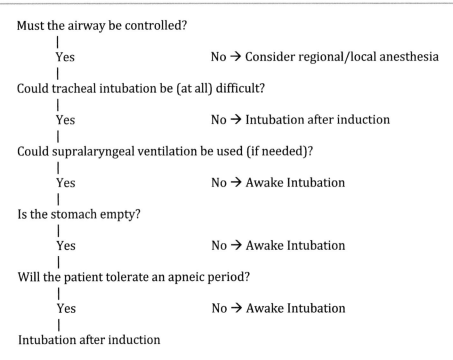

Must the airway be controlled?
|
Yes — No → Consider regional/local anesthesia
|
Could tracheal intubation be (at all) difficult?
|
Yes — No → Intubation after induction
|
Could supralaryngeal ventilation be used (if needed)?
|
Yes — No → Awake Intubation
|
Is the stomach empty?
|
Yes — No → Awake Intubation
|
Will the patient tolerate an apneic period?
|
Yes — No → Awake Intubation
|
Intubation after induction

Using the AAA, if it has been determined that the airway does need to be controlled, there are only two possible answer choices left: (1) awake intubation or (2) intubation after induction. These two choices correspond to the entry points in the ASA Difficult Airway Algorithm (the top of each box in the diagram).

Would you attempt an awake intubation?

Based on the pre-intubation assessment (physical exam, history), the likelihood of encountering difficulty with intubation or mask ventilation must be assessed.

Indications for an awake intubation include the following:

- Previous history of difficult intubation
- Anticipated difficult mask ventilation
- Physical examination consistent with difficult intubation
- Trauma to the face, neck, upper airway, cervical spine
- High risk of aspiration
- Cervical spine disease
- Hypotension, shock
- Respiratory failure

This patient is in a cervical immobilization collar and also has a facial laceration as well as a distracting injury (lower extremity open fracture), so there is an index of suspicion of cervical spine trauma in this case. In general, with regard to cervical spine disease or trauma to the cervical spine, an awake intubation allows for a focused neurologic exam after intubation prior to the induction of general anesthesia. This exam can be compared to the pre-intubation neurologic exam and documented in the record. This patient would also be considered a full stomach and, therefore, at higher risk of aspiration.

If the airway exam on this patient is more reassuring with respect to likelihood of success with direct laryngoscopy, then another approach to patients such as this with a potentially unstable cervical spine is manual in-line stabilization (MILS).

Would a nasal approach to tracheal intubation be better than an oral approach?

For fiberoptic intubation using the nasal approach may be considered in some cases for reportedly less neck movement during intubation. In addition, the nasal fiberoptic approach to the glottic opening is more of an arc, compared to oral fiberoptic approach which is more of a right angle, therefore some argue this makes the view of the glottis easier to obtain.

However, a nasal approach would not be favored in this patient due to the evidence of facial trauma (which is a relative contraindication to nasal intubation) and also consideration of prior sinus surgery.

How would you manage the cervical collar when proceeding to intubate?

The goal of the cervical collar is to restrict neck movement in a patient with known or suspected neck injury. Its presence also restricts the patient's mouth opening, which is in direct conflict with what is customarily needed for successful direct laryngoscopy. For direct laryngoscopy wherein MILS is planned, the front of the collar may be removed while a dedicated trained individual applies the stabilization (without applying traction).

For fiberoptic intubation, the collar may be left in place if sufficient mouth opening is available to insert the fiberoptic bronchoscope (and a bite block to protect the scope).

Would you administer a drying agent before topicalizing the airway?

When airway topicalization is warranted prior to an awake fiberoptic intubation, administration of an antisialogogue should be considered. Of the anticholinergics, glycopyrrolate (0.2 mg IV) is most commonly chosen. It has a rapid onset of action (2–4 min) and, compared to atropine, it reduces the risk of delirium from central anticholinergic effects since it does not cross the blood-brain barrier.

Antisialogogues decrease oral secretions which improves visibility for the anesthesiologist. Additionally, when the oropharyngeal mucosa is dry, the application of topical anesthetic is more effective, thus less local anesthetic need to be applied and the risk of local anesthetic toxicity is reduced.

This patient is tachycardic on presentation, the etiology of which is likely multifactorial (pain, anxiety, hypovolemia, etc.). Nonetheless, another consideration of administering anticholinergics in this setting is the side effect of increased heart rate. Clearly, some patients would tolerate the heart rate increase from anticholinergic administration better than others.

For patients who are not good candidates for antisialogogues, other options for drying the oral cavity and mucosa may be considered. Gentle suctioning with a Yankauer suction or soft-tip endotracheal suction catheter may decrease secretions; however, it is important to bear in mind the potential for eliciting the gag reflex when doing so. Alternatively, manual drying of the tongue and oral mucosa is an option—for instance, using a gauze pad wrapped around a tongue depressor and applied directly (again with the caveat of not eliciting a gag reflex).

How would you topicalize the airway with local anesthetic? What are the risks or side effects of topicalizing the airway?

Numerous techniques are available for topicalization of the airway including atomizers, nebulizers, ointments and transtracheal instillation. Lidocaine or benzocaine are commonly used, each with their own set of risks.

Topical anesthesia can be time-consuming and may hinder next steps in the patient's care. If secretions are present it may be difficult to achieve adequate topicalization, and with repeated application of anesthetic the risk of toxicity increases. Finally, topicalization (especially of the vocal cords) may induce coughing or vomiting, which in turn can accelerate the timeline for needing to secure the airway if aspiration or desaturation ensues. Instillation of local anesthetic in smaller aliquots ($\sim$1–2 mL) is likely to yield less of a cough reflex compared to larger volumes.

In the contemporary training and practice of anesthesiology, the idea of calling for help when difficulty is encountered is encouraged. Would you call for help *before* attempting an awake intubation on this patient?

In general, anesthesia practice relies on the ability of the anesthesiologist to be largely independent in the performance of carrying out their tasks, but it is recognized that they function as part of a larger team and will call for help appropriately when conditions dictate.

In the ASA Difficult Airway Guidelines, one of the dictums about calling for help is that at least one additional individual will be immediately available to assist with management. It is not specified what level of training or experience this person should have, so this apparently is left up to the judgment of the individual anesthesiologist as to whom to appoint.

The patient's SpO_2 is 96% on a nonrebreather mask. How will you maintain oxygenation during airway management?

Preoxygenation with a facemask before initiating management of the difficult airway is recommended to delay the onset of desaturation should additional time be required to secure the airway. This laudable goal, however, may be derailed by an uncooperative/combative or a pediatric patient, and in these instances it is recognized that success with this part of the process may not be complete. Otherwise, for a cooperative patient that cannot tolerate application of the facemask due to claustrophobia or anxiety, simply removing the mask and having them breathe from the circuit connector may be better tolerated and would lead to at least some preoxygenation (compared to not using the mask at all).

Delivery of supplemental oxygen throughout the process of difficult airway management is also an important part of managing the difficult airway. For delivering oxygen *before* intubation, this can include (but is not limited to) nasal cannula, facemask or both. For delivering oxygen *after* extubating a patient with a difficult airway, options include (but again are not limited to) facemask, blow-by oxygen, or nasal cannula.

Under which circumstances would you call ENT to the bedside to be immediately available, or even have the neck prepared for surgical airway?

It must be acknowledged that there is at least some overlap between the airway management aspect of anesthesia practice and that of our colleagues in related specialties (e.g., emergency medicine, otorhinolaryngology), and collaboration is welcomed in the interest of better patient care.

If invasive airway access is a likely possibility, prudence would dictate taking measures to be ready for that eventuality, and this would include a gowned-and-gloved ENT surgeon with scalpel at the ready to operate on a surgically prepped neck. In clinical practice this is a rare instance, yet it is appropriate when indicated. Whether or not the patient in this case would require such preparation would depend on if she is deemed low likelihood for successful intubation (orotracheal or nasotracheal), and low likelihood for success with supraglottic ventilation (mask ventilation or LMA), and unable to cooperate with an awake intubation or awake tracheostomy. Should all of these conditions exist, this patient is veering on a path to emergency invasive airway access if the low-likelihood scenarios mentioned above actually do come to pass.

The "end point" of the ASA Difficult Airway Algorithm in terms of establishing a definitive airway when all other modes have been unsuccessful and the patient cannot be otherwise oxygenated and ventilated is the emergency invasive airway access. Ironically, though this technique is delineated on the algorithm published *by* the ASA *for* anesthesiologists, almost all the training with respect to this procedure is geared toward how to *avoid* getting into a situation where it is needed. This is because the failure rate is high and the complication rate is high. Therefore, having immediate availability of a practitioner who is accustomed to operations on the trachea is of great utility. The algorithm does not mandate that this procedure (invasive airway access) be performed by the anesthesiologist.

If you elect to do an awake fiberoptic intubation for this patient, how would you prepare her—what would you tell her?

In truly urgent situations, it can seem that counterproductive to spend time informing a patient who has a difficult airway about the risks and procedures that are planned for managing it. For one reason, it can seem that this time is detracting from getting on with the task at hand, and secondly it would be very unlikely that any such discussion would change the approach to management. However, the premise of good communication (with the patient or their health care proxy/representative) is worth considering for such an important and potentially life-threatening procedure, and having the patient understand the need for cooperation will benefit them as well as the practitioner. When a patient presents with a difficult airway, the ASA Guidelines do in fact recommend informing them (or their proxy) about the special risks and procedures related to managing their difficult airway.

The patient tells you she is very anxious and asks if she could receive some sedation for the intubation? How would you answer her?

The key concept in this situation is "judicious use," for the reason that there are many risks involved with administering sedatives to this patient.

In this case, the patient is described as being awake and alert; however, she does not remember the accident itself, which does raise some concern. Clinically, it appears she is relatively stable but her cervical spine has not been cleared. If an awake intubation approach is chosen, the ideal situation is for topicalization of the airway with local anesthetic, which should require little to no analgesia or anxiolysis.

If the decision is made to administer anxiolytics in order to improve patient cooperation and, thereby, the likelihood of success with the intubation, several options are available:

Midazolam is relatively short-acting, provides anxiolysis and amnesia, and can be reversed with flumazenil. Given the synergistic effects of benzodiazepines with opioids, respiratory depression is a concern, of course, and it would be worth determining if the patient received any opioids up to this point in her clinical course.

Dexmedetomidine is another option, with its beneficial properties of maintaining respiratory drive while providing anxiolysis; however, it lacks a reversal agent.

Ketamine, though it can be used for sedation in certain situations, has some unwanted side effects such as dysphoria and increased salivation which would not be of use in a situation such as this.

After the sedation medication that you just administered, the patient appears less anxious. A few minutes later you note the patient's respiratory rate has significantly declined and she is less arousable. What would you do now?

There are several things that could be done at this point, but the most crucial is recognizing that the situation requires immediate attention. Delivery of supplemental oxygen must be assured. Verbal or tactile stimulation should be used to attempt to increase level of consciousness. If a reversal agent for the sedation that was administered has not been given it should be considered at this point.

The next steps would involve bag mask ventilation with supplemental oxygen to combat the decline in respiratory rate.

When attempting to mask ventilate, you do not see end-tidal CO_2 on the monitor. What would you do now?

The answer lies, at least in part, in the level of confidence the practitioner has regarding the adequacy of facemask ventilation. Signs of inadequate facemask ventilation include:

- Insufficient or absent chest movement
- Absent or inadequate breath sounds
- Audible signs of airway obstruction, gastric insufflation/dilatation
- Inadequate or decreasing oxygen saturation
- Cyanosis
- Absent, inadequate or elevated end-tidal carbon dioxide
- Absent or inadequate exhaled gas flow (spirometry)
- Hemodynamic consequences of hypercarbia or hypoxemia (e.g., tachycardia, hypertension, dysrhythmias)

In some cases, the monitoring technology may falsely indicate no $ETCO_2$ (for instance, an extension on the CO_2 sampling tubing can lead to a delay in the sampled gas reaching the monitor, or perhaps a loose connection somewhere along the course of the circuit). Another possibility is extremely low cardiac output which may present as imperceptibly low $ETCO_2$.

This is clearly of immediate concern. In any case, reestablishing ventilation is required, either through improving attempts at mask ventilation or proceeding to intubation immediately.

Could this difficulty with bag mask ventilation have been predicted?

As this situation involves an urgent intubation, the circumstances for mask ventilation are not ideal, and the cervical collar can easily interfere with mask fit as well as jaw thrust and repositioning maneuvers that may be available under normal circumstances. The patient does have at least one risk factor for difficult mask ventilation, which is her BMI. Though "obesity" is often quoted as a risk factor for difficult mask ventilation, this is not entirely accurate, as a BMI of greater than >26 kg/m^2 was quoted in the original article by Langeron [3], and this actually corresponds to "overweight" in conventional metabolic classification.

It is also not known from the reported case information if the patient snores or not (as discussed earlier, this is not always a clear finding from the patient-reported history, and only infrequently gets listed as a medical condition in the chart). As such, this may or may not be a contributing factor, but should be a consideration, especially in a patient with an elevated BMI.

The commonly cited risk factors for difficult mask ventilation are the following:

- Presence of a beard
- Body Mass Index >26 kg/m^2
- Lack of teeth
- Age > 55 years old
- History of snoring

When you go to chart the intubation on this patient in the anesthetic record, how would you describe the difficulty you encountered with mask ventilation?

Documenting sufficient detail about the experience and degree of success (or not) with mask ventilation is important for future care delivery, and commonly used descriptors are usually adequate. Han and colleagues developed a useful grading scale to characterize the ease or difficulty associated with mask ventilation, presented below:

DIFFICULT MASK VENTILATION SCALE

Grade 0	Ventilation by mask not attempted (24%)
Grade 1	Ventilated by mask (54%)
Grade 2	Ventilated by mask with oral airway or other adjuvant (20%)
Grade 3	Difficult mask ventilation* (1.2%)
Grade 4	Unable to mask ventilate (0.05%)

*In this scale "Difficult Mask" is defined as "inadequate, unstable, or requiring two providers" and "with or without the use of muscle relaxant."

How common is it to encounter problems with mask ventilation?

Generally speaking, difficult mask ventilation is likely to occur about 1–2 times per 100 general anesthetics. Impossible mask ventilation (i.e., no success despite standard ventilation, oral airway, two-person mask ventilation, etc.) may be encountered approximately 1–2 times per 1000 general anesthetics. These numbers are gross estimates, of course, as the actual incidence is higher in the subgroups of patients who have more risk factors for difficult mask ventilation.

Defining inadequate mask ventilation has some challenges. Some definitions relate to adequacy of breath sounds, chest movement, oxygen desaturation below a certain percentage, development of cyanosis, etc. Compared to tracheal intubation, there is more of a continuum of adequacy of mask ventilation rather than a binary "yes/no" of success.

With newer technology and training with more advanced airway devices (video laryngoscopes in particular), it may be less reliable to depend on a patient's report that there were no airway problems with prior anesthetics. It may very well be that there were no problems because the difficult airway was anticipated and planned for with specialized equipment available.

How common is it to encounter a patient who is a difficult intubation?

In contrast to difficult mask ventilation, defining difficult intubation is straightforward—the trachea is either intubated or not intubated; there is no ambiguity. The incidence of difficult intubation by direct laryngoscopy ranges from 0.1 to 13%. For failed intubation, the incidence is about 0.5–2.5%.

How common is it to encounter a patient who is both a difficult mask ventilation and difficult intubation?

This combination of a patient being a difficult mask as well as a difficult intubation is very rare, luckily. Reports estimate the incidence of this to be approximately 0.01–2 per 10,000 general anesthetics.

What are the options for invasive airway access?

Again, the ASA Difficult Airway Algorithm must be referenced; there are only three options on this list:

1. Surgical or percutaneous airway
2. Jet ventilation
3. Retrograde intubation

For an elective case, it may be reasonable to cancel surgery because of repeated failed airway attempts as there may be concern for airway edema, vocal cord trauma or potential for causing unnecessary trauma. In the case presented here, cancellation is not a viable option.

What are the contraindications to cricothyrotomy?

Preexisting laryngeal disease

Acute inflammation
Chronic inflammation
Malignancy

Coagulopathy
Distortion of normal airway anatomy
Infants and children < 6-years old
Inexperience in cricothyrotomy procedure (experience decreases complications)

Would you consider this patient to be high risk for extubation?

Admittedly, most of the focus on difficult airway management is on intubation. However, if a good management plan is required for intubation, the corollary to this is that a good management plan is also required for extubation.

Deciding whether a patient who was initially difficult to intubate may also present difficulty when it is time for extubation is a judgment call, and again many factors must be considered. If the conditions that made intubation a challenge are no longer present (e.g., cervical collar no longer in place, or an airway tumor that has now been excised), it could be argued that the risk of extubation is actually lower. Conversely, if the patient now has a surgically fused cervical spine, or now has more airway edema, the risk of extubation is likely higher.

Other clinical situations that may indicate higher risk for extubation include the following:

Medical conditions:

Tracheomalacia (dynamic airway obstruction)
Paradoxical vocal cord motion (VC adduction with inspiration or expiration)
Parkinson's Disease (tremor: abnormal glottic opening/closing, aspiration risk)
Rheumatoid Arthritis (baseline difficult neck extension, cricoarytenoid arthritis)
OSA (airway obstruction at baseline, worse with sedatives/anesthetics)
Obesity (accelerated oxygen desaturation, ±airway obstruction)
Burns (impaired clearance of secretions, increased CO_2 production)

Surgical procedures:

ENT surgery
Laryngeal surgery (glottic edema)
Thyroid surgery (SLN or RLN injuries, local hematoma)
Deep neck infections (edema)
Tracheal resections (guardian suture limits access for reintubation)
Uvulopalatopharyngoplasty (preexisting OSA, obesity, airway edema)
Maxillofacial surgery (mandibular surgery, wiring of mandible)
Cervical spine surgery (decreased ROM, +/−prone position —airway swelling)

Posterior fossa surgery (CN or VC injury, respiratory control center injury)
Carotid endarterectomy (hematoma, nerve injury)

Would you take any special precautions when attempting to extubate this patient? Would you have the ENT surgeon at the bedside?

The same recommendations of the ASA Guidelines that apply to intubation also apply to extubation (e.g., preoxygenation, delivery of supplemental oxygen when the airway is not secured, availability of additional personnel to assist in management).

Being able to re-intubate in a timely fashion if necessary should be part of the plan, so having a defined plan in place and specialized equipment available would be indicated.

Consideration of short-term use of a device that can serve as a guide for expedited re-intubation is recommended, and the ASA Guidelines endorse two different types of such devices: a *stylet* (intubating bougie) or a *conduit*:

A *stylet* (intubating bougie) is inserted through the endotracheal tube and into the trachea before extubation so that re-intubation, if needed, could occur by inserting an ETT over the stylet. Examples of such devices would include an airway exchange catheter or a bougie. The fundamental difference between these two devices is that the hollow core of the airway exchange catheter allows at least some ability to oxygenate and ventilate (requires using an adapter that can attach to a bag mask or anesthesia circuit or jet ventilator), whereas this is not possible with the solid bougie. Another difference is that the bougie has a coude tip (40° bend), whereas the airway exchange catheter does not.

A *conduit*, on the other hand, would include devices such as an LMA or intubating LMA, which would allow for supraglottic ventilation and intubation.

Should this patient be told she has a difficult airway?

A patient with some risk factors for difficult airway may or may not turn out to be a difficult airway upon attempting intubation. The actual clinical experience of intubation will yield reliable information as to how challenging it was to secure the airway. Also, the clinical situation (i.e., emergency vs. elective) or patient characteristics (e.g., cervical collar, patient positioning) may make a patient "difficult" in that situation but not so if those elements were changed or no longer relevant in the event of a subsequent intubation.

In cases where a patient has some or several risk factors for difficult intubation but ultimately proves to be straightforward (by conventional methods of bag mask ventilation and/or direct laryngoscopy), it is perhaps more important that this information be documented in the record and passed on to the patient so that the extra clinical resources and potential psychological impact on the patient are not invoked unnecessarily in the future.

The ASA Guidelines do suggest that details about any airway difficulties encountered be recorded in the patient's chart. This would naturally include information on techniques and devices used and the extent to which each was successful or detrimental. Some hospital record systems may also employ a system to flag the charts of such patients should they present for care in the future.

It is also recommended that such important information be communicated to others. Principally, of course, this would mean informing the patient (or, if incapacitated, the patient's healthcare representative). Toward this end, a "difficult airway letter" may be issued to them, and possibly a recommendation that they obtain an alert bracelet to warn others of the presence of this condition. Perhaps an alert bracelet may be more useful for patients who may not outwardly appear to be a difficult airway (an "unanticipated difficult airway" patient).

The surgeon and primary care provider should also be informed of any airway difficulties encountered.

What are the principal adverse outcomes associated with the difficult airway?

A difficult airway presents high risk in several respects, even when it is anticipated and when there is time to plan for it. There are few instances in medicine when cause and effect of a devastating outcome are so closely related temporally than when trying to secure the difficult airway. When it is not successfully secured in a timely fashion, adverse outcomes are possible and some would say likely. These adverse outcomes include airway trauma (including bleeding, edema, esophageal perforation, tracheal perforation, pneumothorax), damage to teeth or airway, aspiration, death, brain injury, cardiopulmonary arrest, and unnecessary surgical airway.

What are the top reasons for airway complications and management failures?

- Inaccurate or incomplete preoperative airway assessment
- Incorrect prediction of easy mask airway
- Incorrect prediction of direct laryngoscopy guided intubation
- Incorrect prediction of uncomplicated extubation
- Unwillingness to abandon failed airway management plan
- Failure to call for help early, when difficult airway is first apparent
- Incomplete preparation of backup plan

- Deterioration of performance under stress
- Failure in judgment

References

1. Practice Guidelines for Management of the Difficult Airway. American Society of Anesthesiologists. Anesthesiology. 2013;128 (2):1–19.
2. The Airway Approach Algorithm. Rosenblatt WH. J Clin Anesth. 2004;16(4):312–6.
3. Langeron O, Masso E, Huraux C, et al. Prediction of difficult mask ventilation. Anesthesiology. 2000;92:1229.
4. Han R, Tremper K, Kheterpal S, O'Reilly M. Grading scale for mask ventilation. Anesthesiology 2004;101:267.

Suggested Reading

5. Atlee JL. Complications in Anesthesia. Chapter: Elsevier/Saunders; 2007 40.
6. ASA (2005) Management of the difficult airway—a closed claims analysis.
7. Glick DB, Cooper RM. The Difficult Airway. 2013.
8. Hagberg, CA. Benumof and Hagberg's airway management, 3rd Ed.; 2013.
9. Hung OR, Murphy MF. Management of the difficult and failed airway, 2nd Ed. McGraw-Hilll; 2011.
10. Rosenblatt WH, Popescu, WM. Master techniques in upper and lower airway management; 2015.

Pediatric Tonsillectomy and Adenoidectomy 38

Makara E. Cayer

Case:

A 4-year-old 17-kg male with Down syndrome presents for tonsillectomy and adenoidectomy.

Medications: none

Allergies: NKDA

Past Medical History:

Trisomy 21
Obstructive sleep apnea
Tonsillar and adenoid hypertrophy

Physical Exam:

VS: within normal limit for age; BMI 25
Oropharynx: tonsils 3+, otherwise normal
Otherwise insignificant

1. **What are the most common indications for tonsillectomy and adenoidectomy?**

In 2006, there were approximately 530,000 pediatric tonsillectomies (with or without adenoidectomy) performed in the United States [1]. Common indications for tonsillectomy are obstruction (including OSA), infection (including chronic tonsillitis), and tonsil mass. Common indications for adenoidectomy include nasopharyngeal obstruction, Eustachian tube dysfunction and recurrent otitis media, chronic sinusitis, obstructive sleep apnea (OSA), and chronic or recurrent adenoiditis [2].

M.E. Cayer (✉)
Department of Anesthesiology, Massachusetts Eye and Ear Infirmary, 243 Charles Street, Suite 712, Boston, MA 02114, USA
e-mail: Makara_Cayer@meei.harvard.edu

© Springer International Publishing AG 2017
L.S. Aglio and R.D. Urman (eds.), *Anesthesiology*,
DOI 10.1007/978-3-319-50141-3_38

2. **What is OSA and how is this disorder classified differently in pediatric patients than in adults?**

OSA is defined as a syndrome having various degrees of upper airway obstruction during sleep, from partial to complete. It is the most severe form of sleep-disordered breathing. These episodes can lead to oxygen desaturation, hypercarbia and cardiac dysfunction. Signs and symptoms include poor sleep, frequent arousals, daytime sleepiness, snoring, and observed apnea. In children, symptoms also include hyperactivity or distractibility [3]. OSA is classified by sleep study into severities: mild, moderate and severe (though different sleep study centers use different classification systems). In children, an obstructive apnea index greater than one is abnormal. The obstructive apnea index is the number of obstructive efforts that include more than two obstructive breaths. A saturation nadir less than 92% is abnormal [2]. In children, an apnea–hypopnea index greater than 10 per hour and an oxygen saturation nadir less than 80% is often categorized as severe [4].

3. **What are symptoms of OSA in children?**

Symptoms of sleep apnea include loud snoring, gasping while sleeping, pausing while sleeping, night terrors, restless sleep, confused arousal, drooling, mouth breathing, sleep walking, difficult morning wakening, daytime irritability, enuresis, daytime somnolence, poor school performanc, and frequent upper respiratory infections (URIs) [5].

4. **If this child has OSA, is he at risk for cor pulmonale? Why or why not?**

Children with OSA may have hypoxia and hypercarbia. Hypoxia and hypercarbia can result in pulmonary artery constriction. As a longstanding condition this can lead to pulmonary hypertension, right-sided heart failure, and cor pulmonale [2]. This is can be minimized if sleep apnea is treated early.

5. **How is tonsil size evaluated, and what size tonsils could place a child at increased risk of obstruction under general anesthesia?**

Surgical indications include tonsillar hypertrophy, and the size of the tonsils is evaluated by the otolaryngologist. Sizing relates to the percentage of pharyngeal area that is obstructed by tonsillar mass, and is reported on a scale ranging from 0 to 4+.

Rating	Percentage of tonsillar mass obstructing the pharyngeal area
0	None
1+	≤25%
2+	>25% but ≤50%
3+	>50% but ≤75%
4+	≥75%

A rating of 3+ or greater indicates increased risk of obstruction on induction of anesthesia [2].

6. **What if the child has an URI? Will you cancel the case? Why or why not? How will you decide?**

In pediatric anesthesiology, there is frequently the consideration of recent URI. History of recent URI should be elicited. There has been evolution of the treatment of children with URIs and anesthesia. In the past, many practitioners would cancel a case in a child who had a current or recent respiratory infection within 4 weeks prior to surgery. This decision was based on the evidence that children with URIs or recent URIs had greater incidence of respiratory adverse events compared to children without URIs or who had a URI more than 4 weeks prior [6, 7]. Independent risk factors for respiratory adverse events in these children included endotracheal tube (ETT) in children <5 years of age, parental smoking, copious secretions, prematurity, reactive airway disease, nasal congestion and surgery on the airway [7]. However these children had no long-term adverse morbidity. Because of this, most children can undergo anesthesia in the presence of a URI or recent URI, taking into consideration the independent risk factors above. A review by Tait and Malviya [8] proposes an algorithm for pre-anesthetic decision-making for a child with URI symptoms. This algorithm takes into account the urgency of the surgery, the severity of the signs and symptoms (and whether or not they are indicative of an infectious etiology), the anesthetic plan (general versus regional). Other independent risk factors are also considered, such as the need for an ETT in a patient less than 5 years old, parental smoking, copious secretions, nasal congestion, history of prematurity, and any history of reactive airway disease. Still other considerations include whether or not the case has been canceled in the past, if there is an expedient need for surgery, if the patient and family have traveled a long distance, and the anesthesiologist's comfort level with anesthetizing a child with a URI. After taking these factors into account and discussing any concerns with the surgeon and the patient's family, make a decision. If the decision is made to proceed with surgery, some measures can be taken to mitigate the risks, including consideration of avoiding an ETT if possible, hydrating the child, or the administration of an anticholinergic to decrease secretions, or the use of humidified oxygen [8].

7. **Should this patient have a sleep study?**

Polysomnography (sleep study) is the gold standard for diagnosing and characterizing severity of OSA. However, there are half a million pediatric tonsillectomies performed yearly in the United States, and resources to perform sleep studies in this number of patients are not available [4]. A 2011 Clinical Practice Guideline on polysomnography prior to pediatric tonsillectomy recommends sleep study for children with obesity, craniofacial abnormalities, Down syndrome, neuromuscular disorders, sickle cell disease or mucopolysaccharidoses. This patient falls into the category recommended to have a sleep study prior to tonsillectomy. A sleep study allows for better characterization of OSA, and its severity. This allows for appropriate perioperative planning for these patients, including need for overnight admission, and site of overnight admission (intensive care versus a less intensive care setting), and can help determine need for surgery in the first place [9].

8. **What special considerations should be made for a child with trisomy 21 (also called Down syndrome) undergoing anesthesia?**

Children with trisomy 21 are at a higher risk of OSA than the general population, with a prevalence of approximately 30–50% [10, 11]. Thus, children with Down syndrome and OSA will have risks associated with OSA. Children with trisomy 21 are at risk of atlantoaxial instability (AAI), may have congenital heart disease (CHD), hypotonia, and hypothyroidism. Children with trisomy 21 often have had thorough cardiac evaluation and repair of CHD prior to presenting for tonsillectomy or adenoidectomy. If these patients are not stable from a cardiac standpoint the surgery should not proceed. If the patient has certain cardiac defects or repairs, preoperative antibiotics may be needed for endocarditis prophylaxis.

9. **How common is AAI in the trisomy 21 population? How is it evaluated? What are current recommendations for evaluation? What are the symptoms? What should be done to protect patients with trisomy 21 in relation to AAI during anesthesia and surgery?**

10–30% of those with trisomy 21 have radiographic evidence of AAI. Of those, only 1–2% are symptomatic [12].

Recommendations for evaluation and care of trisomy 21 patients in relation to AAI have changed over the past decades. In the past, the Down Syndrome Medical Interest Group recommended screening radiographs between the age of 3–5 years, again at the age of 12 and as an adult if participating in the Special Olympics, and prior to elective surgeries [12]. In 2011, the American Academy of Pediatrics updated its guidelines for children with Down syndrome, including an update to guidelines for AAI [13]. These new guidelines for trisomy 21 emphasize that screening radiographs do not predict future risk of AAI, and underscore the importance of health checks with physical exam, questions about symptoms and anticipatory guidance for patients and parents about symptoms and cervical spine protection. Anticipatory guidance for parents should begin at birth to one month of age for correct cervical spine positioning and continuing forward. Parents should be educated on the signs and symptoms of myelopathy throughout the first year of life. Cervical spine films are no longer recommended for asymptomatic children. People with trisomy 21 and their families should be cautioned about participating in full contact sports or sports that could cause injury to the cervical spine.

Sudden symptoms can develop after otolaryngology procedures. This may be due to manipulation by the anesthesia or surgical team. Continued anticipatory guidance should continue through late childhood, adolescence, and adulthood [12].

Symptomatic patients should have radiographic films in the neutral position only. If these films are normal, only then should flexion and extension films be performed. If an abnormality is found, urgent referral should be made to a neurosurgeon or orthopedists for management [13].

On preoperative evaluation, the patient and family should be questioned for signs or symptoms of AAI (e.g., neck pain, gait disturbance, or signs of paralysis). If no signs or symptoms of AAI are elicited, then surgery may proceed, with maintenance of neutral cervical spine position throughout the anesthetic and surgical procedure.

10. **Should the patient get a CBC and coagulation studies? What about a type and screen?**

Unless there is reason to suspect anemia, a complete blood count need not be performed. Unless a patient has a history of abnormal hemostasis, either a formal diagnosis or by symptoms including unusually easy bruising or bleeding, or a family history of a bleeding disorder, no coagulation studies need to be performed [14]. Coagulation screening is not cost-effective [15]. In addition, type and screens need not be performed because the transfusion rate after tonsillectomy or adenotonsillectomy is low. This type of preoperative testing in patients who are unlikely to require transfusion increases costs [16].

If a patient does have a coagulopathy, this should be appropriately treated preoperatively. Perioperative plans should be made preoperatively with the assistance of a hematologist.

11. **This patient is having surgery because of severe sleep apnea. Would you give the patient oral midazolam prior to the operating room?**

Parental presence and distraction may be safer methods to attempt to calm a child with severe sleep apnea. In combination with pain medications in children with OSA, midazolam can lead to increased respiratory depression. If non-pharmacologic methods are ineffective, and a benzodiazepine is used for preoperative sedation, an anesthesia provider or preoperative nurse should stay with the patient and monitoring with pulse oximetry should be used. Having flumazenil immediately available would also be a prudent measure to take.

12. **Would you proceed with induction of anesthesia without intravenous (IV) access in a patient with severe OSA?**

It would be preferable to have an IV in place prior to induction. OSA patients can have obstruction occur after anesthetic induction that may make mask ventilation difficult if not impossible [2]. In children, induction is often inhalational via mask as many patients are not amenable to intravenous placement without prior sedation. Although having IV access prior to induction is preferable, proceeding with an inhalation induction in this patient may be considered with the following conditions:

1. Patient is not a known difficult mask ventilation or difficult intubation
2. Patient does not have other risk factors for difficult mask ventilation and difficult intubation. As noted above, OSA due to tonsillar hypertrophy can make mask ventilation difficult, but intubation is not usually difficult.
3. Assistance is available for IV placement immediately after induction.

If these conditions are not met, an IV should be placed prior to induction, even in an uncooperative child.

13. **After a mask induction with sevoflurane, the child becomes bradycardic. What do you think is happening? What would you do?**

First, it should be confirmed that the patient is oxygenating and ventilating well, as hypoxia can lead to bradycardia. If oxygenation and ventilation are adequate, then bradycardia secondary to inhaled anesthetic should be next on the differential diagnosis. In patients with Down syndrome, bradycardia can be a complication of induction with volatile agents including sevoflurane and halothane, regardless of history of CHD. Impairment of autonomic cardiac regulation may explain this bradycardia [17]. This can be ameliorated by decreasing volatile anesthetic concentration and by airway adjustments including oral airway insertion, jaw thrust, chin lift, and improved mask seal [17, 18]. If bradycardia is severe and does not respond to the above measures, atropine or epinephrine administration may be required. If necessary, cardiopulmonary resuscitation and pediatric advanced life support protocols should be performed.

14. **Efforts to improve mask ventilation have been successful, and an IV has now been placed. What type of airway device do you plan to place at this point—an ETT (cuffed or uncuffed) or Laryngeal Mask Airway (LMA)?**

Adenotonsillectomy procedures have been safely carried out with the use of either an ETT or LMA; however, each choice has benefits and risks.

The surgical procedure uses electrocautery in the oropharynx which represents an airway fire risk. An uncuffed ETT does not protect against this risk. Therefore, if an ETT is used it should be cuffed to isolate gases in the airway. Additionally, avoiding an enriched oxygen environment will further decrease the fire risk, so a low fraction of inspired oxygen (FiO_2) (e.g., lower than 30%) is also advisable.

LMAs can be used safely for adenotonsillectomy; however, an LMA may need to be converted to an ETT. In this patient with tonsillar hypertrophy, LMA insertion may prove more difficult. Also, if this patient becomes apneic during the case, positive pressure ventilation may be required. Positive pressure ventilation has been found to increase rate of complications with LMA during pediatric tonsillectomy. Surgeon comfort with LMA for this procedure should also be taken into consideration [19].

15. **You are careful to have the FiO_2 at 28%, but the patient's oxygen saturation decreases to the low 1980s when the ETT is right main-stemmed. You turn the FiO_2 to 100%. You pull the ETT back and have bilateral breath sounds. You forget to turn down the oxygen fraction. The surgeon uses electrocautery. There is a flame in the airway. What components are necessary to start a fire?**

There are three components necessary for a fire to start; oxygen, heat and fuel. In the operating room, the oxidizer is the oxygen, air or nitrous oxide, the heat source is often electrocautery, a light source, or laser, and the fuel can be an ETT, a drape, a gauze pad, patient hair or skin [20].

16. **How can operating room fires be prevented?**

Before a procedure begins, fire safety should be discussed among the operating room team. The surgeon, anesthesiologist, and rest of operating room team should know roles for prevention and treatment of fire.

Any flammable skin preparation should dry before draping. Oxidizer should not be allowed to build up under drapes, and discussion of use of oxidizer and use of heat source should continuously take place between surgeon and anesthesiologist. Use of ignition source should be announced, the anesthesiologist should reduce oxygen concentration, and nitrous oxide should be stopped. Moistened sponges should be used near ignition sources. Use cuffed ETTs for surgery in the airway. In addition, look for early warning signs of fire including pop, flash, heat or smoke. Stop the procedure if these signs are seen and evaluate for fire [21].

17. **What would you do now that fire is present?**

I would remove the airway device (ETT or LMA) and stop all airway gas flows. Flammable material should be removed from the airway. Saline should be poured into the airway. If fire is not extinguished a CO_2 fire extinguisher should be used.

Next, ventilation must be reestablished. If able to avoid high FiO_2, this should be done. Inspect the removed ETT for damage to see if fragments may be left behind. Bronchoscopy should be considered. Next, the patient's pulmonary and hemodynamic status should be assessed and further management plan should be discussed with the surgeon [21].

18. **Assume that the fire never took place. The patient is intubated and the surgeon has begun the tonsillectomy. Would you give dexamethasone? Why would you give it or why not?**

The American Academy of Otolaryngology-Head and Neck Surgery (AAO-HNS) strongly recommends an intraoperative dose of intravenous dexamethasone for children undergoing tonsillectomy [22]. Intraoperative dexamethasone results in decreased postoperative nausea and vomiting (PONV) in the first 24 h. Patients who received intraoperative dexamethasone are more likely to advance to a soft or solid diet on postoperative day one. A dose of 0.5 mg/kg is the most common dose used in studies, but lower doses may be effective. According to AAO-HNS, there is little evidence that administration for one intraoperative dose of dexamethasone causes harm. One study found evidence of increased bleeding after one intraoperative dose of 0.5 mg/kg dexamethasone [23]. Further research needs to be conducted in this area.

19. **Would you give ondansetron?**

The rate of PONV after tonsillectomy in children is greater than 70% if no antiemetic prophylaxis is received. This increases overnight admissions, need for intravenous fluid administration, and increases resource utilization. A dose of dexamethasone decreases the risk of PONV, and adding a serotonergic antagonist such as ondansetron can further decrease this risk [22, 24].

20. **Would you give promethazine to prevent or treat PONV?**

In 2004, the FDA issued a "black box warning" For promethazine regarding its use in children under the age of 2 years, and an increased warning for use in children older than the age of two [25]. Promethazine is associated with adverse events including fatal respiratory depression and it should not be used in children under the age of two. There should be a very strong reason for use in children over 2 years of age, especially when given with other respiratory depressants such as opiates or anesthetics. If it is given in a child postoperatively, apnea monitoring should be strongly considered, at least in the form of continuous pulse oximetry.

21. **Will you give intraoperative opioids? How might opioid dosing in this patient differ from a 10-year old without OSA having tonsillectomy for chronic tonsillitis?**

Risk of serious respiratory complications including death after adenotonsillectomy is increased in the following populations: children less than 3 years old, children with severe OSA and children with Down syndrome or neuromuscular disease. This patient falls into this increased risk group. In a retrospective study of children undergoing adenotonsillectomy with severe sleep apnea, reducing opioid administration and giving dexamethasone decreased the incidence of a major respiratory medical intervention by more than 50%. Decreased doses of opioids should be used in patients with OSA, with approximately 50% reduction in dose compared to those without OSA [4, 26, 27].

In addition, acetaminophen should be given either preoperatively as an oral premedication or intraoperatively as a suppository as part of a multimodal analgesic plan.

22. **Would you give any non-steroidal anti-inflammatory drugs (NSAIDs) for postoperative pain control?**

Though NSAIDs are effective in treating pain in the post-tonsillectomy patients [28], theoretically NSAIDs may increase bleeding by their effect on platelet function. A 2013 Cochrane Database Systematic Review could not include or exclude an increased risk of bleeding with the use of NSAIDs in the pediatric post-tonsillectomy population. Of particular note in this review, ketorolac was not found to increase risk of bleeding compared to other NSAIDs, as had been found in past reviews [29]. An earlier practice guideline from the American Academy of Otolaryngology—Head and Neck Surgery recommends avoiding ketorolac because of bleeding risks [22]. However, ibuprofen may be part of an opiate-sparing postoperative pain management plan, but this decision should be discussed with the surgeon in advance. Questions still remain about NSAID use in this population.

23. **Does dexmedetomidine have a role in these cases? What is dexmedetomidine and how can its pharmacology be used to your advantage perioperatively? What common side effects must you take into account? Can it be used in the recovery room?**

Dexmedetomidine can be used as part of a multimodal pain regimen. It may decrease required dose of postoperative opioids [30]. It also decreases emergence delirium in children and can be useful in the immediate postoperative period [31].

Dexmedetomidine is a centrally acting selective alpha-2 agonist. Compared with clonidine, it is seven times more selective for alpha-2 receptors than clonidine.

It has sedative and analgesic effects with little respiratory depression. Some notable side effects include hypotension and bradycardia [20].

In addition, it can be used in the post-anesthesia care unit as both an analgesic and as a treatment for emergence delirium and agitation. Recovery room nursing staff should be educated about the side effects of dexmedetomidine (including bradycardia and hypotension, as mentioned) though these are not commonly symptomatic in routine administration and dosing.

24. **Should this patient be extubated awake or under a deep plane of anesthesia?**

Extubating children under a deep plane of anesthesia is a practice undertaken to decrease risk of bleeding after tonsillectomy. However, many children are extubated awake without an increased risk of post-tonsillectomy bleeding. One might expect that in patients with sleep apnea, an increased risk of respiratory complications would be found with deep extubation. Post-tonsillectomy, these patients are still at risk of obstruction on extubation, and this risk would be increased under a deep plane of anesthesia. The risk of laryngospasm would also likely be higher.

However, one study did not demonstrate increased complications with deep versus awake extubation post-tonsillectomy in children, even in patients with comorbidities including Down syndrome, craniofacial abnormalities, OSA, or presence of URI within two weeks, among other factors. The only increased risk of perioperative respiratory complications in this study was with children weighing less than 14 kg [32]. Preoperative diagnosis and symptoms of OSA, ability to mask ventilate and intubate the patient should be taken into account when considering deep versus awake extubation.

25. **In the recovery room, the patient is comfortable and sleeping. His oxygen saturation is on pulse oximetry is in the mid-1990s. The parents ask you if the surgeon will give them a prescription for codeine postoperatively for pain. Do you think codeine is an appropriate postoperative analgesic for this patient?**

Codeine is not an appropriate postoperative analgesic for this patient. In 2013, the Food and Drug Administration issued a "boxed warning" and a "contraindication" for codeine use in children after tonsillectomy and/or adenoidectomy. Codeine is converted to morphine by the liver. Some patients are "ultra-metabolizers" of codeine, converting codeine into "life-threatening" or "fatal amounts of the drug. This boxed warning was issued as a result of deaths and other serious adverse events in children after tonsillectomy and/or adenoidectomy who had taken codeine [33].

26. **The surgeon had planned to give codeine to the patient for postoperative pain control. What would you recommend to the surgeon for postoperative pain control?**

According to the 2011 AAO–HNS guideline, it is important to educate the caregiver to communicate with the child about pain severity, pain medications, hydration, regularly scheduled pain medication, rectal administration of acetaminophen if oral medication is refused, and normal pain increase in the mornings [22]. Acetaminophen on a scheduled basis is recommended as first-line post adenotonsillectomy pain treatment. Ibuprofen may be safe as a second line medication, and can be discussed with the surgeon. Ibuprofen should not be given to the dehydrated patient because of concern for renal injury. Hydrocodone and oxycodone can be cautiously administered, but not codeine. The lowest effective dose should be chosen. Any child who is excessively sleepy should not receive opioids [34]. As above, a one time intraoperative dose of dexamethasone reduces postoperative nausea, vomiting, and pain, but may increase postoperative bleeding severity, though not incidence of postoperative bleeding [35].

27. **Should the patient be discharged home on the same day of the surgery?**

This patient has risk factors for postoperative respiratory complications and he should stay overnight and have apnea monitoring. Severe OSA is an indication for inpatient monitoring after tonsillectomy [4]. Patients with preoperative OSA continue to have OSA on the first postoperative night, and those with preoperative severe OSA have the most severe postoperative OSA events [36]. According to AAO-HNS: Clinical Practice Guidelines for children with OSA documented by sleep study, these patients should be admitted overnight for monitoring after tonsillectomy if they are less than 3 years old or have severe sleep apnea [9].

28. **You are on call, and a 10-year old who had a tonsillectomy 5 days ago arrives from the emergency department with post-tonsillectomy hemorrhage for planned surgical intervention. Describe the time frame and causes of post-tonsillectomy bleeding.**

There are two periods of post-tonsillectomy bleeding. The first is known as primary hemorrhage and occurs within the first 24 h of bleeding. It is suspected to be the result of inadequate surgical hemostasis. The second time frame is referred to as secondary bleeding, and most commonly occurs 5–12 days postoperatively as a result of premature eschar separation. Rates of primary bleeding range from 0.2 to 2.2% and secondary bleeding rates range from 0.1 to 3% [37].

29. **What are your concerns in this patient at this time and how will you address them?**

This patient may be hypovolemic as a result of large volume blood loss, reduced intake from vomiting (swallowed blood can cause gastric irritation and induce vomiting). In addition, the patient may be acutely anemic, depending on the volume of blood loss and crystalloid replacement. The patient has likely swallowed blood, and thus is not fasted, and risk of pulmonary aspiration is increased. Blood in the oropharynx and supraglottic area can make visualization on intubation difficult.

A rapid preoperative assessment should be performed, including signs and symptoms of hypovolemia such as orthostatic hypotension or dizziness. Other medical history should be reviewed and previous anesthetic record reviewed if available, with attention to past intubation and airway information [2].

The operating room should be prepared with intubation equipment including more than one direct laryngoscope, styletted ETTs in multiple sizes, and multiple ETTs. If possible, more than one anesthesia provider should be present for assistance. Blood should be cross-matched and at least 2 units should be prepared. If large volume bleeding has taken place or is ongoing, or if the patient is hemodynamically unstable, blood should be available in the operating room, or even infusing while being transported to the OR. Prior to induction, standard monitoring should be applied and large bore IV access obtained. Two suction sets should be available, in the event that one suction becomes obstructed or non-functional for any reason.

Intravenous access should be established prior to induction of anesthesia for both administration of fluids and blood, and medication administration.

Preoxygenation of the patient should take place in the left lateral decubitus position to allow blood to drain away from the airway. The patient should be turned supine and rapid sequence induction should be performed. Cricoid pressure may be applied, though this may not prevent aspiration.

Induction medications should include a hypnotic in a decreased dose, as a standard dose may lead to severe hypotension in the hypovolemic patient. If the patient is already hypotensive and hypovolemic, vasopressor administration may be necessary prior to induction. Unless contraindicated, succinylcholine should be used in doses of 1.5–2 mg/kg with atropine 200 mcg/kg. The rationale for the use of atropine is that succinylcholine alone can stimulate cholinergic autonomic receptors and cause arrhythmias including bradycardia and asystole. A cuffed ETT should be rapidly placed to secure the airway.

After surgical control of bleeding is complete, the patient's oropharynx and stomach should be suctioned. The patient should be extubated awake in the left lateral decubitus position to promote drainage of secretions or residual blood [2].

References

1. Cullen KA, Hall MJ, Golonsky A. Ambulatory surgery in the United States, 2006. Natl Health Stat Report. 2009;11:1–25.
2. Raafat SH, Brown KA, Verghese ST. Otorhinolaryngologic procedures. In: Cote CJ, Lerman J, Anderson BJ, editors. A practice of anesthesia for infants and children. 5th ed. Philadelphia: Elsevier Saunders; 2013.
3. American Society of Anesthesiologists. Practice guidelines for the perioperative management of patients with obstructive sleep apnea: a report by the American Society of Anesthesiologists Task Force on Perioperative Management of Patients with Obstructive Sleep Apnea. Anesthesiology. 2006;104:1081–93.
4. Brown KA, Brouilette RT. The elephant in the room: lethal apnea at home after adenotonsillectomy. Anesth Analg. 2014;118:1157.
5. Cote CJ, Posner KL, Domino KB. Death or neurologic injury after tonsillectomy in children with a focus on obstructive sleep apnea: Houston, we have a problem! Anesthesia Analgesia. 2013;118 (6):1276–83.
6. Cohen MM, Cameron CB. Should you cancel the operation when a child has an upper respiratory tract infection? Anesth Analg. 1991;72:282–8.
7. Tait AR, Malviya S, Voepel-Lewis T, et al. Risk factors for perioperative adverse respiratory events in children with upper respiratory tract infections. Anesthesiology. 2001;95:299–306.
8. Tait AR1, Malviya S. Anesthesia for the child with an upper respiratory tract infection: still a dilemma? Anesth Analg. 2005;100(1):59–65.
9. American Academy of Otolaryngology—Head and neck surgery: clinical practice guideline: polysomnography for sleep-disordered breathing prior to tonsillectomy in children. http://oto.sagepub.com/content/145/1_suppl/S1.full. Accessed 29 July 2015.
10. Stebbens VA, Dennis J, Samuels MP, Croft CB, Southall DP. Sleep related upper airway obstruction in a cohort with Down's syndrome. Arch Dis Child. 1991;66:1333–8.
11. de Miguel-Diaz J, Villa-Asensi JR, Alvarez-Sala JL. Prevalence of sleep-disordered breathing in children with down syndrome: polygraphic findings in 108 children. Sleep. 2003;26:1006–9.
12. Dedlow ER, Siddiqi S, Fillipps DJ, Kelly MN, Nackashi JA, Tuli SY. Symptomatic atlantoaxial instability in an adolescent with trisomy 21 (Down's syndrome). Clin Pediatr. 2013;52(7):633–8.
13. Bull MJ. The COMMITTEE ON GENETICS. Clinical report-health supervision for children with down syndrome. Pediatrics. 2011;128:393–406.
14. American Academy of Otolaryngology-head and neck surgery; clinical indicators: tonsillectomy, adenoidectomy, adenotonsillectomy in childhood. https://www.entnet.org/sites/default/files/TA-Adenotonsillectomy-CI%20Updated%208-7-14.pdf. Accessed 29 July 2015.

15. Werner EJ. Preoperative hemostatic screening for pediatric adenotonsillar surgery: worthwhile effort or waste of resources? Pediatr Blood Cancer. 2010;55(6):1045–6.
16. Fernández AM, Cronin J, Greenberg RS, Heitmiller ES. Pediatric preoperative blood ordering: when is a type and screen or crossmatch really needed? Paediatr Anaesth. 2014;24(2):146–50.
17. Kraemer FW, Stricker PA, Gurnaney HG, McClung H, Meador MR, Sussman E, et al. Bradycardia during induction of anesthesia with sevoflurane in children with Down syndrome. Anesth Analg. 2010;111(5):1259–63.
18. Bai W, Voepel-Lewis T, Malviya S. Hemodynamic changes in children with Down syndrome during and following inhalation induction of anesthesia with sevoflurane. J Clin Anesth. 2010;22 (8):592–7.
19. Lalwani K, Ritchins S, Aliason I, Milczuk H, Fu R. The laryngeal mask airway for pediatric adenotonsillectomy: predictors of failure and complications. Int J Pediatr Otorhinolaryngol. 2013;77:25.
20. Ehrenwerth J, Seifert HA. Electrical and Fire Safety. In: Barash PR, Cullen BF, Stoelting RK, Cahalan MK, Stock MC, editors. Clinical anesthesia. 6th ed. Philadelphia: Lippincott Williams and Wilkins; 2009.
21. American Society of Anesthesiology. Practice advisory for the prevention and management of operating room fires. Anesthesiology. 2008;108:786–801.
22. Baugh RF, Archer SM, Mitchell RB, et al. Clinical practice guideline: tonsillectomy in children. Otolaryngol Head Neck Surg. 2011;144:S1.
23. Czarnetzki C, Elia N, Lysakowski C, Dumont L, Landis BN, Giger R, et al. Dexamethasone and risk of nausea and vomiting and postoperative bleeding after tonsillectomy in children: a randomized trial. JAMA. 2008;300:2621–30.
24. Bolton CM, Myles PS, Nolan T, Sterne JA. Prophylaxis of postoperative vomiting in children undergoing tonsillectomy: a systemic review and meta-analysis. Br J Anaesth. 2006;97:593.
25. Starke PR, Weaver J, Chowdry BA. Boxed warning added to promethazine labeling for pediatric use. N Engl J Med. 2005;352:2653.
26. Raghavendran S1, Bagry H, Detheux G, Zhang X, Brouillette RT, Brown KA. An anesthetic management protocol to decrease respiratory complications after adenotonsillectomy in children with severe sleep apnea. Anesth Analg. 2010;110(4):1093–101.
27. Brown KA, Laferriere A, Moss IR. Recurrent hypoxemia in young children with obstructive sleep apnea is associated with reduced opioid requirement for analgesia. Anesthesiology. 2004;100:806.
28. Kelly LE, Sommer DD, Ramakrishna J, Hoffbauer S, Arbab-Tafti S, Reid D, et al. Morphine or Ibuprofen for post-tonsillectomy analgesia: a randomized trial. Pediatrics. 2015;135(2):307–13.
29. Lewis SR, Nicholson A, Cardwell ME, Siviter G, Smith AF. Nonsteroidal anti-inflammatory drugs and perioperative bleeding in paediatric tonsillectomy. Cochrane Database Syst Rev. 2013;7.
30. Pestieau SR, Quesado ZM, Johnson YJ, Anderson JL, Cheng YI, McCarter RJ, et al. High-dose dexmedetomidine increases the opioid-free interval and decreases opioid requirement after tonsillectomy in children. Can J Anaesth. 2011;58(6):540–50.
31. Ibacache ME, Munoz HR, Brandes V, Morales AL. Single-dose dexmedetomidine reduces agitation after sevoflurane anesthesia in children. Anesth Analg. 2004;98:60–3.
32. Baijal RG1, Bidani SA, Minard CG, Watcha MF. Perioperative respiratory complications following awake and deep extubation in children undergoing adenotonsillectomy. Paediatr Anaesth. 2015;25(4):392–9.
33. FDA Drug Safety Communication: Safety review update of codeine use in children; new Boxed Warning and Contraindication on use after tonsillectomy and/or adenoidectomy. http://www.fda.gov/Drugs/DrugSafety/ucm339112.htm.
34. Yellon RF, Kenna MA, Cladis FP, McGhee W, Davis PJ. What is the best non-codeine post adenotonsillectomy pain management for children? Laryngoscope. 2014;124(8):1737–8.
35. Plante J, Turgeon AF, Zarychanski R, et al. Effect of systemic steroids on post-tonsillectomy bleeding and reinterventions: systematic review and meta-analysis of randomized controlled trials. BMJ. 2012;345:e5389. doi:10.1136/bmj.e5389.
36. Nixon GM, Kermack AS, McGregor CD, Davis GM, Manoukian JJ, Brown KA, Brouillette RT. Sleep and breathing on the first night after adenotonsillectomy for obstructive sleep apnea. Pediatr Pulmonol. 2005;39:332–8.
37. Windfuhr P, Chen YS, Remmert S. Hemorrhage following tonsillectomy and adenoidectomy in 15,218 patients. Otolaryngol Head Neck Surg. 2005;132(2):281–6.

Laser Surgery of the Airway

39

Dongdong Yao

Clinical case:

A 57-year-old female with 40-pack-year smoking history presents with voice hoarseness due to laryngeal cancer and laryngeal stenosis. She is scheduled for direct laryngoscopy, suspension microscopy, and laser treatment.

Medications:	Amlodipine 50 mg oral daily
	Tiotropium (Spiriva®) 2 puffs twice daily
	Albuterol 2 puffs PRN difficulty breathing
Allergies:	NKA
Past medical history:	
	Cardiac: hypertension
	Pulmonary: chronic obstructive pulmonary disease (COPD)
Physical Exam:	
	VS: BP 132/84 mmHg HR 75 bpm RR 20/min SpO_2 95% on room air
	HEENT: no stridor
	Cardiac: within normal limits
	Pulmonary: no wheezing
	Airway exam: Mallampati class II
	Otherwise: insignificant

1. **What is a laser and what are the advantages of using laser in airway procedures?**

Though often seen written as "laser," the term "LASER" is actually an acronym for "**L**ight **A**mplification by **S**timulated **E**mission of **R**adiation." Lasers emit a narrow, parallel beam of coherent monochromatic light that can be reflected by mirrors and focused with lenses. These characteristics allow surgeons to direct high-energy laser beams onto focal spots, sometimes in difficult-to-reach narrow spaces, for precise lesion resection, with minimal bleeding, edema, and damage to surrounding tissue.

Since its introduction into medical practice, laser use and applications have been expanded rapidly into many specialties, including otolaryngology, urology, dermatology, ophthalmology, etc. Otolaryngologists are among the pioneers to develop and optimize this tool in treating various upper airway pathologies, such as laryngeal stenosis, benign laryngeal polyps, vocal cord nodules, cysts, granulomas, recurrent respiratory papillomatosis, and malignant laryngeal lesions.

2. **What are the most commonly used lasers in airway procedures? What are the major differences between these lasers?**

Different types of laser technologies are used in otolaryngeal procedures today, and each type has characteristic benefits and drawbacks. The operators should find the balance between tissue efficacy and thermal damage when choosing a particular laser for any given case.

Since the 1970s, the carbon dioxide (CO_2) laser has been the most commonly used laser in otolaryngeal procedures. The wavelength of CO_2 lasers is 10,600 nm, corresponding to the infrared light. The energy emitted by CO_2 lasers is completely absorbed by water in the first few layers of cells, and then transformed into thermal energy, causing instantaneous tissue vaporization. In addition, CO_2 lasers can be delivered through a microscope for accurate and efficient operation on small lesions. These features make CO_2 lasers the ideal cutting/ablating tool for minimally invasive procedures, with excellent hemostasis. However, one limitation of the traditional CO_2 laser is that it does not allow for fiberoptic transmission. It needs an articulated light guide to reflect light to the surgical site, thus it can only be used in areas that can be aligned directly. This line-of-sight

D. Yao (✉)
Department of Anesthesiology, Perioperative and Pain Medicine, Brigham and Women's Hospital, 75 Francis Street, Boston, MA 02115, USA
e-mail: dyao1@partners.org

© Springer International Publishing AG 2017
L.S. Aglio and R.D. Urman (eds.), *Anesthesiology*,
DOI 10.1007/978-3-319-50141-3_39

requirement limits the use of the CO_2 laser to the operating room (OR) setting as general anesthesia is employed to enable patient positioning for full direct laryngoscopy.

Other commonly used lasers are the Pulsed Dye Laser (PDL) and Potassium Titanyl Phosphate–Neodymium–Yttrium aluminum garnet laser (KTP-Nd-Yag). Different from the CO_2 laser, these lasers emit green light with the wavelength of approximately 500 nm and selectively target hemoglobin. Thus, they can selectively heat up blood vessels, causing eradication of vascular lesions while preserving overlying epithelium. In addition, both PDL and KTP-Nd-Yag lasers are readily transmitted via a fiberoptic bundle. Photoangiolysis of the microvasculature has been found to be an effective treatment strategy for laryngeal conditions such as recurrent papillomatosis, dysplasia, and microvascular angiomata, especially in the office-based setting, without the need for general anesthesia.

Lasers are a relatively new component of surgical equipment for airway procedures. The unique characteristics of lasers pose potential challenge for anesthesia providers. Sharing airway with surgeons makes the situation even more complicated. Mutual understanding and intensive cooperation between different disciplines is crucial for successful and safe operations.

3. **What are the key considerations of airway evaluation/management for this patient?**

Airway evaluation and difficult airway management are essential skills for anesthesia providers. This is especially crucial for airway diseases, because they may pose significant challenges for airway management.

A detailed history and meticulous physical exam is always a good starting point. A thorough investigation of the voice and breathing pattern may elucidate useful information regarding laryngeal stenosis. Usually the supraglottic stridor occurs on inspiration; glottic stridor may be inspiratory or expiratory (depending on the type of lesion); subglottic lesions presents with biphasic stridor. A hoarse voice indicates the lesion is likely at the level of vocal cords. If the patient has developed dyspnea, this can be an indication that laryngeal stenosis may be severe. Furthermore, if the reclining position worsens the patient's dyspnea, this finding is particularly ominous for airway compromise—complete airway obstruction may ensue if general anesthesia is induced. In this scenario, awake fiber optic intubation, or even awake tracheostomy, may be warranted instead.

Radiation therapy may be part of the regimen for some laryngeal cancer patients. This treatment modality may produce anatomical alterations in the upper and lower airways, and potentially make the tracheal intubation more difficult. Special attention should be given to assessing head/neck mobility, soft tissue edema and fibrosis, mouth opening, dentition, etc.

Imaging studies are another set of useful tools to evaluate the laryngeal tumor. They can be a great resource to identify the anatomical characteristics of the tumor, including its size, exact location, relationship with vocal cords and other airway structures, etc.

Many patients may have undergone indirect laryngoscopy by the surgeon in clinic prior to surgery. Surgeons may provide valuable information, such as the severity of laryngeal stenosis, the motility and bleeding potential of the tumor, etc. The importance of discussing the findings and plans with surgeons preoperatively cannot be overemphasized.

4. **What is your recommendation for preoperative smoking cessation?**

Smokers require special care when undergoing anesthesia for surgery because smoking is associated with numerous perioperative comorbidities. The most common perioperative risks associated with smoking are impaired wound healing, wound infection, and pulmonary complications.

Within 20 min after quitting smoking, the heart rate and blood pressure drop. Within 12 h after quitting, the blood carbon monoxide level returns to normal. Abstinence starting 3–8 weeks before surgery will significantly reduce the incidence of smoking-related complications. The American Society of Anesthesiologists (ASA) advocates that all patients presenting for surgery should be questioned regarding smoking, and provided with an appropriate consult for smoking cessation. Patients should abstain from smoking for as long as possible both before and after surgery, and they should obtain help in doing so.

5. **Is there more preoperative testing indicated for this patient before the scheduled procedure?**

For patients with well-compensated mild-to-moderate diseases undergoing low-risk elective surgical procedure, and if the procedure is not associated with significant intraoperative blood loss, routine preoperative testing is generally not indicated. Instead, a complete history and thorough physical examination are essential to ensure patient safety. Based on the findings obtained, some relevant lab tests may be considered accordingly.

COPD is the most frequently identified risk factor for postoperative pulmonary complications. When COPD patients undergo noncardiothoracic surgeries, pulmonary function testing results are generally not predictive of perioperative outcomes.

For this case, no further testing is warranted.

6. **How would you monitor this patient?**

Standard ASA monitoring should be sufficient for this case. This is a relatively healthy patient with good functional status, coming for a low-risk procedure. No significant blood loss or fluid shift is expected. Therefore, no additional or more invasive monitoring is indicated.

Standard ASA monitoring includes:

Oxygenation. An oxygen analyzer with a low-oxygen concentration limit alarm is recommended. During the laser airway procedure, a low fraction of inspired oxygen (FiO_2) is delivered to the patient to reduce the potential for airway fire. The oxygen analyzer ensures the patient is receiving clinically safe concentration of oxygen throughout the procedure. A quantitative method of measuring body oxygenation such as pulse oximetry is also required.

Ventilation. Every patient receiving general anesthesia shall have the adequacy of ventilation continually evaluated. Continual monitoring for the presence of expired CO_2 should be employed.

Circulation. The basic monitoring requirements to ensure adequacy of circulatory function are continuous electrocardiogram (EKG), arterial blood pressure (either by noninvasive blood pressure monitor or arterial line), and heart rate. In addition to these, patients undergoing general anesthesia should also have their circulatory function continually evaluated by at least one of the followings: palpation of a pulse, auscultation of heart sounds, monitoring or a tracing of intra-arterial pressure, ultrasound peripheral pulse monitoring, or pulse plethysmography or oximetry.

Body temperature. Esophageal temperature may be impractical for airway procedures. Other sites such as forehead or axilla may be considered, although they may not reflect the core temperature as accurately.

Other routine monitoring, such as neuromuscular blockade monitor, may be considered if clinically indicated (see question #17).

7. **What are the options for airway management in laryngeal laser surgery?**

There are two options to ventilate the patient during laryngeal laser surgeries: general anesthesia via endotracheal intubation with intermittent apnea, or jet ventilation.

The advantages of endotracheal intubation are as follows:

(1) It provides a secured airway that prevents aspiration and allows for controlled ventilation.
(2) It provides surgeons with better access to some areas.
(3) It poses less time constraints to surgeons or anesthesiologists.
(4) It presents completely immobilized vocal folds, which afford surgeons more stable working environment.

The disadvantages of endotracheal intubation are as follows:

(1) It may limit the access to parts of the larynx, and require intermittent withdrawal of the endotracheal tube for optimal surgical exposure and resection. This technique may pose a potential desaturation risk to patients.
(2) It poses a potential fire risk.

The advantages and disadvantages of jet ventilation will be discussed later in the text.

8. **What is your plan to induce general anesthesia for this patient?**

The detailed plan of the anesthesia induction should be formulated based on the condition of the airway with special consideration of the patient's pathology. If a difficult intubation and/or difficult mask ventilation is suspected, awake fiberoptic intubation is often the most prudent choice, with minimal or no pre-induction sedation. Suction should be readily available for potential bleeding from the laryngeal tumor during the instrumentation of the airway. If the patient is not a known or suspected difficult airway, and is completely free from any symptoms or signs of airway compromise, any routine induction technique is considered safe.

9. **What are the key components required for surgical fire?**

A surgical fire is defined as a fire that occurs on or in a patient. An airway fire is a surgical fire that occurs in a patient's airway. It may or may not include a fire in the attached breathing circuit. There are estimated 550–650 surgical fires annually in the United States including airway and non-airway fires. Laser surgeries of the airway pose a significant and sometimes deadly risk of fire. Three key components are required for any surgical fire (sometimes referred to as the surgical fire triangle):

1. Ignition sources. Electrosurgical units and lasers, using energy to cut and coagulate tissue, present particular risks during airway surgeries. Other ignition sources include fiberoptic bronchoscopes, burrs and drills (due to the extreme thermal energy that they can create).

2. Oxidizers. Oxygen and nitrous oxide are commonly used gases in the OR. They are oxidizers that can increase the likelihood and intensity of combustion.
3. Fuels. There are a variety of materials in the OR that are combustible, including endotracheal tubes, sponges/gauzes, surgical drapes, face masks, nasal cannulae, and alcohol-containing solutions.

10. **How would you prevent an airway fire?**

Airway fire often causes devastating complications. The best way to deal with airway fire is through prevention. Close communication among OR personnel is essential to airway fire prevention. Many institutions incorporate fire risk assessment into the surgical pause before airway surgeries. This should include a plan for preventing an airway fire as well as a plan for dealing with an airway fire should it occur intraoperatively, so that all OR team members know in advance what to do and what resources are needed.

Several strategies have been developed to tackle the three components required for surgical fire.

(1) Ignition source/laser. Surgeons should notify the entire OR crew before each of the laser use so that they can take preventive measures accordingly. A warning sign should be placed on the OR entry door to warn of this risk. The anesthesiologist must keep close communication with surgeons, and maintain special vigilance while laser is activated. Laser output should be used with the lowest clinically acceptable power and duration. The laser apparatus should be deactivated and put in standby mode before removing from the surgical site.
(2) Oxidizers. Before surgeons initiate the laser, nitrous oxide should be stopped if in use for procedure, and oxygen concentration should be reduced to the minimum needed to avoid hypoxia.
(3) Fuels. The traditional polyvinyl chloride endotracheal tubes (ETT), as well as red rubber and silicone tubes, are easily ignited when exposed to intense heat, and the byproducts of combusting these materials are potentially toxic. Specially designed laser-resistant ETTs should always be used for laser airway surgeries. The U.S. Food and Drug Administration (FDA) has approved a number of these such ETTs specifically for laser surgery. Commonly a size 5.0 (with the inner diameter of 5 mm) laser-resistant ETT is used for adult patients, for the reason that it will minimize obstruction of the operative field. The ETT cuff should be filled with saline tainted with a dye (such as methylene blue) for the purpose of identifying a rupture of the ETT cuff by the laser. The gauzes and sponges used in procedure should be soaked wet.

11. **How would you manage an airway fire?**

Although airway fire is rare, when it happens, it requires immediate action. The ASA Task Force on Operating Room Fires has developed guidelines and an algorithm to manage OR fires. Anesthesiologists should take the leading role in managing the airway fire.

First, the surgery should be aborted, and the laser should be turned off or put in standby mode.

Second, the flow of all airway gases should be stopped, and the ETT and any other flammable materials such as sponges and gauzes should be removed to minimize potential thermal and chemical damage to the airway. Disconnecting the breathing circuit usually is the quickest way to stop the gas flow. By removing the oxidizers, the fire intensity can be significantly decreased or even eliminated.

Third, saline should be poured into the airway to extinguish the fire. If the fire does not extinguish on the first attempt, a CO_2 fire extinguisher may be used on the patient if necessary. If the fire still persists, the OR personnel should consider activating the fire alarm, evacuating the patient, closing the OR door, and turning off gas supply to the room.

Fourth, the anesthesiologist should reestablish the airway and resume ventilation, preferably with room air if tolerated. An oxidizer-enriched atmosphere should be avoided if clinically appropriate. The ETT should be examined to see if any fragments may have been left behind in the airway. Then the anesthesiologist should carefully assess the airway for the extent of damage and treat the patient accordingly. Bronchoscopy may be considered. Findings and further management plan should be discussed with surgeons. Depending on the extent of damage, re-intubation or tracheotomy may be indicated.

12. **What are other potential hazards in laser surgery and how to protect the patient from these hazards?**

Laser has its unique advantage when used in surgical procedures. However, it also presents potentially serious and sometimes fatal risks to both patients and OR personnel. Its clinical use is subject to some degree of federal regulation and to voluntary consensus standards to minimize these possible risks. The FDA has suggested a set of regulations that have been adopted and modified by several states. The American National Standards Institute (ANSI) has published the American National Standard for the Safe Use of Lasers in Health Care Facilities (Z136.3-2011). These standards and guidelines should be followed to the maximal extent possible.

Other than surgical fire, several other potential hazards are associated with laser use in the OR:

- Atmospheric contamination by laser fumes

Laser beams vaporize tissue with intense energy. During this process, a smoke byproduct along with fine particulates of debris is often produced. The amount of smoke produced varies with the type of surgery, the type of disease, the amount of lasing employed, and the surgeon's technique. Research studies have confirmed that this smoke plume can contain toxic gases and vapors such as benzene, hydrogen cyanide, formaldehyde, bioaerosols, dead and live cel lular material (including blood fragments). At high concentrations the smoke causes ocular and upper respiratory tract irritation. The laser plume may also be mutagenic, teratogenic, or a vector for viral infection. These airborne contaminants generated by laser procedures can be effectively controlled by a combination of general room and local exhaust ventilation. The latter can be achieved with an efficient smoke evacuator at the surgical site. In addition, special high-efficiency masks are strongly recommended for OR personnel during laser surgeries.

- Energy transfer to an inappropriate location

The laser system should be put on standby whenever the laser beam is not being aimed at the target tissue. Occasionally, inadvertent exposure to laser emission does cause injury to either patients or OR staff. Ocular tissues are especially susceptible. CO_2 lasers can induce serious corneal damages, while KTP-Nd-Yag, argon, or ruby lasers may precipitate retina burn. The use of eye protection for both patients and OR staff during laser surgeries is required according to the ANSI standards. For the patient, eyes are shut closed and taped, and then wet gauze pads are applied on top to avoid any unintentional exposure from laser beams. OR staff should wear laser safe protective goggles. In addition, all windows of the OR should be shielded, and warning signs should be posted on all doors leading to the OR to alert anyone entering that this danger exists.

Unintentional tissue damage, blood vessel perforation, or venous gas embolism are other possible complications associated with laser surgeries.

13. **What is the intermittent apnea technique? What is the special consideration during the apnea phase?**

Sometimes even small-size ETTs may still obstruct the surgical field. The intermittent apnea technique may be applied to achieve the best surgical exposure.

The patient is first hyperventilated with anesthetic agent in oxygen. Then the ventilation is paused, and surgeons remove the laser-resistant ETT from the patient to operate on the airway lesions. When the patient's oxygen saturation starts to decline, surgery will be stopped, and the ETT is reinserted into the trachea under direct visualization via the operating laryngoscope. The patient is then hyperventilated again to allow for the next apnea phase. The intermittent apnea technique removes the ETT and all the other flammable materials from the airway during the laser treatment, thus minimizing the fire risk.

The advantages of the intermittent apnea technique are excellent visibility of the surgical field, and minimal fire risk while using lasers in the airway. The disadvantages include time constraint of surgery for each apnea phase, potential airway trauma through multiple extubation/re-intubation cycles, inadequate ventilation, aspiration risk, and variable anesthesia level if using inhalational anesthesia technique.

Close communication between anesthesiologist and surgeon provides the key for safe transition between apnea and ventilation phases.

14. **What is jet ventilation? What are the advantages of this technique?**

Jet ventilation was developed in the 1960s to reconcile the practical problems of maintaining adequate ventilation and good surgical exposure during rigid bronchoscopy. It applies pulsed gas jet into the airway without airtight connection of the patient to the ventilator.

For patients without airway concern, general anesthesia is induced with routine pre-oxygenation and intravenous medication such as propofol. After the confirmation of mask ventilation, neuromuscular relaxant agent is administered, and the airway is secured with either ETT or laryngeal mask airway (LMA). Then the operational laryngoscope and jet ventilator are positioned. Alternatively, the patient remains apneic while setting up the instruments. Once aligned with the trachea, jet ventilation is initiated, and chest excursion is monitored to ensure sufficient ventilation. Supraglottic jet ventilation provides a complete surgical field. However, it is not possible to accurately monitor airway pressure or end-tidal CO_2 with this approach. On the other hand, although airway pressure and end-tidal CO_2 monitoring is achievable with subglottic jet ventilation, a catheter is usually required for this approach. This may impede surgical access, and pose potential fire risk as well.

Compared to the ETT, the advantages of jet ventilation are enhanced surgical exposure, less direct laryngotracheal mucosal trauma, and lower risk of airway fire.

In some cases, the intermittent apnea technique is combined with jet ventilation, so that the instrumentation can be removed temporarily to further expose the surgical field.

15. **What are the potential complications of jet ventilation? What are the contraindications to this technique?**

The potential complications associated with jet ventilation include the following:

- Gastric distension, without definitive airway protection. Thus, there is a higher risk of pulmonary aspiration.
- Inadequate ventilation and/or oxygenation. Capnometry can be greatly inaccurate and usually underestimates the true end-tidal CO_2 value during jet ventilation. The gas exchange for CO_2 becomes insufficient when very high jet frequencies are used. Intraoperative pulse oximetry monitoring is mandated.
- Barotrauma, pneumothorax, pneumomediastinum, or crepitus.
- The passive movement of the vocal cords during ventilation makes surgery more difficult.
- Mucosal desiccation. Prolonged exposure to dry gases under pressure can cause mucosal inflammation, excessive mucous and airway plugging, loss of ciliated epithelium, or even necrotizing tracheobronchitis.

The contraindications for jet ventilation include the following:

- Obesity. Reduced chest wall compliance may cause inadequate ventilation and inadvertent gastric distention.
- COPD. Inadequate expiratory phase may cause breath stacking and auto-positive end-expiratory pressure (PEEP), thus increasing the risk of barotrauma. It is especially dangerous if bullous emphysema is present.
- Retrognathia or overbite. This condition is associated with challenging oropharyngotracheal alignment.
- Glottic lesions, significant pharyngolaryngeal scarring, and laryngospasm. Obstructed airways make the complete passive exhalation more difficult, which may lead to inadequate ventilation and/or barotrauma.

16. **What is your plan of anesthesia maintenance for laser surgery of the airway?**

Either the total intravenous anesthesia (TIVA) or inhalational anesthesia is suited for laser surgeries of the airway. The choice of one technique or the other depends on many factors, such as ventilation via ETT versus jet ventilator, patient medical condition, or the anesthesia provider's personal preferences and experience.

For jet ventilation, inhalational anesthetic technique is not preferred. Because there is no secured conduit to deliver volatile agents, it is difficult to control their alveolar concentration to achieve a stable anesthesia depth. In addition, overflow of volatile agents will cause OR pollution.

Even for ETT-controlled ventilation, if frequent apnea is expected during the procedure, TIVA is also recommended. With TIVA, the delivery of anesthetic agents is relatively constant, and not affected by intermittent interruption of ventilation, thus ensure the patient's stability.

TIVA for laser surgeries in the airway is usually achieved by combining a hypnotic agent such as propofol with a short-acting opioid agent such as remifentanil or alfentanil. Assessing the depth of anesthesia, such as Bispectral index (BIS^{TM}) monitoring, is recommended for TIVA to guide anesthetic administration.

17. **Is neuromuscular relaxant indicated for this procedure?**

Neuromuscular blockade is generally not required for laser surgeries in the airway, except for intubation, introduction of the operating laryngoscope, and jet ventilation.

Inserting the suspension laryngoscopy is highly stimulating to the patient. Adequate muscle paralysis provides masseter muscle relaxation and facilitates the optimal positioning of the laryngoscope. A deep anesthetic and profound analgesia are further required for this process. Muscle relaxation is also desirable for jet ventilation; it can improve chest wall compliance, and minimize the airway obstruction, thus decreasing the chance for barotrauma.

To achieve satisfactory intraoperative muscle relaxation, either a continuous succinylcholine infusion or intermittent boluses of intermediate-acting non-depolarizing neuromuscular blockade (NDNMBs) agents are suitable. Succinylcholine is associated with cardiac arrhythmias, hyperkalemia, malignant hyperthermia, and histamine release. In addition, succinylcholine infusion may cause phase II block during unexpectedly long procedures. On the other hand, for short procedures, intermediate-acting NDNMBs may not be readily reversible at the end, causing delayed extubation. Therefore, vigilant monitoring of neuromuscular function with nerve stimulator is required if NDNMBs are in use.

18. **What are the common complications observed in the recovery room after airway laser surgeries?**

- Dental, lip, and other soft tissue injuries. These are the most common complications associated with laryngeal microsurgery. Careful dental and oral inspection is warranted before and after intubation, as well as before and after instrumentation with the surgical laryngoscope.

- Sore throat and difficulty with swallowing are other common postoperative complications. Usually no special treatment is needed other than careful observation. If these problems arise but do not show improvement over the first couple of days after surgery, or worsen over that time, the patient should be referred for consultation with the ENT specialist.
- Postoperative airway edema. Although lasers can potentially reduce its incidence, postoperative mucosal edema is not uncommon for airway surgeries. Patients usually present with inspiratory stridor in the recovery room. Intravenous corticosteroids such as dexamethasone are routinely used as a preventive method. Racemic epinephrine is the first-line treatment option. Rarely tracheotomy may be indicated for severe postoperative airway obstruction.
- Postoperative hemorrhage. Just as lasers can be effective in limiting postoperative airway edema, they can also potentially decrease postoperative bleeding. However, secondary hemorrhage can occur, especially after extensive tissue resection. If significant bleeding persists, emergent re-intubation and surgical exploration may be indicated.
- Pneumothorax and subcutaneous emphysema are rare complications. Thorough physical examination and chest X-ray can help with the diagnosis. Re-intubation should be considered if the patient's breathing becomes compromised.
- Laryngospasm. Laryngospasm is first treated with positive pressure ventilation with 100% oxygen. If laryngospasm persists, small doses of intravenous anesthetic agent (such as propofol with 0.5–1 mg/kg) or succinylcholine (0.1–0.5 mg/kg) are treatment options unless any contraindications exist.

Further Reading

1. American Society of Anesthesiologists (2008) HOD statement of smoking cessation. http://www.asahq.org/resources/clinical-information/hod-statement-of-smoking-cessation.
2. American Society of Anesthesiologists (2010) Standards for basic anesthetic monitoring. http://www.asahq.org/~/media/Sites/ASAHQ/Files/Public/Resources/standards-guidelines/standards-for-basic-anesthetic-monitoring.pdf.
3. Apfelbaum JL, et al. Practice advisory for the prevention and management of operating room fires: an updated report by the American Society of Anesthesiologists Task Force on Operating Room Fires. Anesthesiology. 2013;118(2):271–90.
4. Jaquet Y, et al. Complications of different ventilation strategies in endoscopic laryngeal surgery: a 10-year review. Anesthesiology. 2006;104(1):52–9.
5. Macias AA, et al. Lasers, airway surgery, and operating room fires. In: Vacanti CA, et al., editors. Essential clinical anesthesia. New York: Cambridge University Press; 2011. p. 708–12.
6. Rampil IJ. Anesthesia for laser surgery. In: Miller RD, editor. Miller's anesthesia. 7th ed. Philadelphia: Churchill Livingstone; 2009. p. 2405–18.
7. Smetana GW, et al. Preoperative pulmonary risk stratification for noncardiothoracic surgery: systematic review for the American College of Physicians. Ann Intern Med. 2006;144(8):581–95.
8. Steiner W, Ambrosch P. Endoscopic laser surgery of the upper aerodigestive tract: with special emphasis on cancer surgery. New York: Thieme Stuttgart; 2000.
9. Surgeon General's Reports (2004) The Health Consequences of Smoking: A Report of the Surgeon General.
10. Tonnesen H, et al. Smoking and alcohol intervention before surgery: evidence for best practice. Br J Anaesth. 2009;102(3):297–306.
11. Yan Y, et al. Use of lasers in laryngeal surgery. J Voice. 2010;24(1):102–9.

Part VIII

Blood/Hematologic System

Section Editor: Charles P. Plant

Charles P. Plant
Department of Anesthesia, Tufts Medical Center, Boston, MA, USA

Transfusion Reactions

40

Charles P. Plant and Jonathan H. Kroll

Case An 18 y/o man presents with a deep laceration on his right forearm sustained upon breaking a plate glass window with his fist. He has no other injuries.

Medications:	Adderall (amphetamine/dextroamphetamine)				
Allergies:	NKDA				
Past Medical History:	Attention Deficit Hyperactivity Disorder (ADHD)				
Physical Exam:	BP 110/40	HR 150		RR 25	oxygen saturation: 95% on room air

He appears well developed and of normal height and weight for his age. His is alert and oriented and cooperative. He is in moderate distress owing to anxiety and arm pain. Diaphoresis is apparent on the forehead. He is extremely tachycardic with a vigorous cardiac impulse. He has no other injuries. His exam is otherwise unremarkable.

An IV is placed in the uninjured arm. Labs are sent. The hematocrit is 35%. He is given 3 L of normal saline while waiting for cross-matched blood. The hematocrit is now 25%. Cross-matched blood is being transfused. The orthopedic surgeon has been summoned.

What is urticarial transfusion reaction (UTR)?

A UTR is minor allergic reaction associated with the transfusion of a blood product. The reaction is limited to the appearance of hives. None of the more serious allergic findings occur; i.e., there is no wheezing, hypotension and angioedema. It is caused by an antigen/antibody interaction upon exposure to donor blood product. A number of donor serum protein antigens have been implicated.

What is the treatment?

When a UTR occurs, the transfusion can be paused while the patient is evaluated. Once the more serious finding are ruled out, the transfusion can be restarted. Antihistamine can be given. Prophylactic antihistamine can be considered but is not routinely recommended.

What are the signs and symptoms of an anaphylactic reaction?

Cutaneous manifestations such as urticaria, erythema, pruritus, and/or angioedema are almost always present. Wheezing and hypotension usually develop which can be severe. Gastrointestinal symptoms such as nausea, vomiting, and diarrhea may be present. The patient may have the feeling of impending doom. The onset is typically 5–30 min after intravenous exposure.

What is the treatment?

Anaphylaxis is a medical emergency. The transfusion should be stopped. Help should be summoned. High-flow oxygen should be administered. Adequate IV access should be obtained. If warranted, IO can be considered. Begin aggressive fluid resuscitation with NS. The patent should be monitored by continuous ECG and pulse oximetry. Blood pressure should be checked with a cuff, or if necessary, by direct palpation. Anaphylaxis is due to the release of inflammatory mediators such as histamine and cytokines from mast cells and basophils. Epinephrine slows the release of these mediators; hence, rapid administration of epinephrine is a key intervention. Intramuscular (IM) epinephrine administration is favored but IV should be considered if there are immediate life-threatening manifestations. H1 antihistamines such as diphenhydramine should be administered.

C.P. Plant (✉)
Department of Anesthesia, Tufts Medical Center,
800 Washington Street, Boston, 02111, MA, USA
e-mail: cplant@tuftsmedicalcenter.org

J.H. Kroll
Department of Medicine, MedStar Union Memorial Hospital
201 E University Parkway, 33rd Street Building
Suite 405, Baltimore, 21218, MD, USA
e-mail: jkrollmd@gmail.com

© Springer International Publishing AG 2017
L.S. Aglio and R.D. Urman (eds.), *Anesthesiology*,
DOI 10.1007/978-3-319-50141-3_40

H2 blockers such as cimetidine can also be given. If bronchospasm is present, inhaled beta-adrenergic agonist should be administered. A high-dose IV corticosteroid should be administered early but the benefits of corticosteroids will not manifest for several hours. The blood product should be sent back to the lab for reanalysis.

What is an acute hemolytic transfusion reaction?

An acute hemolytic transfusion reaction is a life-threatening emergency caused intravascular hemolysis of transfused erythrocytes. The most common cause is a clerical error resulting in transfusion of mismatched blood. The patient may complain of chills, anxiety, nausea, shortness of breath, and flank pain. Patients may develop a fever, hypotension, and brown urine. The signs and symptoms usually begin within 15 min of starting the transfusion. If not recognized, life-threatening hyperkalemia can develop owing to the on-going release of potassium from the on-going hemolysis. If a patient is under anesthesia, the findings can include hypotension, urticaria, wheezing, hyperkalemia, ECG changes, blood-tinged urine, and abnormal bleeding. The hemolyzed erythrocytes release hemoglobin and other proteins into the serum. These proteins precipitate in the renal tubules where they can cause blockage and eventual renal failure. The coagulation cascade can become activated (by erythrocytin and other factors) thereby consuming platelets and clotting factors including fibrinogen. This can progress to the disseminated intravascular coagulation syndrome.

What is the treatment?

An acute hemolytic transfusion reaction is a medical emergency. The transfusion should be stopped. Help should be summoned. The patent should be monitored by continuous ECG looking for manifestations of hyperkalemia such as peaked T-waves. Fluids should be changed to NS from LR if necessary to minimize the potassium load. Treatment includes aggressive hydration and diuresis. The blood product should be sent back to the lab for reanalysis. Coagulation labs should be checked frequently for evidence of a coagulopathy. The complete blood count should be checked frequently for thrombocytopenia and anemia. Uncontrolled bleeding in the face of thrombocytopenia and coagulopathy is an indication for emergency transfusion of blood products to replace deficient blood components.

What is a febrile non-hemolytic transfusion reaction?

A febrile non-hemolytic transfusion reaction is a diagnosis of exclusion. Patents develop a fever during or shortly after a transfusion, but the manifestations of a more severe reaction such as acute hemolytic transfusion reaction, anaphylaxis, transfusion-associated sepsis, transfusion-related lung injury are absent. Occasionally, the fever is accompanied by chills, rigors, tachypnea, anxiety, and/or headache. It is caused by leukocytes in the blood product which release cytokines when exposed to recipient blood. The now common use of leukocyte reduced packed red blood cells has reduced the frequency to less than 1%.

What is the treatment?

Management is symptomatic. Itching and/or a minor rash can be treated with an antihistamine. Febrile reactions can be treated with an antipyretic such as acetaminophen. Premedication with these agents can prevent or ameliorate febrile non-hemolytic transfusion reactions.

What is a delayed hemolytic transfusion reaction?

A delayed hemolytic transfusion reaction (by definition) has an onset 24 h after administration of an erythrocyte-containing blood product. Failure to detect an allo-antibody on blood-product screening is usually the cause. The offending allo-antibody is usually an IgG. Some are well known; for example, Kidd, Duffy, and Kell. After a first exposure, the antibodies eventually dissipate, but upon subsequent exposure, an anamnestic response ensues. There is a rapid rise in recipient allo-antibody levels. These allo-antibodies bind to donor erythrocytes causing a hemolytic reaction. Presentation can be delayed for 1–4 weeks. The findings include fever, chills and jaundice. Labs reveal a pattern consistent with hemolysis; i.e., elevated serum bilirubin (unconjugated), elevated urinary urobilinogen, reduced plasma haptoglobin (haptoglobin binds free hemoglobin and is thereby consumed), elevated serum lactic dehydrogenase (LDH), hemosiderinuria, methemalbuminemia and reticulocytosis.

How is it treated?

Treatment is usually unnecessary. Evidence of on-going hemolysis should be absent on follow-up testing. Post-reaction screening will reveal the offending allo-antibody. Delayed reactions are usually less severe that acute reactions. Indeed, the diagnosis might be missed entirely—particularly if the patent has been discharged home. The severity depends on the pathologic potency of the offending allo-antibody (e.g., affinity and titer). Allo-immunization is of particular concern in pregnancy. In particular, an Rh negative mother can potentially be allo-immunized by an Rh positive fetus. Consequently, Rh negative mothers are routinely given Rho

(D) immune globulin prophylactically. Sickle cell patients with a history of transfusions who develop a delayed transfusion reaction are at increased risk for a vaso-occlusive crisis. Hematologic testing including allo-antibody screening may be warranted if repeat pregnancy is planned or surgery is anticipated.

What is transfusion-related circulatory overload (TACO)?

TACO is a syndrome of pulmonary edema that includes dyspnea, orthopnea, peripheral edema, and hypertension, occurring in the context of transfusion. It is caused by an excess volume causing a circulatory overload. Risk factors include age greater than 60 years, congestive heart failure, pulmonary failure, anemia, and transfusion of a large volume over a short period of time. Notwithstanding, TACO can occur in victims of trauma, who are otherwise healthy, who receive a transfusion using a rapid infusion device. TACO can be distinguished from TRALI by blood pressure: TRALI includes hypotension in contrast to the hypertension seen with TACO.

What is the treatment?

Prevention is preferable to treatment. TACO can be prevented by giving transfusion products slowly and careful monitoring so that early intervention is possible. Treatment includes pulmonary support typically with supplementary oxygen and diuresis. Bi-level positive airway pressure (BiPAP) ventilatory support can be considered. Intubation is rarely required.

What is transfusion-associated bacterial sepsis (TABS)?

TABS is caused by bacteria present in transfused blood components. Fortunately, TABS is rare, but when it occurs, it is often life-threatening. Typically, the contamination occurs during a substandard collection procedure. Signs and symptoms include fever, chills, and hypotension. In contrast to typical sepsis, TABS has no localized source of infection. Notwithstanding, such a source should be carefully ruled out. Of particular concern, is the possibility that a large inoculum of endotoxin can be infused, if the blood product contains gram negative organisms.

What is the treatment?

TABS is treated with broad-spectrum antibiotics and hemodynamic support. The provenance of the blood product under suspicion should be investigated.

What is transfusion-related acute lung injury (TRALI)?

Transfusion-related acute lung injury (TRALI) is a potentially life-threatening syndrome of pulmonary distress occurring after transfusion of blood product. It is caused by activation of recipient neutrophils by antibodies from the donor. (Other immunopathologic mechanisms have been postulated.) Thus, blood products rich in donor plasma (e.g., platelets and fresh frozen plasma) are more potent triggers than plasma depleted blood products (e.g., packed red blood cells). The activated neutrophils cause injury to the pulmonary vascular endothelium. The endothelium becomes "leaky" and pulmonary edema results. By definition, pulmonary edema must occur within six hours of receiving blood product. Other causes of respiratory distress should be ruled out; in particular, volume overload and congestive heart failure. Indeed, it may not be possible to distinguish TRALI from other causes of respiratory distress. TRALI typically presents with the sudden onset of dyspnea, tachypnea, cyanosis ($sPO2 < 90\%$) and fever. Hypotension is usually present. Rales are usually present. Chest radiography reveals bilateral, patchy infiltrates; which in severe cases, can progress to "complete white out." By definition, if the respiratory distress can be attributed to another coexisting condition, TRALI cannot be diagnosed.

What is the treatment?

The treatment of TRALI includes supplemental oxygen, intravenous fluids, and vasopressors. Bi-level positive airway pressure (BiPAP) ventilatory support can be considered. Intubation may be required in severe cases. In either case, a lung-protective strategy should be implemented; e.g., use of low/protective tidal volumes. Corticosteroids can be beneficial. Generally, diuretics are avoided owing to hypotension. The recipient should not receive any more products from the implicated donor. The donor of the implicated blood product should be identified so that the donor can be excluded from future donations.

The AABB technical manual provides an extensive reference [1]. Hart et al. [2] provide a more compact reference tailored to anesthesia providers.

Reference

1. Fung MK, Grossman BJ, Hillyer C, Westhoff CM editors. AABB technical manual. 18th ed. Bethesda, MD: American Association of Blood Banks Press; 2011.
2. Hart S, Cserti-Gazdewich CM, McCluskey SA. Red cell transfusion and the immune system. Anaesthesia. 2015;70(Suppl 1):38–45.

Intraoperative Coagulopathies

41

Alimorad G. Djalali and Anil K. Panigrahi

Case Scenario A 40-year-old Asian female presents for an elective revision of breast implants. She has previously had a bilateral mastectomy due to breast cancer. At that time, she was evaluated for coagulopathy after excessive intra- and post-operative bleeding (>1000 ml). Excessive bleeding was also reported after her two cesarean sections.

Her daughter has a chromosomal 22q deletion syndrome. She denies any history of epistaxis or gum bleeding.

Her coagulation workup demonstrates:

- Normal PT and aPTT, sufficient activity of Factors VIII, IX, XII.
- Ristocetin cofactor activity is normal. Normal Von Willebrand antigen level.
- Normal platelets aggregation and function studies.
- Factor V clotting activity and D-dimer levels are pending.
- Fibrinolytic activity studies are ordered.

1. **Is there a role for routine coagulation testing in preoperative patients?**

Routine preoperative coagulation testing has not been proven to help identify patients at risk for intra- and postoperative bleeding [1, 2]. Multiple factors contribute to the low positive predictive value of routine coagulation screening in operative patients.

- A low prevalence of bleeding disorders in the general population which when combined with indiscriminant testing can increase the frequency of false positive results [3].
- Normal values for coagulation laboratory tests are defined by values encompassing results from two standard deviations of the general population. As a result, 2.5% of normal individuals will have prolonged coagulation times.
- Coagulation studies are designed primarily to assess the coagulation system in patients suspected to have hereditary or acquired deficiencies in coagulation factors, which can lead to significant false negative and false positive results when applied indiscriminately [4].
  - PT and aPTT will demonstrate normal values in individuals with deficiencies in Factor XIII or α2-antiplasmin deficiency, both of which can result in significant surgical bleeding.
  - Normal parameters are also observed in patients taking platelet inhibitors such as aspirin.
  - States of pregnancy, stress, or trauma result in increases in Factor VIII levels which can normalize PTT values and mask mild Hemophilia A or von Willebrand disease (VWD).
- False positive testing can result from technical problems such as heparin contamination of blood samples (drawn through heparin-locked catheter) or insufficient blood in tube (elevated citrate concentration), but also can be due to factor deficiencies that are clinically insignificant, such as Factor XII deficiency which is found in 2% of the general population but does not confer an increased bleeding risk [5].

Consequently, a detailed clinical history, family history, and physical examination continue to be the most sensitive methods for identifying patients at risk for significant perioperative bleeding.

A.G. Djalali (✉) · A.K. Panigrahi
Department of Anesthesiology, Perioperative, and Pain Medicine, Stanford University Medical Center, 300 Pasteur Drive, Room H3589, Stanford, CA 94305-5640, USA
e-mail: adjalali@stanford.edu

A.K. Panigrahi
e-mail: anilpani@stanford.edu

© Springer International Publishing AG 2017
L.S. Aglio and R.D. Urman (eds.), *Anesthesiology*,
DOI 10.1007/978-3-319-50141-3_41

2. **How would you assess coagulopathy in your patient?**

Abnormal hemostasis resulting in clinical bleeding can be categorized into two groups:

- Failure of primary hemostasis—Defects of the vascular endothelium or dysfunctional or insufficient platelets.
- Failure of secondary hemostasis—Clotting factor deficiency or defect.

Defects in primary hemostasis generally present as mucosal or cutaneous bleeding and manifest as petechiae (capillary hemorrhage), ecchymoses, or menorrhagia. These platelet or endothelial disorders result in immediate bleeding after vascular injury and rarely present as delayed bleeding. Alternatively, coagulation disorders usually present as large ecchymoses or diffuse deep soft tissue hematomas. Bleeding in these conditions can often be delayed from the inciting trauma.

Understanding the different presentation of these disorders along with a detailed medical history (including medications) and physical exam can help focus diagnostic evaluation to appropriate laboratory tests [6].

3. **What are the major steps of the coagulation cascade?**

Hemostasis is achieved through the coordination of cellular interactions and enzymatic reactions. Primary hemostasis refers to the action of platelets and occurs after injury to the endothelium resulting in exposure of collagen. As circulating platelets come into contact with the exposed collagen, they slow and begin to adhere to the vessel endothelium. Release of von Willebrand factor (VWF) by endothelial cells enhances platelet adhesion by binding to collagen as well as the platelet receptor glycoprotein (GP) Ib/FIX/FV complex [7]. Subsequently, platelets become activated, releasing the contents of their storage granules, which in turn recruits additional platelets and promotes platelet aggregation. This initial platelet plug serves as a substrate for further clotting factor reactions which has been termed secondary hemostasis.

Clotting reactions have historically been described as an ordered cascade of serial events divided into the intrinsic system, extrinsic system, and the common pathway. Although, current evidence indicates that clotting begins with the generation of tissue factor (TF)/Factor VIIa (FVIIa) complexes which then activates Factor IX (FIX) to FIXa [8], the original cascade model is helpful for diagnosing defects identified by coagulation screening tests, as the tests were designed with this organization in mind.

- The intrinsic system includes coagulation Factors XII, XI, IX, and VIII, and prekallikrein and high molecular weight kininogen. The intrinsic system begins with activation of Factor XII from exposure to a negatively charged surface and is monitored using the activated partial thromboplastin time (aPTT) assay.
- The extrinsic system is comprised of tissue factor (also known as tissue thromboplastin) and Factor VII.
- The intrinsic and extrinsic systems converge to the common pathway consisting of Factors X, V, II, and fibrinogen. The final step of the common pathway involves the formation of fibrin from fibrinogen by activated Factor II (thrombin).

4. **What do aPPT and PT assess?**

The two primary tests used to screen for coagulation disorders are the activated partial thromboplastin time (aPTT) and the prothrombin time (PT) which measure the intrinsic and extrinsic coagulation pathways, respectively.

- The aPTT assay is used as screening test for deficiencies in factors of the intrinsic system, monitoring heparin therapy, and detecting lupus anticoagulant.
  - The aPTT will be prolonged in patients with decreased levels of intrinsic and/or common pathway components.
- The PT assay is used to screen for deficiencies in extrinsic system and common pathway components and to monitor oral anticoagulant therapy.
  - The PT will be prolonged with decreased levels of fibrinogen, Factors II, V, VII, or X.

5. **How are the aPTT and PT tests performed?**

The activated partial thromboplastin assay is performed by first incubating patient plasma with contact activators, namely phospholipid and silica or kaolin for several minutes. This incubation results in the autoactivation of Factor XII, which with the cofactors prekallikrein and high-molecular-weight kininogen, activates Factor XI. Factor XIa then converts Factor IX to IXa. Next calcium is added to facilitate Factors IXa/VIII activation of Factor X. Factors Xa/V convert Factor II to IIa (thrombin) which then cleaves fibrinogen to fibrin. The time for clot formation is measured. The preincubation step with contact activators is the reason the assay is termed *activated* partial thromboplastin time.

The prothrombin time is performed by incubating patient's plasma with thromboplastin (recombinant tissue factor/phospholipid/calcium mixture). After incubation, calcium is added to the mixture and the time to fibrin formation is measured.

6. **Why is the INR value used?**

Due to variations in thromboplastin formulations, prothrombin times will vary from lab to lab. In order to provide a value to monitor warfarin anticoagulation that would be comparable between labs, the international normalized ratio (INR) was designed. It is calculated by dividing the patient's PT by the mean normal PT for the local lab. This ratio is then raised to the power of the international sensitivity index (ISI) which is a measure of how a specific labs tissue factor formulation compares to an international reference tissue factor.

7. **What conditions would cause an increase in PT, PTT, or both?**

- Isolated PT prolongation—Factor VII inhibition/deficiency
- Isolated aPTT prolongation—Heparin therapy, Factor VIII deficiency, Factor IX deficiency, Factor XI deficiency. Deficiencies in Factor XII, prekallikrein, high molecular weight kininogen, or presence of lupus anticoagulant (anti-phospholipid antibody) will prolong aPTT without clinically significant increase in bleeding risk.
- Prolongation of PT and aPTT—Liver disease, vitamin K deficiency, anticoagulant therapy, DIC, massive transfusion, deficiencies or defects in Factors X, V, or II, dysfibrinogenemia.

8. **What co-morbidities can cause coagulation abnormalities?**

- Hepatic dysfunction
- Renal insufficiency
- Sepsis (crosstalk of inflammation and coagulation pathways)
- Severe thyroid dysfunction
- Amyloidosis
- Connective tissue disease
- Neoplastic and paraneoplastic diseases
- Malnutrition
- Inflammatory bowel disease
- Envenomation (e.g., snake bite).

9. **What are the major causes of intraoperative coagulopathy?**

- Inherited bleeding disorders
  - Bleeding diathesis—VWD (most common), Hemophilia A & B
  - Prothrombotic—antithrombin deficiency, Protein C or S deficiency, antiphospholipid syndrome, Factor V Leiden, dysfibrinogenemia
- Acquired bleeding disorders
  - Medications—anticoagulants and antiplatelet agents
  - Liver disease
  - Renal disease (uremic platelet dysfunction)
  - Disseminated intravascular coagulation (DIC)
  - Prothrombotic—heparin induced thrombocytopenia, malignancy, immobilization, acquired dysfibrinogenemia (e.g., secondary to liver disease or multiple myeloma)
- Coagulopathy associated with trauma (acute traumatic coagulopathy)

10. **Coagulopathy of trauma, brain trauma and massive bleeding**

The different types of trauma may have different impacts on the coagulation system. A minor brain injury may create a more severe coagulopathy than a femur fracture with some hundred milliliters of blood loss. In general, the amount of blood lost is a better indicator for the severity of coagulopathy. In this context the following definition of massive transfusion is helpful:

1. Replacement of entire blood volume within a 24-h period (10–12 units of packed red blood cells, PRBC's).
2. Replacement of 50% of total blood volume within 3 h (5–6 units of PRBC's).
3. Need for at least 4 units of PRBC's within 4 h with continued major bleeding.
4. Blood loss exceeding 150 ml/min.

The definitions of massive transfusion may slightly vary based on different guidelines.

During the resuscitation of a trauma patient, significant deficits are encountered: decrease in concentration and activity of plasma coagulation factors, thrombocytopenia, and anemia [9]. Ordering coagulation screening studies during the active bleeding phase is unlikely to yield useful information. In addition, conventional coagulation tests (aPTT, PT) need some time to be completed and will not reflect the real-time situation during active bleeding.

The treatment of massive blood loss is as complex as the trauma presentation in the operating room. Assessment and monitoring of fibrinogen levels, platelet count, anemia, and core body temperature are important factors to consider when treating a trauma patient [10].

11. **What are the effects of temperature and pH on coagulation?**

Hypothermia compromises fibrinogen synthesis and reduces the activity of many coagulation factors which depend on adequate temperature (>35 °C) for optimal enzymatic function [11]. In addition, lower body core temperature contributes to platelet dysfunction [12, 13]. Notably, standard coagulation assays will not demonstrate the effects of hypothermia, as samples are generally warmed to 37 °C prior to analysis.

A physiologic milieu is necessary for coagulation factors to function. As a result they are less effective in the setting of acidosis. Clotting dysfunction is observed at pH < 7.2 and is thought to be due to the inhibition of calcium-dependent clotting factor complex formation. Specifically, activity of the prothrombinase complex (Factor Xa, Va, phospholipid, and prothrombin) progressively decreases as acidosis worsens [14]. In addition, clot formation and its strength is reduced in an acidotic environment.

12. **Which coagulation factor has the shortest half-life and what is the relevance of it?**

Factor VII is the coagulation factor with the shortest half-life in vivo of 3–6 h. Factors V ($t_{1/2}$ 36 h) and VIII ($t_{1/2}$ 10–14 h) are labile and are the factors most affected during storage of plasma. Factors V and VIII also appear to be most commonly deficient in patients with trauma associated coagulopathy [15]. As a result of these findings and more recent studies demonstrating morbidity and mortality benefits, early treatment of severe trauma associated coagulopathy by resuscitation of blood products in a 1:1:1 ratio of PRBCs, FFP, and platelet units is recommended [16, 17].

13. **What is activated Factor VII?**

Recombinant activated human Factor VII (rFVIIa) can be administered in situations where Factor VII deficiency is suspected to contribute to coagulopathy. Activated Factor VII was initially developed and approved for use to treat hemophilia in patients who have developed inhibitors to Factors VIII or IX, acquired hemophilia, or individuals with isolated Factor VII deficiency. Since its introduction, however, several off label indications have emerged. In particular, given the short half-life of Factor VII and its synthesis by the liver, rFVIIa has been administered to correct coagulopathy in patients with liver dysfunction, especially those who may be unable to tolerate large volume loads from FFP transfusion. Additionally, rFVIIa has been used to reduce microvascular bleeding after trauma and surgery that is not responsive to standard blood product transfusion.

14. **What are fibrinogen degradation products and what do they affect?**

When fibrin polymers are cleaved by plasmin, fibrin degradation products are released. Tissue plasminogen activator initially activates plasminogen to form plasmin. Plasmin is the primary enzyme responsible of fibrinolysis. In addition to fibrin, plasmin also degrades fibrinogen, and other coagulation factors. Its action on fibrin polymers liberates dimerized D-domains of fibrin into the circulation. The crosslinking of D-dimers is the result of Factor XIII activity during the process of fibrin clot formation. As a result, an increase in circulating D-dimers suggests fibrinolysis of an intravascular clot.

15. **What are the indications for transfusion of FFP?**

According to the updated ASA Practice Guidelines on Perioperative Blood Management [18], plasma should be transfused in the following situations:

- Excessive microvascular bleeding in the setting of an INR greater than 2.0 without the presence of heparin.
- Excessive microvascular bleeding due to suspected clotting factor deficiency in patients transfused greater than 1 blood volume (when coagulation studies are not readily available).
- Urgent reversal of warfarin when prothrombin complex concentrates are unavailable.
- Correction of known clotting factor deficiencies when specific factor concentrates are unavailable.

Notably, plasma transfusion is not indicated when PT/INR and aPTT are normal, nor is it indicated to increase intravascular volume.

16. **How is cryoprecipitate made and what coagulation factors does it contain?**

Cryopreciptate is generated by thawing fresh frozen plasma at 1–6 °C. Proteins insoluble at cold temperatures precipitate and can be collected via centrifugation. This precipitate is resuspended in a small amount of plasma (usually 10–15 mL). Each unit contains 200–250 mg fibrinogen, ≥80 IU FVIII, 80–120 IU vWF, 40–60 IU FXIII, and fibronectin. The usual adult dose is 10 units often administered as a 10-pack. Cryoprecipitate is a poor source of vitamin K-dependent factors (II, VII, IX, X). Thus, cryoprecipitate should not be used to reverse warfarin-induced anticoagulation; instead, FFP should be used. Similarly, cryoprecipitate should not be used to treat Hemophilia B (FIX deficiency); instead, recombinant human factor IX (rFIX) should be used.

17. **How can platelet activity be monitored?**

Platelet activity is commonly monitored by aggregometry. This process involves incubation of a platelet suspension (platelet-rich plasma) with specific agonists such as collagen, ADP, epinephrine, or ristocetin. The time and degree of platelet aggregation is measured by monitoring light transmission through the suspension which increases as the platelets aggregate.

An alternative is the Platelet Function Analyzer, PFA-100. This test can be run on whole blood anticoagulated with citrate and stored at room temperature. Platelets within the blood are subjected to high flow rates within a capillary tube and are exposed to a collagen-coated membrane. An aggregation agonist (ADP or epinephrine) is added to provoke platelet aggregation. The resulting decrease in flow rate is monitored as a platelet plug is formed. This time is reported as the closure time (CT) and is prolonged in the setting of platelet dysfunction.

18. **What is the thromboelastograph?**

The thromboelastograph (TEG) is an assay of the dynamics of clot formation from whole blood. The TEG device measures viscoelastic properties of the clot during formation and lysis which are then analyzed and plotted. Although TEG technology has been available for some decades, it has not yet established itself as a routine intraoperative analysis of coagulation. A recent Cochrane review found insufficient evidence to support use of TEG to guide transfusion practice in adult trauma patients; however, the authors note that this conclusion is likely due to a lack of consensus over how TEG measurements should influence patient management [19].

19. **What drugs could cause intraoperative coagulopathy?**

The number of therapeutic drugs interfering with normal hemostasis is ever increasing.

Anticoagulants:

- Vitamin K-antagonists—Warfarin reduces the production of essential factors such as II, VII, IX and X. Protein C and S concentrations, both anticoagulation factors, are also reduced.
- Unfractionated heparin (UFH): UFH is a mixture of glycosaminoglycans of various lengths. UFH functions by complexing with antithrombin (AT, formerly known as antithrombin III) and accelerating its inactivation of thrombin and Factor Xa. UFH easily dissociates from AT upon protamine administration.
- Low molecular weight heparin (LMWH): LMWH is a purified and smaller molecule than unfractionated heparin with greater anti-Xa activity and little inactivation of thrombin. LMWH has a longer half-life, which can increase with diminishing kidney function. Unlike UFH, LMWH cannot be completely reversed by protamine.
  - Fondapariunux and danaparoid are two LMWH-related compounds with higher specific anti-Xa activity and long half-lives.
- Direct Xa inhibitors—Rivaroxaban ($t_{1/2}$ 7–17 h), apixaban ($t_{1/2}$ 5–9 h), and edoxaban ($t_{1/2}$ 6–11 h) act to inactivate circulating and clot-bound FXa. They are administered orally and do not have a specific reversal agent.
- Thrombin inhibitors—There are many new formulations of compounds which inactivate circulating and clot-bound thrombin (factor IIa).
  - Parenteral—bivalirudin ($t_{1/2}$ 25 min), argatroban ($t_{1/2}$ 40–50 min), desirudin ($t_{1/2}$ 2 h)
  - Oral—dabigatran ($t_{1/2}$ 12–17 h); there is no reversal available for dabigatran.

Antiplatelet Agents:

- Aspirin—Aspirin irreversibly inhibits the platelet cyclooxygenase and thromboxane A2. Other non-steroidal anti-inflammatory drugs such as ibuprofen and celecoxib inhibit the cyclooxygenase in a mostly reversible fashion. The risk of significant intraoperative bleeding after aspirin or NSAIDs therapy is low.
- ADP receptor blockers—These agents block the platelet $P2Y_{12}$ receptor which is responsible for binding of adenosine diphosphate (ADP), thereby limiting platelet aggregation.
  - Clopidogrel, ticlopidine, prasugrel, ticagrelor, and cangrelor are examples of ADP receptor blockers.
- GP IIb/IIIa Inhibitors—Agents in this class inhibit platelet aggregation by preventing crosslinking mediated by GP IIb/IIIa binding of fibrinogen.
  - Abciximab, tirofiban, or eptifibatide are currently used GP IIb/IIIa Inhibitors.

Medications with bleeding side effect:

- Selective Serotonin Reuptake Inhibitors can reduce platelet activity by depletion of serotonin from platelet granules.

- Valproic acid decreases levels of factors VII, VIII, XIII, platelets, vWF, fibrinogen, protein C, and antithrombin.

20. **What causes HIT?**

Heparin induced thrombocytopenia (HIT) results from the autoantibodies recognizing heparin complexes with platelet factor 4 (PF4), a protein present in platelet granules. The autoantibodies recognize PF4 epitopes exposed when it is bound by heparin, therefore the clinical activity of these antibodies generally requires heparin exposure. Thrombocytopenia occurs due to clearance of antibody coated platelets by the reticuloendothelial system (spleen, liver), as well as, platelet consumption through formation of arterial and venous thrombi. Thrombus formation is felt to be a result of platelet activation caused by antibody binding. Onset of thrombocytopenia usually occurs within 5–10 days of beginning heparin therapy, as this correlates with the timeframe for antibody formation; however, it can occur within the first 24 h of exposure if the patient has been previously exposed to heparin and the antibodies are still present (1–3 months). The latter is an anamnestic immune response. Thrombosis can occur in up to 50% of patients with HIT and can result in skin necrosis, limb gangrene, and organ infarction [20]. HIT is diagnosed by new onset thrombocytopenia (counts <150,000/μL) or $a \geq 50\%$ decrease in platelet count beginning 5–10 days after initiation of heparin therapy along with the presence of platelet activating antibodies. The ability of these antibodies to activate platelets can be measured by a serotonin release assay (SRA) or by heparin-induced platelet aggregation assay (HIPA). If these tests are not available, enzyme-linked immunosorbent assays (ELISA) can be used, although they have higher false positive and false negative rates compared to functional assays. If HIT is suspected, all heparin containing products should be immediately stopped. Suitable anticoagulation should be initiated. Initially, the direct thrombin inhibitors should be used (e.g., argatroban and bivalirudin). Eventually, patients can usually be transitioned to warfarin. Direct FXa inhibitors have been used off label.

21. **What is VWD and what is its clinical presentation?**

VWD is the most common bleeding disorder, being present in approximately 1% of the general population [21]. It affects men and women in equal proportion. VWD encompasses several subtypes that present with different features reflecting either qualitative or quantitative defects in von Willebrand factor (VWF) resulting in varying therapeutic implications [22]. VWF circulates as large multimeric proteins, which through interactions with platelet receptors and sub-endothelial proteins, facilitate binding of platelets to sites of vessel injury. VWF also binds Factor VIII thereby increasing its half-life and promoting fibrin clot formation. Patients with reduced VWF concentration or activity may present with mucosal bleeding, epistaxis, or gingival bleeds. Interestingly, the level of VWF depends to some extend on race, blood type, age, and inflammatory status. For instance, the type O blood group is associated with decreased levels and half-life of VWF, whereas African Americans seem to have higher levels.

VWD is classified into three main types:

- Type 1—partial quantitative deficiency of VWF
- Type 2—qualitative VWF variant
  - Type 2A—decrease in large VWF multimers; decreased platelet adhesion
  - Type 2B—increased affinity for platelet glycoprotein Ib
  - Type 2M—decreased platelet adhesion, but normal multimer distribution
  - Type 2N—decreased binding of Factor VIII
- Type 3—severe (near complete deficiency of vWF)

Perioperative therapy of VWD includes 3 strategies:

1. Increasing the plasma concentration of VWF by promoting release of the endogenous reserves.
2. Increasing the level of VWF by exogenous administration of the factor (rFVIII-VWF complex or cryoprecipitate).
3. Improve hemostasis with other agents.

22. **What is the utility of DDAVP in patients with VWD?**

DDAVP (desmopressin) promotes the release of VWF from the endothelial reservoirs, and is useful in VWD type 1 and some subgroups of type 2. It increases the concentration of FVIII at the same time. Tranexamic acid, an antifibrinolytic agent, is of some benefit in therapy of intraoperative VWD. Desmopressin is a synthetic analog of vasopressin that is mostly devoid of pressor activity, but retains antidiuretic activity.

23. **What are the different types of Hemophilia?**

There are two major types of Hemophilia, A and B. Hemophilia A is the most common form (1 out of 5000 live births) and more likely to be severe. Hemophilia B, also known as Christmas disease, is less common (1 out of 30,000 live births) [23].

- Hemophilia A—Congenital deficiency of Factor VIII
- Hemophilia B—Congenital deficiency of Factor IX

Both hemophilias are observed in all ethnic groups and demonstrate an X-linked recessive pattern of inheritance. Albeit rare, females can be affected if both alleles are affected; i.e., both X chromosomes. The severity of hemophilia is graded into three categories:

- Severe hemophilia—<1% of normal factor activity (<0.01 IU/mL)
- Moderate hemophilia—≥1 to <5% of normal factor activity (0.01 to <0.05 IU/mL)
- Mild hemophilia—≥5 to <40% of normal factor activity (≥0.05 to <0.40 IU/mL)

Up to 2/3 of hemophilia A and 1/2 of hemophilia B patients have severe disease.

24. **What factor level is required for operative procedures in patients with Hemophilia?**

For early joint or muscle bleeding, factor levels of 30–40% are sufficient. For dental procedures or development of intramuscular hematomas, a factor level of 50% is desired. For severe bleeding (intracranial or intraabdominal hemorrhage) factor levels of 80–100% are required. Similarly, for orthopedic and other major surgeries, factor levels of 80–100% are to be achieved preoperatively. Once bleeding is controlled, a prophylactic level of 30–50% is maintained in the post-operative period (10–14 days).

25. **How do you dose recombinant Factor VIII (rFVIII) and IX (rFIX)?**

One international unit (IU) of clotting factor is defined as the amount of factor in 1 ml of normal plasma. Therefore 100% of normal factor level is equal to 1 IU/mL. Due to differences in volume of distribution, the calculation of rFVIII and rFIX dosage differs.

- Dose of factor VIII (international units) = weight (kg) × (desired percent increase) × 0.5.
- Dose of factor IX (international units) = weight (kg) × (desired percent increase) × *F*.
  - *F* = correction factor for volume of distribution that differs with rFIX formulation and varies from 1 to 1.2.

References

1. Chee YL, Greaves M. Role of coagulation testing in predicting bleeding risk. Hematol J. 2003;4(6):373–8. doi:10.1038/sj.thj.6200306.
2. Kitchens CS. To bleed or not to bleed? Is that the question for the PTT? J Thromb Haemost. 2005;3(12):2607–11. doi:10.1111/j.1538-7836.2005.01552.x.
3. Eisenberg JM, Clarke JR, Sussman SA. Prothrombin and partial thromboplastin times as preoperative screening tests. Arch Surg. 1982;117(1):48–51.
4. Levy JH, Szlam F, Wolberg AS, Winkler A. Clinical use of the activated partial thromboplastin time and prothrombin time for screening: a review of the literature and current guidelines for testing. Clin Lab Med. 2014;34(3):453–77. doi:10.1016/j.cll.2014.06.005.
5. Halbmayer WM, Haushofer A, Schon R, Mannhalter C, Strohmer E, Baumgarten K, Fischer M. The prevalence of moderate and severe FXII (Hageman factor) deficiency among the normal population: evaluation of the incidence of FXII deficiency among 300 healthy blood donors. Thromb Haemost. 1994;71(1):68–72.
6. Kozek-Langenecker SA, Afshari A, Albaladejo P, Santullano CA, De Robertis E, Filipescu DC, Fries D, Gorlinger K, Haas T, Imberger G, Jacob M, Lance M, Llau J, Mallett S, Meier J, Rahe-Meyer N, Samama CM, Smith A, Solomon C, Van der Linden P, Wikkelso AJ, Wouters P, Wyffels P. Management of severe perioperative bleeding: guidelines from the European Society of Anaesthesiology. Eur J Anaesthesiol. 2013;30(6):270–382. doi:10.1097/EJA.0b013e32835f4d5b.
7. Brass LF. Thrombin and platelet activation. Chest. 2003;124(3 Suppl):18S–25S.
8. Gailani D, Broze GJ Jr. Factor XI activation in a revised model of blood coagulation. Science. 1991;253(5022):909–12.
9. Murray DJ, Pennell BJ, Weinstein SL, Olson JD. Packed red cells in acute blood loss: dilutional coagulopathy as a cause of surgical bleeding. Anesth Analg. 1995;80(2):336–42.
10. Levy JH, Dutton RP, Hemphill JC 3rd, Shander A, Cooper D, Paidas MJ, Kessler CM, Holcomb JB, Lawson JH, Hemostasis Summit P. Multidisciplinary approach to the challenge of hemostasis. Anesth Analg. 2010;110(2):354–64. doi:10.1213/ANE.0b013e3181c84ba5.
11. Martini WZ. The effects of hypothermia on fibrinogen metabolism and coagulation function in swine. Metabolism. 2007;56(2):214–21. doi:10.1016/j.metabol.2006.09.015.
12. Michelson AD, MacGregor H, Barnard MR, Kestin AS, Rohrer MJ, Valeri CR. Reversible inhibition of human platelet activation by hypothermia in vivo and in vitro. Thromb Haemost. 1994;71(5):633–40.
13. Martini WZ. Coagulopathy by hypothermia and acidosis: mechanisms of thrombin generation and fibrinogen availability. J Trauma. 2009;67(1):202–8 discussion 208-209.
14. Engstrom M, Schott U, Romner B, Reinstrup P. Acidosis impairs the coagulation: a thromboelastographic study. J Trauma. 2006;61(3):624–8. doi:10.1097/01.ta.0000226739.30655.75.
15. Rizoli SB, Scarpelini S, Callum J, Nascimento B, Mann KG, Pinto R, Jansen J, Tien HC. Clotting factor deficiency in early trauma-associated coagulopathy. J Trauma. 2011;71(5 Suppl 1):S427–34. doi:10.1097/TA.0b013e318232e5ab.
16. Holcomb JB, del Junco DJ, Fox EE, Wade CE, Cohen MJ, Schreiber MA, Alarcon LH, Bai Y, Brasel KJ, Bulger EM, Cotton BA, Matijevic N, Muskat P, Myers JG, Phelan HA, White CE, Zhang J, Rahbar MH, Group PS. The prospective, observational, multicenter, major trauma transfusion (PROMMTT) study: comparative effectiveness of a time-varying treatment with competing risks. JAMA Surg. 2013;148(2):127–36. doi:10.1001/2013.jamasurg.387.
17. Holcomb JB, Tilley BC, Baraniuk S, Fox EE, Wade CE, Podbielski JM, del Junco DJ, Brasel KJ, Bulger EM, Callcut RA, Cohen MJ, Cotton BA, Fabian TC, Inaba K, Kerby JD, Muskat P,

O'Keeffe T, Rizoli S, Robinson BR, Scalea TM, Schreiber MA, Stein DM, Weinberg JA, Callum JL, Hess JR, Matijevic N, Miller CN, Pittet JF, Hoyt DB, Pearson GD, Leroux B, van Belle G, Group PS. Transfusion of plasma, platelets, and red blood cells in a 1:1:1 vs a 1:1:2 ratio and mortality in patients with severe trauma: the PROPPR randomized clinical trial. JAMA 2015;313 (5):471–82. doi:10.1001/jama.2015.12.
18. American Society of Anesthesiologists Task Force on Perioperative Blood M. Practice guidelines for perioperative blood management: an updated report by the American Society of Anesthesiologists Task Force on Perioperative Blood Management*. Anesthesiology. 2015;122(2):241–75. doi:10.1097/ALN.0000000000000463.
19. Hunt H, Stanworth S, Curry N, Woolley T, Cooper C, Ukoumunne O, Zhelev Z, Hyde C. Thromboelastography (TEG) and rotational thromboelastometry (ROTEM) for trauma induced coagulopathy in adult trauma patients with bleeding. Cochrane Database Syst Rev. 2015;2:CD010438. doi:10.1002/14651858.CD010438.pub2.
20. Greinacher A. Clinical practice. Heparin-Induced Thrombocytopenia. N Engl J Med. 2015;373(3):252–61. doi:10.1056/NEJMcp1411910.
21. Mannucci PM. Treatment of von Willebrand's Disease. N Engl J Med. 2004;351(7):683–694. doi:10.1056/NEJMra040403, 10.1097/TA.0b013e3181a602a7.
22. Nichols WL, Hultin MB, James AH, Manco-Johnson MJ, Montgomery RR, Ortel TL, Rick ME, Sadler JE, Weinstein M, Yawn BP. von Willebrand disease (VWD): evidence-based diagnosis and management guidelines, the National Heart, Lung, and Blood Institute (NHLBI) Expert Panel report (USA). Haemophilia. 2008;14(2):171–232. doi:10.1111/j.1365-2516.2007.01643.x.
23. Carcao MD. The diagnosis and management of congenital hemophilia. Semin Thromb Hemost. 2012;38(7):727–34. doi:10.1055/s-0032-1326786.

Hemophilia

42

Shamsuddin Akhtar

Case A 23-year-old man with history of moderate hemophilia A is scheduled to undergo repair of an incarcerated right inguinal hernia. His past medical history is significant for easy bruising and hematomas. His past surgical history is significant for dental extractions under general anesthesia. Medications: none.

Clinical Aspects of Hemophilia

What Is Hemophilia? What Are the Different Types of Hemophilia?

Hemophilia is a disorder characterized by congenital deficiency or low levels of Factor VIII (FVIII), Factor IX (FIX), or Factor XI [1]. There are three types of hemophilia: FVIII deficiency is called hemophilia A, FIX deficiency is called hemophilia B (formerly known as Christmas disease), and deficiency of Factor XI is called hemophilia C.

Hemophilia is the most common, severe inherited bleeding disorder recognized in humans. Almost all patients with hemophilia A and B have a mutation in the gene that produces FVIII or FIX, respectively. Multiple types of gene mutations have been described [2]. Because the gene for FVIII and FIX are located on the X chromosome, hemophilia A and B typically follow an X-linked recessive inheritance pattern and thus affects mostly males [1]. Females with both X chromosomes affected will manifest the disease. Such patients are rare. About 30% of hemophilias are caused by a sporadic mutations and present without a family history of the disorder [1]. The prevalence of hemophilia A is approximately 1 in 10,000 males and for hemophilia B is 1 in 50,000 males. The clinical signs and symptoms and inheritance patterns for hemophilia A and B are identical [1]. Hemophilia C is rare (1 case per 100,000 persons), and is typically seen in Ashkenazi Jews. Unlike Hemophilia A or B, it is an autosomal recessive disorder.

What Is Acquired Hemophilia A (AHA)?

Acquired hemophilia A (AHA) is a rare autoimmune disease caused by immunoglobulin G antibodies that bind to specific domains on the FVIII molecule, partially or completely neutralizing its coagulant function [3]. The incidence of AHA increases with age, with more than 80% of those affected are age 65 years and older. Half of the cases are idiopathic, while the remaining cases are associated with pregnancy, autoimmune disorder, malignancy, or a drug/allergic reaction.

What Is Von Willebrand Disease?

Von Willebrand (vWD) disease is a disorder of reduced level or abnormal function of von Willebrand Factor (vWF). vWF is stored and secreted by the vascular endothelium and megakaryocytes [2]. vWF has 2 functions: (1) it promotes platelet adhesion to the sub-endothelium, and; (2) vWF is a carrier molecule for FVIII and protects it from proteolysis by activated protein C. Without this interaction, plasma half-life of FVIII is reduced from 12 h in the presence of vWF, to only 2 h in it absence [4]. Decreased plasma half-life leads to low FVIII levels, causing a bleeding disorder simulating FVIII deficiency [1]. The normal plasma concentration of FVIII is 100–200 ng/mL, while the concentration of vWF is approximately 10 μg/mL [1]. The molar ratio of FVIII to vWF is 1:50. Thus, vWF concentration normally exceeds FVIII concentration. Six different types of Von Willebrand disease have been described [2]. As vWF and FVIII are intimately linked functionally, patients suspected with FVIII deficiency are also evaluated for von Willebrand disease [2].

S. Akhtar (✉)
Department of Anesthesiology and Pharmacology, Yale University School of Medicine, 333 Cedar Street, TMP #3, P.O. Box 208051New Haven, CT 06520-8051, USA
e-mail: shamsuddin.akhtar@yale.edu

© Springer International Publishing AG 2017
L.S. Aglio and R.D. Urman (eds.), *Anesthesiology*,
DOI 10.1007/978-3-319-50141-3_42

How Do FVIII and FIX Participate in Coagulation?

FVIII has structural similarities to coagulation Factor V (FV). Both are serine protease enzymes in the coagulation cascade [1]. FVIII plays a critical role in the amplification of the coagulation cascade. The physiological activator of FVIII is thrombin, which cleaves FVIII at 3 sites, releasing FVIII from vWF and resulting in activated FVIII (aFVIII). FXa and FIXa can also activate FVIII. aFVIII, in association with FIX, causes activation of thrombin. This reaction takes place on antiphospholipid surface (activated platelets), and is enhanced by the presence of aFVIII by about 200,000-fold. That is the reason that severe FVIII deficiency profoundly reduces the rate of FXa generation and adversely affects coagulation [1]. Deficiency of FVIII or FIX affects the intrinsic pathway and leads to prolongation of activated partial thromboplastin time (aPTT). Prothrombin time and platelet function test (PFA 100) are usually normal in hemophilia [2].

FVIII is principally synthesized in the liver and vascular endothelium. Patients with liver failure usually have adequate levels of factor VIII owing to extrahepatic production including the pulmonary vasculature [1, 5]. It has long been known that hemophilia can be cured by liver transplantation.

When and How Is Hemophilia Diagnosed?

Evaluation for hemophilia begins with a family history. In patients with family history of hemophilia, diagnosis can be made in utero, or in early neonatal life. Either chorionic villous sampling or amniocentesis can make prenatal diagnosis. In contrast, when there is no family history, the diagnosis is often made after an episode of bleeding. Initial workup will show a normal platelet count and PT with an abnormally elevated aPTT. Suspicion of a deficiency of clotting factor is evaluated by measurement of FVIII or FIX concentrations in the plasma. FIX levels are below normal in newborns, thus it is advisable to wait for one month after birth to test for hemophilia B. Isolated low plasma levels of FIX are almost always caused by congenital hemophilia B [1].

DNA analysis can also be used. Specific genetic mutations can be identified in up to 98% of the cases of hemophilia [1]. Determination of the specific hemophilia genotype is now the standard of care in comprehensive hemophilia management. As vWF and FVIII are intimately linked functionally, patients suspected with FVIII deficiency are also evaluated for von Willebrand disease [2].

How Is Hemophilia a Categorized?

Hemophilia A is categorized into three levels based on severity. Patients with *severe* hemophilia A have <1% of normal FVIII, patients with *moderate* hemophilia have 1–5% of normal FVIII, and patients with *mild* hemophilia may have up to 5–40% levels of normal FVIII. In severe deficiency, the diagnosis is often made in the first 2 years of life, when the child becomes active. In case of moderate disease the diagnosis may be made later, typically in the first two decades. In some cases of mild hemophilia, the diagnosis may be delayed until later in life, when bleeding occurs after a surgical intervention [2].

What Is the Clinical Manifestations of Hemophilia (A and B)?

The clinical features of hemophilia A and B are identical. Baseline levels of clotting factors determine the bleeding tendency in hemophilia. In severe cases (with <1% of FVIII level), intracranial hemorrhage can develop during difficult childbirth. Spontaneous bleeding episodes occur multiple times each year. Soft tissue or joint bleeding presents itself between the age of 6–18 months when the child becomes more mobile and active. In moderate cases (1–5% of FVIII level), spontaneous bleeding is rare but easy bruising is reported. Excessive and prolonged bleeding can occur with dental procedures, trauma, and surgical procedures. In case mild cases (5–40% of FVIII level) excessive bleeding is usually noted with trauma or invasive procedures.

In severe hemophilia, hemarthrosis is a classical clinical sign. Typically the ankles, knees and elbows are affected, but hemarthrosis can occur in any joint. Hemarthrosis leads to swelling, reduced mobility, synovial hypertrophy and chronic pain [6]. Bleeding into the joints account for 75% of all bleeding events in hemophilia patients [1, 2]. Subsequently, decreased mobility leads to muscle wasting of the affected limbs.

In addition to hemarthrosis, patients with hemophilia are prone to excessive and prolonged soft tissue and mucocutaneous bleeding. Muscle bleeds are quite common in hemophilia patients and they occur in calves, thighs, buttocks and forearm. If the bleeding is severe, surgical decompression and fasciotomy may be indicated, since bleeds into these locations can lead to compartment syndrome, entrapment neuropathy and ischemic necrosis. Neurovascular compromise requires urgent factor replacement and potentially surgical decompression. Chronically, muscle and soft tissue hematomas become encapsulated "hemophiliac pseudotumors" and may require surgical drainage. A large proportion of patients with hemophilia suffer from chronic pain [6].

Intracranial hemorrhage can occur after trauma. Before the advent of modern medicine, 75% of these intracranial hemorrhages caused death [6]. Occasionally, spontaneous hematuria and GI hemorrhage can occur [2].

What Is the Clinical Presentation of Acquired Hemophilia A (AHA)?

The usual clinical presentation of AHA is spontaneous or provoked bleeding and an unexplained, prolonged aPTT, in patients without family history of hemophilia. Spontaneous subcutaneous hematomas and extensive bruising are common in AHA. Curiously, hemarthrosis is uncommon [3].

What Level of FVIII Is Necessary for Hemostasis? What Are the Current Guidelines in the Nonoperative Setting for Managing Patients with Hemophilia?

The FVIII level necessary for normal hemostasis are described in Table 42.1. In the nonoperative setting, severe hemophiliacs are typically treated after an episode of bleeding (on-demand) with FVIII or FIX. Prophylactic therapy, (three times/week), with the aim of keeping the trough levels above 1% of normal, has been shown to prevent arthropathy associated with bleeding episodes [2, 7, 8]. Many different prophylactic dosing regimens have been developed for patients with hemophilia [9, 10].

How Much FVIII and FIX Is Present in Fresh Frozen Plasma, Cryoprecipitate, and Prothrombin Complex Concentrate [PCC]? How Is Factor VIII or FIX Replenished?

Fresh frozen plasma (FFP) typically contains 0.7–0.9 U/ml of FVIII clotting activity [11]. FVIII is most labile, and its activity falls by approximately 40% in 5 days after thawing [12]. Cryoprecipitate contains 5–13 U/ml of FVIII clotting activity. Generally, cryoprecipitate is only be used to treat Hemophilia A when Factor VIII concentrate is unavailable. Cryoprecipitate also contains vWF, Factor XIII, and fibrinogen [11]. Cryoprecipitate does not contain FIX, thus should not be used to treat hemophilia B. On the other hand, three and four factor prothrombin complex concentrate (PCC) have 20–30 IU/ml of FIX, but do not contain factor VIII, thus should not be used to treat hemophilia A [12].

A typical bleeding episode is treated with FVIII replacement therapy especially if it is within 2 h of the injury. Spontaneous bleeding is typically controlled if FVIII levels are raised to >50% of normal levels. However, for major surgery, spontaneous bleeding in critical sites (enclosed spaces, central nervous system) or severe posttraumatic bleeding, FVIII levels need to be elevated to 100%, (or >125% for FIX, see Table 42.1) and normal levels are maintained until healing occurs. After a major bleed or surgery, FVIII levels need to be maintained for 10–14 days. This can be achieved by bolus dosing or infusion. A bolus dose that achieves 100% of the desired level, then is followed by half the initial dose every 8–12 h, with close monitoring of the factor levels, with the aim of keeping the factor levels above 50% in the postoperative period. Alternatively, replacement therapy is administered by continuous infusion at the rate of 3 U/kg/h after an initial bolus dose [1].

Table 42.1 Recommendations for clotting factor replacement (from Ref. [1])

Site of bleed	Level desired (%)	Hemophilia A (rFVIII) (U/kg)	Hemophilia B (rFIX) (U/kg)
Oral mucosa	>30	20	40
Epistaxis	>30	20	40
Joint or muscle	>50	30	50
Gastrointestinal	>50	30	50
Genitourinary	>50	50	75
Central nervous system	>100	75	125
Trauma or surgery	>100	75	125

Administration of 1 U/kg of FVIII should increase the plasma concentration by 2% relative to the normal level. Similarly, administration of 1 U/kg of FIX should increase its concentration by 1%. Therefore, in patients with severe hemophilia A, to achieve a desired level 100% of normal, FVIII should be administered at 50 U/kg. The desired concentration of FVIII and FIX in different clinical situations is shown in Table 42.1.

What Is the Half-Life of FVIII? FIX?

All plasma-derived factors have similar pharmacokinetics. The half-life of FVIII is the shortest. The half-life of FVIII (recombinant or plasma derived) is 12 h, while for FIX is 24 h.

Preoperative Management

What Specific Information Would You Like to Know or Prepare for Before Elective Surgery?

Many patients (30%) with severe hemophilia A, who are treated with FVIII, develop alloantibodies to FVIII at some stage in their lives. It is important to know about the presence of these antibodies, since their presence can render a patient refractory to replacement with exogenous FVIII. Autoantibodies against factor IX are extremely rare [1]. If a patient has a low titer, additional FVIII infusion can potentially overcome the antibody effect temporarily. If a patient has a high titer, administration of rFVIIa may be necessary to control bleeding. This bypasses the defect in the clotting cascade. Before the advent of rFVIIa and aPCC, elective surgery was contraindicated in these patients.

Factor supplementation is required for many days after surgery. It is important to confirm availability of specific factor concentrates, not only for the immediate postoperative period, but also for the period until wound healing is complete [13].

What Other Diseases Should Be Considered in Patients with History of Hemophilia?

Until the late 1980s, the only sources for factor replacement products were FFP or cryoprecipitate. Many hemophilia patients were inadvertently infected with viral diseases like HIV, and hepatitis B and C. Thus, older hemophilia patients are at higher risk for acquired immunodeficiency syndrome (AIDS), chronic hepatitis, cirrhosis, or hepatoma. Liver disease may lead to thrombocytopenia which can exacerbate bleeding episodes [2]. Fortunately, recognition of these potential complications lead to the development of a safer blood product supply chain. Donors are screened and every unit is tested. Protocols for viral inactivation have been developed. Some recombinant replacement products are now available (rFVIII, rFIX, and rFVIIa).

To What Extent Should the Patient's Coagulation Status Be Corrected Before Surgery?

Excessive bleeding is almost inevitable in patients with severe or moderate hemophilia who undergo surgery. Bleeding causes pain that leads to poor wound healing and increases risk of infection. Correction by administration of specific replacement therapy is mandatory before surgery. With appropriate multidisciplinary management intra- and postoperative hemorrhages can be prevented.

The exact factor level required for hemostasis and the duration of clotting factor replacement after surgery is not known. A calculated dose of the required factor concentrate (FVIII or FIX), which will bring the factor levels to 100% of the normal, should be administered within 10–20 min of starting the procedure. Trough levels should be maintained at 80–100% level for the first 3 days after surgery. Between day 4 and 6, trough level should be between 60 and 80%, and after day 7 it should be maintained at 40–60% range [13].

What Is the Role of Desmopressin (DDAVP) in Patients with Hemophilia?

DDAVP provides an alternate means of increasing plasma FVIII levels in patients with *mild* hemophilia. DDAVP causes the release of endogenous vWF from the endothelial cells and increases the level of FVIII complex by two- to fourfold [1, 2]. The levels remain high for 8–10 h [14]. The rise in FVIII level is proportional to the resting level. DDAVP also increase platelet adhesiveness independent of its effect on FVIII complex levels. However, repeated doses of DDAVP leads to tachyphylaxis due to depletion of endogenous stores and should not be given for more than 3 consecutive days [1]. Typical intravenous dose is 0.3 μg/kg, infused over 30 min. The maximum effect is seen after 30–60 min of intravenous infusion. Because it is a vasopressin analog, it can cause hyponatremia. DDAVP can be administered intravenously, subcutaneously, or intranasal. It can be administered immediately after accidental trauma and hemorrhage in patients with mild hemophilia A [2]. It can also be used in cases of acquired hemophilia and is potentially effective in patients with low antibody titers.

In contrast to factor VIII, factor IX levels do not rise in response to DDAVP, thus DDAVP has no role in the management of hemophilia B. Preoperative administration of factor IX is needed to raise plasma concentration to the desired level for surgery [13].

Intraoperative Management

Was a Role Off Activated Recombinant Factor VII (RFVIIa) in Patients with Hemophilia? How Should It Be Administered?

Recombinant activated Factor VII (rFVIIa) or activated PCC (aPCC) can be useful in the treatment of bleeding episodes in patients with hemophilia, [10] acquired hemophilia A [3] and with inhibitors against exogenous FVIII [10]. They are considered bypass drugs, because FVIIa directly complexes with the tissue factor exposed at the site of tissue injury, activates Factor X and produces local hemostasis, while activated PCC have enough FXa to activate prothrombin to thrombin. The pathway is independent of FVIII to FIX and is not affected by their inhibition. As FVIIa has a short half-life (approximately 2 h), it may need to be administered frequently, [2] while aPCC has a longer half-life of about 7 h [3, 15, 16].

What Is the Role of Antifibrinolytics in the Management of Patients with Hemophilia?

Antifibrinolytics (tranexamic acid or epsilon aminocaproic acid) can decrease mucosal bleeding in hemophilia patients and are most commonly used in the context of oral or dental surgery. For major surgery, tranexamic acid can be administered intravenously (typically 1 g) shortly before induction of anesthesia. Alternatively, oral administration (1 g, 3–4 times daily) may be started, a day or 2 days before surgery, to ensure adequate blood levels are present at the time of operation [13]. Tranexamic acid should be continued for 7–10 days. A longer time may be needed after tonsillectomy, as the eschar typically falls off 7 days afterwards [1]. Simultaneous use of tranexamic acid and FVIII increases clot resistance to fibrinolysis [10].

Is It Safe to Administer Intramuscular Injection in Patients with Hemophilia?

Theoretically, intramuscular injection is safe if the FVIII activity is greater than 30%. The smallest gauge needle possible should be used. However, in current practice, it is unlikely that a patient will require an intramuscular injection. Most patients will already have an established intravenous access, temporary or long-term central venous device that can be used during the intraoperative period.

Is It Advisable to Conduct Neuroaxial Block for Inguinal Hernia Repair in This Patient?

Neuroaxial anesthesia is contraindicated in patients with coagulation disorder. However, regional anesthesia can be conducted in patients who have been appropriately replenished with factor concentrates and have adequate coagulation status. However, in vast majority of cases general anesthesia would be the anesthetic of choice.

What Precautions Should Be Taken in Intubating the Patient with Hemophilia?

Though these patients are prone to bleeding, endotracheal intubation is not a contraindication. Extreme care should be exercised during laryngoscopy and intubation. Gentle handling of tissues and avoiding unnecessary manipulation is advised.

Are There Any Specific Considerations in Choosing a Particular Anesthetic Drug in Patients with Hemophilia?

Patients with hemophilia may have coexisting liver disease. Based on the extent of liver dysfunction, drugs that are metabolized by the liver should be used with caution [17]. Aside from avoiding neuroaxial anesthesia/analgesia, no particular anesthetic technique can be recommended in patients with hemophilia.

Postoperative Management

Should This Patient Be Sent Home the Same Day, After Open Inguinal Hernia Repair?

Inguinal hernia surgery is one of the common surgeries performed in patients with hemophilia [13]. However, as discussed above, intraoperative is not the only time when significant bleeding can happen. High levels of FVIII or FIX have to be maintained for 7–10 days after surgery, until the wound is healed. Based on the severity of disease, extent of surgery, bleeding risk, and resources available, these patients are typically cared for by a multidisciplinary team, in the hospital or specialized hemophilia centers.

How Should a Patient with Hemophilia Be Managed Postoperatively?

Aspirin, non-steroidal anti-inflammatory drugs (NSAIDS) that can induce platelet dysfunction, should be avoided in patients with hemophilia. Pain is typically managed with opioids.

Special Considerations

Management of Hemophilia Patient for Emergency Surgery or with Trauma?

Management of patient with hemophilia for emergency surgery or trauma can be extremely challenging. Specific clotting factors have to be replenished to 100% the normal level. Hematologist and blood bank should be involved as soon as possible. Patient may require adjunctive therapy with, rFVIIa or aPCC and antifibrinolytics with frequent monitoring of coagulation status and maintenance of appropriate factor levels.

References

1. Carcao M, Moorehead P, Lillicrap D. Hemophilia A and B. In: Hoffman R, Benz EJ, Silberstein LE, Heslop HE, Weitz JI, Anastasi J, editors. Hematology: basic principles and practice. 6th ed. Philadelphia: Elsevier; 2013. p. 1940–60.
2. Hoffbrand AV, Moss PAH. Coagulation disorders. Essential haematology. Singapore: Wiley-Blackwell; 2011. p. 345–61.
3. Janbain M, Leissinger CA, Kruse-Jarres R. Acquired hemophilia A: emerging treatment options. J Blood Med. 2015;6:143–50. doi:10.2147/JBM.S77332. eCollection 2015.
4. Lenting PJ, van Mourik JA, Mertens K. The life cycle of coagulation factor VIII in view of its structure and function. Blood. 1998;92(11):3983–96.
5. Jacquemin M, Neyrinck A, Hermanns MI, Lavend'homme R, Rega F, Saint-Remy JM, et al. FVIII production by human lung microvascular endothelial cells. Blood. 2006;108(2):515–7.
6. Young G, Tachdjian R, Baumann K, Panopoulos G. Comprehensive management of chronic pain in haemophilia. Haemophilia. 2014;20(2):e113–20. doi:10.1111/hae.12349 Epub 2013 Dec 23.
7. Manco-Johnson MJ, Abshire TC, Shapiro AD, Riske B, Hacker MR, Kilcoyne R, et al. Prophylaxis versus episodic treatment to prevent joint disease in boys with severe hemophilia. N Engl J Med. 2007;357(6):535–44.
8. Oldenburg J, Brackmann HH. Prophylaxis in adult patients with severe haemophilia A. Thromb Res. 2014;134(Suppl 1):S33–7. doi:10.1016/j.thromres.2013.10.019 Epub 4 Sep 26.
9. Carcao M. Changing paradigm of prophylaxis with longer acting factor concentrates. Haemophilia. 2014;20(Suppl 4):99–105. doi:10.1111/hae.12405.
10. Berntorp E, Shapiro AD. Modern haemophilia care. Lancet. 2012;379(9824):1447–56.
11. American Society of Anesthesiologists Task Force on Perioperative. Blood T, Adjuvant T. Practice guidelines for perioperative blood transfusion and adjuvant therapies: an updated report by the American Society of Anesthesiologists Task Force on Perioperative Blood Transfusion and Adjuvant Therapies. Anesthesiology. 2006;105(1):198–208.
12. Tanaka KA, Mazzeffi M, Durila M. Role of prothrombin complex concentrate in perioperative coagulation therapy. J Intensive Care. 2014;2(1):60. doi:10.1186/s40560-014-0060-5. eCollection 2014.
13. Mensah PK, Gooding R. Surgery in patients with inherited bleeding disorders. Anaesthesia. 2015;2015(70 Suppl 1):112–20.
14. Svensson PJ, Bergqvist PB, Juul KV, Berntorp E. Desmopressin in treatment of haematological disorders and in prevention of surgical bleeding. Blood Rev. 2014;28(3):95–102. doi:10.1016/j.blre.2014.03.001 Epub Mar 22.
15. Villar A, Aronis S, Morfini M, Santagostino E, Auerswald G, Thomsen HF, et al. Pharmacokinetics of activated recombinant coagulation factor VII (NovoSeven) in children vs. adults with haemophilia A. Haemophilia. 2004;10(4):352–9.
16. Varadi K, Negrier C, Berntorp E, Astermark J, Bordet JC, Morfini M, et al. Monitoring the bioavailability of FEIBA with a thrombin generation assay. J Thromb Haemost. 2003;1(11):2374–80.
17. Leff J, Shore-Lesserson L, Kelly RE. Hemophilia and coagulation disorders. Yao and Artusio's Anesthesiology. Philadelphia: Wolters Kluwer; 2012. p. 793–811.

Sickle Cell Disease: Anesthetic Management

43

Gustavo A. Lozada

Case

A 27-year-old African-American man presents with a left ankle fracture sustained the previous day when he slipped on ice. He has a mild cough. He is anxious. The surgical plan is an open reduction and internal fixation.

Medications	Oxycodone 5 mg: 10 mg PO q4 h Acetaminophen 650 mg PO q6 h Hydroxyurea Folic acid
Allergies:	NKDA
Past Medical History:	Sickle Cell Disease Pain crises Pneumonia Acute chest syndrome Multiple transfusions
Past Surgical History	Laparoscopic cholecystectomy Tonsillectomy Incision and drainage of hip abscess

Physical Exam

VS: BP 132/79	HR 100	RR 18	Temp 36.8 °C O_2 Saturation: 98%
Height: 5 ft. 9 in.	Weight: 71 kg		

GEN: AAOx3, anxious
CHEST: RRR, Bilateral lung fields clear to auscultation
ABD: three small incision scars consistent with trocar placement
Ext: cast in left lower extremity
Otherwise: insignificant
Labs
Hemoglobin 8 g/dL
WBC 10
Platelets 215
INR 1.0
Glucose 89

1. What is sickle cell disease?

Sickle cell disease is a congenital, autosomal-recessive, hemoglobinopathy that is characterized by deformed (sickle-shaped) erythrocytes. It is caused by a single point mutation in codon 6 of exon 1 in the β-globin gene, which results in the substitution of the amino acid valine for glutamic acid. The resultant mutant hemoglobin, hemoglobin S, differs from normal adult hemoglobin A in the structure of the β-chains. The homozygous state, hemoglobin SS, causes the most severe form of the disease. The heterozygous state, hemoglobin AS, primarily results in a benign carrier state.

2. What are the pathophysiological implications of hemoglobin S?

Hemoglobin S is unstable and degrades more rapidly than hemoglobin A. Due to the instability of this hemoglobin, iron is released causing oxidative damage to the cell membrane of the erythrocyte and subsequent hemolysis. Resultant free iron in circulation consumes free nitric oxide and exposes the vascular endothelium to oxidative damage. Nitric oxide transport within the erythrocyte is also impaired due to loss of intracellular intact hemoglobin. These events contribute to the development of a chronic inflammatory microangiopathy.

In the deoxygenated form, hemoglobin S is insoluble and precipitates. Precipitated hemoglobin polymerizes, which deforms the cell. Pathologic cellular dehydration due to oxidative membrane damage associated with the breakdown of unstable hemoglobin S also contributes to deforming the cell. Consequently, the erythrocyte acquires primarily its characteristic "sickle" shape.

G.A. Lozada (✉)
Department of Anesthesiology, Tufts Medical Center, 800 Washington Street, Boston, MA 02111, USA
e-mail: glozada@tuftsmedicalcenter.org

© Springer International Publishing AG 2017
L.S. Aglio and R.D. Urman (eds.), *Anesthesiology*,
DOI 10.1007/978-3-319-50141-3_43

3. What is the incidence of sickle cell disease?

Sickle cell disease is one of the most common inherited hemolytic anemias. It affects about 50,000–70,000 people in the United States [1].

4. What are the clinical manifestations of sickle cell disease?

Sickle cell disease is characterized by chronic hemolytic anemia, acute painful vaso-occlusive exacerbations, vascular disease, evolving end-organ damage, and shortened life span. Manifestations of the disease process include pulmonary disease, progressive neurological damage, including intracranial hemorrhage and thrombotic stroke, renal disease, deep vein thrombosis, and leg ulcers. Pain crises and acute chest syndrome are the most common acute complications and are pathognomonic features of sickle cell disease.

5. What is a sickle cell pain crisis?

Sickle cell pain crisis, also referred to as vaso-occlusive crisis (VOC), manifests predominantly as bone pain and/or abdominal pain. VOC is a complex process believed to involve leukocyte adhesion and migration, vasoconstriction, platelet activation and adhesion, and coagulation. Bone pain is thought to be caused from either cortical or marrow infarction, which produces cortical pressure from inflammation and edema. The most common sites of pain are the lumbar spine, femoral shaft, and knee. Abdominal pain can arise from abdominal distention, gastrointestinal dysfunction, and organ infarction or can be referred from the ribs.

6. What is the acute chest syndrome?

The acute chest syndrome (ACS), which has similar features to pneumonia, consists of a new lobar infiltration on chest radiography with chest pain, fever greater than 38.5 °C, and respiratory distress (wheezing, cough, or tachypnea). Possible precipitants of ACS include infection, pulmonary infarction, fat embolism after bone marrow infarction, and surgical procedures.

Treatment of ACS includes antibiotics, bronchodilators, supplemental oxygen, incentive spirometry, and consideration of transfusion.

7. What are the leading causes of morbidity and mortality in sickle cell disease patients?

The leading causes of morbidity and mortality in this patient population are pulmonary and neurologic disease. Chronic renal disease is also an important cause.

Sickle cell disease causes chronic progressive lung disease. It can initially present as lower airway obstruction and reactive airway disease in children and adolescents and progress to fibrosis and restrictive lung disease in later stages. Recurrent episodes of ACS can accelerate the progression of lung disease. Neurologic disease in sickle cell patients can include stroke, either hemorrhagic or infarctive. Renal diseases include glomerular disease and papillary necrosis.

8. What is the normal hemoglobin level in a patient with sickle cell disease?

Most sickle cell disease patients are anemic. Their baseline hemoglobin levels are usually in the range of 5–10 g/dL.

9. Why is hydroxyurea used in sickle cell disease patients?

Hydroxyurea increases the production of fetal hemoglobin, reduces the expression of adhesion molecules, and improves NO delivery. It has been shown to reduce pain episodes and hospitalizations.

10. What are the most commonly performed surgical procedures in sickle cell disease patients?

Cholelithiasis secondary to chronic hemolysis is common in these patients. Hence, cholecystectomy is the most commonly performed surgical procedure. Splenectomy, hip arthroplasty from avascular necrosis of the femoral head, and drainage of bone infections are also common. The most common neurosurgical procedure performed in sickle cell disease patients is intracerebral aneurysm ablation.

11. How will you preoperatively assess this patient?

The history should identify the frequency, pattern, and severity of sickle cell exacerbations. It is important to know when the patient had the last exacerbation and the length of his hospital admission. Longer hospitalizations usually reflect more severe exacerbations. Establish the presence and extent of organ damage. The most commonly affected organs are the lungs, kidneys, and brain.

A baseline hemoglobin level, chest X-ray, and urinalysis should be obtained on all patients. Further studies, including pulmonary function tests, electrocardiogram, arterial blood gas, and neurologic imaging should be obtained if warranted based on the history and extent of organ damage established and the anticipated surgical stress.

12. Are pulmonary function tests necessary?

Assessment of pulmonary status is essential. More extensive testing depends on the severity of disease. A chest X-ray should be obtained for all patients. If extensive lung involvement is suspected, then pulmonary function tests can be considered.

13. Is a preoperative electrocardiogram necessary?

Obtaining an electrocardiogram on this 27-year-old should be based on history and not ordered reflexively. If the history or clinical presentation warrants it, then it should be obtained prior to proceeding with the surgery.

14. Is preoperative neuroimaging necessary?

The brain is one of the most affected organs in sickle cell disease. Progressive neurological damage, including intracranial hemorrhage and thrombotic stroke are common in sickle cell patients. However, the decision to order neuroimaging studies in this patient should be based on the history. Unless the history warrants it, these studies should not be ordered.

15. Is urinalysis needed prior to surgery?

The kidneys are commonly affected by sickle cell disease. The preoperative workup of the sickle cell patient includes urinalysis to assess for renal disease. It should be ordered in this case.

16. Is a preoperative arterial blood gas required for this patient?

Unless there is a clinical reason, i.e., the patient shows signs and symptoms of pulmonary dysfunction (e.g., hypoxia), an arterial blood gas is not necessary.

17. Will you order a preoperative hemoglobin level?

Most sickle cell disease patients are anemic with baseline hemoglobin levels of 5–10 g/dL. It is essential to know the preoperative hemoglobin level.

18. Can the surgical procedure be performed under regional anesthesia?

Sickle cell disease is not a contraindication for regional anesthesia, including neuraxial anesthesia. There are various options for this patient. The surgery can be performed under spinal, epidural, combined spinal/epidural, or with a combined popliteal (sciatic) and saphenous (femoral) peripheral nerve block, either single shot or with catheters. The peripheral block can also be offered for postoperative pain control even if general anesthesia is chosen. Regional anesthesia has certain advantages, including better pain control, narcotic sparing effect with less side effects, and earlier discharge.

19. What will be your anesthetic modality for this case?

This surgery can be performed either under general anesthesia or regional anesthesia. There are certain benefits to doing the case under regional anesthesia, including enhanced pain control. If performing an epidural or peripheral block with the insertion of a catheter, good pain control can be established and maintained for a few days.

20. Would you provide premedication for this patient?

Traditionally, concern of causing respiratory depression, hypoxia, and sickling has resulted in the avoidance of premedication. However, patients with sickle cell disease have endured much suffering due to the chronic nature of their disease. Avoidance of anxiolytic premedication would be inappropriate if the patient is highly anxious.

Patients with sickle cell disease often have a high level of opioid tolerance, especially if they have had recent recurrent episodes of severe pain, which were treated with high doses of opioids. Therefore opioids should be titrated up to an appropriate level to avoid unnecessary suffering.

Following administration of any premedication, the same principle of monitoring the patient for over sedation and respiratory depression, with pulse oximetry, for instance, should be employed just as in the general population.

21. The surgeon would like to use a tourniquet for the procedure and asks for your opinion. What do you tell her?

The uneventful use of occlusive arterial tourniquets for orthopedic procedures has been described in a series of 37 patients in three reports [2–4] Clinical reports confirming that the use of a tourniquet is contraindicated in this patient population are lacking. Therefore, the surgeon can use a tourniquet for the procedure.

22. What are the anesthetic management goals for patients with sickle cell disease?

The goals include providing adequate hydration (normovolemia), good oxygenation, good analgesia, avoiding hypothermia, acidosis, and venous stasis.

23. What are your fluid management goals in this patient?

There are no studies assessing perioperative fluid balance in sickle cell disease patients. There are data to support modification of standard, routine fluid management. Therefore, normovolemia should be the goal.

24. What intravenous fluid will you use during the surgery?

Any of the commonly used intravenous fluids, such as lactated ringers, plasmalyte, or normal saline can be used for fluid maintenance. A colloid, such as albumin can also be used if indicated.

25. Does hypothermia increase perioperative complications in sickle cell disease patients?

There are no case reports or studies concluding that perioperative hypothermia causes perioperative vaso-occlusive crisis or other sickle cell disease complications. Hypothermia has been induced in sickle cell patients during cardiopulmonary bypass without consequence.

However, the avoidance of hypothermia is a basic objective of most anesthetics. Therefore, just as it is for the general patient population, normothermia should be maintained and core body temperature should be monitored. An active warming device such as a forced-air warming blanket should be applied unless contraindicated.

26. Are there any implications of sickle cell disease for transfusion therapy?

Red cell alloimmunization, the development of non-ABO erythrocyte antibodies, has a high incidence in sickle cell disease patients. Therefore, extensive cross-matching should be routine. If warranted, a type and screen should be done well before surgery (a day or two) to give the blood bank time to find compatible blood products.

In patients with sickle cell disease, there is also a higher incidence of delayed transfusion reactions, development of new antibodies, and shortened life span of transfused erythrocytes.

27. Would you transfuse this patient preoperatively?

Preoperative transfusion is controversial as there is no consensus on whether there is a benefit. For minor surgical procedures and patients at lower risk, e.g., younger patients and patients with milder symptoms, postoperative risks of sickle cell complications are low, thus the risks outweigh the benefits. Vis-à-vis. for patients undergoing an extensive surgical procedures or who are at higher risk, the benefits of preoperative transfusion are not clear, as there are no studies that definitively support this practice. There is one small study that recommended transfusing to a preoperative hemoglobin level of 10 g/dL, but the study closed early and had a small number of participants [5]. A discussion of the risks and benefits with the patient and surgeon is warranted. Specifically: What is the severity of the patient's sickle cell disease? What is their baseline hemoglobin level? What end organ damage has already occurred? What is the risk for blood loss? Will a tourniquet be used?

28. Is an arterial line needed for the surgery?

Unless the patient has underlying cardiac disease that warrants more invasive monitoring, an arterial line is not needed. A blood pressure cuff is adequate.

29. Is a central venous pressure catheter necessary?

Unless there is a separate indication, monitoring central venous pressures is not necessary in this patient.

30. How will you induce anesthesia in this patient?

A standard induction will suffice. An intravenous anesthetic, such as propofol or etomidate, can be combined with an opioid, such as fentanyl. Any of the commonly used non-depolarizing neuromuscular relaxants, such as atracurium, vecuronium, or rocuronium, can be used. There is no contraindication to using succinylcholine unless the patient has advanced renal disease.

31. How will you secure the airway?

Either standard endotracheal intubation or use of a laryngeal mask airway is acceptable for this case. However, the patient experienced a trauma the day before and it can be argued that he should be treated as a full stomach.

32. What is your plan for anesthetic maintenance?

As in any other patient, a balanced anesthetic can be delivered. Isoflurane, sevoflurane, or desflurane can be used. Adequate analgesia can be accomplished using fentanyl with either morphine or hydromorphone. Given the chronic use of narcotics in sickle cell disease, adjuvants should be considered. For instance, ketamine can be used as part of the anesthetic. Muscle relaxant can be administered as needed.

If an epidural is in place, it can be used for the case, either by intermittent bolus or as an infusion.

33. How will you manage the patient's pain during the surgical procedure?

Sickle cell patients potentially have a high tolerance to opioid analgesics, thus higher doses may be required.

Adjuvants should be considered; for example, ketamine which has a narcotic sparing effect and has been found to decrease the hyperalgesic state caused by chronic, long-standing opioid consumption. And ideally, the patient should receive a preoperative nerve block.

34. Will your extubation criteria be different for this patient?

The extubation criteria for patients with sickle cell disease are the same as for patients in the general population.

35. What are the postoperative management goals?

Postoperative management should include standard supportive care plus any interventions appropriate for sickle cell patients. These include oxygen supplementation as needed, sufficient analgesia and hydration, early mobilization, and incentive spirometry.

36. Would you provide supplemental oxygen?

Oxygen supplementation should be employed as in any other patient; however, since hypoxemia can induce sickling, this is especially important in sickle cell patients.

37. How would you manage the patient's pain in the PACU?

Multimodal analgesia should be the goal in this sickle cell disease patient just as it is for the general population patient. Patients with sickle cell disease have a high tolerance to narcotics. Some patients may also have problems with addiction. Dosing of narcotics should therefore be appropriate, taking care not to under medicate the patient and cause unnecessary suffering. A hydromorphone or morphine PCA should be considered. There are various non-narcotic adjuvants that can be used in managing postoperative pain. Among these are pregabalin, gabapentin, acetaminophen, clonidine, ketamine, and nonsteroidal anti-inflammatory drugs. These are meant to be adjuvants and not alternatives to opioid analgesics. If a patient did not get a preoperative peripheral nerve block, a single shot or continuous popliteal and saphenous nerve block can be offered.

38. What are possible sickle cell disease associated postoperative complications?

A higher rate of postoperative complications is seen in patients with more severe sickle cell disease and with more extensive surgeries. Two complications, vaso-occlusive crisis and acute chest syndrome, are specific for the sickle cell disease patient. Vaso-occlusive crisis can result in excruciating pain. Administration of hydromorphone, morphine, fentanyl, or meperidine is the standard for treating the severe pain of a sickle cell pain crisis. Consider using a combination of opioid analgesia with non-opioid adjuvants. Patient-controlled analgesia or a fentanyl patch is recommended. The acute chest syndrome is a significant complication of sickle cell pain crises. On average, it develops 3 days after surgery and lasts 8 days. To decrease its progression, bronchodilators, broad-spectrum antibiotics, supplemental oxygen, incentive spirometry, and appropriate analgesia are recommended.

39. Is meperidine contraindicated in patients with sickle cell disease?

Meperidine is not contraindicated in sickle cell disease. However, because of the accumulation of the epileptogenic metabolite normeperidine, it should be used with caution, especially in patients with renal impairment or seizure foci.

40. One hour after arrival in the post anesthesia care unit (PACU), the patient experiences respiratory distress. You are called to assess the patient. What do you do?

In addition to disease-specific postoperative complications, sickle cell disease patients can experience the same postoperative complications as patients in the general population. Your assessment for postoperative respiratory distress should include a physical exam with auscultation of the chest, establishing how alert, awake, and oriented the patient is, and assessing the vital signs. The cycle of: 1. Evaluate, 2. Identify, and 3. Intervene, should be followed. Ordering a chest X-ray and arterial blood gas may be warranted. Supplemental oxygen may be necessary. Treat with bronchodilators as needed. If the condition of the patient continues to deteriorate, you might consider bag-mask ventilation or intubation. Sickle cell disease patients are at an increased risk of developing acute chest syndrome; hence, respiratory distress requires immediate, aggressive treatment.

41. Will your post PACU discharge criteria be different for this patient?

PACU discharge criteria for sickle cell disease patients are the same as for patients in the general population. These include spontaneous respiration without support, stable vital signs, normothermia, and adequate pain control.

References

1. Hassell KL. Population estimates of sickle cell disease in the U.S. Am J Prev Med. 2010;38(Suppl. 4):S512–21.
2. Stein RE, Urbaniak J. Use of the tourniquet during surgery in patients with sickle cell hemoglobinopathies. Clin Orthop Relat Res. 1980;151:231–3.

3. Adu-Gyamfi Y, Sankarankutty M, Marwa S. Use of a tourniquet in patients with sickle-cell disease. Can J Anaesth. 1993;40(1):24–7.
4. Oginni LM, Rufai MB. How safe is tourniquet use in sickle-cell disease? Afr J Med Med Sci. 1996;25(1):3–6.
5. Howard J, Malfroy M, Llewelyn C, Choo L, Hodge R, Johnson T, Purohit S, Rees DC, Tillyer L, Walker I, Fijnvandraat K, Kirby-Allen M, Spackman E, Davies SC, Williamson LM. The transfusion alternatives preoperatively in sickle cell disease (TAPS) study: a randomized, controlled, multicenter clinical trial. Lancet. 2013;381:930–8.

Part IX
Orthopedic Surgery

Section Editor: Kamen Vlassakov

Kamen Vlassakov
Department of Anesthesiology, Perioperative
and Pain Medicine, Brigham and Women's Hospital,
Boston, MA, USA

Total Hip Replacement

44

Vijay Patel, Kamen Vlassakov, and David R. Janfaza

Case: THR for end stage arthritis (OA/RA)

1. Preoperative care and coordination (PRE)—assessment, tests, and medical optimization
2. Day of surgery (DOS)—premedication, monitors, choice of anesthesia techniques
3. Postoperative care (POST)

CASE:

A 65 y/o man presents for right total hip replacement. He has intractable right hip pain secondary to end stage arthritis (RA/OA). Activity severely limited secondary to pain.

Medications: • simvastatin 20 mg oral daily • clopidogrel 75 mg oral daily • oxycodone 5–10 mg oral every 4 h for pain • lisinopril 20 mg oral daily • atenolol 50 mg po daily	
Allergies:	NKA
Past Medical History:	
Cardiac:	
• coronary artery disease—s/p drug eluting stent LAD 2 years ago • hypertension • hypercholesterolemia	

(continued)

Physical Exam:	
VS:	BP 160/80 mmHg HR 60 RR 12 oxygen saturation: 98%

1. PRE

A. What are the preoperative considerations for a patient with OA/RA? Does this patient require any further evaluation? [1]

Preoperative considerations regarding the anesthetic management in a patient with RA or OA include review of possible systemic or multi-organ involvement of the primary disease, secondary effects of treatments on end organs, as well as coexisting diseases.

(1) Airway: Evaluation must include careful history and examination of the cervical spine with concerns for underlying atlanto-axial subluxation or other cervical instability. Undiagnosed cervical instability and manipulation of the cervical spine during direct laryngoscopy can result in potential neurological injury. A thorough neurologic examination, as well as an evaluation of the airway with range of motion of the neck should be performed. It would be prudent to obtain cervical X-rays if symptoms or physical findings of instability are present. Difficulties in intubation may be complicated by a narrow glottis resulting from direct involvement of the disease at the cricoarytenoid joint. Patients should be assessed for any symptoms indicating airway involvement, including hoarseness, which may necessitate otolaryngology consult. Disease at the TMJ may severely limit mouth opening and an awake FOB may also be considered.

(2) Cardiac: rheumatoid arthritis (RA) patients are prone to pericardial effusion and tamponade. They are also at

V. Patel (✉)
Department of Anesthesiology, Lenox Hill Hospital, 100 E 77th St., New York, NY 10065, USA
e-mail: vjpatel8@gmail.com

K. Vlassakov · D.R. Janfaza
Department of Anesthesiology, Perioperative and Pain Medicine, Brigham and Women's Hospital, 75 Francis St., Boston, MA 02115, USA
e-mail: djanfaza@partners.org

© Springer International Publishing AG 2017
L.S. Aglio and R.D. Urman (eds.), *Anesthesiology*,
DOI 10.1007/978-3-319-50141-3_44

increased risk for CAD. In the face of an abnormal EKG or CXR, a cardiology consult should be considered.

(3) Pulmonary: Fibrosis and restrictive lung disease are a result of chronic disease and should be assessed with pulmonary function testing and a pulmonology consult.

(4) Renal/Gastrointestinal (GI): As a result of chronic NSAID use patients with RA and osteoarthritis (OA) often develop chronic renal failure and PUD and GI bleeding.

(5) Infectious/Hematologic: Immunosuppression from disease modifying drugs (DMDs) and steroids may predispose patients not only to infection but to anemia and platelet dysfunction.

B. Does the patient's history of CAD have any implications? Would this affect your choice of anesthesia/monitoring? Is he at an increased risk for cardiac complications intra/post op? What further tests would you like to assess his cardiac function? Is the patient's hypertension a concern? What about the history of drug eluting stents? Would you delay the case?

A history of CAD in a patient with rheumatoid arthritis is not uncommon. While drug-eluting stents (DES) delay the epithelialization and neointimal thickening associated with coronary artery dilatation, they also carry a longer term risk of thrombosis. Therefore, patients are routinely placed on anticoagulants, most commonly a glycoprotein IIb/IIIa inhibitor like clopidogrel and or aspirin. Current recommendations for dual therapy with stenting are typically 4 weeks with bare metal stents and up to 6 months with drug eluding stents (depending on the type of stent used). Although there are no prospective comparative studies reporting the relative cardiovascular risk of deliberately stopping antiplatelet medication preoperatively, maintaining dual antiplatelet therapy is the mainstay of early stent thrombosis prevention. However, short-term discontinuation of clopidogrel one-week prior to surgery might be associated with relatively low risk if aspirin therapy is maintained.

It can be difficult to assess the cardiac status of these patients based on functional status alone because mobility is often limited by pain from joint disease. Poor exercise tolerance associated with chest pain, or any other cardiac symptomology should warrant further workup. In most patients, total hip arthroplasty is performed as an elective procedure and there should be sufficient time to optimize the patient's general medical condition prior to surgery.

Patients with poor exercise tolerance at baseline secondary to underlying disability need to be appropriately screened for coronary disease. Patients with known risk factors for CAD but no known disease may be appropriate for cardiac stress testing. Traditional treadmill stress test is likely not feasible and consideration for alternative methods assess cardiac function and reserve should be considered.

C. What are the implications of clopidogrel on surgery/anesthetic technique? What further blood tests would you order? What is the appropriate amount of time to wait (GA vs. RA is there a difference)? [2]

Clopidogrel (Plavix) is a thienopyridine drug that prevents platelet aggregation by inhibiting ADP receptor-mediated platelet activation. This results in irreversible blockade that extends for the life of the platelet (which is typically 7–9 days). In the setting of elective surgery, the discontinuation of clopidogrel for 7 days prior to the day of surgery is generally recommended because the degree of inhibition can only be overcome by platelet transfusion or by the generation of new platelets. If surgery is performed without holding medication, bleeding risk is increased and the potential for higher transfusion requirements should be discussed and prepared for. Neuraxial anesthesia in a patient on clopidogrel carries the risk of epidural hematoma. Therefore, if a spinal injection is to be performed on a patient prior to 7 days of discontinuation of the drug.

D. What premedication would you consider/would you order? Are preoperative/perioperative prophylactic antibiotics necessary? [3, 4]

Pain control for major joint surgery often incorporates a "multimodal approach" that begins with the administration multiple synergistic medications. Studies have shown that a mulimodal approach has the potential to reduce of opioid related side effects, improve analgesia, and lead to better patient satisfaction. Typically, a combination of NSAIDS, COX-2 inhibitors, and anticonvulsants are employed and continued in the postoperative period.

The use of preoperative/perioperative antibiotics has become a standard of care for orthopedic surgeries. They have been proven to reduce the incidence of surgical site and prosthesis site infection. Prosthetic site infections incur staggering costs with the potential need for multiple reoperations. Therefore, it is recommended that all total joint replacement patients receive antibiotics prior to any arthroplasty. The primary agent used in the United States is typically a 1st generation cephalosporin. The addition of vancomycin as a second agent is also very common. Appropriate antibiotic prophylaxsis includes adequate dosing based on ideal body weight, timing of administration with respect to surgical incision and appropriate re-dosing.

2. INTRA

1) Does the surgeon's approach (anterior vs. posterolateral) have any implications or concerns? [5]

The type of patient positioning for total hip replacement surgery varies with the surgical approach.

The most common approach is the posterior approach (lateral decubitus position), where the incision is made from the lateral aspect of the thigh with the patient in the lateral recumbent position. The anesthesiologist, together with the surgical and nursing teams, must be vigilant in maintaining the legs and spine in a neutral position and properly padding all pressure points to prevent nerve-related damage and compression injury. In the lateral position, there is a risk of excessive lateral neck flexion and pressure on the dependent limbs. Furthermore, if an anterior stabilizing peg is used to hold the patient in the lateral position, adequate padding must be ensured to avoid compression of the femoral triangle. The dependent eye should be free of compression and both eyes should be taped prior to positioning. A chest roll (often called "axillary roll") is placed just caudal to the axilla, ensuring that weight is not distributed into the axilla and preventing brachial plexus and vascular compression in the dependent arm. The dependent arm is placed perpendicular to the body and the nondependent arm is suspended on a padded arm board with the shoulder and elbow at less than 90° angles.

Surgeries utilizing an anterior approach are typically performed in the supine position with the arm on the surgical side placed across the chest to allow for surgical access to the operative field as well as positioning of a fluoroscopy unit used for the surgery. The arm on the nonoperative side is placed in standard position at less than 90° abduction to protect the brachial plexus. Access of the necessary fluoroscopy unit needed for this surgery should be considered when positioning both the arm on the operative side as well as the nonoperative side. Appropriate padding of arm boards and the arm placed across chest should be utilized to protect pressure points as well as the ulnar nerves. The most common nerve injury from positioning is ulnar neuropathy and the use of padded arm boards, limiting arm abduction to 90°, positioning the forearm in a neutral or supinated position, and frequent position and pressure points checks are critical in preventing this injury.

2) What monitors would you use for this case? Arterial line? CVP?

All patients undergoing surgery with RA or GA should be monitored with blood pressure (usually noninvasive), ECG, and pulse oximetry. If hypotensive anesthesia is to be attempted, invasive arterial blood pressure monitoring should be performed. Capnography, inspired oxygen, volatile agent analysis, and airway pressure monitoring are standard for general anesthesia. A central line is not necessary in most hip replacement surgery, but large bore intravenous access is necessary (two large bore IV catheters are recommended). For patients undergoing surgery in the lateral position, placement of IV lines in the lower arm has the advantages of better flow and keeping the upper arm free for noninvasive blood pressure cuff. Regardless of anesthetic choice, patient normothermia should be pursued with forced air warming if available and temperature should be monitored throughout. Actively warming the patient may reduce intraoperative blood loss. In addition, hypothermia may cause poor wound healing, infection and cardiovascular dysfunction.

(3) What anesthetic technique would you use for this patient? Does one have an advantage over the other?

Total hip replacement can be performed under general, spinal, or epidural anesthesia, and often a combination of techniques is used. Although there are many opinions on what choice of anesthetic is superior, currently, there is no evidence of a difference in mortality between the techniques and significant difference in perioperative morbidity is difficult to confirm independently. When finalizing the anesthetic choice for hip replacement surgery, one should consider the risks and benefits of either technique. However, recent studies show several distinct advantages to using regional anesthesia over general anesthesia.

(4) What are advantages of regional anesthesia [6]?

- The use of regional anesthesia, and neuraxial anesthesia in particular, has shown a decrease in intraoperative blood loss and need for intraoperative and postoperative transfusion
- Decreased bleeding at the operative site, improved cement bonding, as well as shorter surgical time are all reported advantages to regional anesthesia
- Reduced incidence of deep venous thrombosis (DVT) and pulmonary embolism (PE) in the postoperative period
- Avoids the effects of general anesthesia and mechanical ventilation on pulmonary function
- Provides good early post operative analgesia and leads to decreased length of hospital stay
- Lower overall cost.

The reduced blood loss observed with regional anesthesia, as compared with general anesthesia is likely due to the reduction in arterial and venous pressures resulting from sympathetic blockade, which gives rise to notably less venous oozing of blood in the surgical field.

(5) What if the patient has: heart valve disorder (AS), low platelets, COPD?

Although regional anesthesia can provide a safe anesthetic in most cases, there are both absolute and relative contraindications to neuraxial, and particularly, spinal, anesthesia.

Absolute Contraindications

- Patient refusal
- Bacteremia or sepsis
- Infection at the site of needle insertion
- Coagulopathy, anticoagulation or extreme platelet dysfunction.

Relative Contraindications

- Preexisting neurological deficits and increased ICP
- Heart disease and valvular disorders
- Inability to cooperate, failure to respond
- Hypovolemia.

Although valvular disorders, such as aortic stenosis, are not an absolute contraindication to spinal anesthesia, the decrease in afterload that results from even a modest sympathectomy can have potentially disastrous effects on coronary perfusion. Careful monitoring of arterial blood pressure should be considered as well as adequate maintenance (and monitoring) of intravascular volume (preload) and early aggressive vasoactive treatment (common first-line agent is phenylephrine) as indicated.

COPD is not a contraindication for regional anesthesia, in fact, regional anesthesia is often preferred in situations where endotracheal intubation and mechanical ventilation are less than desirable.

While a decreased platelet count could potentially increase the risk of epidural hematoma, it does not represent an absolute contraindication for regional anesthesia. What becomes more important than the absolute platelet count is the pathophysiology and nature of the thrombocytopenia itself, as well as platelet function.

(6) The patient develops hypotension shortly after induction … and midway through surgery

Causes/differential diagnosis:

- Venous thromboembolism (VTE) is the most reported morbidity for THR during the perioperative period
- What are the earliest signs and symptoms of VTE?
- Blood loss and the determinants of CO, CPP. Controlled hypotension-risks benefits?
- Methyl methacrylate/fat embolism - risk factors?

- Bone cement implantation syndrome: Methyl methacrylate is an acrylic polymer that has been used extensively in orthopedic surgery for 30 years. Its use is associated with the potential for hypoxia, hypotension, and cardiovascular collapse including cardiac arrest. The most likely cause is fat embolization resulting from raised intramedullary pressure due to the cement expanding as it hardens. Direct toxic effects of the cement are also possible. Such problems typically occur soon after cement insertion, but may sometimes also present at the end of the operation when the hip joint is reduced (relocated) and emboli are dislodged from a previously obstructed femoral vein.

Prevention and treatment

- Ensure adequate blood volume prior to cementing

Increased inspired oxygen concentration prior to cementing

- Frequent monitoring of blood pressure and capnography
- Cessation of N_2O anesthesia
- Pressors to treat hypotension
- Suction applied to the bone cavity by the surgeon to evacuate air and fat during cement insertion dramatically reduces the incidence of complications
- Thorough pulse lavage of the medullary space by the surgeon can significanlty reduce the debris displaced subsequently by the increased intramedullary pressure
- It may be appropriate to avoid the use of cement in patients with severe cardiac disease, and this should be discussed with the surgeon beforehand.

(7) What intraoperative methods can be used to reduce intraoperative blood loss during THR? What are the contraindications for using TXA? What are the contraindications for using cell salvaging techniques?

The reduction of intraoperative blood loss remains a central goal for surgeons and anesthesiologists during total joint surgery. Hypotensive anesthesia and blood-salvaging techniques have been used to prevent blood loss and blood transfusion with varying success.

Recently, intravenous tranexamic acid (TXA) has been employed with data showing that it is not only clinically efficient but cost-efficient as well. Tranaxemic acid is a relatively weak antifibrinolytic that competitively inhibits the activation of plasminogen to plasmin. It is roughly 8 times more powerful than its predecessor, aminocaproic acid. Multiple studies have shown the ability of TXA to reduce intraoperative and postoperative blood loss in total joint replacement.

The intraoperative administration of TXA does carry a theoretical increased risk for thromboembolism, but reports of such events have been limited and require further validation. Patients who are at increased risk for thromboembolism or conditions that could be further complicated by thromboembolism, should not receive TXA for prevention of blood loss during elective surgery.

Patients with the following conditions should be excluded from elective TXA use:

- History of active arterial or venous thromboembolic disease
- Coronary stents placed within 1 year
- History of severe ischemic heart disease or MI
- Pregnancy
- Significant renal impairment
- Recent subarachnoid hemorage (SAH)
- Cerebrovascular accident (CVA) within 3 months
- Acquired defective color vision.

(Source: BWH guidelines on TXA administration)

Autologous blood transfusion as a means to reduce the need for allogenic transfusion typically takes place in the form of intraoperative cell savaging techniques and preoperative blood donation. Preoperative donation typically takes place within 2 weeks prior to surgery and no less than 72 h prior to surgery and requires adequate iron supplementation and considerable cost to the hospital. While preoperative autologous donation has the benefit of absolving patient concern about transfusion acquired infection, it is limited in the volume of blood that can be donated and by the patients preexisting medical conditions. Patients with active infection, and those with cardiovascular disease that could be potentially worsened by donating blood (e.g., ischemic heart disease) should not participate in preoperative autologous blood donation.

Blood-salvaging techniques provide a more cost-effective and-efficient way to provide autologous transfusion during the intraoperative period without the need for preoperative donation. It should be considered for all surgeries that anticipate a greater than 1 L blood loss and has proven to reduce transfusion requirements for joint replacement surgeries.

However, blood-salvaging techniques are not acceptable when blood in the surgical field encounters substances that can damage red blood cells including hypotonic fluids, and in the presence of topical coagulants and surgical bone cement. Cell-saver blood salvage techniques have very limited role in total hip arthroplasty since the quality of the collected blood is also compromised by debris, including a considerable amount of fat that is difficult to wash or filter out.

Controlled hypotension and normovolemic hemodilution are both methods used to reduce blood loss by actively decreasing perfusion to the bleeding site through different mechanisms. Controlled hypotension is primarily achieved intraoperatively using anesthetic and vasodilatory substances with a goal of reducing MAP to approximately 30% below baseline. It has been proven effective in reducing blood loss in a variety of orthopedic procedures and enhancing surgical field visualization, but it is not without its drawbacks. Ischemia to organs that are already stressed can lead to end organ damage and increase mortality and morbidity.

Acute normovolemic hemodilution (ANH) is a technique that entails the removal of whole blood from a patient shortly after induction of anesthesia, and maintaining normovolemia using crystalloid and/or colloid replacement. The effectiveness in ANH reducing the need for allogenic transfusion is debatable, and the safety of the technique is dependent on practitioner experience. Therefore, the technique should be only reserved for patients with an adequate starting hematocrit and for whom other options are not feasible. The contraindications for ANH include poor cardiac function with impaired or hindered cardiac output, a starting Hg of <11 g/dL, baseline kidney dysfunction, and underlying platelet or clotting disorders [7–10].

3. POST

(1) What are the most common complications after LE total joint replacement? Does one technique have better outcomes than the other in mortality and specific outcomes?

- Thromboembolism

Venous thromboembolism is serious but decreasing risk following total hip replacement surgery. Patients are routinely placed on thromboprophylactic regimens in the immediate postoperative period. Chemoprophylactic therapy is the preferred method, however, much emphasis is placed on early ambulation to prevent the formation of DVT.

- Pain and pain control—patient has to be on anticoagulation (AC) with epidural? When to resume AC? Are there any regional techniques that could offer pain control?

The hip joint is innervated by the femoral, sciatic and obturator nerves with skin and superficial tissues receiving branches from the lower thoracic nerves T10–T12. The gluteal nerves and other small branches from the sacral plexus may also contribute to the joint innervation. Because of the complex innervation of the hip, no single peripheral nerve block is sufficient for hip replacement. A lumbar plexus block that blocks the nerve roots of T12–L5, may provide effective analgesia which extends into the postoperative period (with the exception of the skin dermatomes of T10–T11). Furthermore, this block should only be performed after appropriate training due to the technical difficulties and propensity for complications. The femoral 3 in 1 block, which is technically easier with fewer complications, may be used as an alternative to lumbar plexus block with the intention of blocking the nerves more distally. However, both of these nerve blocks do not cover the sciatic innervation of the joint, do not reliably cover the obturator nerve and may provide less effective pain control than lumbar epidural analgesia.

The use of continuous lumbar epidural anesthesia for postoperative pain control has proven to be an effective choice, however, it is challenged by the widespread use of chemical thromboprophylaxis. Most importantly, postoperative lumbar epidural analgesia interferes with early mobilization.

References

1. Miller RD, et al. Miller's anesthesia, 7th ed. Churchill Livingstone: p 1034–5; 2009 (1172).
2. Horlocker TT, et al. Regional anesthesia in the patient receiving antithrombotic or thrombolytic therapy: American Society of regional anesthesia and pain medicine evidence-based guidelines, Vol. 35(Issue 1). 3rd ed. Regional Anesthesia and Pain Medicine; 2010. p 64–101.
3. Gandhi K, Viscusi E. Multimodal pain management techniques in knee and hip arthroplasty. J N Y Sch Reg Anesthesia. 2009;13: 1–10.
4. Southwell-Keely JP, Russo RR, March L, et al. Antibiotic prophylaxis in hip fracture surgery: a metaanalysis. Clin Orthop Relat Res. 2004;179.
5. Cheney FW, Domino KB, Caplan RA, Posner KL. Nerve injury associated with anesthesia: a closed claims analysis. Anesthesiology. 1999;90:1062–9.
6. Mauermann WJ, Shilling AM, Zuo Z. A comparison of neuraxial block versus general anesthesia for elective total hip replacement: a meta-analysis. Anesth Analg. 2006;103:1018–25.
7. Jashvant Poeran, Rehana Rasul, Suzuko Suzuki, Thomas Danninger, Madhu Mazumdar, Mathias Opperer, et al. Tranexamic acid use and postoperative outcomes in patients undergoing total hip or knee arthroplasty in the United States: retrospective analysis of effectiveness and safety. BMJ. 2014;349:g4829.
8. Huang F, Wu D, Ma G, Yin Z, Wang Q. The use of tranexamic acid to reduce blood loss and transfusion in major orthopedic surgery: a meta-analysis. J Surg Res. 2014;186:318–27.
9. Thompson GE, et al. Hypotensive anesthesia for total hip arthroplasty: a study of blood loss and organ function (brain, heart, liver, and kidney). Anesthesiology. 1978;48(2):91–6.
10. Bennett J, Haynes S, Torella F, Grainger H, McCollum C. Acute normovolemic hemodilution in moderate blood loss surgery: a randomized controlled trial. Transfusion. 2006;46(7):1097.

Local Anesthetics

45

Cyrus A. Yazdi

Case A 65-year-old 280 lbs woman is brought to the operating room for open reduction and internal fixation of right displaced radial fracture. She presents to the ER with a closed distal radius fracture and the orthopedic surgeon is unable to reduce the fracture under sedation.

History of Present illness: The patient suffers from a long-standing, severe osteoarthritis and has fallen the previous day in her kitchen while cooking. She is complaining of right wrist pain and paresthesia. She does not remember what exactly has happened. Her son has found her on the floor and brought her to ER.

Medication: Diltiazem, furosemide, Naproxen, Aspirin, and Tylenol PRN.
Past Medical History:
Hypertension since age 33.
Old MI 5 years ago without subsequent symptoms.
Obesity
Past Surgical History:
Tonsillectomy and Adenoidectomy in Childhood
Removal of Gallbladder when she was 40
Foot surgery for fracture 10 years ago, reportedly "under local anesthesia"—record unavailable.
Allergies: Latex causes rash and itching
Physical Exam: P 100, BP 165/70 mmHg, R 25, T 36.7 °C
Alert and Oriented. Anxious appearing obese lady in pain
Airway: restricted mouth opening, full dentition, unable to visualized base of uvula.
Lungs: reduced breath sounds bilaterally. Heart: regular rate and rhythm.
Mild peripheral edema.
CXR: LV concentric hypertrophy.
ECG: NSR, Q waves—lead II, III, AVF; nonspecific ST-T wave changes.
LABS:
Blood sugar 180 mg/dL; Hgb 12.0 gm/dL; SpO2 (room air) 91%.
The patient has a 18 gauge peripheral IV catheter.

1. **What are the possible benefits of regional anesthesia in this patient?**

Regional anesthesia could be used as the primary mode of anesthesia to avoid airway manipulation; potential risks of general anesthesia such as airway trauma, respiratory complications, nausea, and vomiting and DVT could be avoided. Regional anesthesia can provide better postoperative analgesia when compared with intravenous opioids; it can also contribute to faster postoperative recovery and can facilitate rehabilitation by providing pain control and increased passive joint mobility.

Other benefits include increased patient satisfaction, increased patient responsiveness, reduction of delirium and better pain control, especially in chronic pain patients. There is some evidence that it can reduce hospital cost by shortening of the postoperative hospital stay [1].

2. **What are the contraindications for regional anesthesia?**

Absolute:

- Patient refusal
- Allergy to local anesthetics
  - Amide allergies are usually due to the methylparaben used as a preservative in the multiple dose vials.
  - Ester local anesthetics are associated with a higher incidence of allergic reactions due to one of their metabolites, para-aminobenzoic acid (PABA).

C.A. Yazdi (✉)
Department of Anesthesiology/Pain Medicine, Umass Memorial Medical Center, 119 Belmont St, Worcester, MA 01605, USA
e-mail: yazdic@gmail.com

© Springer International Publishing AG 2017
L.S. Aglio and R.D. Urman (eds.), *Anesthesiology*,
DOI 10.1007/978-3-319-50141-3_45

Relative:

- Local site infection—alternative distant site for blocking the relevant nerves may be chosen.
- Bleeding: Restrictions, identical to those for neuraxial techniques, are observed for anticoagulated patients with noncompressible vasculature near the nerve block site [2].
- Preexisting nerve injury: There is no evidence that properly conducted regional anesthesia can worsen preexisting neuropathy. However, the ability to elicit paresthesias or electrical nerve stimulation, may both be altered unpredictably. This would logically compromise nerve localization by these methods, including their potential for detection of intraneural needle placement and injection. Also, there is a hypothetical concern about possible "double-crush" complication compounding, i.e., combining preexisting injury with chemical neurotoxicity or mechanical trauma, especially when the block location and the area of the preexisting injury are anatomically close.
- Perioperative neurological examination: If immediate and/or serial postoperative neurological assessments are required, regional anesthesia should be avoided; alternatively, a nerve block with short-acting local anesthetics can be considered [3].
- High suspicion and predilection for acute compartment syndrome—need for neurovascular monitoring. The role of regional anesthesia in such situation is controversial and still debated.

3. **What are the possible complications of regional anesthesia?**

- Local anesthetic systemic toxicity (LAST) due to accidental intravascular injection, rapid/accelerated absorption or abnormal threshold/sensitivity. Frequent aspiration and using ultrasound technique reduces the rate of intravascular injections. Patients need to be monitored during and for at least 30 min after performing regional anesthesia for signs and symptoms of systemic local anesthetic toxicity.
  - Local anesthetics toxicity should be considered in any patients with any neurological symptoms or cardiovascular instability.
  - CNS signs include: excitatory (confusion, agitation, muscle twitching and seizures), depressive (sleepiness, obtundation and coma) or nonspecific—metallic-like taste, tinnitus or dizziness.
  - Cardiovascular signs include: initially, hyperdynamic states with hypertension and tachycardia, followed by hypotension, conduction block, ventricular arrhythmias, and asystole [4].
- Peripheral nerve injury (PNI): The traditional mechanisms of PNI have been described in animal models as mechanical, injection-related, ischemic, and/or neurotoxic. Forceful needle-to-nerve contact and/or injection into the nerve are believed to set in motion a series of events that might lead to ischemia or neurotoxicity. Needle trauma to or rupture of the perineurium is believed to disrupt the fascicle's protective environment, which then becomes a crucial contributory factor in determining the likelihood and severity of subsequent PNI. Direct application of (otherwise innocuous) local anesthetic to denuded axons can cause acute inflammatory reactions or neurotoxicity. Such insults are magnified in the setting of a disrupted perineurium and prolonged exposure to the local anesthetic (as might occur with vasoconstrictive adjuvants, which reduce drug clearance or cause ischemia). If the needle does not completely disrupt the perineurium, injection can transiently elevate intraneural pressure and lead to ischemia. Bleeding around the nerve or microhematoma within the nerve can also lead to ischemia. Finally, nonspecific inflammatory responses can affect single or multiple nerves and at sites close to or distant from the surgical site. Such inflammatory changes have been observed during surgical nerve bypass procedures for permanent phrenic nerve injuries associated with interscalene block. The incidence of PNI has remained stable in recent decades, despite the introduction of ultrasound guidance. The reported rate of long-term injury is in the 2–4 per 10,000 blocks range. Risk of peripheral nerve injury depends on surgical, anesthetic, and patient related factors, and sometimes, it is very hard to pinpoint the exact cause of nerve injury. Axillary or musculocutaneous nerve injuries are more likely after shoulder surgery. Postoperative ulnar neuropathy persists in up to 10% of elbow replacement patients. The frequency of nerve injury after total hip arthroplasty (THA) varies widely but generally falls in the 1% range. The common peroneal nerve is most frequently injured during THA (0.08–3.7%). Injuries to the femoral and superior gluteal nerves occur less often. Most of the nerve injuries will recover without any intervention within 3–6 months. Neurology consultation is recommended if persistent sensory or motor deficits are encountered [5].
- Vascular puncture: hematoma.

4. **What monitors and equipment are required to perform regional anesthesia safely?**

Standard monitors, including EKG, blood pressure and pulse oximetry, and appropriate resuscitation equipment (oxygen, suction catheter, bag-mask, and emergency intubation equipment) are critical when performing regional anesthesia. Also, immediate access to an emergency response cart and lipid emulsion is strongly recommended.

5. **What type of regional anesthesia will you choose for this patient? Would you do interscalene brachial plexus block? Could you list the complications that might happen after this block?**

Interscalene brachial plexus block can often miss C8 and T1 root distribution (the entire ulnar nerve, but also the entire medial antebrachial cutaneous and medial brachial cutaneous nerves, and parts of the radial and median nerves) so for this patient with distal radius fracture, a more distal technique, such as axillary brachial plexus block is more appropriate.

Complications of interscalene brachial plexus block include:

- Phrenic nerve paralysis in nearly 100%—occurs as phrenic nerve runs just anterior to the anterior scalene muscle.
- Hoarseness, due to recurrent laryngeal nerve block.
- Horner's syndrome with upside-down ptosis, anhidrosis, nasal stuffiness, miosis and enophthalmus due to spread of local anesthetic to the cervical sympathetic chain [6] and very rarely.
- Pneumothorax by direct needle injury to the pleura.
- Spinal or epidural block by injecting directly or channeling into an intervertebral foramen or epidural space.
- Injury or injection into the vertebral artery.

Axillary block The brachial plexus finally evolves into the peripheral nerves of the upper extremity once it exits from under the lateral border of the pectoralis minor muscle. The radial, median, and ulnar nerves surround the axillary artery, with the musculocutaneous nerve located between the bellies of the biceps and coracobrachialis muscles.

The axillary block is a good choice for patients having surgery distal to the elbow. This technique requires the patient to be placed supine with the ipsilateral arm abducted 90° at the shoulder. The forearm is often flexed at the elbow such that the hand is almost behind the patient's head.

The axillary approach to the brachial plexus was developed primarily as a means to provide anesthesia to the forearm and hand, while avoiding the risk of pneumothorax and phrenic nerve block. The drawback, however, is that the musculocutaneous nerve can be missed and that placement of the block requires several needle passes, which has shown to reduce patient satisfaction. Ultrasound guidance has made identifying and blocking the musculocutaneous nerve relatively easy.

When compared with the supraclavicular approach, the axillary block is considered by many to require more time and more needle passes, with decreased fidelity and the higher likelihood of needing a "rescue block" distal to the elbow. This may arguably contribute to a decrease in patient satisfaction. However, the axillary block is still practiced widely and offers a safe alternative for patients in whom supraclavicular or infraclavicular block is not a viable option [6].

6. **Most commonly used local anesthetics—basic pharmacology**

All local anesthetics consist of three components:

1. Aromatic benzene ring
2. Tertiary amine
3. Intermediate hydrocarbon linkage

The amino esters are hydrolyzed in the plasma by cholinesterase enzyme, whereas the amino amide compounds undergo enzymatic biotransformation in the liver.

Potency, duration of the block and onset of action
Local anesthetics inhibit electrical conduction of nerves by blocking the voltage-gated sodium channels within the nodes of Ranvier. To reach these targets, local anesthetics must cross the lipid bilayer of the nerve sheath. Local anesthetic molecules, which are highly lipophilic, easily penetrate nerve cell membranes and become intracellular, resulting in channel blockade. Graphs of the potency of local anesthetics against the oil/water partition coefficients demonstrate a clear correlation between potency and lipid solubility [7].

The protein binding capacity of a local anesthetic correlates with the duration of block. Protein binding is also related to lipid solubility. In general, agents with greater protein binding have a greater affinity for receptor sites and attach to sodium channels for a longer period of time. This means that agents with higher protein binding capacity are associated with a longer duration of action.

A major determinant of local anesthetic onset is pKa. The pKa of a local anesthetic molecule is the pH at which 50% of the agent exists in its ionized and 50% is in its non-ionized form. The pKa determines the agent's onset of action. The onset is related to the concentration of the local anesthetic molecules present in the non-ionized form, which is associated with penetration of the nerve cell membrane. The pKa of most local anesthetic agents is higher than physiologic (7.7–9.0) [8].

Based on their chemical structure, local anesthetics are classified into two major groups: esters and amides. Commonly used (amino) ester local anesthetics include benzocaine, 2-chloroprocaine, cocaine, procaine, and tetracaine. Since ester links are more easily broken, these drugs are unstable in solution. Commonly used (amino) amide local anesthetics include bupivacaine, etidocaine, levobupivacaine, lidocaine, mepivacaine, prilocaine, and ropivacaine. Amide solutions are very stable and can be autoclaved [9].

Commonly used (amino)ester local anesthetics are:

1. **Procaine** (fast onset, very short duration)

Procaine was the first synthetic local anesthetic agent introduced into clinical practice. It is a relatively weak local anesthetic with a short duration of action. It has low systemic toxicity because of rapid plasma hydrolysis. Procaine is hydrolyzed to p-aminobenzoic acid, which is responsible for the allergic reactions associated with repeated use of procaine. Procaine is used primarily for infiltration anesthesia, diagnostic differential spinal blocks in certain pain states, and obstetric spinal anesthesia.

2. **Chloroprocaine** (fast onset, very short duration)

Chloroprocaine has short onset and short duration of action, as well as low systemic toxicity. It undergoes hydrolysis by human plasma esterases approximately 4 times faster than procaine. Chloroprocaine is primarily employed for epidural analgesia and anesthesia in obstetrics because of its rapid onset and low systemic toxicity in the mother and fetus. However, frequent injections are required to provide adequate pain relief during labor. Sometimes, epidural analgesia is established in the pregnant patient with Chloroprocaine, followed by a longer-acting agent such as bupivacaine. Chloroprocaine has also proved of value for various regional anesthetic procedures in ambulatory surgical patients for whom surgery is not expected to exceed 30–60 min and no lasting analgesia is desired. Concerns about potential myotoxicity and neurotoxicity have limited chloroprocaine use, but for a recent resurgence of use for spinal anesthesia in ambulatory patients.

3. **Tetracaine** (slow onset, long duration)

Tetracaine has been used primarily for spinal anesthesia. It may be employed as an isobaric, hypobaric, or hyperbaric solution for spinal blockade, although hyperbaric solutions of tetracaine are probably used most often. Tetracaine provides a relatively rapid onset of spinal anesthesia, adequate sensory anesthesia and profound block of the motor function. Plain solutions of tetracaine produce an average duration of spinal anesthesia of 2–3 h, whereas the addition of epinephrine can extend anesthesia to 4–6 h. Tetracaine is rarely used for other forms of regional anesthesia because of its extremely slow onset of action and the potential for systemic toxic reactions when larger doses are employed. It is no longer available in the USA.

4. **Benzocaine**

This local anesthetic is used exclusively for topical anesthesia. Benzocaine is available in a variety of proprietary and nonproprietary preparations. The most common forms used in an operating room setting are aerosol solutions for oropharynx and larynx, and ointments for oral/gingival application and lubrication of endotracheal tubes. One should remember that benzocaine can also cause methemoglobinemia [9].

5. **Cocaine**

Cocaine was the first agent successfully employed clinically to produce local and regional anesthesia. It has limited use in modern anesthesia practice because of its relatively high potential for systemic toxicity and addiction liabilities. It is listed as a schedule II drug in the United States. Cocaine is an excellent topical anesthetic agent, and it produces vasoconstriction at clinically useful concentrations. As a result, it is still sometimes employed to anesthetize and constrict the nasal mucosa before nasotracheal intubation, and otolaryngologists sometimes use cocaine during nasal surgery because of its vasoconstrictor and topical anesthetic properties. It is the only local anesthetic that inhibits the reuptake of catecholamines in the central and peripheral nervous systems.

Commonly used (amino)amide local anesthetics are:

1. **Lidocaine** (fast onset, short to intermediate duration)

Lidocaine remains the most versatile and most frequently used drug in this category. It is popular because of its inherent potency, rapid onset, moderate duration of action, topical anesthetic activity and relatively low toxicity. Available and commonly used concentrations are 1.0–2% for regional (conduction) anesthesia and 0.5% for intravenous regional anesthesia (Bier block). Lidocaine is ideal for painful/surgical procedures of less than two-hour duration. However, these properties are also its main weakness. It is not the best option for long procedures or for postoperative pain control. Typically, 2% lidocaine is the concentration selected for profound short duration surgical anesthesia. In addition, lidocaine is still used for short duration spinal anesthesia, but is associated with high incidence of transient neurologic symptoms. Lidocaine is also used in ointment, jelly, viscous, and aerosol preparations for a variety of topical anesthetic procedures. Lidocaine is currently the only agent officially approved in the United States for IV regional anesthesia.

Lidocaine is administered intravenously as an analgesic for certain chronic pain states, as an antiarrhythmic, and as a supplement to general anesthesia, but is rarely employed as an antiepileptic agent in very low doses (dose-dependent effect).

2. **Mepivacaine** (fast onset, intermediate duration)

Mepivacaine structure is very similar to that of lidocaine. Mepivacaine onset is similar to lidocaine; however, its duration of action is longer. Mepivacaine may be used for infiltration, peripheral nerve blocks and epidural anesthesia, and in some countries, 4–5% hyperbaric solutions of mepivacaine are also available for spinal anesthesia. The most commonly available concentrations are 1%–1.5%–2%—a good choice for surgical procedures, when two to three hours of block duration is needed, but quick postoperative return of limb function is necessary and severe postoperative pain is not anticipated.

Unfortunately, mepivacaine is not an effective topical anesthetic agent. Although toxicity appears to be similar to lidocaine, the metabolism of mepivacaine is prolonged in fetus and newborn, and as a result, mepivacaine is not used for obstetric anesthesia. Mepivacaine has less vasodilator property than lidocaine; this seems to be particularly useful for brachial plexus blocks when large volumes of local anesthetics are administered.

3. **Bupivacaine** (slow onset, long duration)

Bupivacaine is a popular, generic and low-price local anesthetic, available as a racemic mixture of its two enantiomers. It remains an appropriate choice for peripheral nerve blocks placed for postoperative pain control or surgical anesthesia for procedures that are expected to be longer than several hours. It is available in concentrations of 0.25–0.5% (0.75% is also available, but recommended for spinal anesthesia only), and it has a slow onset and long duration of action. Its duration of action is significantly enhanced by the addition of epinephrine and can be up to 24 h and longer for peripheral nerve blocks, with appropriate volumes and placement. Higher volumes and concentrations of bupivacaine may cause a profound block that can be used as a surgical anesthetic if given enough time for achieving full effect. Typically, 0.5% bupivacaine is used for surgical anesthesia, while 0.0625–0.25% for continuous catheter infusion; 0.25–0.5% bupivacaine single-shot injections are employed for postoperative pain control, with the lower concentration spectrum providing some motor function sparing.

4. **Ropivacaine** (slow onset, long duration)

Ropivacaine is very close in chemical structure to bupivacaine and exhibits similar properties; it is available in its S-enantiomer only. Potential advantages of ropivacaine when compared to bupivacaine include lower cardiotoxicity and slightly lower potency (with slightly less motor block for equianalgesic doses), as well as mild vasoconstrictive properties. It is a good and widely preferred choice for nerve blocks where high volumes/doses are necessary and significant absorption is expected.

5. **Levobupivacaine** (slow onset, long duration)

The clinical profile of levobupivacaine, the S-enantiomer of bupivacaine, is essentially the same as the profile of racemic bupivacaine except for its wider therapeutic index for cardiac toxicity and systemic toxicity. Not currently available in the USA, levobupivacaine is used increasingly in Europe.

6. **Prilocaine**

The clinical profile of prilocaine is similar to that of lidocaine. Prilocaine has a relatively rapid onset of action while providing a moderate duration of anesthesia and a profound depth of conduction blockade. Because this agent causes significantly less vasodilatation than lidocaine, it can be used without epinephrine.

Prilocaine biotransformation produces aminophenols that oxidize hemoglobin to methemoglobin thus limiting its clinical use. The primary use of prilocaine is in EMLA cream, a eutectic mixture of prilocaine and lidocaine for topical application.

7. **Etidocaine**

Etidocaine is characterized by very rapid onset and prolonged duration of action. It has a significantly quicker onset of action than bupivacaine. Concentrations of etidocaine required for adequate sensory anesthesia produce more profound motor blockade. As a result, etidocaine is primarily useful as an anesthetic for surgical procedures in which muscle relaxation is required. Consequently, this agent is of limited use for obstetric epidural analgesia and postoperative pain relief, as it does not provide a differential blockade favoring sensory over motor fibers. The drug was used infrequently in North America and was subsequently discontinued.

8. **Dibucaine**

Dibucaine is only available for topical anesthesia in the United States. It is more potent than tetracaine, although the onset of action of the two agents is similar. The duration of spinal anesthesia is slightly longer with dibucaine. The degree of hypotension and depth of motor blockade appear to be less with intrathecal dibucaine than with intrathecal tetracaine, although the spread of sensory anesthesia is similar in the two groups.

7. **What factors contribute to local anesthetics plasma levels?**

- **Site of Injection**: Absorption is dependent on the blood supply at the site of the block. Highly vascular areas are the higher risk of systemic absorption.
  From Fastest systemic absorption to the slowest: Intravenous > Intercostal > Caudal, Epidural > Lumbar Epidural > Brachial plexus > Subcutaneous
- **Dose of Local Anesthetics**: Risk of toxicity increases with higher concentrations and doses of the local anesthetic agent (See Table 1).
- **Choice of Local Anesthetic**: high tissue binding (prilocaine) and high protein binding capacity (bupivacaine) or large volume of distribution may result in lower measurable plasma levels, but not predictably diminish systemic toxicity.
- **Metabolism**: Amide local anesthetics are metabolized in the liver and esters are degraded by plasma esterases.
- **Adding Epinephrine** reduces the local anesthetic plasma levels and also increases the time to achieve the peak plasma concentrations [10].

8. **Are you going to add any other medication to your local anesthetics mix?**

Epinephrine is probably one of the most commonly used local anesthetic additives in peripheral nerve blocks. It is typically added in proportions of 1:200,000 to 1:400,000 parts per solution (5–2.5 μg/mL). It reduces the local anesthetic absorption by causing vasoconstriction at the site of injection, thus prolonging the duration of regional blocks when added to the local anesthetic solutions. Epinephrine should be avoided in distal extremity blocks, as it is a potent vasoconstrictor. Also, if injected intravascularly, it can cause systemic hypertension and tachycardia, so it should be used with caution in patients with cardiac disease. However, it has been traditionally added to local anesthetic solutions as an indicator for intravascular injection because of these very properties [10].

Alkalization of local anesthetic solutions by the addition of sodium bicarbonate has also been practiced and reported to decrease the onset of conduction blockade. An increase in the pH of the local anesthetic solution increases the amount of drug in the uncharged base form, which should enhance the rate of diffusion across the nerve sheath and nerve membranes [11].

Clonidine is an α2-agonist that has been shown to prolong peripheral nerve block duration when used in doses between 10 and 150 μg. Dexmedetomidine is a newer, more specific α2-agonist that is showing promise as a local anesthetic adjunct, also increasing block duration. Dexamethasone in doses from 1 to 4 mg has been used as adjunct to

Table 1 Maximum dose and duration of action of commonly used local anesthetic agents

Agents	Maximum dose (mg/kg)	Duration of effects (hours)
Esters		
2-chloroprocaine	12	0.5–1
Procaine	12	0.5–1
Cocaine	3	0.5–1
Tetracaine	3	1.5–6
Amides		
Lidocaine	4.5 (7*)	0.75–1.5
Mepivacaine	4.5 (7*)	1–2
Prilocaine	8	0.5–1
Bupivacaine	2–2.5 (3*)	1.5–8
Ropivacaine	3	1.5–8

*Maximum if mixed with Epinephrine [10]

local anesthetics for peripheral nerve blocks—its block enhancing effects; its optimal doses and safety are still debated.

Different opioids have also been added to peripheral nerve blocks for their presumed synergistic effects; however, only buprenorphine has been shown to increase the duration, onset, and quality of the block.

9. **What are Transient Neurologic Symptoms (TNS) after spinal anesthesia? Are there any risk factors for developing TNS? What would you advise patient with similar complaints?**

Transient Neurologic Symptoms (TNS) define a syndrome consisting of variable pain and paresthesias mainly in the buttocks that radiate to the legs and are self-limited, resolving in several days to one week. TNS is much more common after spinal anesthesia with hyperbaric lidocaine, especially in higher doses. Bupivacaine is four times less likely to cause TNS than lidocaine.

Possible causes of TNS include specific local anesthetic toxicity, needle trauma, neural ischemia, secondary to sciatic stretching, patient positioning, pooling of local anesthetics secondary to small gauge pencil-point needles and hyperbaric solutions, deep muscle spasms, myofascial pain, early mobilization, and irritation of the dorsal root ganglion [12].

Risk factors, including lidocaine spinal anesthesia, lithotomy position and ambulatory surgical status, have all been determined to be important predictors for the development of TNS. Additional factors that may contribute to TNS incidence are arthroscopic knee surgery and obesity. None of the patients with TNS should have abnormal neurologic exams or motor weakness. Therefore, if a patient presents with sensory or motor deficits, other possible etiologies, necessitating emergent intervention, such as epidural hematoma, neuraxial infection or nerve root damage, must be considered and excluded first. Often, imaging studies such as spine CT with contrast and/or MRI are needed to complement diagnostically a very thorough neurological exam.

Current therapeutic options include nonsteroidal anti-inflammatory drugs (NSAIDs), opioids, muscle relaxants and other symptomatic therapy. Patients generally report good pain relief with NSAIDS. If patients do not respond to these therapies, treatment with oral opioids, muscle relaxants, physical therapy, or transcutaneous electrical nerve stimulation (TENS) may be added. For the patient willing to return to the hospital because of intense and disabling discomfort, trigger point injections may be performed. Most of the symptoms are self-limiting and resolve in 1–4 days [13].

10. **What are the signs and symptoms of local anesthetics systemic toxicity (LAST)?**

To produce local and regional anesthesia, local anesthetics inhibit voltage-gated sodium channels in the axons of peripheral nerves and decrease action potential conduction velocity. These agents can block potassium and calcium channels as well. LAST occurs usually as a result of inadvertent intravascular injection and rarely follows injection of an excessive amount of local anesthetic into an appropriate site.

Central Nervous System Initially, the patient might report some nonspecific signs like circumoral paresthesias, metallic taste in mouth, dizziness, and lightheadedness. These symptoms are followed by auditory and visual changes like tinnitus, diplopia, and nystagmus. Anxiety and sense of “impending doom” have been reported. As the plasma levels increase, agitation, muscle twitches, confusion progress to tonic-clonic seizures and could be followed by EEG activity slow down as patient loses consciousness and becomes comatose. In the concomitant presence of other CNS depressant drugs (e.g., premedication), CNS depression can develop without the preceding excitatory phase. The potency of local anesthetics is directly related to CNS toxicity.

Cardiovascular Local anesthetic cardiotoxicity can initially present with and evolve into life-threatening conduction delay (PR interval prolongation to complete heart block, sinus arrest and asystole) and ventricular dysrhythmias (from simple ventricular ectopy to torsades de pointes and fibrillation). The negative inotropic effect of local anesthetics is dose dependent and consists of myocardial contractility depression and a resulting decrease in cardiac output. Dysrhythmias, due to local anesthetic overdose may be recalcitrant to traditional therapies; the reduced myocardial contractility and low output state further complicate the treatment.

The sequence of cardiovascular events is usually as follows: lower level of local anesthetics usually causes a small increase in cardiac output, heart rate and blood pressure because of increase in sympathetic activity and increase in systemic vascular resistance. As the plasma levels increase, hypotension ensues as a result of peripheral vasodilation and reduction in systemic vascular resistance and/or malignant and refractory arrhythmias. These may eventually progress to a cardiac arrest.

Plasma and tissue pH play an important role in the setting of local anesthetics toxicity. Hypercarbia increases cerebral blood flow and as a result may worsen CNS toxicity.

Diffusion of carbon dioxide across the cell membrane also worsens the intracellular acidosis. Intracellular acidosis converts the local anesthetics to cationic or active form. Because cationic form cannot travel through cell membranes, ionic trapping occurs, worsening further CNS toxicity [14].

11. **Is there any way that you could prevent LAST?**

Prevention of toxicity is the key to safe practice and it starts with making sure that the work environment is optimized for performing regional anesthesia. Monitoring, vigilance, and trained personnel availability are critical (simulation training is strongly recommended). Emergency resuscitation equipment must be functioning and readily available to be immediately deployed in case of local anesthetics toxicity including cardiac arrest.

A judicious selection of the type, dose, and concentration of the local anesthetic, and the choice and safe practice of regional anesthesia techniques are critical. Pretreatment with benzodiazepines is commonly used, but their effects are often debated. Benzodiazepines raise the seizure threshold and can mask early signs of CNS toxicity. A heavily sedated patient is not able to reliably communicate to the physician initial signs and symptoms of LAST.

The presence of premedication or general anesthesia is not perceived to increase the risk of local anesthetic toxicity, but may delay or deny early diagnosis. Considerable research has been dedicated to the subject of the ideal test for detecting intravenous injection and to what constitutes an ideal test dose. Epinephrine (5–15 μg) is still widely in use as a marker of intravascular injection. An increase in heart rate >10 bpm, increase in systolic blood pressure by >15 mm Hg, or a 25% decrease in lead II T-wave amplitude signify a positive test dose. However this test is not reliable in elderly, in patients on beta-blockers or with low cardiac output.

Regardless of whether epinephrine is used as a marker of an intravascular injection, it is of utmost importance to use slow, incremental injections of local anesthetic, with frequent aspirations (every 3–5 mL) between injections while monitoring the patient for signs of toxicity. A slow rate of injection of divided doses at distinct intervals can decrease the possibility of summating inadvertent intravascular injections. With a rapid injection, the seizures may occur at higher blood level because there is no time for distribution of the drug as compared to a slow infusion where the seizure occurs at a lower drug level because of the distribution [14].

12. **Is pregnancy associated with higher risk of local anesthetics toxicity? Why?**

Yes, plasma concentrations of alpha 1-acid glycoprotein (AAG) are decreased in pregnant women. This effectively increases the free fraction of bupivacaine in plasma, and it might be responsible for the bupivacaine toxicity and the number of cardiac arrests that have been reported with inadvertent overdoses with bupivacaine in pregnant women. However, with intermediate duration LAs (e.g., lidocaine and mepivacaine), smaller changes in protein binding occur during pregnancy, and the use of these LAs is not associated with an increased risk of cardiac toxicity during pregnancy [15].

13. **More about allergic reaction to local anesthetics?**

The amino esters, such as chloroprocaine, are all derivatives of the Paraaminobenzoic acid (PABA). Accordingly, the local anesthetics belonging to the ester group may cause positive skin reactions, ranging from toxic eruptions in situ to generalized rash or urticaria. True allergic reactions to the local anesthetics of the amino amide group are extremely rare. By and large, preparations of amide anesthetics do not cause allergic reactions, unless they contain the preservative methylparaben, which is in its chemical structure virtually the same as PABA. For patients who report an allergy to amino amides, one may be able to safely use a preservative-free amide anesthetic unless a well-documented allergy reports point to an unambiguous allergy. Anaphylaxis due to local anesthetics remains a rare event, even within the ester group. It should be considered if the patient starts wheezing or develops respiratory distress instantly following injection.

Management of local anesthetic triggered allergic reactions is very similar to the treatment algorithms for other more common allergic reactions. Intravenous lidocaine can result in paradoxical airway narrowing and bronchospasm in patients with asthma. The mechanism of this reaction is not well understood.

Some patients may react to preservatives, such as methylparaben, included with LAs. In the allergy and immunology literature, several recent studies have shown that patients referred for evaluation of apparent LA allergy, even after exhibiting signs or symptoms of anaphylaxis, almost never demonstrate true allergy to the LA that was administered.

A unique side effect of some local anesthetics is methemoglobinemia. It has been associated with the topical, epidural, and intravenous administration of prilocaine. Prilocaine is the local anesthetic for which there appears to be greatest risk for this to occur. A dose–response relationship exists between the amount of prilocaine administered and the degree of methemoglobinemia. In general, doses of prilocaine of 600 mg are required for the development of clinically significant levels of methemoglobinemia in an adult. The formation of methemoglobin is believed to be related to prilocaine's chemical structure. The metabolism of prilocaine in the liver results in the formation of O-toluidine, which is responsible for the oxidation of hemoglobin to methemoglobin. The methemoglobinemia caused by prilocaine is self-limiting and reversible. Reversal can be accelerated with the administration of methylene blue intravenously (1 mg/kg) [16].

14. **How do you manage LAST?**

Early recognition and early discontinuation of the administration is of crucial importance. The administration of local anesthetics should be stopped immediately. The airway should be maintained at all times, and supplemental oxygen should be provided while ensuring that the monitoring equipment is functional and properly applied. Neurologic parameters and cardiovascular status should be assessed until the patient is completely asymptomatic and stable [17].

Administration of a benzodiazepine to offset or ameliorate excitatory neurological symptoms or a potential tonic-clonic seizure is indicated. Early treatment of convulsions is particularly meaningful because convulsions can result in respiratory and metabolic acidosis, thus aggravating the toxicity. Anti-seizure treatment consists of halting the seizure by administering a benzodiazepine (midazolam 0.05–0.1 mg/kg) or a small dose of propofol (0.5–1.0 mg/kg) while preventing the detrimental effects of hypoxia and hypercarbia by ventilating with 100% oxygen [18].

In case reports and animal studies, lipids have been shown to increase the success rate of resuscitation from LAST. Intralipid® is a 20% lipid emulsion solution most commonly used as part of total parenteral nutrition. It contains soybean oil, glycerol, and egg phospholipids. It is theorized that these lipids act as a "sink" that binds lipid-soluble local anesthetics, reducing their free fraction and decreasing availability in the myocardium and other critical sites. Lipid therapy should be implemented based on the severity and rate of progression of toxicity. Early use during prolonged seizures may prevent cardiac toxicity [19, 20].

The recommended bolus dose is 1.5 mL/kg IV (lean body mass) followed by an infusion of 0.25 mL/kg/min. If cardiovascular instability persists, the bolus may be repeated up to two more times and the infusion rate may be doubled. The infusion should be continued for a minimum of 10 min after a perfusing rhythm is restored [21]. Refractory arrhythmias and asystole are managed using slightly modified standard cardiopulmonary resuscitation protocols—recommended epinephrine dose is significantly reduced and vasopressin administration is advised against. Acknowledging that a prolonged effort may be needed to increase the chance of survival, the nearest cardiopulmonary bypass capable facility should be alerted and arrangements made. The rationale of this approach is to maintain the circulation until the local anesthetic is redistributed or metabolized below the level associated with cardiovascular toxicity, at which time spontaneous circulation should resume. Because the contractile depression is a core factor underlying severe cardiotoxicity, it would be intuitive to believe that the use of sympathomimetics should be helpful. However, epinephrine can induce dysrhythmias or exacerbate the ongoing arrhythmia associated with local anesthetic toxicity. Consequently, significantly reduced epinephrine doses are recommended during LAST resuscitation. In ACLS protocols not related to local anesthetic toxicity, vasopressin may be appropriate to maintain the blood pressure, support coronary perfusion, and facilitate local anesthetic metabolism [22]. However, the ASRA Practice Advisory [21] recommends against the use of vasopressin in LAST. The current advanced cardiac life support algorithm emphasizes amiodarone as the mainstay drug for treatment of arrhythmias. Also, for ventricular arrhythmias prompted by local anesthetic overdose, current data favor amiodarone as drug of choice [23]. The use of bretylium is no longer endorsed. Occurrence of Torsades des Pointes with bupivacaine toxicity may require overdrive pacing if that rhythm predominates [24, 25].

Recovery from local anesthetic–induced cardiac arrest can take enduring resuscitation efforts for more than an hour. Propofol is a direct cardiodepressant and is not an adequate alternative to treatment with intralipid, although judicious administration to control seizures in small divided doses may be appropriate. Because Lipid Rescue is still an innovative therapy, future laboratory work and clinical experience are needed for a better understanding of the mechanisms and a further refinement of the treatment protocols.

The following are some recommendations for the management of local anesthetic toxicity and other adverse reactions:

- Bronchospasm and generalized edema, sometimes associated with allergic reactions, may require use of bronchodilators, antihistamines, and corticosteroids.
- Avoiding hypoxia and hypercarbia; airway management and tracheal intubation decision should be individualized.

- Chest compressions and defibrillation may be required to restore organ perfusion and should be instituted based on patient hemodynamics.
- Lipid emulsion intravenous therapy can be lifesaving in LAST and should be administered as soon as possible. Lipid emulsion should be available in locations where local anesthetics are used in potentially toxic doses.
- Seizures should be controlled with benzodiazepines (e.g., midazolam 0.05–0.1 mg/kg), but Propofol (0.5–1.5 mg/kg) can also be used
- Severe hypotension can occur in both allergic reactions and systemic toxicity and usually responds well to vasopressors (e.g., epinephrine) and volume expanders. However, very small doses of epinephrine are recommended in LAST (<1 mcg/kg).
- Epinephrine can exacerbate malignant dysrhythmias, occurring with bupivacaine toxicity. Same is reported experimentally with vasopressin. Therapeutic agents that are less arrhythmogenic have been investigated, including phosphodiesterase inhibitors such as milrinone and amrinone, though their use still needs to be validated clinically in LAST.
- In addition to lipid treatment, ventricular arrhythmias should be suppressed primarily with amiodarone 300 mg IV, with repeat administration of up to 150 mg 3–5 min later.
- Effective resuscitation in this setting is difficult, and atrioventricular pacing and cardiopulmonary bypass are additional options in refractory cases [26].

References

1. Barash MD, Paul G, Bruce F, Cullen MD, Robert K, Stoelting MD. editors. Clinical anesthesia. 5th ed. Philadelphia: Lippincott Williams & Wilkins; 2006, p. 718–45, 1118–26.
2. Horlocker TT, Wedel DJ, Rowlingson JC, Enneking FK, Kopp SL, Benzon HT, Brown DL, Heit JA, Mulroy MF, Rosenquist RW, Tryba M. Regional anesthesia in the patient receiving antithrombotic or thrombolytic therapy: american society of regional anesthesia and pain medicine evidence-based guidelines. Reg Anesth Pain Med. 2010;35(1):64–101.
3. Hadzic A. Textbook of regional anesthesia and acute pain management. New York: McGraw-Hill Professional; 2006, p. 144–65, 403–543.
4. Finucane, BT. editor. Complications of regional anesthesia. New York: Springer; 2007, p 39–52, 74–86.
5. Neal JM, et al. The second ASRA Practice Advisory on neurologic complications associated with regional anesthesia and pain medicine: executive Summary 2015. Reg Anesth Pain Med. 2015;40(5):401–30.
6. Casati A, Putzu M. Multi stimulation techniques for peripheral nerve blocks. In: Hadzic A. editor. NYSORA textbook of regional anesthesia and acute pain management. New York, NY: McGraw-Hill; 2007. Chapter 46.
7. Catterall WA, Mackie K. Local anesthetics. In: Brunton LL, Chabner BA, Knollmann BC. editors. Goodman & gilman's the pharmacological basis of therapeutics, 12e. New York, NY: McGraw-Hill; 2011. Chapter 20.
8. Butterworth J. Clinical pharmacology of local anesthetics. In: Hadzic A. editor. NYSORA textbook of regional anesthesia and acute pain management. New York, NY: McGraw-Hill; 2007. Chapter 6.
9. Wallace A. Local Anesthetics. In: Johnson KB, editor. Clinical pharmacology for anesthesiology. New York, NY: McGraw-Hill; 2015.
10. Albert J, Lofstrom B. Bilateral ulnar nerve blocks for the evaluation of local anaesthetic agents. Acta Anaesth Scand. 1965;9:203–11.
11. Ca DiFazio, Carron H, Grosslilght KR, et al. Comparison of pH-adjusted lidocaine solutions for epidural anesthesia. Anesth Analg. 1986;65:760–4.
12. Pollock JE. Transient neurologic symptoms: etiology risk factors, and management. Reg Anesth Pain Med. 2002;27(6):581–6.
13. Hoefnagel A, Yu A, Kaminski A. Anesthetic complications in pregnancy. Crit Care Clin. 2016;32(1):1–28.
14. Hadzic A, Carrera A, Thomas B. Hadzic's peripheral nerve blocks and anatomy for ultrasound-guided regional anesthesia (New york school of regional anesthesia). New Delhi: McGraw-Hill; 2004.
15. Bern S, Weinberg G. Local anesthetic toxicity and lipid resuscitation in pregnancy. Curr Opin Anaesthesiol. 2011;24(3):262–7.
16. Becker DE, Reed KL. Local anesthetics: review of pharmacological considerations. Anesthesia Progress. 2012;59(2):90–102.
17. Weinberg GL. Treatment of local anesthetic systemic toxicity (LAST). Reg Anesth Pain Med. 2010;35(2):188–93.
18. Weinberg G, Hertz P, Newman J. Lipid, not propofol, treats bupivacaine overdose. Anesth Analg. 2004;99:1871–82.
19. Cave G. Harvey M Intravenous lipid emulsion as antidote beyond local anesthetic toxicity: a systematic review. Acad Emerg Med. 2009;16(9):815–24.
20. Ozcan MS, Weinberg G. Intravenous lipid emulsion for the treatment of drug toxicity. J Intensive Care Med. 2014;29(2): 59–70.
21. Neal JM, Bernards CM, Butterworth JF IV, Di Gregorio G, Drasner K, Hejtmanek MR, Mulroy MF, Rosenquist RW, Weinberg GL. ASRA practice advisory on local anesthetic systemic toxicity. Reg Anesth Pain Med. 2010;35(2):152–61.
22. Felice KL, Schumann HM. Intravenous lipid emulsion for local anesthetic toxicity: a review of the literature. J Med Toxicol. 2008;4(3):184–91.
23. Wolfe JW, Butterworth JF. Local anesthetic systemic toxicity: update on mechanisms and treatment. Curr Opin Anaesthesiol. 2011;24(5):561–6.
24. Weinberg GL. Current concepts in resuscitation of patients with local anesthetic cardiac toxicity. Reg Anesth Pain Med. 2002;27(6): 568–75.
25. Krismer AC, Hogan QH, Wenzel V, et al. The efficacy of epinephrine or vasopressin for resuscitation during epidural anesthesia. Anesth Analg. 2001;93:734–42.
26. Mayr VD, Raedler C, Wenzel V, Lindner KH, Strohmenger H-U. A comparison of epinephrine and vasopressin in a porcine model of cardiac arrest after rapid intravenous injection of bupivacaine. Anesth Analg. 2004;98:1426–31.

Spinal Anesthesia

46

Benjamin Kloesel and Galina Davidyuk

Case 1

A 67-year-old man presents for elective primary right total knee replacement.

Medications:	aspirin 81 mg oral daily
	clopidogrel 75 mg oral daily
	amlodipine 10 mg oral daily
	metoprolol 25 mg oral twice daily
	hydrochlorothiazide 25 mg oral daily
	albuterol inhaler as needed
	fluticasone/ salmeterol 250/50 mcg inhaler 1 puff twice daily
	omeprazole 20 mg oral daily
	atorvastatin 20 mg oral daily
Allergies:	NKA
Past Medical History:	
Cardiac:	Hypertension
	Hypercholesterolemia
	Coronary artery disease s/p DES to LAD and LCx (4 years ago)
	Severe COPD (FEV1 of 32%)
	GERD

(continued)

Physical Exam:	
vs:	BP 140/98 HR 80 RR 16 oxygen saturation: 98%
Heart:	regular rate and rhythm, 2/6 systolic murmur
Lungs:	distant breath sounds, mild bilateral end-expiratory wheezing
Otherwise:	insignificant

What are possible indications for spinal anesthesia?

Spinal anesthesia can provide anesthesia, analgesia, and muscle relaxation. It has been successfully employed for procedures involving the abdomen, perineum, lower extremities, and urogenital tract as well as obstetric surgeries [1, 2].

What are landmarks that can be used to identify the correct intervertebral space for placement of spinal anesthesia?

Palpation of the neck reveals a prominent spinous process that belongs to the 7th cervical vertebra, called vertebra prominens. Palpation of the scapula reveals the root of the spine of the scapula commonly corresponding to a T3 level. The lower border of the scapula ends in a tip that usually is at the T7 level. At the lumbar spine level, a line drawn between the top of the bilateral iliac crests typically crosses the body of the 4th lumbar vertebra or the L4/5 interspace. This line is called Tuffier's line. While those landmarks are considered "traditional teaching,", studies have highlighted that their use frequently results in inaccurate determination of the intervertebral space, yet at a degree that still allows safe neuraxial placement in clinical practice. For patients whose anatomical landmarks are difficult or impossible to identify, imaging modalities such as fluoroscopy or ultrasound can assist in proper identification of the intervertebral space and additionally provide information that improve safety during placement (fluoroscopy shows real-time

B. Kloesel
Department of Anesthesiology, Perioperative and Pain Medicine, Boston Children's Hospital, 300 Longwood Avenue, Boston, MA 02115, USA
e-mail: Benjamin.kloesel@childrens.harvard.edu

G. Davidyuk (✉)
Department of Anesthesiology and Perioperative Pain Medicine, Brigham and Women's Hospital, 75 Francis street, BWH, Anesthesia Dept, CWN bld, L1, Boston, MA 02115, USA
e-mail: gdavidyuk@partners.org

© Springer International Publishing AG 2017
L.S. Aglio and R.D. Urman (eds.), *Anesthesiology*,
DOI 10.1007/978-3-319-50141-3_46

needle advancement while ultrasound allows identification of the midline and measurement of the epidural space depth) [1, 2].

What anatomy is important for the placement of a spinal anesthetic?

The spinal cord is continuous with the brainstem cranially and extends down to the L1 level in adults and L3 level in infants where it terminates as the conus medullaris. It is enveloped by a dural sac, which terminates more caudally, at the S2 level. The subarachnoid space between L1/L3 (adults and infants, respectively) and S2 is filled by the filum terminale internum (an extension of the pia mater) and spinal nerve roots originating from the conus medullaris (called cauda equina). The cauda equina harbors the L2–L5, S1–S5, and coccygeal nerve pairs, which innervate the lower limbs, pelvic organs, and perineum. After reaching the termination of the dural sac at the S2 level, the filum terminale internum continues as filum terminale externum to the back of the first segment of the coccyx.

Three distinct layers surrounding the spinal cord (from innermost to outermost) are called pia mater, arachnoid mater, and dura mater. The pia mater is highly vascularized and closely attaches to the spinal cord. Between the arachnoid mater and the pia mater, a small space called the intrathecal (subarachnoid) space is found which contains the cerebrospinal fluid (CSF). It is the target area for local anesthetic deposition in spinal anesthesia. The dura mater is attached to the arachnoid mater. Between them, a potential space exists, the subdural space. Outside of the dura mater, another small space called the epidural space is found which serves as the target area for deposition of local anesthetics in epidural anesthesia. The epidural space contains fat, lymphatics, and blood vessels (venous plexus). The arachnoid is a nonvascular membrane that offers the most resistance (90%) to drug migration.

The spinal cord itself has 31 segments (8 cervical, 12 thoracic, 5 lumbar, 5 sacral, 1 coccygeal) with their respective spinal nerves and is composed of the inner gray matter and the surrounding white matter.

During spinal anesthetic placement using a midline approach, multiple ligaments are traversed after entering the skin and subcutaneous tissue: the first ligament encountered is the supraspinous ligament, followed by the interspinous ligament. The following ligamentum flavum has a distinct feel that may alert the anesthesiologist to the proximity of the epidural space. After passage through the ligamentum flavum, the needle crosses the epidural space and pierces through the dura mater and the arachnoid mater into the subarachnoid space where CSF is encountered. When using a paramedian approach, the supraspinous and interspinous ligaments are bypassed [1, 2].

Describe the blood supply of the spinal cord

The spinal cord is supplied by a single anterior spinal artery that originates from the vertebral arteries and a pair of posterior spinal arteries that are formed by the inferior cerebellar arteries. These three arteries receive contributions from intercostal and lumbar arteries via segmental spinal arteries. The largest of those tributaries is the artery of Adamkiewicz (Arteria radicularis magna). In 75% of individuals, the artery of Adamkiewicz originates on the left side between T8 and L1. The anterior spinal artery supplies the anterior 2/3 of the spinal cord while the posterior spinal arteries cover the posterior 1/3.

Venous blood drains into three anterior and three posterior spinal veins that connect to the internal venous plexus located in the epidural space [1, 2].

What is the mechanism of action of local anesthetic injected into subarachnoid space?

Local anesthetics reversibly bind to voltage-gated sodium channels and block sodium conduction. By decreasing sodium currents, the initiation and propagation of action potentials is interrupted. Local anesthetics cause a "state-dependent" block: while sodium channels can be found in three states (resting-closed, activated-open, inactivated-closed), local anesthetics have the greatest affinity for channels in the activated-open state (less so for the inactivated-closed state).

Local anesthetics injected into the spinal space gain access to the spinal nerve roots and dorsal root ganglia.

Traditional teaching states that smaller, unmyelinated fibers are blocked first while larger, myelinated fibers take a longer time for complete blockade. As a result, onset of blockade follows a temporal progression, starting with preganglionic sympathetic conduction supplied by B-fibers, followed by cold temperature sensation conveyed by C-fibers, pinprick sensation transmitted via A-delta fibers, touch sensation through A-beta fibers and, finally, motor function provided by A-alpha fibers. Recovery follows in reverse order. The differences in sensitivity account for a phenomenon called differential sensory block: the peak block height of a given anesthetic may vary according to the sensory modality that is being tested. Typically, the highest block level (largest dermatomal spread) is attained for cold sensation, followed by sensation to pinprick (1–2 levels lower) and touch (3–4 levels lower). Sympathetic block height can reach 2–6 dermatomes above sensory block level while motor block height is found to be 2–3 dermatomes below sensory block level.

The term "differential sensory block" was introduced based on studies in the 1950s. Since then, multiple investigators have reported conflicting results. Some were able to reproduce a difference in block height extension for different modalities while others did not find this effect. These differences also vary between the different local anesthetics. Another layer of complexity is added when contrasting basic and clinical science results. Experimental studies on rat sciatic nerves, for example, have shown a higher susceptibility to lidocaine-induced blockade in A-gamma/delta/alpha and beta fibers compared to C-fibers [1, 2].

What level of spinal anesthesia is required for different surgeries and what are surface landmarks for the respective levels?

Upper abdominal surgery (cholecystectomy) and C-section require a T4–5 level corresponding to the nipple line (T4). While the uterus is located in the lower abdomen, a T4 level is necessary to blunt stimuli caused by traction on the peritoneum and uterine exteriorization. Lower abdominal surgery requires a T6–8 level, with T6/7 being at the level of the xiphoid process. Anesthesia extending to the level of the umbilicus, corresponding to the T10 dermatome, is adequate for TURP, hip surgery, and vaginal delivery. Thigh surgery and lower limb surgery are covered by a level extending at least to the inguinal ligament which corresponds to T12/L1, while foot surgery only requires a L2/3 level (except in cases that use a tourniquet); the area under the tourniquet corresponds to L1–L4 dermatomes. Taking temporal regression of the block into account, one should factor in a safety margin. An anesthetic level involving the S2–5 dermatomes adequately covers hemorrhoidectomy and perineal surgery.

What physiologic alterations are caused by successful administration of a spinal anesthetic?

<u>Cardiovascular system:</u>

In the cardiovascular system, spinal anesthesia causes a decrease in cardiac output and systemic vascular resistance. Blockade of sympathetic fibers inhibits vasoconstriction and leads to pooling of blood in the splanchnic system and the lower extremities. A decrease in venous return (~preload) results in a decrease in cardiac output. If local anesthetic spread reaches T1–T4 levels, blockade of the cardiac accelerator fibers occurs causing a decrease in heart rate, which further lowers cardiac output [3, 4].

In addition to those changes, three reflexes are associated with spinal anesthesia which can worsen bradycardia and even lead to cardiac arrest:

(1) the pacemaker reflex involves cells in the sinoatrial node that respond to stretch with depolarization (proportional to the degree of stretch). A sudden decrease in venous return leads to a decrease in stretch and depolarization of sinoatrial cells, lowering the heart rate.
(2) The baroreceptor reflex involves receptors located in the wall of the right atrium and the vena cava–atrial junction. Increases in venous return trigger signals transmitted to the cardiac accelerator fibers via the vagus nerve and cause an increase in heart rate. Conversely, a decrease in venous return decreases stimulation of the baroreceptors.
(3) The Bezold–Jarisch reflex binds a decrease of left ventricular volume to an increase in vagal output through the vagus nerve resulting in bradycardia.

<u>Pulmonary system:</u>

Overall, the direct effects of spinal anesthesia on the respiratory system are minimal. Even with mid- to high-thoracic levels of anesthesia, respiratory indices including minute ventilation, tidal volume, and mean inspiratory flow rate are unaffected. The same is true for pulmonary gas exchange. A small decrease in vital capacity and maximal expiratory pressure and flow has been observed and is attributed to weakness of the abdominal muscles [3, 4].

<u>Central nervous system:</u>

Spinal anesthesia has consistently been found to reduce hypnotic and sedative requirements through yet poorly understood mechanisms. Theories to explain this finding include de-afferentiation phenomenon (blockade of the spinal nerves reduces afferent input to the brain, making the reticular activating system more sensitive to sedative/hypnotic drugs), rostral spread of local anesthetics within the CSF (with direct blocking effects of local anesthetics on brain centers), and absorption of local anesthetics leading to increased systemic levels [3, 4].

<u>Urinary system:</u>

Bladder and urethral sphincters are controlled via the sacral spinal nerves (S2–S4). Blockade of those segments abolishes the urge to void, creating the risk of bladder overdistention and postoperative urinary retention in the setting of long-acting local anesthetics. Bladder overdistention can cause pain and hypertension, and stimulation of vagal afferents can also lead to bradycardia and hypotension. Therefore, consideration should be given to placement of an indwelling urinary catheter or ultrasound bladder volume monitoring with as-needed in-and-out catheterization [3, 4].

<u>Gastrointestinal system:</u>

Ablation of sympathetic stimuli to the gastrointestinal tract generated at T6–L1 levels results in hyperperistalsis from unopposed parasympathetic stimulation. Nausea and vomiting can be secondary to this effect (or, in other cases, related to hypotension and hypoperfusion) [1, 2].

<u>Thermoregulation:</u>

In general, the body thermo-regulative capabilities are more impaired by general anesthesia than by spinal anesthesia; nevertheless, vasodilation from sympathetic blockade causes a re-distribution of heat from core tissues (head, trunk, internal organs) to skin, upper and lower extremities.

Also, shivering thresholds are reduced in the blocked segments, thereby reducing the ability to generate heat [3, 4].

What factors influence the block level/distribution during spinal anesthesia?

Block level in spinal anesthesia is determined by drug, patient, and procedure factors [1, 2].

(1) Drug factors
  (a) Baricity (isobaric/hypobaric/hyperbaric): baricity of the drug and patient body position are important in influencing and predicting the injected drug's behavior. Baricity is defined as the density of the local anesthetic relative to the density of CSF measured in mass/volume at 37 °C—isobaric solutions have density virtually equal to that of CSF, hyperbaric have higher, and hypobaric have lower densities relative to CSF. Gravity distributes hyperbaric drugs to the dependent areas, while hypobaric drugs move to non-dependent areas. Depending on the body position, a hypobaric solution could, for example, be used to produce a predominantly left spinal anesthesia for a left hip surgery when injected in a right lateral decubitus position. For supine patients who have received a hyperbaric solution, it is important to consider the natural curvature of the spine (lumbar lordosis, thoracic kyphosis) when trying to predict the spread. In the supine patient, the highest spine vertebra is L3 (L4) while the lowest point is T5–T6.
  (b) Dose: the dose [mg] of a local anesthetic can be calculated by multiplication of volume [ml] and concentration [mg/ml]. It is the most important factor that determines block spread and duration.

(2) Patient factors
  (a) CSF volume and composition
  (b) Age: advanced age correlates with increased block height based on a decrease in CSF volume and increased sensitivity to local anesthetics
  (c) Pregnancy and other conditions leading to increased intraabdominal pressure and epidural vein engorgement.

(3) Procedural factors
  (a) Patient position
  (b) Site of injection

What local anesthetics are being used for spinal anesthesia?

The following local anesthetics are successfully used for spinal anesthesia: procaine*, chloroprocaine (short-acting); mepivacaine, lidocaine, prilocaine* (intermediate-acting); ropivacaine, bupivacaine, levobupivacaine*, and tetracaine* (long-acting). (*presently not available in the USA)

Lidocaine and mepivacaine have largely fallen out of favor due to concerns regarding a higher incidence of side effects. Chloroprocaine used to be associated with a high incidence of neurologic injury. As more recent evidence has identified the preservative as the etiologic factor, new preservative-free preparations of chloroprocaine are increasingly used for short procedures [5].

What problems can arise when using lidocaine or mepivacaine for spinal anesthesia?

The use of lidocaine for spinal anesthesia has been associated with transient neurological symptoms (TNS), also called transient radicular irritation or transient neurologic toxicity. Symptom onset occurs within a few hours up to 24 h after successful spinal anesthetic and includes pain in the gluteal region with radiation to both lower extremities. A distinguishing feature to cauda equina syndrome is the absence of weakness, neurologic deficiencies, and pathologic findings on imaging (CT/MRI). While TNS can occur with other local anesthetics, a Cochrane analysis of trials found that the likelihood of TNS after lidocaine administration was four times higher (RR = 7.31) than compared to bupivacaine, prilocaine, procaine, levobupivacaine, ropivacaine, and 2-chloroprocaine. Mepivacaine might carry a similar risk for TNS as lidocaine. Another factor that increases the risk for TNS is surgery in lithotomy position [4, 6].

What adjuvants can be added to local anesthetics?

Multiple drugs have been tested as "additives" to local anesthetics. The followings are commonly used in clinical practice [4]:

(a) Opioids (discussed below)
(b) Vasoconstrictors (epinephrine, phenylephrine): cause local vasoconstriction and thereby prolong duration of local anesthetics (reduced uptake into blood vessels and clearance from CSF). The magnitude of those effects varies between local anesthetics. The most pronounced effect is seen with tetracaine. In addition, adrenergic agents have antinociceptive effects via stimulation of alpha-adrenergic receptors in the dorsal horn of the spinal cord.
(c) Alpha-2-agonists (clonidine, dexmedetomidine): prolong duration of sensory and motor blockade and thereby reduce analgesic requirements
(d) Acetylcholinesterase inhibitors (Neostigmine): prolong duration of sensory and motor blockade and thereby reduce analgesic requirements but may have significant side effects (nausea, emesis, bradycardia)

Other agents such as ketamine, magnesium, adenosine, tramadol, NSAIDs, and midazolam are being investigated as possible additives.

How do intrathecal opioids work?

Intrathecally administered opioids work at the spinal cord level, specifically in the substantia gelatinosa in the gray matter of the spinal cord dorsal horn (lamina II). Less lipophilic opioids (morphine, hydromorphone) are 100–200 times more potent when administered intrathecally as compared to intravenous administration, and are associated with pronounced rostral spread, carrying the risk for delayed respiratory depression. In contrast, more lipophilic opioids (fentanyl, sufentanil) are only 10–20 times more potent intrathecally than intravenously; rostral migration occurs to a lesser extent as more lipophilic opioids are absorbed faster into the systemic circulation.

Another important point to recognize is the spinal opioid receptor bioavailability of the respective opioid. Intrathecally administered morphine and hydromorphone have high spinal opioid receptor bioavailability, whereas fentanyl and sufentanil have only moderate spinal opioid receptor bioavailability [7]. This is based on the location of opioid receptors. Spinal cord opioid receptors are situated in the gray matter which is surrounded by white matter. More lipophilic opioids partition into the white matter and are subsequently cleared into the plasma so that only a minor fraction reaches the gray matter. Less lipophilic opioids tend to reside in the CSF for a longer time. While they do not partition to the white matter in a great extent, they can diffuse through the aqueous extracellular space of the white matter to the opioid receptors in the gray matter.

What is the underlying pathophysiology of respiratory depression with intrathecal opioid administration?

For a long time, different views have prevailed about the ability and speed of rostral spread of intrathecally administered opioids. The current understanding is that every opioid (less lipophilic or more lipophilic) moves at the same speed within the CSF. This movement is secondary to diffusion and CSF bulk flow produced by pulsatile movement of blood into the brain which creates intermittent swelling. When brain mass increases, a plunger effect occurs that pushes CSF downward the dorsal surface and upward on the ventral surface of the spinal cord [7]. The explanation why less lipophilic opioids seem to have a much larger rostral spread lies in the fact that they remain in CSF much longer than their more lipophilic counterparts, which are absorbed and re-distributed into the systemic circulation. While both opioid groups can cause respiratory depression and other supraspinal effects, less lipophilic opioids cause it by reaching brainstem centers via rostral spread in the CSF while more lipophilic opioids reach those centers via the bloodstream [1, 2].

What are typical side effects of intrathecal opioids?

Pruritus, early respiratory depression (fentanyl, sufentanil), delayed respiratory depression (up to 24 h for morphine and hydromorphone), urinary retention, nausea, and vomiting

What are absolute and relative contraindications to spinal anesthesia?

Absolute contraindications include patient refusal, untreated systemic infection (sepsis), local infection at the planned injection site, raised intracranial pressure, and allergy to the drug planned for administration.

Relative contraindications include spinal stenosis, aortic stenosis, hypovolemia, and coagulopathy.

What are side effects of spinal anesthesia?

Local anesthetic blockade of sympathetic fibers causes vasodilation and hypotension of varying severity depending on dose, intrathecal spread, and patient factors. Many studies have examined the value of pre- or periprocedural intravenous fluid administration and vasopressor/inotrope use.

Patients can experience nausea and emesis from either administration of intrathecal opioids or hypotension from sympathectomy. The unopposed parasympathetic stimulation of the gastrointestinal tract with subsequent hyperperistalsis may also play a role. In case of hypotension, nausea is often relieved with administration of phenylephrine and/or ephedrine. Otherwise antiemetics can be used.

Pruritus is the most common side effect of intrathecal opioid administration and can be treated effectively with mu-receptor antagonists such as naloxone, naltrexone, or nalbuphine (the latter being a partial agonist–antagonist). A salutatory effect of diphenhydramine is mainly attributed to its sedating effect as opioid-induced pruritus is not mediated via histamine release.

Bradycardia can occur secondary to blockade of cardioaccelerator fibers originating from T1 to T4 in cases of intrathecal spread to those levels.

Urinary retention is related to blockade of the sacral nerve fibers. It resolves after the local anesthetic effect wears off and is, in the interim, managed with urinary catheterization [1, 2].

What are possible complications of spinal anesthesia?

Cardiac arrest during spinal anesthesia is a rare but disastrous complication. Presumed mechanisms include the blockade of sympathetic fibers, including the cardiac accelerator fibers originating from T1 to T4, and vasodilation leading to a decrease in venous return. The combination of bradycardia and decreased preload causes a drop in cardiac output. Elicitation of the Bezold–Jarisch reflex further decreases the already low heart rate. Development of bradycardia during spinal anesthesia is on a continuum with cardiac arrest; hence, patients with high vagal tone are at higher risk. Factors associated with the development of moderate bradycardia (heart rate <50 beats/minute) during spinal anesthesia include baseline heart rate <60, ASA status I versus III/IV, use of beta-blockers, sensory level at or above T5, age <50 years, and prolonged PR interval. Factors associated with spinal anesthesia-induced hypotension include sensory level at or above T5, age >40 years, baseline systolic blood pressure <120 mmHg, combined spinal/general anesthesia, spinal puncture at or above L2/3 interspace, and addition of phenylephrine to local anesthetic. A common suggestion is to avoid hemodynamic instabilities to maintain adequate preload during the procedure. If bradycardia occurs, the patient should be placed in Trendelenburg position and treated with atropine and/or ephedrine. Phenylephrine can be used to address hypotension but care should be given to avoid exaggeration of bradycardia [8].

A rare but serious complication of spinal anesthesia is CNS infection. Meningitis has been reported to occur in less than 1 in 50,000 spinal anesthetics. It requires prompt diagnosis and treatment with antibiotics. Other infectious complications include spinal abscess and localized skin infections at the needle insertion site.

Arachnoiditis is a meningeal inflammation that can be secondary to multiple etiologies such as infection, blood, local anesthetics, preservatives, and other irritants. Recently, questions have been raised whether inadvertent introduction of alcohol and chlorhexidine used for skin site disinfection during performance of spinal anesthesia could be a cause for reports of severe neurologic complications.

Bleeding complications range from commonly occurring, less concerning local hematomas at the needle insertion site to space occupying spinal hematomas that require prompt diagnosis with imaging and possible surgical decompression to avoid paralysis. Most spinal hematomas have been reported in patients that were either taking anticoagulants or had documented hematologic abnormalities such as thrombocytopenia or coagulopathies. Prompt diagnosis is key as studies have shown that spinal cord ischemia secondary to a hematoma is typically reversible when addressed with laminectomy within 8 h of onset of neurologic symptoms.

Nerve injuries secondary to spinal anesthesia are rare (reported incidence between 0.03 and 0.1%). Fortunately, most nerve injuries are transient and function recovers in the majority of cases. Some authors have reported catastrophic sequelae (cauda equina syndrome, paraplegia); most of those outcomes were in the setting of injection of local anesthetics despite patient report of pain or paresthesia, highlighting the importance of performance of neuraxial techniques in the awake or lightly sedated patient. Historically, such grave complications have also been reported with "pooling" of hyperbaric high-concentration lidocaine delivered by spinal microcatheters, as well as with different preservatives, such as bisulfites.

Patients can manifest allergic reactions to local anesthetics, preservatives, or additives. Local anesthetics more commonly implicated in allergic reactions are of the ester type due to their metabolism to the known allergen para-aminobenzoic acid (PABA). The preservative methylparaben is also metabolized to PABA and should not be present in local anesthetic preparations intended for spinal injection. Allergies to amide local anesthetics are rare.

Total spinal anesthesia refers to inadvertent excessive cephalad spread of the injected local anesthetics, producing blockade that includes the cervical spinal segments. The ensuing extensive vasodilation results in hypotension, bradycardia, respiratory arrest, and loss of consciousness or a "locked-in" state. Treatment includes cardiopulmonary support (intubation, fluids, vasopressors/inotropes) and administration of amnestics until the local anesthetic effect subsides [1, 2].

How do you diagnose a post-dural puncture headache?

Post-dural puncture headache (PDPH) can occur in the setting of penetration of the dura mater, either accidentally (e.g., during performance of an epidural placement) or intentionally (during performance of spinal anesthesia or spinal tap). Central to the diagnosis is a headache with a prominent positional component. While 90% of PDPH cases occur within 72 h of dural puncture, rare instances have been reported in which onset was reported to be hours to months after the event. Based on the International Classification of Headache Disorders Diagnostic Criteria for Post-Dural Puncture Headache, the diagnosis of PDPH can be made if the following four criteria are met: (1) Headache that worsens within 15 min after sitting or standing and improves within 15 min after laying with at least one additional criterion of (a) neck stiffness, (b) tinnitus, (c) hypacusia, (d) photophobia, or (e) nausea; (2) Dural puncture has been performed; (3) Headache develops within 5 days of dural puncture; and (4) Headache resolves either (a) spontaneously within 1 week of (b) within 48 h of effective treatment of the spinal fluid leak [9].

What are the incidence, risk and modifying factors for post-dural puncture headache after spinal anesthesia?

Risk factors for the occurrence of PDPH are divided into non-modifiable and modifiable. Non-modifiable risk factors include (1) age (highest risk at age 20–30, rare over the age of 60), (2) female gender, (3) low BMI, (4) history of prior

PDPH, and (5) history of chronic headache. Modifiable risk factors include (1) size of the spinal needle, (2) needle shape, (3) bevel orientation and angle of insertion, (4) stylet replacement, and (5) operator experience.

In regards to spinal needles, small atraumatic needles (Sprotte, Whitacre) have the lowest likelihood of causing PDPH, while larger cutting needles (Touhy, Quincke).

Insertion of a spinal catheter after unintentional dural puncture during epidural placement has been found to reduce the incidence of PDPH [9].

What are treatment options for PDPH?

Conservative treatment consists of hydration and PO caffeine, Fioricet (Butalbital 50 mg/Acetaminophen 300 mg/Caffeine 40 mg) and NSAIDs. Fioricet is administered as 1–2 tablets every 4 h as needed, not to exceed 6 tablets (this is based on the maximum daily dose of Butalbital, which is 300 mg). Since January 2014, the Acetaminophen content of Fioricet tablets has been reduced from 325 mg to 300 mg to avoid unintentional overdoses. For prolonged and severe PDPH, an epidural blood patch can be performed [10].

Additional case scenarios:

1. **10 min after successful identification of the spinal space and injection of 1.6 ml of hyperbaric bupivacaine, 0.75% the patient complains of shortness of breath and becomes mildly tachypneic with normal pulse oximetry readings. What is happening?**

The local anesthetic has migrated cranially and blocked spinal nerves that innervate the abdominal muscles. While most respiratory indices and pulmonary gas exchange remain unchanged, the patient can experience subjective dyspnea due to impaired proprioceptive input from abdominal and chest wall muscles, resulting in the feeling of breathlessness. Anxiety-related tachypnea can ensue leading to hypocapnea. Treatment includes reassurance and prevention of further cranial migration of the local anesthetic if a hyperbaric solution was used.

2. **10 min after successful identification of the spinal space and injection of 1.6 ml of hyperbaric bupivacaine, 0.75% the patient becomes hypotensive and apneic. What is happening?**

The local anesthetic has migrated cranially to such an extent that the resulting blockade of sympathetic fibers resulted in significant hypotension that caused brainstem hypoperfusion. A previously hypothesized mechanism of local anesthetic-mediated blockade of the respiratory center has been disproven.

3. **A spinal anesthetic is performed on a 56 y/o male patient for right total hip replacement. After identification of the L3/4 spinal space, 2 ml of isobaric, 0.75% bupivacaine is injected. After 10 min, a level is checked and is noted to be patchy, with extension to about T12 on the left and L1 on the right. The patient has insufficient anesthesia for the procedure. The spinal attempt is declared a failure and the anesthetic is converted into general endotracheal anesthesia. What is a possible explanation of this finding?**

Besides abnormal/atypical anatomy and manufacturing error resulting in decreased local anesthetic efficacy, the most likely explanations are inadvertent subdural injection, epidural injection, or partial dose delivery into the subarachnoid space. Subdural injections rarely occur during spinal anesthesia attempts and are more concerning in the setting of epidural anesthesia due to the larger volume of injected local anesthetic that can lead to high or total spinal anesthesia. Doses used for spinal anesthesia more commonly result in unsatisfactory block levels and insufficient or patchy anesthesia.

The interface between the dura mater and the arachnoid is characterized as a potential space that can be expanded by a local anesthetic injection if the spinal needle is malpositioned and does not completely enter the spinal canal. Whitacre and Sprotte needles, for example, have a side hole that can be malpositioned in a way that part of the hole reaches the spinal space, rendering a positive spinal fluid return, while the other part juxtaposed against the interface of the dura and arachnoid. Part of the injected local anesthetic reaches the spinal space while the rest opens up the subdural space [11].

What is a "saddle block"?

To achieve a saddle block, a hyperbaric solution is injected into the spinal space. The patient remains in a sitting position after the injection in order to allow the "heavy" local anesthetic solution to migrate downwards and pool in the caudal part of the dural sac. Alternatively, a hypobaric solution can be injected after which the patient needs to be placed prone in a jackknife position. The local anesthetic spreads to affect the sacral and low lumbar dermatomes only, leading to anesthesia and analgesia of the buttocks, inner thighs, and perianal region in a dose-dependent fashion. The technique can be successfully employed for perineal and anal surgeries.

What is the lumbosacral approach to the spinal space?

The lumbosacral approach to the spinal space, also called Taylor approach, is used if usual approaches fail. It targets the largest interlaminar space of the spinal cord, L5-S1. To further improve chances of successful access to the spinal space, the needle is advanced from a paramedian position. To find the correct insertion site, identify the posterior superior iliac spine and insert the needle 1 cm lateral and 1 cm caudal with a cephalad orientation of 45–55° along with a slight medial angulation.

What are some of the implications of pregnancy on spinal anesthesia?

The physiologic changes of pregnancy influence spinal anesthesia in multiple ways. Uterine enlargement leads to an increase in intraabdominal pressure, compression of abdominal vessels leading to epidural vein engorgement. CSF is displaced and its low volume in the thoracolumbar region accounts for a decreased dose requirement of local anesthetics. Increased progesterone levels account for an increased sensitivity to the blocking effects of local anesthetics.

Hormonal changes in the pregnant women also induce softening of the spinal ligaments making it more challenging to identify the ligamentum flavum. As for palpatory landmarks, pregnancy causes pelvic rotation that displaces Tuffier's line above the typical L4/L5 level. A study in 45 women showed a wide range of anatomic variation: the median level of intersection was immediately below the L2–L3 interspace, with a range from immediately above L1–L2 to immediately above L4–L5 [12].

What are current recommendations for treatment of hypotension during spinal anesthesia for cesarean sections?

Hypotension in the setting of spinal anesthesia for cesarean section is common, and multiple studies have examined possible treatments, including fluid administration either before or during spinal anesthesia, use of colloids versus crystalloids, and use of vasopressors and inotropes. A review by Loubert published in 2012 states that strategies using a crystalloid co-load, a colloid preload, or a colloid co-load yield equivalent results in terms of decreased hypotension and vasopressor requirements. A crystalloid preload regimen has been shown to be inferior. Co-loading strategies refer to fluid administration immediately after the spinal anesthetic has been placed. In regards to vasoactive medications, phenylephrine has a more beneficial profile as ephedrine was noted to increase $PaCO_2$, decrease pH, and oxygen content in cord blood from newborns whose mothers received large doses of ephedrine. Therefore, phenylephrine administered either in bolus form or as a continuous infusion is considered the first-line agent [13].

What are implications of antiplatelet agents and anticoagulants for performance of spinal anesthesia?

Hematology is an evolving field and new drugs are constantly being developed that aim to influence the coagulation cascade. It is therefore prudent for the practicing clinician to follow the most up-to-date practice guidelines, practice advisories, and drug information. In addition, different institutions may modify existing recommendations, again making the practicing clinician responsible for keeping current with institutional policies.

In general terms, coagulopathy (inherited and acquired) as well as use of antiplatelet agents/anticoagulants is a contraindication to neuraxial techniques. An exception is the use of NSAIDs (including aspirin), which have been found to be safe when used alone.

The use of twice-daily subcutaneous unfractionated heparin (daily doses of 10,000 IU or less) does not limit the use of neuraxial anesthesia; three-times per day dosing schedules have not yet been evaluated and guidelines state that the safety of neuraxial block in those patients is unknown.

Subcutaneous administration of low molecular weight heparins (LMWH) is a well-established risk factor for formation of spinal hematomas; guidelines recommend 12 and 24 h of discontinuation prior to neuraxial block placement for prophylactic and therapeutic LMWH, respectively.

For the oral anticoagulant warfarin, a period of 3–5 days of discontinuation is recommended, followed by documentation of a normal INR.

Guidelines recommend discontinuation of antiplatelet agent use before neuraxial blockade to allow recovery of platelet function. Depending on the agent, different discontinuation timeframes are reported (ticlopidine—14 days; clopidogrel—5–7 days; prasugrel—7–10 days; eptifibatide/tirofiban—8 h; abciximab—48 h).

In the setting of fibrinolytic therapy, guidelines recommend against the performance of neuraxial anesthesia.

The direct thrombin inhibitor dabigatran should be discontinued 5 days before neuraxial anesthesia. The direct factor Xa inhibitor rivaroxaban should be withheld for 3 days [14].

The understanding of these interactions is a dynamic process and frequent updates of our collective knowledge are just as critical for patient safety as sound risk–benefit consideration.

References

1. Bernards CM, Hostetter LS. Epidural and spinal anesthesia. In: Barash PG, Cullen BF, Stoelting RK, Cahalan MK, Stock MC, Ortega R, editors. Clinical anesthesia. 7th ed. Philadelphia, PA: Lippincott Williams & Wilkins; 2013. p. 905–33.
2. Brull R, Macfarlane AJR, Chan VWS. Spinal, epidural, caudal anesthesia. In: Miller RD, Cohen NH, Eriksson LI, Fleisher LA, Wiener-Kronish JP, Young WL, editors. Miller's anesthesia. 1. 8th ed. Philadelphia, PA: Elsevier; 2015. p. 1684–720.
3. Salinas FV, Sueda LA, Liu SS. Physiology of spinal anaesthesia and practical suggestions for successful spinal anaesthesia. Best Pract Res Clin Anaesthesiol. 2003;17(3):289–303.
4. Liu SS, McDonald SB. Current issues in spinal anesthesia. Anesthesiology. 2001;94(5):888–906.
5. Goldblum E, Atchabahian A. The use of 2-chloroprocaine for spinal anaesthesia. Acta Anaesthesiol Scand. 2013;57(5):545–52.
6. Zaric D, Christiansen C, Pace NL, Punjasawadwong Y. Transient neurologic symptoms after spinal anesthesia with lidocaine versus other local anesthetics: a systematic review of randomized, controlled trials. Anesth Analg. 2005;100(6):1811–6.
7. Bernards CM. Understanding the physiology and pharmacology of epidural and intrathecal opioids. Best Pract Res Clin Anaesthesiol. 2002;16(4):489–505.
8. Pollard JB. Cardiac arrest during spinal anesthesia: common mechanisms and strategies for prevention. Anesth Analg. 2001;92(1):252–6.
9. Bezov D, Lipton RB, Ashina S. Post-dural puncture headache: part I diagnosis, epidemiology, etiology, and pathophysiology. Headache. 2010;50(7):1144–52.
10. Bezov D, Ashina S, Lipton R. Post-dural puncture headache: part II–prevention, management, and prognosis. Headache. 2010;50(9):1482–98.
11. Agarwal D, Mohta M, Tyagi A, Sethi AK. Subdural block and the anaesthetist. Anaesth Intensive Care. 2010;38(1):20–6.
12. Margarido CB, Mikhael R, Arzola C, Balki M, Carvalho JC. The intercristal line determined by palpation is not a reliable anatomical landmark for neuraxial anesthesia. Can J Anaesth. 2011;58(3):262–6.
13. Loubert C. Fluid and vasopressor management for Cesarean delivery under spinal anesthesia: continuing professional development. Can J Anaesth. 2012;59(6):604–19.
14. Horlocker TT, Wedel DJ, Rowlingson JC, Enneking FK, Kopp SL, Benzon HT, et al. Regional anesthesia in the patient receiving antithrombotic or thrombolytic therapy: American Society of Regional Anesthesia and Pain Medicine Evidence-Based Guidelines (Third Edition). Reg Anesth Pain Med. 2010;35(1):64–101.

Brachial Plexus Block

47

Nantthasorn Zinboonyahgoon and Kamen Vlassakov

A 65-year-old male patient, arriving to the hospital by ambulance after a fall, is complaining of severe pain in his right elbow. Upper extremity radiography reveals a complex fracture of the right distal humerus and the right proximal radius. The orthopedic trauma team recommends an open reduction and internal fixation (ORIF) of the right elbow; Informed consent is obtained and anesthesiology consult is called.

Past medical history:	Atrial fibrillation, COPD, CHF
Medications:	Coumadin 3 mg PO daily, Albuterol MDI 2 puffs prn for shortness of breath, Spiriva 2 puffs daily, furosemide 20 mg PO daily, metoprolol ER 100 mg PO daily
Allergies:	NKDA
Physical exam:	
Vitals:	BP 110/60, HR 65, RR 16, oxygen saturation 98% on nasal cannula at 3 L/min
	Weight 160 lbs., Height 67 in.
Alert and oriented ×3, no focal neurological deficit	
Irregular HR, no murmur; lungs—clear to auscultation	
Visible deformity of the right elbow	
Otherwise: non-contributory	

1. What are some relevant preoperative concerns and recommended work up?

This patient has a complicated medical history and has suffered trauma from a fall. Besides the general concerns, the preoperative evaluation for this patient should specifically include:

1.1 Clarifying the cause of the fall: a mechanical fall or a fall associated with other medical problems such as neurological (TIA, stroke) or cardiovascular (syncope, orthostatic hypotension, arrhythmia) deficits and/or events.

1.2 Assessing for concomitant injuries, especially cervical spine fractures and head injuries. If such injuries cannot be excluded by history and physical examination, a CT or MRI scan of the head and neck are recommended and the patient's neck should be temporarily immobilized and supported in a collar.

1.3 Details of patient's comorbidities:
   - Heart disease—obtain a 12-lead ECG; focus on active cardiac conditions, baseline functional class and cardiac work up, including review of recent echocardiography results if available. If active symptoms or suspicion of cardiovascular fall etiology, recommend a preoperative echocardiography exam to assess current function and rule out signs of ischemia.
   - COPD—assess stage of disease by history, severity and frequency of exacerbations, medication use, (including steroids), and home oxygen therapy.
   - Laboratory tests should include CBC, coagulation status, electrolytes, BUN, and creatinine.

2. What are the anesthesia choices for this patient? What are the risks and benefits for each choice?

N. Zinboonyahgoon
Department of Anesthesiology, Siriraj Hospital, 2 Phranok Road, Siriraj, Bangkoknoi, Bangkok, 10700, Thailand
e-mail: nantthasorn@gmail.com

K. Vlassakov (✉)
Department of Anesthesiology, Perioperative and Pain Medicine, Brigham and Women's Hospital, 75 Francis Street, CWN-L1, Boston, MA 02115, USA
e-mail: kvlassakov@partners.org

© Springer International Publishing AG 2017
L.S. Aglio and R.D. Urman (eds.), *Anesthesiology*,
DOI 10.1007/978-3-319-50141-3_47

ORIF of the elbow can be conducted under general anesthesia, regional anesthesia, or a combination of both. However, each choice has considerations as follows:

(a) Brachial plexus block (BPB)
 Benefits/advantages include:
 - Minimal hemodynamic changes
 - Superior pain control
 - Safer positioning (awake)
 - No cognitive effects
 - No need to manipulate the airway
 - Faster recovery

 Risks/disadvantages include:
 - Diaphragmatic weakness—BPB, especially interscalene block, is strongly associated with ipsilateral hemidiaphragmatic block (weakness), which may be poorly tolerated by patients suffering from COPD or other chronic lung disease
 - Limited ability for postoperative assessment of neurologic function—this patient has a complex fracture, which is associated with a higher risk for acute compartment syndrome (ACS). There is still controversy about the role of nerve blocks in potentially complicating/"masking" the clinical picture of ACS delaying diagnosis of ACS (discussed below)
 - Lack of airway/ventilation control in (heavily) sedated patients
 - Difficult to guarantee a completely immobilized extremity

(b) General anesthesia
 Benefits/advantages include:
 - High success rate (100%)
 - Initiated faster
 - Reliable
 - No need for specialized regional anesthesia skills or equipment

 Risks/disadvantages include:
 - Significant hemodynamic changes, especially in sitting position
 - General anesthesia is associated with higher cardiovascular and pulmonary complication risks
 - Risks of airway manipulation

 The choice of anesthesia should be based on a discussion of risks and benefits of each option and possible complications between anesthesiologist, patient and surgeon, in the immediate context of the patient's medical conditions, their severity, and the procedure urgency. Surgeon's preference and availability of regional anesthesia-trained personnel and equipment, all contribute to the choice of anesthesia

3. What are the contraindications for a brachial plexus block?
 - Absolute contraindications: Patient's refusal.
 - Relative contraindications include:
   - Allergy to local anesthetics
   - Preexisting nerve deficit or need to test/monitor nerve function after the surgery
   - Infection at the block site
   - Coagulopathy for deep (noncompressible space) nerve block
   - Patients at high risk for acute compartment syndrome
   - Patient with severe restrictive or obstructive pulmonary disease (except axillary block)
   - Severe time constraints—emergency surgery (if immediate anesthesia induction is indicated, block can still be performed postoperatively or intraoperatively)

4. What are the regional anesthesia limitations and recommendations in anticoagulated patients?

According to the 2010 ASRA practice advisory on regional anesthesia in patients receiving antithrombotic or thrombolytic therapy [1], the same strict guidelines recommended for neuraxial blocks, should be also applied for deep noncompressible space blocks. For example, the procedure should be performed at least 12 h after a prophylactic dose of low-molecular weight heparin, and INR should be normal.

Even though there is no conclusive definition, deep noncompressible space blocks include paravertebral blocks, lumbar plexus block, and possibly the parasacral and transgluteal sciatic nerve blocks and infraclavicular blocks. For other brachial plexus block techniques, the threshold can be more liberal due to the ability to control the bleeding/hematoma by compression and especially with the added ability of ultrasound imaging to detect and more predictably avoid vascular structures. No specific consensus recommendations are available, regarding the coagulation status for superficial blocks, and the clinical decision rests upon the anesthesiologist's clinical experience, judgment and meaningful discussion of risks, and benefits with the patient and the multidisciplinary team.

5. Explain the anatomy relevant to brachial plexus blocks and discuss common approaches. How to choose a specific approach for a specific patient and procedure? What is the potential risk of each approach?

The brachial plexus is formed by the ventral primary rami of the C5-T1 spinal nerves (also called nerve roots) [2]. Five

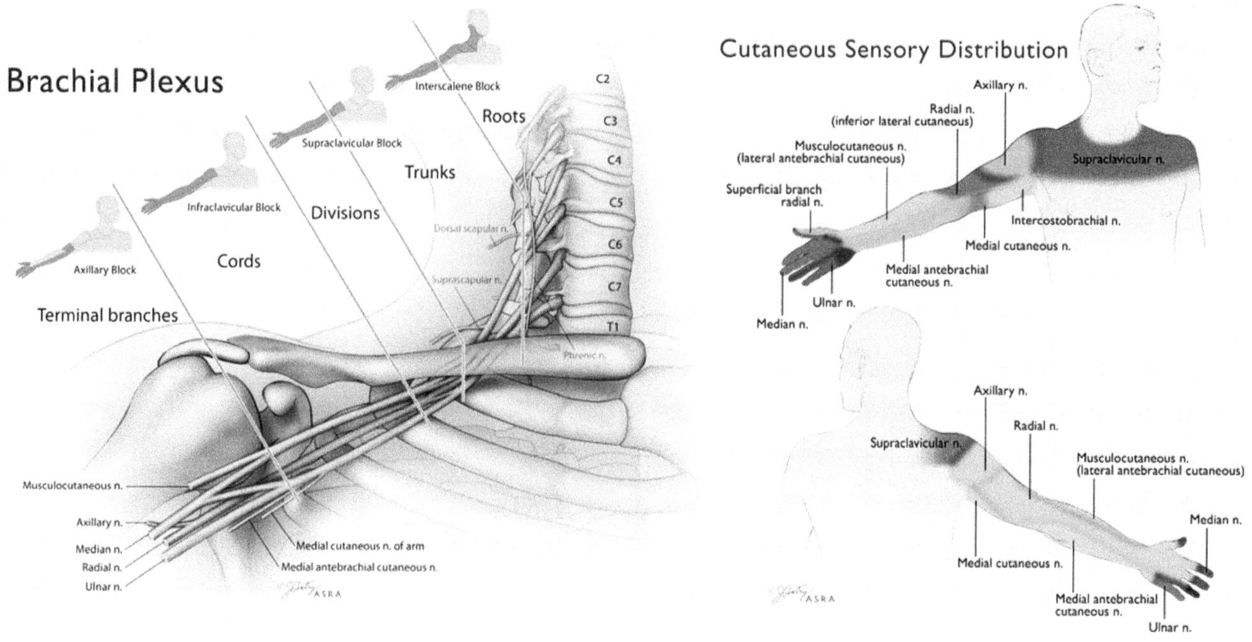

Fig. 47.1 Anatomy of brachial plexus and cutaneous nerve supply [2]. With permission of Wolters Kluwer

Table 47.1 Common brachial plexus blocks—surgical area and specific complications

Common brachial plexus blocks	Area of injury/surgery	Specific complications
Interscalene (roots and trunks)	Shoulder, upper arm	Diaphragmatic paralysis (phrenic nerve), recurrent laryngeal nerve block, intraarterial injection (vertebral artery), intrathecal injection, Horner's syndrome, C8-Th1 sparing
Supraclavicular (trunks and divisions)	Arm, forearm	Pneumothorax, diaphragmatic paralysis (phrenic nerve), bleeding (rich vasculature)
Infraclavicular/Retroclavicular (cords)	Arm, forearm, hand	Pneumothorax, bleeding (noncompressible), discomfort during placement
Axillary block (terminal branches)	Forearm, hand	Hematoma (superficial), musculocutaneous nerve spare (anterolateral aspect of forearm)

nerve roots unite, divide, and form trunks, divisions and cords as they travel through the neck and form terminal branches (Fig. 47.1).

The plexus provides motor and sensory innervation to the upper extremity, except for part of the cutaneous sensory innervation to the inner surface of the upper arm (intercostobrachial nerve—T2-3 intercostal nerves) and sensory cutaneous innervation to the top of the shoulder and the medial clavicle (cervical plexus C2-4).

The brachial plexus blocks are classified by the approach (anatomysite) of needle access to the plexus (Table 47.1).

The choice of technique is primarily dependent on the area of injury and surgery, but is also influenced by the inherent specific risks and individual patient anatomy. Logically, the proximal approaches (e.g., interscalene block) cover more predictably the proximal upper extremity (shoulder), whereas the more distal ones (e.g., axillary block) cover the forearm and hand more completely. Notably, the proximal part of the brachial plexus is in close proximity to many vital structures such as the phrenic nerve, vertebral artery, and pleura, and blocks at that level may be associated with rare, but serious complications such as pneumothorax, intraarterial injection or permanent hemidiaphragmatic paralysis. At the same time, transient deficits such as short-lived phrenic nerve block, Horner's or voice hoarseness are common and usually tolerated well. Logically, the most distal approach, which still covers the surgical area, is usually chosen to avoid such complications (Table 47.1).

Beside specific complications, brachial plexus blocks still also carry the general risks of peripheral nerve blocks including nerve injury, systemic local anesthetic toxicity, infection, hematoma, pain/discomfort during the block, and block failure.

6. Why most BPB are relatively contraindicated in severe pulmonary disease? What is the alternative choice of nerve block for postoperative analgesia?

Most proximal BPB approaches are associated with variable incidence of transient hemidiaphragmatic paralysis (phrenic nerve block), resulting in up to 30% reduction of pulmonary function [2]. Healthy individuals may experience mild shortness of breath, but usually tolerate these subclinical changes well. However, in patients with limited pulmonary reserve, such as severe COPD, this may lead to respiratory failure.

The interscalene brachial plexus block is associated with close to 100% incidence of hemidiaphragmatic paralysis. Even the supraclavicular and infraclavicular blocks are also associated with 34–50% and 14% reported incidence of hemidiaphragmatic block, respectively [3, 4]. The safest approach for patients with respiratory compromise is the axillary block, which carries no such risk. For shoulder surgery, a study showed that suprascapular nerve block provides significant shoulder analgesia and opioid sparing [5] without diaphragmatic function involvement. Even though its analgesic effect is not as complete as interscalene block, the suprascapular nerve block is a safe alternative technique for postoperative analgesia after shoulder surgery.

7. What should be communicated with the surgical team before proceeding to the block? What are some relevant perioperative concerns?

Interdisciplinary communication is essential for best patient care. Specific details that should be addressed before the block (and before the case, in general) include:

- Need for postoperative neurological tests, especially for fractures, surgical interventions, and hardware placement in immediate proximity to nerves and major blood vessels. If preexisting or iatrogenic nerve injury is a likely concern, the regional anesthesia block could be performed postoperatively, after a neurological examination. However, a postoperative block may be more challenging due to patient position, discomfort and cooperation, surgical dressing, and tissue edema. Preoperative catheter placement without local anesthetic injection and bolus with local anesthetics after the operation and satisfactory examination may be considered, especially in anatomically challenging patients.
- Need for intraoperative nerve stimulation—sometimes, especially in cases where injury or/and subsequent scarring has disrupted normal anatomy, intraoperative nerve stimulation could be helpful in identifying nerve structures. Proximal plexus block does not impair the ability to obtain motor response from stimulation distal to the level of the block. Logically, in such cases, neuromuscular blockers should be avoided.
- Concerns for postoperative acute compartment syndrome (ACS). Early signs and symptoms of acute compartment syndrome include disproportional pain, paresthesia, and paresis before developing limb ischemia. Neural blockade intends to produce analgesia, numbness and motor weakness—signs and symptoms similar to these of ACS, which may make such diagnosis more difficult. The anesthesiologist should discuss the specific risks and benefits with the surgical team, especially in high-risk patients, which include patients with fractures of leg or forearm, younger patients (age <35 years) and male patients [6, 7]. The use of peripheral nerve blocks for patients at risk for ACS remains controversial and is the subject of an ongoing debate. To mitigate the risks of "masking" warning signs and symptoms, nerve blocks should be followed by vigilant monitoring for ACS, including compartment pressure monitoring, and close communication with the surgical team should be maintained. Short-acting local anesthetics may be used for anesthesia/analgesia while allowing for rapid recovery of nerve function, continual testing, and monitoring. Low concentrations of local anesthetics should be used for analgesia to avoid "dense" motor blocks [8].

8. Would you perform a brachial plexus block with ultrasound (US) guidance, nerve stimulator (NS), or landmark with paresthesia? What is the evidence in support of US utilization over NS?

- Ultrasound-guided peripheral nerve blocks are associated with higher success rate, quicker block onset, reduced number of needle passes, lower local anesthetic dose requirements/use, and improved detection and avoidance of intraneural and intravascular injection [9]. However, since the incidence of nerve injury is extremely low (1.5:10,000), studies have failed to prove a difference between ultrasound-guided and conventional techniques [10].

9. Is it safe to perform peripheral nerve blocks outside the OR? Is there any benefit to perform the block in the block room?

Peripheral nerve blocks can be performed safely outside the operating room as long as the environment meets the minimal standard requirements to perform regional anesthesia. The designated area (block room) must have standard equipment not only to perform the block, but also for monitoring for and resuscitation from potential complications such as oversedation or local anesthetics systemic toxicity (LAST). The block room should also be staffed by a nurse or other medical personnel with perioperative experience and training to monitor the patient's vital signs and mental status after the block. According to ASRA recommendations, patients should be monitored (standard ASA monitoring—noninvasive blood pressure, oxygen saturation, and electrocardiography) during the block and for at least 30 min after the injection due to the risk of immediate (from intravascular injection) and delayed (from uptake, overdose) local anesthetic systemic toxicity [11]. Resuscitation equipment (oxygen, suction, and airway equipment) and medications, including 20% lipid emulsion (Intralipid), should be at hand and preferably organized in a cart or kit.

Block rooms allow the surgeon and anesthesiologist to perform parallel work without excessive production pressure. Moreover, evidence shows the availability of block room and dedicated regional anesthesia service not only improves OR efficiency, but may also lead to decreased OR cost and decreased hospital length of stay in ambulatory patients [12], while enhancing residency education due to more teaching time and increased residents' exposure to regional anesthesia by more than 400% [13].

10. If the patient develops ventricular tachycardia and cardiovascular collapse within seconds after supraclavicular block with 0.5% bupivacaine 30 ml, what should the differential diagnosis, immediate management, and prevention be?

Classic manifestations of local anesthetics systemic toxicity (LAST) begin with CNS toxicity (agitation, auditory change, drowsiness, mental status change, and progressing to generalized clonic-tonic seizures) before CVS toxicity (hypertension, tachycardia, ventricular arrhythmias, conduction block, decreased contractility, and asystole). However, some commonly used local anesthetics such as bupivacaine, ropivacaine, and even levobupivacaine have a narrow window of transition from CNS to CVS toxicity (low CC/CNS ratio); therefore, manifestations of cardiac toxicity without prodromal signs and symptoms of CNS toxicity or simultaneous presentation of CNS and CVS toxicity can also occur, especially in the context of sedatives administration. **LAST** should be considered **first** and should determine the initial response and treatment, if cardiac arrhythmia, cardiovascular instability and cardiac arrest happens during or immediately after nerve block.

Management [11]:
- Prompt and effective airway management to prevent hypoxia and acidosis
- Seizure control with benzodiazepine or low dose propofol
- Start lipid emulsion therapy at the first sign of LAST
  Dose:
  - 1.5 ml/kg 20% lipid emulsion bolus and 0.25 ml/kg/min infusion at least 10 min after circulatory stability is attained
  - If circulatory stability is not attained, consider rebolusing and double infusion rate
  - Approximately 10 ml/kg lipid emulsion for 30 min is recommended as the upper limit for initial dosing
- If cardiac arrest occurs, initiate ACLS. If epinephrine is used, small initial doses (10–100 mcg) are preferred, due to concern for arrhythmogenicity and animal studies, which showed and epinephrine had poorer outcomes with usual doses of epinephrine and vasopressin in local anesthetics induced cardiac arrest, when compared to lipid emulsion (vasopressin is not recommended)

Prevention:
Two major mechanisms of LAST are excessive uptake (overdose) or inadvertent intravascular injection; the risk of these can be diminished by
- observing the maximum recommended doses for the different local anesthetics, for example total bupivacaine dose should not exceed 2.5 mg/kg [14]
- taking into consideration the vascularity of the block site and the anticipated local anesthetic absorption (e.g., intercostal > caudal > brachial plexus) to modify local anesthetic dose and timing
- minimizing the risks of intravascular injections:
  - incremental injection of local anesthetic, 3–5 ml at a time, with continuous weak aspiration while advancing needle and before each injection
  - adding epinephrine to local anesthetics at 2.5–5 mcg/ml (i.e., 1/400,000–1/200,000) as a marker for intravascular injection
  - ultrasound guidance is shown to decrease the risk of vascular injury and may reduce the likelihood of intravascular injections

11. A patient complains of shortness of breath, 30 min after a supraclavicular BPB:
    - What is the differential diagnosis? What should be done to confirm the diagnosis? What is the recommended management?

If the patient has underlying cardiac and respiratory problems, but develops the symptoms after the procedure, the differential diagnosis can be classified into two broad categories by etiology—procedure-related and comorbidity-related:

- Procedure-related complications
  - Pneumothorax

Signs and symptoms: pleuritic chest pain during a deep inspiration is common; history of a challenging nerve block, multiple needle passes, or difficult needle visualization, cough or positive air aspiration during the block are suggestive clues. Physical examination may reveal decreased breath sounds on auscultation and hyperresonant percussion sounds on the suspected side. However, physical examination may not be able to detect a small pneumothorax

Diagnostic assessment: traditional investigation includes a chest X-ray to find radiolucent area without lung markings, visible visceral pleural line or mediastinal shift, or lung collapse in a severe case. Limitations include the time needed to obtain a quality chest X-rays and their interpretation; chest X-ray may also be insufficiently sensitive to detect a small pneumothorax.

Thoracic ultrasound is another modality that can detect pneumothorax and many lung pathologies. Ultrasound is portable, available in most operating rooms and provides immediate bedside information. Additionally, studies show that apical thoracic ultrasound scans have superior sensitivity (100%) and specificity (100%) for the detection of post-procedure pneumothorax compared to chest X-ray. The positive sign of pneumothorax includes loss of lung sliding of the pleura (B mode) and loss of "seashore" sign (M mode) [15] (Fig. 47.2). However, information from ultrasound is operator-dependent and needs practice for scanning and interpretation.

Management [16]:

- Surgical team should be consulted for evaluation and management, including possible chest tube placement.
- Patient must be observed and monitored for signs and symptoms of respiratory distress and a follow-up chest X-ray should be done in next 2–3 h.
- Oxygen administration may facilitate the air absorption.
- If the patient becomes symptomatic or the size of pneumothorax becomes larger or needs mechanical ventilation, a chest tube placement is required.

Generally, a small closed pneumothorax will be spontaneously absorbed, and a healthy individual may tolerate it well without a chest tube. In fact, there is a suspicion that the incidence of asymptomatic pneumothorax complications related to nerve block and central line placement might be higher than reported, due to lack of routine testing in asymptomatic patients. However, a patient with underlying pulmonary disease may not tolerate pneumothorax to any extent, and a chest tube may be needed earlier before the patient's condition deteriorates.

– Diaphragmatic paralysis:

Signs and symptoms: patients usually complain of shortness of breath in supine position, and paradoxical movements of epigastrium may be observed.

Diagnostic assessment: Radiographic signs of diaphragmatic paralysis include one-sided diaphragmatic elevation on chest X-ray and paradoxical diaphragmatic movement during the inspiration on fluoroscopy.

Thoracic ultrasound at the lower intercostal space can diagnose diaphragmatic paralysis by detecting the absence of excursions with breathing and the presence of paradoxical motion on sniffing [17]. However, information on ultrasound is operator-dependent and needs practice for scanning and interpretation.

Management: Diaphragmatic paralysis will resolve when the effect of local anesthetic wears off. Supportive treatment by positioning patient in a more upright position, administrating oxygen, and observing respiratory status are usually sufficient. However, a patient with underlying pulmonary disease may develop respiratory failure and need ventilation support or intubation.

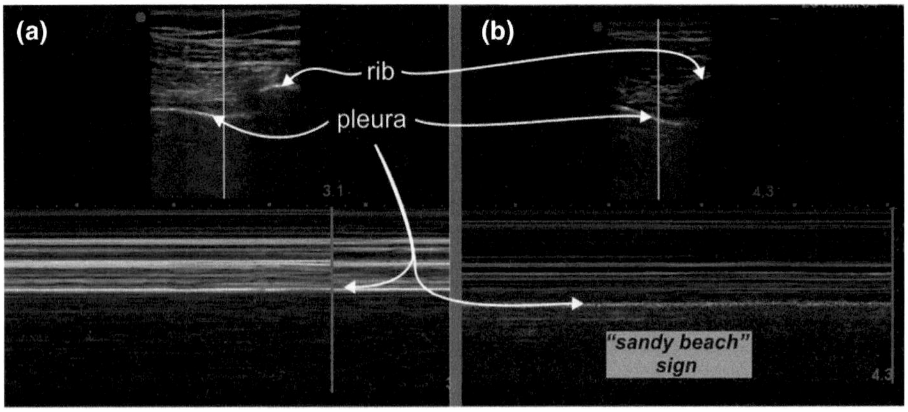

Fig. 47.2 Thoracic ultrasound image in M mode of pneumothorax (*left*) and normal lung (*right*).The normal lung finding (*right*) are streaks of multiple *horizontal lines* running parallel from the top of the screen to the *bright-white pleural line* in the middle of the screen and granular appearing below the pleural line (*sandy beach or seashore sign*). Pneumothorax finding (*left*) are streaks of horizontal lines run above and below pleural line (*barcode sign*). From [27], with permission of Wolters Kluwer

- Comorbidity-related:

In patients with complex underlying cardiopulmonary disease who develop acute distress, the diagnostic considerations should include COPD with acute exacerbation, atelectasis, aspiration, and acute heart failure of ischemic or nonischemic etiology. Detailed knowledge of the patient's history and constructing a comprehensive differential diagnosis is critical for timely treatment, including respiratory and cardiovascular support, while specific options dependent on the potential causative pathology (such as bronchodilators or diuretics) are determined with specialized consultative help.

12. Skin incision made 45 min after a supraclavicular block with 0.5% bupivacaine 30 ml. Patient unable to move his arm, but complaining of pain during incision. What are the differential diagnosis and management?

Onset of Bupivacaine and Ropivacaine for peripheral nerve block is 15–30 min (10–15 min for lidocaine and mepivacaine) [18]. At the 45-min time point, bupivacaine should already attain the full effect. Sensation tests of upper extremities, especially the surgical site, will provide more information about sparing the area as follows:

Cutaneous sensation remains intact in the medial aspect of the upper arm: This area is fully or partially innervated by the intercostobrachial nerve (T2 nerve root) and is not covered by a brachial plexus block. The intercostobrachial nerve is a cutaneous nerve, and a supplemental block can be easily done by subcutaneous infiltration of the skin at the medial aspect of the arm in axilla. If the surgical incision involves the medial aspect of the arm, an intercostobrachial block should be done with a brachial plexus block from the start. However, if the surgical field was already prepped and draped, the surgeon can do supplemental skin infiltration on the medial aspect of arm, either proximal to the incision or at the incision site.

Cutaneous sensation intact in other areas: An incomplete block can occur with an interscalene block (lower plexus-C8, Th1 roots sparing—**ulnar**, medial brachial cutaneous, medial antebrachial cutaneous nerves, plus parts of median and radial nerves) and axillary block (musculocutaneous nerve distribution; anterolateral aspect of forearm). As a supraclavicular block is performed at the divisions over the first rib, where the brachial plexus is relatively compact, it usually results in complete anesthesia of the entire upper extremity. However, many factors, including technical difficulty and anatomical variations, can contribute to an incomplete block or failure. Additional bolus of local anesthetics though an indwelling BPB catheter and supplemental skin infiltration by the surgical team, and systemic analgesic/sedative are usually sufficient for a small area of "block-sparing." A rescue peripheral nerve block can be done, but there is a theoretical concern about nerve injury when performing nerve blocks in an anesthetized area (even if incompletely anesthetized) [19]. Finally, if the rescue management is not sufficient, conversion to general anesthesia may be necessary.

13. The patient has complete analgesia of the right upper extremity. Operation is performed with the application of a tourniquet and is uneventful for the first 2 h, then patient complains of pain in the arm. What is the explanation?

Prolonged application of tourniquet causes tissue ischemia and accumulation of inflammatory mediators such as potassium and hydrogen ions, producing intense nociceptive stimulation, and "tourniquet pain". Unlike somatic surgical pain, which is transmitted both through A-delta and C-fibers, the transmission pathway for ischemic pain is mainly via C-fibers [20, 21].

A-delta are small myelinated fibers and more sensitive to local anesthetic block than non-myelinated C-fibers. In other word, conduction of pain through C-fibers is more resistant to nerve block and will return earlier when the block starts to wear off. This is a plausible explanation of why the patient may experience dull aching pain in the anesthetized area after a prolonged tourniquet application.

Tourniquet pain is ultimately relieved by releasing the tourniquet; however, if critical for the procedure, administration of systemic analgesics or sedation may temporarily alleviate the pain till safe deflation is possible.

14. The operation goes on uneventfully and patient is pain free in the recovery room. The supraclavicular catheter is infused with 0.2% bupivacaine at 6 ml/h. However, 20 h later, the patient complains of severe pain around the elbow. What should the management response be?

The event of adequate anesthesia and analgesia from the initial local anesthetic bolus via the block needle, but failed analgesia from the catheter can be called secondary failure and is not uncommon (reportedly, 10–26% for upper extremity blocks). In one study, a slightly higher incidence of failure was found in supraclavicular catheters (26%), compared to infraclavicular catheters, presumably due to less stable surrounding tissue and more movement [22].

The causes of secondary failure of peripheral nerve catheter include initial catheter malposition, catheter migration, dislodgement, obstruction, leakage, disconnect, or infusion pump malfunction. Troubleshooting should start from checking the infusion pump and catheter site, catheter depth/length markings at skin, followed by sensory and motor testing. If the catheter migrated in, it can be adjusted by pulling it out to minimum depth of 1–3 cm (1 cm for single orifice and 3 cm for multi orifice catheters) beyond the original (needle) depth from skin to plexus (target). If the pump and catheter work properly, but the patient has an area of intact sensation, the catheter can be bolused with 5–10 ml of 0.1–0.2% bupivacaine (analgesic concentration of local anesthetics) and reassess after an appropriate wait period (30 min). If the pain is improved after the bolus, the infusion rate may be increased to prevent pain from an inadequate amount of local anesthetics later.

15. Thirty minutes after adjusting the catheter and a supplemental bolus of 0.2% bupivacaine 10 ml through the catheter, the patient has decreased sensation in the whole upper extremity but still reports worsening severe pain.

What are your concern and pain management response?

Breakthrough pain in the setting of effective regional anesthesia block (sensory and/or motor) indicates serious pathology. Several case reports describe patients with severe pain through functioning peripheral nerve blocks before developing full-scale acute compartment syndrome (ACS) [8, 23–26].

Acute compartment syndrome is a consequence of elevated pressures in confined fascial spaces, leading to neurovascular compromise and ultimately to tissue necrosis. Similar to the ischemic effect from the application of a tourniquet, the intense nociception is resistant to an analgesic dose of local anesthetics. The patient may have complete skin numbness and even motor weakness, but still be in severe pain [8]. Signs and symptoms of ACS include pain, pallor, paresthesia, paralysis and pulselessness. However, only pain out of proportion and pain on passive movement are consistently early signs for diagnosis before irreversible tissue damage starts to occur.

Once ACS is suspected, an orthopedic/trauma surgery team should be called to evaluate the patient with the acute pain team.

In the case of an incipient ACS, initial management includes releasing the cast or circumferential dressing and close monitoring for signs of ischemia and follow-up intracompartmental pressure. Established ACS is an urgent limb-threatening condition, and delays with diagnosis and fasciotomy are associated with poor outcomes. Fasciotomy should be promptly done ideally before or immediately after tissue perfusion is compromised.

A peripheral nerve block for a patient who is at risk for ACS is still a debatable issue, due to concern that the block can mask the pain and delay the diagnosis. However, the pain from ischemic pain originates from the strong noxious stimuli and should not be blocked with an analgesic dose of local anesthetics (0.1–0.2% ropivacaine at 4–6 ml/h) [8]. Moreover, pain through a working nerve block can be an early warning sign of ACS. The best practices for peripheral nerve block for a patient who is at risk for ACS requires close communication and mutual understanding between the surgical team, the anesthesia team and the patient, regarding the risks and benefits of regional anesthesia signs and symptoms of ACS, safe and effective analgesic closes of local anesthetics and other available pain management modalities.

References

1. Horlocker TT, Wedel DJ, Rowlingson JC, Enneking FK, Kopp SL, Benzon HT, Brown DL, Heit JA, Mulroy MF, Rosenquist RW, Tryba M, Yuan CS. Regional anesthesia in the patient receiving antithrombotic or thrombolytic therapy: American Society of Regional Anesthesia and Pain Medicine Evidence-Based Guidelines. 3rd ed. Reg Anesth Pain Med. 2010 Jan–Feb;35(1):64–101.
2. Neal JM, Gerancher JC, Hebl JR, Ilfeld BM, McCartney CJL, Franco CD, Hogan QH. Upper extremity regional anesthesia essentials of our current understanding, 2008. Reg Anesth Pain Med. 2009;34:134–70.
3. Mak PH, Irwin MG, Ooi CG, Chow BF. Incidence of diaphragmatic paralysis following supraclavicular brachial plexus block and its effect on pulmonary function. Anaesthesia. 2001;56 (4):352–6.
4. Petrar SD, Seltenrich ME, Head SJ, Schwarz SK. Hemidiaphragmatic paralysis following ultrasound-guided supraclavicular versus infraclavicular brachial plexus blockade: a randomized clinical trial. Reg Anesth Pain Med. 2015 Mar–Apr;40(2):133–8.
5. Singelyn FJ, Lhotel L, Fabre B. Pain relief after arthroscopic shoulder surgery: a comparison of intraarticular analgesia, suprascapular nerve block, and interscalene brachial plexus block. Anesth Analg. 2004 Aug;99(2):589–92, table of contents.
6. Elliott KG, Johnstone AJ. Diagnosing acute compartment syndrome. J Bone Joint Surg Br. 2003;85(5):625–32.
7. McQueen MM, Gaston P, Court-Brown CM. Acute compartment syndrome. Who is at risk? J Bone Joint Surg Br. 2000;82(2): 200–3.
8. Aguirre JA, Gresch D, Popovici A, Bernhard J, Borgeat A. Case scenario: compartment syndrome of the forearm in patient with an infraclavicular catheter, breakthrough pain as indicator. Anesthesiology. 2013;118:1198–205.
9. Chan V, Abbas S, Brull R, Perlas A. Outcome data. In: Chan V, editor. Ultrasound imaging for regional anesthesia, a practical guide booklet. 2nd ed.
10. Jeng CL, Torrillo TM, Rosenblatt MA. Complications of peripheral nerve blocks. Br J Anaesth. 2010;105(Suppl 1):i97–107.
11. Neal JM, Bernards CM, Butterworth JF IV, Di Gregorio G, Drasner K, Hejtmanek MR, Mulroy MF, Rosenquist RW, Weinberg GL. ASRA practice advisory on local anesthetic systemic toxicity. Reg Anesth Pain Med. 2010 Mar–Apr;35(2):152–61.
12. Armstrong KP, Cherry RA. Brachial plexus anesthesia compared to general anesthesia when a block room is available. Can J Anaesth. 2004;51(1):41–4.
13. Martin G, Lineberger CK, MacLeod DB, El-Moalem HE, Breslin DS, Hardman D, D'Ercole F. A new teaching model for

resident training in regional anesthesia. Anesth Analg. 2002;95 (5):1423–7.
14. Freck E, Braveman F. Local anesthetics. In: Urman R, Vadivelu N editors. Pocket pain medicine. Philadelphia: Lippincott Williams & Wilkins; 2011.
15. Reissig A, Kroegel C. Accuracy of transthoracic sonography in excluding post-interventional pneumothorax and hydropneumothorax. Comparison to chest radiography. Eur J Radiol. 2005;53 (3):463–70.
16. Gupta S, Hicks ME, Wallace MJ, Ahrar K, Madoff DC, Murthy R. Outpatient management of postbiopsy pneumothorax with small-caliber chest tubes: factors affecting the need for prolonged drainage and additional interventions. Cardiovasc Intervent Radiol. 2008 Mar–Apr;31(2):342–8.
17. Sarwal A, Walker FO, Cartwright MS. Neuromuscular ultrasound for evaluation of the diaphragm. Muscle Nerve. 2013;47(3):319–29.
18. Gadsden J. Local anesthetics: clinical pharmacology and rational selection. In: Hadzic A, editor. Hadzic's peripheral nerve blocks and anatomy for ultrasound-guided regional anesthesia. New York, NY: McGrawHill Medical; 2012.
19. Neal JM, Bernards CM, Hadzic A, Hebl JR, Hogan QH, Horlocker TT, Lee LA, Rathmell JP, Sorenson EJ, Suresh S, Wedel DJ. ASRA practice advisory on neurologic complications in regional anesthesia and pain medicine. Reg Anesth Pain Med. 2008 Sep–Oct;33(5):404–15.
20. Kam PC, Kavanagh R, Yoong FF. The arterial tourniquet: pathophysiological consequences and anaesthetic implications. Anaesthesia. 2001;56(6):534–45.
21. MacIver MB, Tanelian DL. Activation of C fibers by metabolic perturbations associated with tourniquet ischemia. Anesthesiology. 1992;76(4):617–23.
22. Ahsan ZS, Carvalho B, Yao J. Incidence of failure of continuous peripheral nerve catheters for postoperative analgesia in upper extremity surgery. J Hand Surg Am. 2014;39(2):324–9.
23. Cometa MA, Esch AT, Boezaart AP. Did continuous femoral and sciatic nerve block obscure the diagnosis or delay the treatment of acute lower leg compartment syndrome? A case report. Pain Med. 2011;12:823–8.
24. Munk-Andersen H, Laustrup TK. Compartment syndrome diagnosed in due time by breakthrough pain despite continuous peripheral nerve block. Acta Anaesthesiol Scand. 2013;57 (10):1328–30.
25. Walker BJ, Noonan KJ, Bosenberg AT. Evolving compartment syndrome not masked by a continuous peripheral nerve block: evidence-based case management. Reg Anesth Pain Med. 2012;37:393–7.
26. Kucera TJ, Boezaart AP. Regional anesthesia does not consistently block ischemic pain: two further cases and a review of the literature. Pain Med. 2014;15(2):316–9.
27. Edrich T, Pojer C, Fritsch G, Hutter J, Hartigan PM, Stundner O, Gerner P, Berger MM. Utility of intraoperative lung ultrasonography. A A Case Rep. 2015;4(6):71–4.

Part X
Obstetrics

Section Editor: Jie Zhou

Jie Zhou
Department of Anesthesiology, Brigham and Women's Hospital,
Boston, MA, USA

48 Labor and Delivery

Vesela Kovacheva

This morning, a 31-year-old nulliparous woman presents for labor after spontaneous rupture of the membranes. Other than mild asthma treated occasionally with an albuterol inhaler, her pregnancy has been unremarkable. Her last meal was 1 h ago. She requests an epidural.

Medications:	Prenatal vitamins, dailyAlbuterol, as needed
Allergies	No known drug allergies
Past Medical History	Mild asthma

Physical exam

Vital signs	Heart rate 86/min, Blood Pressure 98/62 mmHg, Respirations 22/min, Oxygen Saturation 98%
Lungs	Clear to auscultation, no wheezing
Heart	Regular rate and rhythm, no murmurs
Back	No scoliosis

1. **What are the indications/contraindications for labor epidural?**

The epidural is a very safe and efficient technique for pain control during labor.

Indications:

- Patient's request. Historically, the placement of epidural was advised only after the parturient has reached certain cervical dilation, since it was once believed that the procedure may increase the rate of cesarean delivery. Since this belief has never been proven, an epidural can be placed at any stage of the labor [1].
- Established labor, defined as regular contractions, which results in cervical dilation.
- Lack of contraindications.

Contraindications:

- Patient's refusal or inability to cooperate.
- Coagulation disorders—thrombocytopenia, concurrent use of anticoagulants, DIC, or other causes of coagulopathy—which pose increased risk of epidural hematoma.
- Infection—localized, at the site of insertion or untreated systemic infection—which pose risk of introducing the infection to the CNS.
- CNS space-occupying lesion associated with increased intracranial pressure—tumor, cyst, or vascular malformation—which pose risk of brain herniation in the case of dural puncture.
- Lack of training, experience of the personnel, or inadequate staffing—which prevent the safe placement and monitoring 24/7 of parturients with epidural analgesia.

The epidural placement may be technically challenging in patients with lumbar scoliosis, especially in the presence of spinal instrumentation, high BMI, advanced labor and history of previous difficult placement.

2. **What are the advantages/disadvantages of the epidural?**

Advantages:

- The best method for pain control during labor.
- High level of maternal satisfaction.
- Very low fetal exposure to medications.

V. Kovacheva (✉)
Department of Anesthesiology, Perioperative and Pain Medicine, Harvard Medical School, Brigham and Women's Hospital, 75 Francis St. CWN L1, Boston, MA 02115, USA
e-mail: vkovacheva@partners.org

© Springer International Publishing AG 2017
L.S. Aglio and R.D. Urman (eds.), *Anesthesiology*,
DOI 10.1007/978-3-319-50141-3_48

- Ability for fast and safe conversion to anesthesia if urgent/emergent instrumental vaginal or cesarean delivery is needed.

Disadvantages:

- Risk of complications.
- Offered mostly at hospitals that have 24/7 obstetric anesthesia staffing.
- Need to maintain IV access and bladder drainage (usually using Foley catheter) throughout labor.
- Potential confinement of the parturient to the hospital bed due to concern for motor block.
- Recovery period after the delivery for the motor and sensory block to resolve.

3. **What are the complications of epidural analgesia?**

The complications of the epidural include:

- Uneven block, multiple attempts, and failed epidural necessitating replacement. This commonly happens in about 10% of all epidural placements and can be related to technical difficulties (scoliosis, maternal inability to cooperate, inexperienced operator), suboptimal location of the epidural catheter tip (for example, due to migration), and unknown reasons.
- Accidental intrathecal or intravascular placement. This puts the patient at risk for high block and total spinal anesthesia (if intrathecal catheter) or intravascular injection of high dose of local anesthetic (if intravascular catheter). In the case of dural puncture, there is a risk for post-dural puncture headache.
- Extensive or prolonged block. This usually happens if there is a high concentration and high dose of local anesthetic used.
- Neurological injury, epidural abscess, and epidural hematoma. The incidence of these complications is extremely rare, but since any of these can be permanent and devastating, much attention should be paid on proper technique and monitoring for these complications.

4. **What are the side effects of epidural analgesia?**

- Pruritus due to the administration of epidural opioid. The cause of this side effect is largely unknown, but possibly related to central activation of opioid mu-receptors. Usually, this type of pruritus is transient and thus requires no intervention; if necessary it can be treated with opioid antagonists (naloxone), partial agonists–antagonists (nalbuphine), or antihistamines (diphenhydramine).
- Nausea and vomiting. The incidence of nausea and vomiting during labor, even in the absence of epidural analgesia, is quite high due to multiple mediators. However, the presence of epidural opioid elevates the risk even higher. Thus, a possible prevention in patients with prior history of nausea and vomiting due to opioids is omission of the opioid from the epidural solution. Alternatively, if it has already developed, this side effect can be treated with antiemetics in the absence of contraindications.
- Urinary retention commonly results from blockage of the sympathetic and parasympathetic fibers innervating the bladder. Most laboring women are catheterized even if they are not receiving epidural analgesia. However, in the latter case, if there is evidence of bladder distention and no Foley catheter, the bladder should be drained.
- Maternal hypotension due to sympathetic block and decreased systemic vascular resistance. In the case of uteroplacental insufficiency, the maternal drop in blood pressure may also be associated with fetal bradycardia. The incidence of these events depends on the strength and dosage of the epidurally injected compounds and prior fetal well-being. In order to minimize the risk of these events, frequent maternal blood pressure checks are recommended, especially after placement and epidural boluses. Prompt treatment with repositioning of the mother (uterine displacement, Trendelenburg position), intravenous fluids (500–1000 ml crystalloid solution bolus) and/or vasopressor (phenylephrine and/or ephedrine) usually result in quick improvement.
- Fever. Many studies have shown a higher incidence of fever in women receiving epidural analgesia during labor. The cause for this temperature elevation is unknown. However, these patients have a higher incidence of evaluation and treatment of chorioamnionitis and a higher incidence of instrumental vaginal or cesarean delivery.
- Reactivation of Herpes simplex virus. The cause of this is unknown and there are only a few studies reporting association with neuraxial opioids.

5. **Besides the epidural, are there any other options for neuraxial analgesia?**

In addition to epidural, the armamentarium of the obstetric anesthesiologist for labor neuraxial analgesia involves combined spinal epidural (CSE), dural puncture epidural (DPE), and continuous spinal analgesia. CSE is established by finding the epidural space using large, usually

17 gauge epidural needle. With needle through needle technique, the anesthesiologist will insert a smaller, usually 25 or 27 gauge spinal needle through the epidural needle to perform single shot spinal, after which the epidural catheter is threaded. The CSE technique offers fast onset, high quality analgesia, better sacral spread compared to epidural; however, there is a slightly higher incidence of nausea, itching, and hypotension compared to the epidural. In addition, due to the initial comfort provided by the spinal component, the detection of suboptimal epidural catheter may be delayed. DPE is performed similarly to the CSE but without the injection of spinal medication. This technique offers improved sacral spread of the epidural medications and is considered advantageous if the neuraxial analgesia is requested late in labor. Continuous spinal analgesia is used if there is an unintentional dural puncture or if an epidural cannot be placed for technical reasons. It is associated with high quality block, but the disadvantages include higher risk for PDPH, hypotension, pruritus, catheter malfunction and risk for total spinal analgesia.

6. **Are there any alternatives to the neuraxial analgesia?**

The alternatives to neuraxial analgesia are pharmacologic and non-pharmacologic. Pharmacologic agents for labor control include intravenous opioids, ketamine, dexmedetomidine and inhaled nitrous oxide. Opioid analgesics can be administered as a bolus (meperidine, morphine, fentanyl, nalbuphine) or patient-controlled analgesia (fentanyl, remifentanil). The latter may provide a high quality labor analgesia, however, it is still inferior compared to epidural analgesia [2]. Overall, opioids provide temporary pain relief, but their use is limited by maternal and fetal side effects including nausea, somnolence, disphoria, hypoxia, and fetal bradycardia. Dexmedetomidine infusion or bolus has been described and is an option when neuraxial analgesia is not indicated, however, sedation and bradycardia are possible side effects [3, 4]. Nitrous oxide has recently become an option for labor analgesia in the US, but has been used for many years in other countries like Great Britain. It is self-administered by the parturient as an inhaled gas in 50% oxygen mix in the beginning of each contraction. In most cases, it is not potent enough to be used throughout labor [5], but can help in the early stages or while neuraxial anesthesia is being placed.

Non-pharmacologic means of pain control during labor include emotional support by spouse or friend, massage therapy, hypnotherapy, hydrotherapy, and doulas. A doula is an individual that accompanies the parturient during her labor and provides emotional and spiritual support. Most non-pharmacologic methods can safely be used alongside neuraxial anesthesia and enhance the overall satisfaction of the parturient.

7. **What is the basis of the pain in childbirth?**

The origin of labor pain is quite complex and currently an area of active research. During the first stage of labor, as the uterus contracts and the cervix progressively dilates, multiple stretch receptors are activated in the uterine wall. The sensory afferents travel via spinal nerves to T10-L1 segments of in the spinal cord. This pain is visceral, dull, and difficult to localize. During the second stage of labor, the expulsive efforts of the mother result in distention of the perineum and vagina. The stretch receptors in these areas are innervated by S2–S4 spinal cord segments. The pain is somatic, sharp, and easily localized. The perception of labor pain is highly individualized experience, modulated by numerous hormonal, emotional, social, cultural, and religious factors.

8. **In two hours after uneventful epidural placement, you are called in the labor room due to pain. What do you do?**

A bedside pain consult should include assessment of the location, intensity and duration of the pain, the sensory block level using cold or pinprick, maternal vital signs, labor progress, and the fetal well-being. If there is no sensory block and the epidural catheter at the skin is shallower than when placed, it is likely that the catheter has migrated outside of the epidural space and will need to be replaced. If the sensory block level is low or unequal and the location of the epidural catheter at the skin is unchanged, the likely cause of pain may be insufficient amount of anesthetic. A higher volume of local anesthetic in the form of an epidural bolus should be given and the parturient position could be changed so that the side that has the most pain is dependent. If the sensory level is adequate, and the labor is in the early stage, a higher concentration of local anesthetic could be given. If the sensory level is adequate but the labor progression is approaching the second stage, administering a neuraxial opioid, e.g., fentanyl, may be a better choice. Giving local anesthetic at this point may result in a motor block and interfere with maternal expulsive efforts. In all cases, the maternal and fetal well-being will need to be assessed and emergencies like uterine dehiscence, uterine rupture, and placental abruption will need to be excluded. In cases when the epidural is bolused, frequent checks of the maternal vital signs will need to be done to allow for early detection of hypotension.

9. **In one hour after the epidural was optimized, you are called at the bedside due to non-reassuring fetal heart rate (FHR). What is fetal heart rate monitoring (FHM) and what do you do about it?**

FHM is continuous, intrapartum recording of the fetal heart rate in relation to uterine contractions over time. The rationale is to detect changes in fetal heart rate as a sign of deterioration and, via instituting timely interventions, to prevent adverse outcomes. It is believed that various intrapartum events like fetal hypoxemia, hypoperfusion, and hypercarbia lead to fetal acidemia. Acidemia, in turn, activates the carotid chemoreceptors that send impulses to the medulla and lead to vagal activation in the fetus, leading to bradycardia. In this way, change in fetal heart rate can be an early sign of fetal compromise.

When looking at a FHM recording, the following needs to be evaluated:

- Uterine contractions—recorded at the bottom of the strip, normal is less than five contractions over a 10 min period. A higher frequency of uterine contractions is called uterine tachyphylaxis and this usually results from labor augmentation with oxytocin. It can compromise placental perfusion and lead to fetal acidemia.
- Baseline FHR—the mean heart rate over a 10 min period. Normal FHR is between 110 and 160 beats per minute. Fetal tachycardia can be caused by infection, early stages of acidemia, prematurity, multiple gestations, anemia, hyperthyroidism, and fetal heart anomalies. Fetal bradycardia is associated with administration of some medications like beta blockers and opioids, maternal hypotension, profound anemia, and prolonged academia. Sustained fetal bradycardia may result in fetal demise.
- Accelerations—short, transient cycles of FHR increase by 5–10 beats per minute and prompt return to baseline in less than 2 min. These result from the interplay of fetal sympathetic and parasympathetic nervous system and are a sign of well-being.
- Decelerations—short periods of FHR decrease more than 15 beats per minute and prompt return to baseline. In relationship to the uterine contractions, the decelerations can be:
  - Early decelerations—the nadir of the deceleration coincides with the peak of the uterine contraction and usually results from fetal head compression and mild hypoxia.
  - Late decelerations—the nadir of the deceleration happens in about 10 s after the peak of the uterine contraction, commonly a result from maternal hypotension, medications, or uteroplacental insufficiency
  - Variable decelerations—the occurrence of these decelerations is not related to the uterine contractions, these are usually abrupt, can be in the shape of the letters ‘U’, ‘V’, or ‘W’, irregular, have sharp edges and result from umbilical cord compression.

Based on evaluating the significance of all these characteristics of the FHM, the National Institute of Child Health and Human Development in 2008 established three categories to guide further management [6].

- Category one: includes normal baseline FHR, presence of accelerations, presence or absence of early decelerations. It is very reassuring, sign or normal fetal well-being and requires no further intervention.
- Category two: multiple abnormal FHR which do not belong in category one or three, including minimal baseline variability, recurrent variable decelerations and recurrent late decelerations. It is usually not a sign of fetal compromise, but requires careful monitoring, consideration of further tests to assure fetal status, correction of maternal fever, hypotension or bradycardia.
- Category three: includes sustained fetal bradycardia and absence of variability. It necessitates prompt attempts to resolve, as above, and if it still persists, usually instrumental or cesarean delivery will be initiated.

When called at the bedside in the setting of deteriorating FHR, the anesthesiologists can correct contributing maternal factors like hypotension, bradycardia, or hypoxia. If decision for instrumental or cesarean delivery is made, the epidural level needs to be assessed, and, if necessary, optimized to achieve surgical anesthesia. Since the parturient airway can change as the labor progresses [7], preparation for difficult airway should also be considered in case that neuraxial anesthesia is suboptimal.

10. **Four hours after a healthy boy has been delivered via vacuum and the epidural pulled, the obstetrician requests ‘a little sedation’ so that he can do manual exploration due to continued bleeding at the bedside. What do you do?**

The anesthetic considerations will need to be discussed with the obstetrician. The operating room will be a better location for such case since there are more resources and better equipment. Moreover, sedation will not be the best choice in a patient with possible difficult airway and aspiration risk. If feasible, a spinal anesthesia should be considered and if not, the patient will need general anesthesia and rapid sequence intubation.

11. **After uneventful spinal in the operating room, the obstetrician requests help with uterine relaxation for extraction of retained products. Which agents can you use?**

The best choice in this situation is intravenous nitroglycerin 40–100 mcg. It has a fast onset of action, short duration, and excellent safety profile. Alternatively, administering inhalational anesthetic in 2.0–3.0 MAC will be successful, however, this will require endotracheal intubation.

References

1. American College of Obstetricians and Gynecologists, Committee on Obstetric Practice: ACOG committee opinion. No. 339: Analgesia and cesarean delivery rates. Obstet Gynecol 2006;107:1487–8.
2. Stocki D, Matot I, Einav S, Eventov-Friedman S, Ginosar Y, Weiniger CF. A randomized controlled trial of the efficacy and respiratory effects of patient-controlled intravenous remifentanil analgesia and patient-controlled epidural analgesia in laboring women. Anesth Analg. 2014;118:589–97.
3. Palanisamy A, Klickovich RJ, Ramsay M, Ouyang DW, Tsen LC. Intravenous dexmedetomidine as an adjunct for labor analgesia and cesarean delivery anesthesia in a parturient with a tethered spinal cord. Int J Obstet Anesth. 2009;18:258–61.
4. Elterman KG, Meserve JR, Wadleigh M, Farber MK, Tsen LC. Management of labor analgesia in a patient with acute myeloid leukemia. A A Case Rep. 2014;3:104–6.
5. Likis FE, Andrews JC, Collins MR, Lewis RM, Seroogy JJ, Starr SA, Walden RR, McPheeters ML. Nitrous oxide for the management of labor pain: a systematic review. Anesth Analg. 2014;118:153–67.
6. Macones GA, Hankins GD, Spong CY, Hauth J, Moore T. The 2008 National Institute of Child Health and Human Development workshop report on electronic fetal monitoring: update on definitions, interpretation, and research guidelines. Obstet Gynecol. 2008;112:661–6.
7. Kodali BS, Chandrasekhar S, Bulich LN, Topulos GP, Datta S. Airway changes during labor and delivery. Anesthesiology. 2008;108:357–62.

Preeclampsia

49

Dan Drzymalski

Case

A 26-year-old G1P0 parturient at 32 weeks gestation presents to the labor and delivery floor with a severe headache and onset of contractions.

Physical Exam:
Visibly uncomfortable from labor pain
Mild crackles bilaterally on auscultation
Regular rate and rhythm

Vital Signs:
BP: 190/112 mmHg
HR: 115/min
RR: 26/min
O_2: 99% on room air

Labs:
Platelet count: 85,000/mm^3
2 + proteinuria on urinalysis

__Questions__:

What is preeclampsia?

Preeclampsia is a clinical syndrome whose primary distinguishing features include new onset hypertension and proteinuria after 20 weeks' gestation. The disease can be categorized as either mild preeclampsia (BP ≥ 140/90 mmHg, proteinuria 300 mg/24 h) or severe preeclampsia (BP ≥ 160/110 mmHg, proteinuria 5 g/24 h). Other symptoms include headache, visual disturbances, epigastric or right upper quadrant pain, as well as fetal symptoms (e.g., intra-uterine growth restriction) [1].

Is proteinuria necessary for a diagnosis of preeclampsia?

No. The Task Force Report on Hypertension in Pregnancy by The American College of Obstetricians and Gynecologists published in November 2013 reported that the absence of proteinuria should not exclude a diagnosis of preeclampsia. Parturients without proteinuria who present with persistent epigastric or right upper quadrant pain, persistent cerebral symptoms, fetal growth restriction, thrombocytopenia, and elevated serum liver enzyme concentrations should be evaluated for possible preeclampsia. Waiting for development of proteinuria may delay delivery of optimal care [2].

What is HELLP syndrome?

The acronym of HELLP stands for: Hemolysis, Elevated Liver enzymes, and Low Platelets. Hemolysis can be recognized by abnormal peripheral blood smear and anemia. Laboratory studies reveal AST ≥ 70 IU/L and platelet count less than 100,000/mm^3. Parturients with HELLP syndrome are at an increased risk for peripartum morbidity, including DIC, placental abruption, and preterm delivery [1].

What are risk factors for developing preeclampsia?

Risk factors for developing preeclampsia include obesity, chronic hypertension, diabetes mellitus, and metabolic syndrome. The risk of preeclampsia doubles with each 5 to 7 kg/m^2 increase in body mass index from pre-pregnancy values. The presence of preexisting chronic hypertension triples the risk of developing preeclampsia. Diabetes mellitus is associated with a twofold increased risk of developing preeclampsia [3].

D. Drzymalski (✉)
Department of Anesthesiology, Perioperative and Pain Medicine, Brigham and Women's Hospital, 75 Francis Street, Boston, MA 02115, USA
e-mail: dandrzymalski@gmail.com

© Springer International Publishing AG 2017
L.S. Aglio and R.D. Urman (eds.), *Anesthesiology*,
DOI 10.1007/978-3-319-50141-3_49

What might be a good prophylactic medication for preeclampsia?

Preeclampsia is associated with relatively excessive levels of thromboxane compared to prostacyclin. Thromboxane plays an important role in vasoconstriction and one hypothesis suggests that preeclampsia may be caused by excessive placental thromboxane production. It has been suggested that aspirin could prevent preeclampsia because aspirin inhibits synthesis of thromboxane A_2.

Nevertheless, randomized controlled trials have not found aspirin to be superior to placebo in the prevention of preeclampsia [1].

What are your considerations for placing an epidural for labor analgesia?

Since preeclampsia can be associated with thrombocytopenia, it is important to consider the risks and benefits of placing a labor epidural. Mild preeclampsia in the setting of normal platelet count is not a contraindication for neuraxial labor analgesia and early epidural placement may improve uteroplacental perfusion. Women with severe preeclampsia and thrombocytopenia are at an increased risk for epidural or spinal hematoma. It is important to consider, however, that they are also at an increased risk for emergency Cesarean delivery. The decision to place a labor epidural will ultimately have to be based on each individual patient's clinical situation [1].

Would you place a combined spinal–epidural (CSE) for labor analgesia in this patient?

There are many advantages and disadvantages of a CSE in a laboring parturient with preeclampsia. The main advantage of a CSE is rapid onset of analgesia, which can instantaneously help to decrease the hypertensive response to pain. However, the primary disadvantage of a CSE is the inability to evaluate epidural catheter function after resolution of spinal analgesia. Given the increased risk of emergency Cesarean delivery in the preeclamptic patient, a standard epidural technique may be more favorable because it can be immediately verified and provides a means for rapid induction of epidural anesthesia [1].

What is the minimum platelet count for performing a neuraxial technique in the preeclamptic patient?

Simply considering a "minimum" platelet count for performing a neuraxial technique in the preeclamptic parturient is inadequate for assessing the risk of epidural hematoma. Generally speaking, parturients with mild preeclampsia and a platelet count greater than 100,000/mm^3 do not need further evaluation prior to neuraxial technique. Women with a platelet count less than 100,000/mm^3 may require additional coagulation studies, including PT, PTT, and fibrinogen levels. The trend in platelet count is more important than the absolute platelet count. With a rapid decline, the nadir in platelet count is difficult to predict and may complicate the neuraxial technique. Regardless, parturients with HELLP syndrome and a platelet count less than 50,000/mm^3 are at an increased risk of bleeding and general anesthesia may be required [1, 4].

Is delivery of the child a "cure" for preeclampsia?

Although delivery of the child and placenta are often called the "cure" for preeclampsia, the risks of preeclampsia continue for several days postpartum. These risks include pulmonary edema, cerebrovascular accident, venous thromboembolism, and eclampsia. In fact, pulmonary edema is more likely to occur during the postpartum period because of the marked fluid shifts that occur with delivery of the child. Furthermore, approximately 5% of parturients are found to have postpartum onset of preeclampsia. Therefore, preeclamptic patients need to be closely monitored during the postpartum period before discharging them from the hospital [5].

Would you place an arterial catheter in this patient?

Parturients who present with mild preeclampsia may not need an arterial catheter, but these patients should be closely monitored for progression of the disease. Preeclamptic parturients who have poorly controlled blood pressure and require rapid titration of vasodilators will likely require arterial line placement. Parturients with severe preeclampsia, who require induction of general anesthesia for Cesarean delivery or frequent blood gas measurements, may also require invasive blood pressure monitoring [1].

The patient requires a general anesthetic for STAT Cesarean delivery. What are your concerns with laryngoscopy?

Cerebrovascular accident is the leading cause of death in preeclamptic parturients. The risk of intracranial hemorrhage is particularly high during laryngoscopy and intubation due to the hypertensive response to the procedure. Severely hypertensive parturients will require an arterial catheter for close hemodynamic monitoring prior to induction of general anesthesia. Labetalol should be administered prior to induction until the blood pressure is approximately 140/90. If the hemodynamic goal cannot be attained with labetalol alone, additional antihypertensive medications, including infusions of nitroprusside and/or nitroglycerin, should be strongly considered [1].

The patient has been on magnesium sulfate infusion for seizure prophylaxis. What are your concerns?

Because magnesium sulfate decreases the sensitivity of the neuromuscular junction for acetylcholine, one of the primary concerns is prolonged duration of nondepolarizing muscle relaxants. If general anesthesia is required, doses should be decreased and a peripheral nerve stimulator should be used to carefully monitor return of twitches. On the other hand, the duration of action of succinylcholine is not increased and standard doses should be used for intubation [6].

The obstetrician states the uterus is boggy and requests uterotonics. Which medications are contraindicated in preeclampsia?

The preeclamptic patient may exhibit significant peripartum hemorrhage secondary to uterine atony. Methylergonovine maleate (i.e., methergine, an ergot alkaloid) is an excellent medication for uterine contractility. However, methergine can also cause significant increases in both pulmonary and systemic vascular resistance, leading to pulmonary and systemic hypertensive crisis due to its effects on serotonergic, dopaminergic, and alpha-adrenergic receptors. Therefore, methergine is generally contraindicated in preeclampsia [1].

A preeclamptic parturient with HELLP syndrome presents with acute right upper quadrant abdominal pain and severe hypotension. What are your concerns?

Patients with HELLP syndrome are at an increased risk for rupture of subcapsular hematoma of the liver. Ultrasonography can confirm the diagnosis and emergent surgical intervention is required. Since the most common causes of death include coagulopathy and exsanguination, this patient will require transfusions of both red blood cells and fresh frozen plasma. Emergency laparotomy is necessary to save the life of the mother, but the mortality rate is still very high [1].

What is placental abruption?

Placental abruption is an abnormal separation of the placenta from the uterus prior to delivery of the child. Bleeding is a major complication of placental abruption. It is important to remember that the bleeding may be concealed in the uterus, leading to underestimation of blood loss and delayed diagnosis. Placental abruption is also complicated by coagulopathy, further increasing blood loss. Parturients with abruption will require careful monitoring and early transfusion [7].

Does a patient with preeclampsia have an increased risk of placental abruption compared to an otherwise healthy parturient?

The risk of placental abruption in preeclamptic parturients is approximately triple compared to healthy parturients. Given that placental abruption is associated with a higher risk of DIC and that preeclampsia is already associated with coagulopathy, these parturients are at a particularly high risk for large blood loss during the peripartum period [8].

What may be the cause of cerebral edema in a parturient with preeclampsia?

Cerebral edema is a complication of preeclampsia that may be caused by loss of cerebral autoregulation. In the setting of excessive hypertension, endothelial dysfunction results in hyperperfusion and formation of interstitial edema. Intravenous fluids should be minimized to decrease the risk of exacerbating the cerebral edema [1].

References

1. Chestnut DH. Chestnut's obstetric anesthesia: principles and practice. 5th ed, ed. 1 online resource (xiii, 1267 pages) p.
2. American College of O, Gynecologists, Task Force on Hypertension in P. Hypertension in pregnancy. Report of the American College of Obstetricians and Gynecologists' Task Force on Hypertension in Pregnancy. Obstet Gynecol. 2013;122(5):1122–31. PubMed PMID: 24150027.
3. O'Brien TE, Ray JG, Chan WS. Maternal body mass index and the risk of preeclampsia: a systematic overview. Epidemiology. 2003;14(3):368–74.
4. Halpern SH, Douglas MJ. Evidence-based obstetric anesthesia. Malden: BMJ Books: Blackwell Pub.; 2005. xi, 243 p.
5. Matthys LA, Coppage KH, Lambers DS, Barton JR, Sibai BM. Delayed postpartum preeclampsia: an experience of 151 cases. Am J Obstet Gynecol. 2004;190(5):1464–6.
6. Turner JA. Diagnosis and management of pre-eclampsia: an update. International journal of women's health. 2010;2:327–37. PubMed PMID: 21151680. Pubmed Central PMCID: 2990902.
7. Longnecker DE, Brown DL, Newman MF, Zapol WM. Anesthesiology. 2nd ed. ed. 1 electronic text (xxi, 1748 pages) p.
8. Lindqvist PG, Happach C. Risk and risk estimation of placental abruption. Eur J Obstet Gynecol Reprod Biol. 2006;126(2):160–4.

50 Abruptio Placenta and Placenta Previa

Annemaria De Tina and Jie Zhou

CASE Called stat by obstetrician for a 29-year-old female patient who is presenting pregnant at 30 weeks gestation with fetal bradycardia, vaginal bleeding, and complaining of abdominal pain.

Medications:	Prenatal vitamins
	Iron Supplementation
Allergies:	NKA
Past Medical History:	Gestational GERD
	Iron Deficiency anemia
Physical Exam:	Vital Signs: BP 110/60, HR 105 bpm, RR 30/min, oxygen saturation 99%.
	Patient appears anxious, slow trickle of bright red blood from vagina.
Cardiac:	Regular rhythm, grade 2/6 systolic ejection murmur heard only at left sternal boarder
Otherwise:	insignificant

1. **What are the four major causes of antepartum hemorrhage? What are the incidences of each?**

The major causes of antepartum hemorrhage include placenta previa, placental abruption, uterine rupture, and vasa previa. Placenta previa occurs when the placenta implants over the cervical os. This implantation may be marginal, partial, or total in its covering of the os. The incidence of placenta previa is 4.0 per 1000 pregnancies [1]. Placental abruption refers to the complete or partial separation of the placenta from the uterine wall before delivery of the fetus. The incidence of placental abruption varies with the population studied 3–10 per 1000 pregnancies [2]. Uterine rupture following previous vaginal delivery has an incidence of 0.18 per 1000 pregnancies. This increases significantly to 9 per 1000 pregnancies in women who have had a previous cesarean section [3]. When fetal vessels have a velamentous insertion over the cervical os, the fetal vessels are not protected by the umbilical cord or the placenta. This is diagnosed as vasa previa and has a traditionally reported incidence of 1 in 2500 to 1 in 5000 [4, 5].

2. **What are the risk factors for placenta previa, placental abruption, and uterine rupture?**

The risk factors for placenta previa and placental abruption were studied in over 16 million pregnancies, in the United States, from 1995–2000. Risk factors for placenta previa include advanced maternal age, multiparity, and history of Cesarean delivery. Notably, these risk factors exist *prior* to pregnancy. Risk factors for placental abruption include conditions occurring *during* pregnancy: cigarette smoking, alcohol intake, preterm premature rupture of membranes, and chorioamionitis [6–8].

3. **What are the risk factors for uterine rupture?**

The most common risk factor for uterine rupture is previous Cesarean section or uterine surgery [9]. Other reported risk factors include induction of labor, macrosomia ≥4 kg, gestational age greater than 42 weeks, maternal age over 35, and short maternal stature [3]. Uterine rupture is rare but catastrophic and requires prompt identification and management.

4. **What are normal vital signs for a pregnant patient in her third trimester?**

Normal baseline heart rate (HR) increases up to 25% during pregnancy (by 10–20 bpm on average), however maternal tachycardia is still defined as HR ≥100 bpm [10–12]. Blood pressure (BP) slowly decreases from the first to

A. De Tina (✉) · J. Zhou
Department of Anesthesiology, Perioperative and Pain Medicine, Harvard Medical School, Brigham and Women's Hospital, Boston, MA 02115, USA
e-mail: detinaa@mcmaster.ca

J. Zhou
e-mail: jzhou5@partners.org

© Springer International Publishing AG 2017
L.S. Aglio and R.D. Urman (eds.), *Anesthesiology*,
DOI 10.1007/978-3-319-50141-3_50

second trimester but returns to back to baseline by term gestation [13]. Maternal hypertension is defined as BP ≥ 140/90 [14].

Respiratory rate does not increase significantly with pregnancy, despite a 40% increase in tidal volume and a 30–50% increase in minute ventilation. Tachypnea (RR ≥ 20 bpm) should be considered abnormal in the pregnant patient [15]. Oxygen saturation should remain normal in a pregnant patient at sea level and mild altitude [15].

5. **What are the cardiovascular physiologic changes seen in pregnancy and what is the most likely etiology of the murmur?**

The parturient undergoes a number of physiologic changes with impact on the cardiovascular system. There is a notable decrease in afterload as well as increase in cardiac output, heart rate, and stroke volume. These adaptive hemodynamic changes are likely triggered by an early fall in systemic vascular tone in pregnancy [16]. There is no significant change in pulmonary capillary wedge pressure, central venous pressure, left ventricular stroke work index, or mean arterial pressure [11]. In order to accommodate for the increase in plasma and stroke volume, the left ventricle dilates and hypertrophies. There is an increase in myocardial contractility by the second trimester [17].

The 50% increases in cardiac output and plasma volume may be difficult to tolerate if a pregnant patient has valvular heart disease. The increase in cardiac output worsens myocardial oxygen demand, exacerbates CHF, and the low SVR may decrease coronary perfusion, causing myocardial ischemia. The drop in SVR may also be significant in women with shunt pathology or congenital heart defects [18]. Labor contractions can rapidly increase the already increased cardiac output. During the second stage of labor cardiac output can increase by an additional 50% [11].

Up to 90% of women will develop a systolic ejection murmur during pregnancy. They are commonly heard best at the second left intercostal space or along the left sternal border. These murmurs are related to the alterations of blood flow through normal valves and can be attributed to the increase in blood volume, cardiac output, and blood velocity [19].

6. **What are the four classes of hemorrhagic shock and how much blood will this pregnant patient lose before she becomes hypotensive?**

Based on the ATLS hemorrhagic shock classification (Table 50.1) [20], a healthy pregnant patient will not show signs of hypotension until Class III shock, or 30% of blood loss. In a 70 kg term gestation pregnant patient who has a 50% increase in plasma volume this means that the patient may have up to 2 L of blood loss before she displays signs of tachycardia and hypotension.

7. **What are some clinical signs to indicate this patient is in hemorrhagic shock?**

In practice, staff physicians, residents, and nurses are grossly inaccurate at estimating blood loss after vaginal or cesarean delivery. There tends to be an underestimation which only gets worse with increasing blood loss [21]. Care providers should rely on the clinical picture of the patient to guide fluid and resuscitation management. Clinical signs of severe hemorrhagic shock include decreased urine output, altered mental status (confusion, anxiety, and lethargy), tachypnea, decreased pulse pressure and the late signs of tachycardia and hypotension [20].

Table 50.1 The ATLS classification of hypovolemic shock [20]

	Class I	Class II	Class III	Class IV
Blood loss in %	<15	15–30	30–40	> 40
Pulse rate	<100	100–120	120–140	>140
Blood pressure	Normal	Normal	Decreased	Decreased
Pulse pressure	Normal or increased	Decreased	Decreased	Decreased
Respiratory rate	14–20	20–30	30–40	>35
Mental status	Slightly anxious	Mildly anxious	Anxious, confused	Confused, lethargic
Urine output (ml/h)	>30	20–30	5–15	Negligible
Fluid replacement	Crystalloid	Crystalloid	Crystalloid and blood	Crystalloid and blood

With permission of the American College of Surgeons

8. **What are the immediate steps in management of this patient?**

This patient has multiple emergent issues that must be concurrently diagnosed and treated in the immediate management of this patient. Foremost, this patient is having ongoing vaginal bleeding and is showing early signs of hemorrhagic shock including tachycardia (HR > 100), tachypnea (RR > 20), and altered mental status (anxiety). There is also acute abdominal pain which may shed light into the etiology of the bleed. Finally, there are two patients to consider in this clinical scenario—the parturient and the fetus. Fetal bradycardia is an obstetric emergency and may indicate fetal hypoxia and/or impending death.

Obstetric, anesthesia and neonatal teams should be emergently called to the patient's bedside. The patient should be in a monitored setting with BP, HR, SpO_2, and ECG monitoring. 100% O_2 should be applied to this patient and two large bore IV's should be started above the diaphragm with initiation of a crystalloid bolus of 1–2 L. The patient should get urgent bloodwork including a complete blood count, coagulation profile, and type and crossmatch for potential blood transfusion. It may be appropriate at this time to call for blood products. Vital signs should be measured at minimum every 5 min including level of consciousness. Attempts should be made to keep the patient euthermic. The operating suite should be notified and prepared for an emergency cesarean delivery[22].

9. **If this patient's blood type is unknown, which type of blood should be given in an emergency resuscitation?**

This patient should receive type-O negative or uncross-matched packed red blood cells if crossmatched are not immediately available [23]. Type-AB fresh plasma and apheresis platelets should be given in an emergency-release transfusion if the patient's blood group is unavailable [24, 25]. If an Rh negative patient receives Rh positive platelets in an emergency transfusion, she should receive Rho(D) immune globulin afterwards.

The decision on when to transfuse plasma, platelets and cryoprecipitate should be guided by laboratory and clinical factors. Guidelines have recommended transfusion thresholds of platelet count $\leq 50 \times 10^9$/L, INR > 1.5, and fibrinogen < 1.0 g/L [22].

10. **Should this patient receive a general anesthetic or neuraxial anesthetic?**

In many obstetrical emergencies, the type of anesthetic must be individualized to the patient and clinical scenario. If the fetal heart rate is persistently bradycardic despite adequate resuscitation of the mother, or if the vaginal bleeding remains uncontrolled, an emergency "stat" cesarean delivery should be anticipated. In the setting of uncontrolled and uncorrected hypovolemia a general anesthetic may be favored. A neuraxial technique is contraindicated if the maternal hemorrhage persists to the point of suspected coagulopathy or DIC. The anesthesiologist should keep in mind the time required for induction of neuraxial anesthesia; with persistent fetal bradycardia a general anesthetic may be indicated [26].

11. **Which optimization techniques could be considered prior to induction of this patient?**

If time and the clinical situation permits, optimization of both the parturient and fetus should be explored. These optimization techniques should not delay delivery if there are maternal and/or fetal indications for emergency delivery [27, 28]. A 30 week fetus with threatened preterm labor can be optimized with corticosteroid therapy using either betamethasone 12 mg IM two doses 24 h apart or dexamethasone 6 mg IM four doses 12 h apart. This has been shown to reduce perinatal mortality, respiratory distress syndrome, and other morbidities in the infant [29].

Magnesium sulphate ($MgSO_4$) should be considered for women at ≤31 + 6 weeks with imminent preterm birth. It is dosed as 4 g IV load over 30 min then 1 g/hr infusion until birth for a maximum of 24 h. Risks and side effects of magnesium include muscle atony. An ominous sign is the loss of deep tendon reflexes. Uterine atony may lead to further bleeding postpartum. Fetal hypotonia and apnea may have implications for the neonatal care provider [27, 28].

This pregnant patient is at risk for pulmonary aspiration of gastric contents and should be given prophylaxis for aspiration pneumonitis. A combination of antacids (e.g., 30 mL of oral sodium citrate) plus H_2 antagonist (Ranitidine 50 mg IV) have been shown to prevent low gastric pH [30]. All women undergoing elective or emergency Casarean section should receive antibiotic prophylaxis [31].

12. **What are the 4 major classifications of postpartum hemorrhage? Which is the most common?**

A common way to think of the differential for postpartum hemorrhage (PPH) is the '*4 T's*.' **T**one—uterine atony or distended bladder. Uterine atony is the most common cause of PPH. **T**issue—retained tissue from the placenta or blood clots can cause persistent postpartum bleed and can also contribute to poor uterine tone. **T**rauma—lacerations to the vaginal wall, cervix, or uterine injury may contribute a significant amount of blood loss until appropriately repaired. **T**hrombin—a woman may have an undiagnosed coagulopathy presenting for the first time with childbirth, or it may be an acquired or consumptive coagulopathy [32]. DIC has been associated with placental abruption, placenta previa, amniotic fluid embolism, pre-eclampsia, HELLP syndrome, intrauterine fetal demise, intrauterine infection, and acute fatty liver of pregnancy [33].

13. **What are the risk factors for uterine atony?**

Uterine atony can be broken down into sub-categories in order to organize a differential and remember clinical risk factors. Over-distension of the uterus can be caused by polyhydramnios, multiple gestation, or macrosomia. Uterine muscle exhaustion may be secondary to rapid or prolonged labor, high parity and oxytocin use. Intra-amniotic infection should be suspected if there is maternal fever or prolonged rupture of membranes. Uterine abnormality risks include fibroids, placenta previa, bladder distension, or other anomaly. Finally, uterine-relaxing medications can lead to uterine atony including halogenated anesthetics and nitroglycerin [32].

14. **Name four pharmacologic interventions and four mechanical interventions that can be used to treat uterine atony**

Ongoing blood loss with decreased uterine tone requires administration of uterotonics. The following are recommended medications for the management of PPH due to atony:

Oxytocin 10 units IM or 10–40 units in 1 L of crystalloid run in continuously. Rapid undiluted IV boluses should be avoided because they can cause hypotension.

Methylergonovine (Methergine) 0.2 mg IM every 2–4 h can be used but avoided if the patient is hypertensive.

15-methyl PGF-2α (Carboprost or Hemabate) 0.25 mg IM every 15–90 min, 8 doses maximum. This should be avoided in asthmatic patients and is relatively contraindicated in hepatic, renal, and cardiac disease. Common side effects include diarrhea, fever, and tachycardia.

Dinoprostone (Prostaglandin E2) is a vaginal or rectal suppository of 20 mg every 2 h. It should be avoided if the patient is hypotensive. Fever is a common side effect.

Misoprostol (Cyotec, PGE1) 800–1000 mcg rectally [34].

References

1. Faiz AS, Ananth CV. Etiology and risk factors for placenta previa: an overview and meta-analysis of observational studies. J Matern Fetal Neonatal Med. 2003;13(3):175–90.
2. Ananth CV, et al. An international contrast of rates of placental abruption: an age-period-cohort analysis. PLoS ONE. 2015;10(5): e0125246.
3. Kaczmarczyk M, et al. Risk factors for uterine rupture and neonatal consequences of uterine rupture: a population-based study of successive pregnancies in Sweden. BJOG. 2007;114(10):1208–14.
4. Rao KP, et al. Abnormal placentation: evidence-based diagnosis and management of placenta previa, placenta accreta, and vasa previa. Obstet Gynecol Surv. 2012;67(8):503–19.
5. Oyelese KO, et al. Vasa previa: an avoidable obstetric tragedy. Obstet Gynecol Surv. 1999;54(2):138–45.
6. Yang Q, et al. Comparison of maternal risk factors between placental abruption and placenta previa. Am J Perinatol. 2009;26 (4):279–86.
7. Ananth CV, et al. Preterm premature rupture of membranes, intrauterine infection, and oligohydramnios: risk factors for placental abruption. Obstet Gynecol. 2004;104(1):71–7.
8. Ananth CV, et al. Placental abruption in the United States, 1979 through 2001: temporal trends and potential determinants. Am J Obstet Gynecol. 2005;192(1):191–8.
9. Walsh CA, Baxi LV. Rupture of the primigravid uterus: a review of the literature. Obstet Gynecol Sur. 2007;62(5):327–34.
10. Martin SR, Foley MR. Intensive care in obstetrics: an evidence-based review. Am J Obstet Gynecol. 2006;195(3):673–89.
11. Clark SL, et al. Central hemodynamic assessment of normal term pregnancy. Am J Obstet Gynecol. 1989;161(6 Pt 1):1439–42.
12. Sanghavi M, Rutherford JD. Cardiovascular physiology of pregnancy. Circulation. 2014;130(12):1003–8.
13. Iwasaki R, et al. Relationship between blood pressure level in early pregnancy and subsequent changes in blood pressure during pregnancy. Acta Obstet Gynecol Scand. 2002;81(10):918–25.
14. Magee LA, et al. Diagnosis, evaluation, and management of the hypertensive disorders of pregnancy: executive summary. J Obstet Gynaecol Can. 2014;36(7):575–6.
15. Bobrowski RA. Pulmonary physiology in pregnancy. Clin Obstet Gynecol. 2010;53(2):285–300.
16. Duvekot JJ, et al. Early pregnancy changes in hemodynamics and volume homeostasis are consecutive adjustments triggered by a primary fall in systemic vascular tone. Am J Obstet Gynecol. 1993;169(6):1382–92.
17. Robson SC, et al. Serial study of factors influencing changes in cardiac output during human pregnancy. Am J Physiol. 1989;256 (4 Pt 2):H1060–5.
18. Kaplan JA, Reich DL, Konstadt SN. Kaplan's cardiac anesthesia: expert consult premium. Elsevier Health Sciences; 2011.
19. Goldberg LM, Uhland H. Heart murmurs in pregnancy: a phonocardiographic study of their development, progression and regression. Dis Chest. 1967;52(3):381–6.
20. American College of Surgeons. Committee on Trauma. ATLS, advanced trauma life support for doctors: student course manual. American college of surgeons; 2008.
21. Stafford I, Dildy GA, Clark SL, Belfort MA. Visually estimated and calculated blood loss in vaginal and cesarean delivery. Am J Obstet Gynecol. 2008;199(5):519–e1.
22. Lyndon A, Lagrew D, Shields L, Main E, Cape V. Improving health care response to obstetric hemorrhage Version 2.0, in California Maternal Quality Care Collaborative 2015.
23. Main EK, et al. National Partnership for Maternal Safety: consensus bundle on obstetric hemorrhage. Anesth Analg. 2015;121(1):142–8.
24. Quraishy NJ, Cross AR. A compendium of transfusion practice guidelines. Washington DC: American Red Cross; 2010.

25. Gutierrez MC, et al. Postpartum hemorrhage treated with a massive transfusion protocol at a tertiary obstetric center: a retrospective study. Int J Obstet Anesth. 2012;21(3):230–5.
26. Chestnut DH. et al. Chestnut's obstetric anesthesia: principles and practice. Elsevier Health Sciences; 2014.
27. Magee L, et al. SOGC Clinical Practice Guideline. Magnesium sulphate for fetal neuroprotection. J Obstet Gynaecol Can. 2011;33 (5):516–29.
28. ACOG. Committee opinion no. 455: magnesium sulfate before anticipated preterm birth for neuroprotection. Obstet Gynecol. 2010;115(3):669–71.
29. ACOG. Committee Opinion No. 475: antenatal corticosteroid therapy for fetal maturation. Obstet Gynecol. 2011;117(2 Pt 1): 422–4.
30. Paranjothy S. et al. Interventions at caesarean section for reducing the risk of aspiration pneumonitis. Cochrane Database Syst Rev. 2014;2. Cd004943.
31. Smaill FM, Grivell RM. Antibiotic prophylaxis versus no prophylaxis for preventing infection after cesarean section. Cochrane Database Syst Rev. 2014;10, Cd007482.
32. Active management of the third stage of labour: prevention and treatment of postpartum hemorrhage: no. 235 October 2009 (Replaces No. 88, April 2000). Int J Gynaecol Obstet. 2010;108 (3):258–67.
33. Thachil J, Toh CH. Disseminated intravascular coagulation in obstetric disorders and its acute haematological management. Blood Rev. 2009;23(4):167–76.
34. ACOG Practice Bulletin. Clinical management guidelines for obstetrician-gynecologists number 76, October 2006: postpartum hemorrhage. Obstet Gynecol. 2006;108(4):1039–47.

Nonobstetric Surgery During Pregnancy

51

Jeffrey Huang

Case Report

A 26-year-old woman, Gravida 2, Para 1, was referred at 23-week gestation with acute abdominal emergency. Her past medical history was unremarkable. Her last obstetric visit was two weeks ago during her 20-week routine checkup. She had no previous history of any intra-abdominal procedure. The only medications are prenatal multivitamins, folate, and iron sulfate. Physical examination: vital signs were blood pressure 120/60 mmHg, heart rate 80/min, respiratory rate of 16/min and temperature of 97 °F. Her lungs, heart, and general appearance were all within normal limits for her gestation. Airway assessment showed Mallampati score of 2 with intact dentition, full range of neck motion and a thyromental distance of greater than 5 cm. White blood cell count was 18,600; other laboratory values were normal. Abdominal ultrasound showed cholelithiasis and gall bladder inflammation.

What is the incidence of surgery during pregnancy?

The incidence of nonobstetric surgery performed during pregnancy was estimated range from 0.3 to 2.2% [1, 2]. There are significant number of women who receive nonobstetric surgery during pregnancy. As many as 93,000 pregnant women in the United States may require surgery each year [3]. However, this numbers are probably underestimated because pregnancy is often unrecognized by both patient and physician during early pregnancy.

What is the incidence of positive pregnancy tests in women of childbearing age for elective surgery?

The incidence of positive pregnancy tests of menstruating women presenting for orthopedic surgery was 0.002% [4]. The incidence of previously unrecognized pregnancy in menstruating women presenting for ambulatory, nonobstetric surgery was 0.3% [5]. A significant number of women (2.6%) are already pregnant during elective sterilization procedures [6].

Should pregnancy tests offer to all women of childbearing age before surgery?

The UK National Patient Safety Agency documented that women should be offered a pregnancy test "if there is any possibility that a woman could be pregnant." The American Society of Anesthesiologists Task Force on Preanesthesia Evaluation recommended that preanesthesia pregnancy testing, "may be considered for all female patients of childbearing age," ASA advocates physicians and hospitals to implement their own policies and practices with regard to this. Many hospitals routinely carry out pregnancy tests on all women of childbearing age who are scheduled for elective surgery [4].

What is the common nonobstetric surgical procedure performed during pregnancy?

The most common first-trimester procedure was laparoscopy (34%), whereas appendectomy was the most common surgery in the second and third trimesters [1]. The common indications for nonobstetic surgery include acute abdominal disease, malignancies, and trauma [1]. The rate of major postoperative complications (such as infections, reoperation, wound problems, respiratory complications, venous thromboembolism, blood transfusion, maternal death) for nonobstetic surgery during pregnancy was about 6% [7].

The pregnant woman undergoes physiological adaptations to pregnancy. Briefly discuss these physiology changes.

What are the respiratory system changes in pregnancy?

Maternal alveolar ventilation is increased by 30% or more by mid-pregnancy and rises progressively to 70% at term [8].

J. Huang (✉)
Department of Anesthesiology, Anesthesiologists of Greater Orlando & University of Central Florida, 851 Trafalgar Court, Suite 300W, Maitland, FL 32751, USA
e-mail: jeffhuangmd@gmail.com

© Springer International Publishing AG 2017
L.S. Aglio and R.D. Urman (eds.), *Anesthesiology*,
DOI 10.1007/978-3-319-50141-3_51

There is a 20% decrease in functional residual capacity (FRC) at term as the uterus expands, which result in decreases oxygen reserve and potential for airway closure. Oxygen consumption increases significantly due to the development of placenta, fetus, and uterine muscle.

Because of decreased FRC, increased oxygen consumption, pregnancy women can develop rapid hypoxemia and acidosis from hypoventilation or apnea. Anesthetic requirement for inhalational agents is decreased up to 40% by the second trimester [9]. Possibility of anesthetic overdose is increased. Swelling and friability of oropharyngeal tissues can result in difficult intubation. Failed intubation is a leading cause of anesthesia-related maternal death.

What are the cardiovascular system changes in pregnancy?

Early in pregnancy, significant cardiovascular changes are demonstrated. By 8 weeks' gestation, a pregnant woman has a 57% of increase in cardiac output, 78% of the increase in stroke volume, and 90% of decrease in systemic vascular resistance [10]. Pregnant woman also has a 40–50% increase in blood volume and a 20% reduction in hematocrit due to dilution. Anemia begins during the first trimester of pregnancy and is most significant in the mid-second trimester. Inferior vena caval occlusion is also significant during second trimester, which can result in decrease cardiac output 30% [3]. Vena caval compression result in distention of the epidural venous plexus, therefore increase the possibility of local anesthetic toxicity during the administration of epidural anesthesia.

What are the gastrointestinal system changes in pregnancy?

Reduction of gastrointestinal motility and lower esophageal sphincter pressure, distortion of gastric and pyloric anatomy during pregnancy increase the risk for aspiration of gastric content [11]. It is unclear exactly at which point in gestation a pregnant woman becomes more prone to regurgitation and aspiration under anesthesia [3]. Any pregnant woman with acid reflux presentation should be considered at risk for aspiration.

Describe the altered responsiveness of pregnant women to anesthesia.

Intravenous induction agents: The dose of thiopental for anesthesia was 18% less in pregnant women of 7–13 weeks' gestation compared with the dose needed by nonpregnant women [12]. Whether the dose of propofol for anesthesia changed in pregnant women, the data was conflicting.
Muscle relaxants: Duration of action of succinylcholine is not prolonged in term pregnant women, although plasma cholinesterase levels decrease by 25% from early pregnancy until the seventh postpartum day [13]. Duration of nondepolarizing muscle relaxants was prolonged in pregnant women, because of changes of volume of distribution.
Inhalation agents: The minimum alveolar concentration (MAC) for volatile anesthetic agents was reduced 30–40% in pregnant women at early gestation as compared to non-pregnant women [14].
Regional anesthesia: The reduction of the epidural and subarachnoid spaces in pregnant women lead to more extensive spread of local anesthetic agents administered during central neuraxial blockade. Pregnancy increases the response to peripheral neural blockade. During pregnancy, nerve fibers have become more sensitive to the effects of local anesthetics or there is increased diffusion of the local anesthetic to the membrane receptor site.
Other drugs: The increased blood volume produces physiological hypoalbuminemia during pregnancy. Reduction of protein binding due to lower albumin and alpha-glycoprotein concentrations may result in greater chance of drug toxicity. In addition, because of limited information of pharmacokinetic and pharmacodynamics profiles during pregnancy, it is worthwhile to administer the drugs with caution.

What are the concerns for fetus when surgery is performed during pregnancy?

The potential effects of anesthetic agents as teratogens should be considered.

What are teratogens?

Teratogenicity is defined as any significant postnatal change in function or anatomy in an offspring after prenatal treatment [3].

Almost all commonly used anesthetics are teratogenic in some animal species. Anesthetic agents cause reversible decreases in cell motility, prolongation of DNA synthesis, and inhibition of cell division in mammalian cells experiments [3].

However, in order to induce a defect formation, a teratogenic drug must be given in an appropriate dosage, during a particular developmental stage of the embryo, in a species or individual with a particular genetic susceptibility [3]. Most scientists agreed that any drug can be teratogenic in an animal if enough is given at the right time. A small dose of a teratogen may cause structural abnormality or death in the susceptible early embryo, whereas much larger doses may demonstrate benign to the fetus [15].

Describe the systemic anesthetic drugs effect on animal fetus.

When mice were injected pentobarbital or phenobarbital, many anomalies were detected [16]. Thiamylal can cause growth suppressing defects in the offspring of mice [17]. Exposure of the immature brain of rodents to anesthetic agents such as propofol, thiopental, ketamine are related with brain cell apoptosis and functional deficiency [18, 19].

Methadone is teratogenic in mice [20]. In hamsters, the number of abnormal fetus from female injected with single dose of heroin, phenazocine, methadone enlarged when the maternal dose increased [21]. Morphine and meperidine produced an increase in the number of fetal abnormalities only to a certain dose level. The narcotic antagonists, nalorphine, naloxone, and levallorphan blocked the teratogenic effects [21]. Fentanyl, sufentanil, alfentanil were not teratogenic [22, 23].

Muscle relaxants do not cross the placenta. Muscle relaxants are difficult to test in vivo because of their respiratory effects. D-tubocurarine, pancuronium, atracurium, and vecuronium have been shown to be teratogenic only when at dose 30-fold greater than the paralyzing dose in humans [24].

Injection of lidocaine to pregnant rats did not result in an increased incidence of congenital anomalies or poor outcome [25]. Cocaine has been shown to be teratogenic in mice and rats [26].

Describe the systemic anesthetic drugs effects on human fetus.

Induction agents (barbiturates, ketamine, benzodiazepines) have not been shown to be teratogenic in human when they were used in clinical doses during anesthesia [27]. There is no change in the incidence of structural abnormality among offspring of pregnant women who use morphine or methadone [27].

It had been suggested the association between consumption of tranquilizers during pregnancy and an increased risk of cleft palate from three retrospective studies [28–30]. A new prospective study in 854 women who used diazepam during the first trimester did not show a higher risk of cleft palate [31]. The current consensus is that benzodiazepines are not teratogenic and a single dose appears safe. Because of concerns about increased risk of cleft palate, regular use, particularly in the first trimester, should probably be avoided [32].

Describe the inhalation anesthetic agents effects on animal fetus.

Nitrous oxide

Nitrous oxide is a weak teratogen in rodents. Rats continually exposed to 50–70% nitrous oxide for 2–6 days (starting on day 8 of gestation) had an increased incidence of fetal morphological abnormalities [33]. When rats exposed to 70% nitrous oxide or to a similar concentration of xenon for 24 h on day 9 of gestation, fetal resorption, skeletal anomalies, and macroscopic lesions occurred only in the nitrous oxide group [34]. Nitrous oxide resulted in growth retardation and an increased incidence of morphological abnormalities and altered body laterality in rats [35].

The possible mechanism of nitrous oxide teratogenicity is that nitrous oxide inhibits methionine synthetase. Nitrous oxide can affect DNA synthesis. Transmethylation from methyltetrahydrofolate to homocysteine to produce tetrahydrofolate (THF) and methionine is catalyzed by methionine synthase. Therefore, methionine synthase inhibition by nitrous oxide could decrease THF and reduce methionine level. Reduction of THF resulted in decrease in DNA synthesis. However, this description has been questioned. Folinic acid bypasses the effect of methionine synthase inhibition on THF synthesis. Administration of folnic acid partially (not completely) reduced the teratogenic effects of nitrous oxide in the rat [36]. Use of isoflurane or halothane with nitrous oxide prevents almost all of teratogenic effects but does not prevent inhibitory effects of nitrous oxide on methionine synthase activity [37]. Therefore, the etiology of nitrous oxide teratogenicity in rats remained to be determined.

Volatile agents

Halothane: In Mice, 3 h of halothane exposure evidently increased the incidence of cleft palates and paw defects [38]. In hamsters, 3 h of halothane exposure in midgestation increased the number of abortions [39].
Isoflurane: In mice, isoflurane exposure increased the incidence of cleft palate [40].
Sevoflurane or desflurane: Teratogenic effects of sevoflurane and desflurane have been studied. No evidence has suggested reproductive toxicity in clinical dose.

Describe the inhalation anesthetic agents effects on human fetus.

Human studies are more challenging to conduct. Prospective clinical studies are impractical, unethical. Human studies methods included retrospective epidemiologic surveys of adverse reproductive outcomes in groups chronically exposed to low levels of anesthetic gases or in women who have undergone surgery during their pregnancy.

What is the current data regarding the effects of trace concentrations of anesthetic gases on pregnancy?

These epidemiologic surveys had imperfections because of lack of comparable control groups, lack of details on duration and amounts of actual exposure, exposure to multiple environmental factors. These studies were limited by the small sample sizes, lack of a control group, and low response rate. These studies indicated that the incidence of miscarriage among the exposed women is approximately 25–30%

greater than nonexposed women. However this difference is almost insignificant because incidence of spontaneous abortions is increased 250% in pregnant women who take more than three alcoholic drinks daily [41], and 80% in pregnant women who are smokers [42]. A 10-year prospective survey of all female physicians in United Kingdom showed no difference in reproductive outcomes when anesthesiologists were compared with others working female physicians [43]. These epidemiologic studies do not support an increased risk for congenital anomalies with long-term exposure to low levels of anesthetic gases.

What about pregnant women who undergo a surgical procedure under anesthesia?

Studies were conducted in women who had surgery during pregnancy. Review medical records of 9073 obstetric patients showed there were 147 patients who had surgery during pregnancy. These 147 patients were compared to 8926 patients who delivered at the same time. The incidence of congenital anomalies was not significantly different between two groups [44]. Among the patients who had surgery during pregnancy, the incidence of preterm delivery followed surgery was 8.8%, and the incidences of perinatal mortality and low-birth-weight infants were increased [44]. Canada data showed that there was no significant difference in the incidence of congenital anomalies in 2565 women who had undergone surgery during pregnancy. There was an increased risk of spontaneous abortion in women undergoing surgery with general anesthesia in the first or second trimester [45]. Analysis of three Swedish health care registries data showed 5405 operations in the population of 720,000 pregnant women [1]. 2252 were performed in the first trimester, 65% received general anesthesia. The incidence of congenital malformations and stillbirths were not increased in the offspring of women having surgery. However, the incidences of very low and low-birth-weight infants were increased. No specific types of anesthesia were associated with increased incidence.

Anesthesia during pregnancy does not result in an overall increase congenital abnormality, but may increase risk of miscarriage.

During surgery, surgeon requested to perform intraoperative cholangiography. State the adverse effects of radiation on fetus.

Ionizing radiation is a human teratogen that can result in an increased, dose-related risk for the miscarriage, fetal growth restriction, congenital malformation, mental retardation, and increased risk for childhood malignant disease, and fetal death [46]. Radiation is measured as grays (Gy) or milligrays (mGy) and is calculated as cumulative dose throughout the entire pregnancy. Most researchers agree that a dose of below about 50 mGy in humans and animals represents no detectable noncancer risk to the embryo or fetus at any stage of gestation [47]. Direct radiographic examination of abdomen, pelvic, and abdominal imaging studies that include fluoroscopy may cause more significant fetal radiation exposure [48]. Animal study showed that radiation at level of 300–1000 mGy was associated with failure of implantation, abortion, growth retardation and central nervous system (CNS) effects [48]. A practical threshold for congenital effects in the human embryo or fetus is most likely between 0.10–0.20 Gy (10–20 rads) [47]. According to the Center of Disease Control and Prevention (CDC), cancer risk from prenatal radiation exposure is similar to, or slightly higher than, cancer risk from exposure in childhood [47].

However, if radiographic studies are necessary for the mother's condition, no other acceptable imaging study is available, testing should not be denied. Radiologists should follow the ALARA principle (as low as reasonable achievable) [3]. The providers should use the minimum radiation dose, fetal shielding, radiation dose monitoring [48].

Describe the potential adverse effects of ultrasonography on fetus.

Diagnostic ultrasonography during pregnancy has no embryotoxic effects. Prenatal ultrasound in rats showed no consistent evidence of neurobehavioral effects at low exposure ultrasound intensities (up to 20 W/cm^2) [49]. However, higher intensities (>30 W/cm^2) can cause postnatal neurobehavioral effects [50]. Ultrasound can increase the fetal temperature. Hyperthermia is a recognized teratogen in mammalian laboratory animals and is a suspected teratogen for humans. Human epidemiology does not indicate that diagnostic ultrasound presents a measurable risk to the developing embryo or fetus [51]. Because higher exposures of ultrasound can elevate the temperature of the embryo, the use of diagnostic procedures should take into consideration the hyperthermic potential of higher exposures of ultrasound [51]. To prevent hyperthermia, exposure time and acoustic output should be set to the lowest level possible.

Describe Behavioral teratology

Behavioral teratology was described as the adverse effects of a drug on the behavior or functional adaptation of the offspring to its environment [52]. In animal studies, brief intrauterine exposure to halothane resulted in postnatal learning deficit, CNS degeneration and decrease brain weight in rats [53]. Maternal administration of systemic drugs, including barbiturates, meperidine, resulted in behavioral changes in rat offspring [54, 55]. Maternal administration of lidocaine showed no effect on behavioral changes or clinical dysfunction in rat offspring [25].

The researchers administered to 7-day-old infant rats a combination of drugs commonly used in pediatric anesthesia (midazolam, nitrous oxide, and isoflurane) in doses sufficient to maintain a surgical level of anesthesia for 6 h, and have demonstrated that this causes widespread apoptotic neurodegeneration in the developing brain, deficits in hippocampal synaptic function, and persistent memory/learning impairments [56]. However, there is no evidence to prove that anesthesia administered to a pregnant woman has adverse effects on later intelligence, neuromuscular physiology, learning ability, and behavior of her infant [57].

Describe teratogenicity of Hypoxia and hypercarbia.

Animal studies demonstrated that congenital abnormalities have been described after exposure to hypoxia during organogenesis [58]. In humans, brief experience of hypoxia and hypercarbia has not proven to be teratogenic [59, 60]. Common causes of maternal hypoxia in pregnant women during surgery include laryngospasm, airway obstruction, esophagus intubation, inadequate ventilation, low inspired oxygen in anesthetic gas mixture, severe toxic reactions, high spinal or epidural blocks with maternal hypoventilation.

How do anesthesia providers maintain fetal well-being during surgery?

Intrauterine asphyxia can cause serious damage to fetus. It is important to maintain normal maternal arterial oxygen tension, oxygen-carrying capacity, oxygen affinity, and uteroplacental perfusion in pregnant women during surgery [3].

Maternal oxygen tension commonly elevated during anesthesia. Is there any concern about maternal hyperoxia?

It is a concern that elevated maternal oxygen tensions could decrease uteroplacental blood flow and fetal oxygenation. Multiple studies demonstrated that enhancing maternal PaO_2 will increase fetal PaO_2 [61, 62]. No studies show maternal hyperoxia caused fetal hypoxia [61, 62]. Fetal PaO_2 never surpasses 60 mmHg, even maternal PaO_2 increases to 600 mmHg [3]. High oxygen consumption of the placenta and uneven distribution of maternal and fetal blood flow in the placenta cause this large maternal-fetal oxygen tension gradient [3]. Maternal hyperoxia cannot result in utero retrolental fibroplasia or premature closure of the ductus arteriosus.

How does maternal carbon dioxide affect the fetus?

Fetal $PaCO_2$ is directly related to maternal $PaCO_2$. Maternal hypocapnia can increase mean intrathoracic pressure, decrease venous return to the heart, and reduce uteroplacental prefusion [63]. Maternal alkalosis decreases umbilical blood flow, shifts the maternal oxyhemoglobin dissociation curve to the left, increase the affinity of maternal hemoglobin for oxygen, reduce oxygen release to fetus at the placenta [64].

Maternal hypercapnia can cause fetal acidosis. Mild fetal hypercapnia has little consequence, severe hypercapnia can result in fetal myocardial depression and hypotension.

How does maternal hypotension affect the fetus?

Maternal hypotension can cause reduction of uterine blood flow and lead to fetal asphyxia. The most common causes of maternal hypotension include deep general anesthesia, sympathectomy (high levels of spinal or epidural blockade), hypovolemia, and vena caval compression [3].

Which vasopressor is used to treat maternal hypotension: ephedrine or phenylephrine?

In the past, ephedrine is preferred to phenylephrine for the treatment of hypotension during the administration of neuraxial anesthesia in obstetric patients. New conclusions are achieved from a meta-analysis of randomized controlled trials comparing ephedrine with phenylephrine for the treatment of hypotension during spinal anesthesia for cesarean delivery [65]. There was no difference between ephedrine and phenylephrine for the prevention and treatment of maternal hypotension. Women given phenylephrine had neonates with higher umbilical arterial blood pH than those given ephedrine. There was no difference between the two vasopressors in the incidence of true fetal acidosis [65]. Further studies supported that ephedrine increased fetal concentrations of lactate, glucose, and catecholamine [66]. Ephedrine increased metabolic rate, caused fetal acidosis. Therefore the use of phenylephrine to treat maternal hypotension may be preferable to ephedrine.

What kinds of surgical procedure can cause preterm labor?

Several studies of nonobstetric surgery during pregnancy showed a higher incidence of abortion and preterm labor during the postoperative period [1, 67–69]. Ovarian cystectomy in the first trimester has a high incidence of abortion. Neurosurgical, orthopedic, thoracic, or plastic surgery procedures were not associated with preterm labor [3]. After reviewing 778 pregnant women who had surgery between 24 and 36 weeks, 22% of the patients delivered in the week after surgery [69]. In the women whose pregnancy lasted beyond a week after surgery, there was no further enlarge in the incidence of preterm labor [69]. The lowest risk of preterm labor is during the second trimester procedures and operations that do not involve uterine manipulation.

Can anesthesia increase the incidence of preterm labor?

It is unknown whether anesthetic agents or techniques are associated with the risk of preterm labor. However, the volatile inhalation agents can depress myometrial irritability and are theoretically advantageous for abdominal procedure.

What tocolytic agents can be given to prevent preterm labor?

Magnesium sulfate is the most common medication applied in pregnancy as a tocolytic, fetal neuroprotective agent. Magnesium sulfate has been demonstrated to reduce the incidence and severity of cerebral palsy after very preterm birth. However, it can interfere anesthesia such as an increase in onset of neuromuscular blockade, reduction of general anesthetic requirements [70].

A new class of tocolytic agents (atosiban) was developed, which selectively blunts the calcium influx in the myometrium and inhibit myometrial contractility [71]. But it is unknown whether this new drug can reduce the risk of preterm labor after surgery during pregnancy.

When is the good time to perform nonobstetric surgery?

Elective surgery should not be scheduled during pregnancy. Surgery should be avoided during the first trimester, especially during the period of organogenesis. Urgent surgery is indicated for acute abdominal disease, some malignancies, and neurosurgical and cardiac problems [3]. The management of acute surgery should imitate that for nonpregnant patients [72].

What is the incidence of acute abdominal disease during pregnancy?

The incidence of acute abdominal disease during pregnancy is 1/500–1/635 [73]. Causes of acute abdomen in pregnancy include ectopic pregnancy, peduncular torsion of an ovarian cyst or tumor, torsion of a fallopian tube, ovarian bleeding, and pelvic inflammation. Other causes of acute abdomen in pregnancy include acute appendicitis, ileus, cholecystitis, pancreatitis, bowel obstruction, vascular accidents, and peptic ulcer.

Why is acute abdomen more difficult to diagnose in pregnant women than in nonpregnant women?

The diagnostic work up of an acute abdomen may be more difficult in pregnant than in nonpregnant women. Symptoms of both normal pregnancy and acute abdominal disease are similar. The expanding uterus makes a physical examination difficult. The white blood cell count is high during normal pregnancy. Sometimes, the correct diagnosis is concluded only at surgery.

What advantages do laparoscopic surgery offer over open laparotomy in pregnancy patients?

Initially, laparoscopic surgery in pregnancy was felt to be more dangerous. The reasons include uterine or fetal trauma, fetal acidosis from carbon dioxide, decreased maternal cardiac output and uteroplacental perfusion from intra-abdominal pressure. Now more surgeons understand that the benefits of laparoscopic surgery during pregnancy outweigh the risks. These benefits include: shorter length of hospital stay, less postoperative pain, reduction of risk for thromboembolic and wound complications, faster functional recovery, less uterine irritability, and less fetal depression [74].

Human studies showed that there were no differences in the maternal pH, $PaCO_2$, or arterial to end-tidal CO_2 pressure gradients before, during, and after termination of pneumoperitoneum during laparoscopy [75]. There were no differences in maternal and fetal outcomes when compared open and laparoscopic surgery [76]. Therefore the fetal effects from the CO_2 pneumoperitoneum and intra-abdominal pressure during laparoscopic surgery are limited.

The society of American Gastrointestinal Endoscopic Surgeons published “Guidelines for Diagnosis, treatment, and the Use of Laparoscopy for Surgical Problems during Pregnancy” [77]. The indications for laparoscopic surgery during pregnancy do not differ from nonpregnant patients [77]. The procedures may be performed during any trimester of pregnancy [77].

Describe anesthetic management of nononstetric surgery during pregnancy.

Preoperative care

During the preoperative evaluation, the anesthesia providers should make their best effort to ease maternal anxiety. A focused history and physical examination may be associated with reduced maternal, fetal, and neonatal complications [78]. Pregnant women are at increased risk for acid aspiration after 18–20 weeks’ gestation. Fasting, in these patients should follow the ASA guideline and local hospital policy. Preoperative medications to prevent aspiration include dopamine receptors antagonist, metoclopramide; H_2 receptor antagonists, cimetidine, ranitidine, famotidine; and a clear nonparticulate antacid, sodium citrate.

Intraoperative care

No evidence proved that there is an association between improved fetal outcome and any specific anesthetic technique [3]. However, local or regional anesthesia maybe better selection, because it allows the use of drugs with no evidence of teratogenicity from animal studies or human studies. There regional anesthetic techniques are applied for cervical cerclage and urologic or extremity surgeries. Most abdominal procedures require general anesthesia.

Endotracheal intubations is necessary during general anesthesia for pregnant women after 18–20 weeks' gestation or those with full stomach. Rapid sequence induction with cricoid pressure has been utilized for induction of general anesthesia. Systemic drugs include thiopental, propofol, morphine, fentanyl, succinylcholine, and nondepolarizing muscle relaxants.

Anesthesia is maintained with high concentration of oxygen, muscle relaxants, opioid, and inhalation agents. Research data did not support the omission of nitrous oxide during pregnancy, particularly after the sixth week of gestation [79]. End-tidal CO_2 should be maintained in the normal range for pregnancy.

The Trendelenburg position can further reduce FRC and worsen maternal hypoxemia. Pneumoperitoneum, aortocaval compression, or reverse Trendelenburg position can cause hypotension. Therefore a vasopressor may be needed to maintain maternal blood pressure during surgery [80].

During the second and third trimester, the pregnant women should be transferred on her side, and the uterus should be displaced leftward when she is positioned on the operating table to prevent aortocaval compression [3].

Fetal monitoring during surgery

Continuous fetal heart rate monitoring can provide information of abnormalities in maternal ventilation or uterine perfusion. Continuous fetal heat rate monitoring is feasible at 18–20 weeks' gestation [81]. The American College of Obstetricians and Gynecologists (ACOG) has stated that "the decision to use fetal monitoring should be individualized and, if used, should be based on gestational age, type of surgery, and facilities available" [82]. According to a survey, only 43% routinely used intraoperative FHR monitoring [83]. The significant advantage of intraoperative FHR monitoring is that it allows anesthesia providers and surgeons to optimize the maternal condition if the fetus shows signs of compromise [3].

Postoperative care

The FHR and uterine activity should be monitored in PACU. Adequate analgesia is important as pain will cause increased circulating catecholamines which may damage uteroplacental perfusion. Postoperative pain should be managed with systemic opioids, epidural or subarachnoid opioids acetaminophen, neural blockade. Prophylaxis against venous thrombosis is necessary. This should include early mobilization, maintaining adequate hydration, mechanical thromboprophylaxis with well-fitted compression stockings and consideration of pharmacological prophylaxis.

References

1. Mazze RI, Kallen B. Reproductive outcome after anesthesia and operation during pregnancy: a registry study of 5405 cases. Am J Obstet Gyneol. 1989;161:1178–85.
2. Brodsky JB, CohenEN Brown BW Jr, et al. Surgery during pregnancy and fetal outcome. Am J Obstet Gynecol. 1980;138:1165–7.
3. Van de Velde M. Nonobstetric surgery during pregnancy. In: Chestnut DH, Wong CA, Tsen LC, Ngan Kee WD, Beilin Y, Mhyre J, editors. 5th Edition Chestnut's obstetric anesthesia: principles and practice. Philadelphia: Mosby/Elsevier; 2014. pp. 358–79.
4. Kahn RI, Stanton MA, Tong-Ngork S, et al. One year experience with day-of-surgery pregnancy testing before elective orthopedic procedure. Anesth Analg. 2008;106:1127–31.
5. Manley S, de Kelata G, Joseph NJ, et al. Preoperative pregnancy testing in an ambulatory surgery: incidence and impact of positive results. Anesthesiology. 1995;83:690–3.
6. Kasliwal A, Farquharson RG. Pregnancy testing prior to sterilization. BJOG. 2000;107:1407–9.
7. Erekson EA, Brousseau EC, Dick-Biascoechea MA, et al. Maternal postoperative complications after nonobstetric antenatal surgery. J Matern Fetal Neonatal Med. 2012;25:2639–44.
8. Cugell DW, Frank NR, Gaensler EA, Badger TL. Pulmonary function in pregnancy. I. serial observations in normal women. Am Rev Tuberc. 1953;67:568–97.
9. Palahniuk RJ, Shnider SM, Eger EI II. Pregnancy decreases the requirement for inhaled anesthetic agents. Anesthesiology. 1974;41:82–3.
10. Capeless EL, Clapp JF. Cardiovascular changes in early phase of pregnancy. Am J Obstet Gynecol. 1989;161:1449–53.
11. Macfie AG, Magides AD, Richmoond MN, Reilly CS. Gastric emptying in pregnancy. Br J Anaesth. 1991;67:54–7.
12. Gin T, Mainland P, Chan MT, Short TG. Decreased thiopental requirements in early pregnancy. Anesthesiology. 1997;86:73–8.
13. Leighton BI, Check TG, Gross JB, et al. Succinylcholine pharmacodynamics in peripartum patients. Anesthesiology. 1986;64:202–5.
14. Gin T, Chan MT. decreased minimum alveolar concentration of isoflurane in pregnant humans. Anesthesiology. 1994;81:829–32.
15. Wilson JG. Environment and birth defects. New York: Academic Press; 1973. p. 1–82.
16. Setala K, Nyyssonen O. Hypnotic sodium pentobarbital as a teratogen for mice. Naturwissenschaften. 1964;51:413.
17. Tanimural T. The effect of thiamylal sodium administration to pregnant mice upon the development of their offspring. Acta Anat Nippon. 1965;40:223.
18. Fredriksson A, Ponten E, Gordh T, Eriksson P. Neonatal exposure to a combination of N-methyl-D-aspartate and gamma-aminobutyric and type A receptor anesthetic agents potentiates apoptotic neurodegeneration and persistent behavioral deficits. Anesthesiology. 2007;107:427–36.
19. Nikizad H, Yon JH, Carter LB, Jevtovic-Todorovic V. Early exposure to general anesthesia causes significant neuronal deletion in the developing rat brain. Ann N Y Acad Sci. 2007;1122:69–82.
20. Jurand A. Teratogenic activity of methadone hydrochloride in mouse and chick embryos. J Embryol Exp Morphol. 1973;30:449–58.
21. Geber WF, Schramm LC. Congential malformation of the center nervous system produced by narcotic analgesics in the hamster. Am J Obstet Gynecol. 1975;123:705–13.
22. Fujinaga M, Stevenson JB, Mazze RI. Reproductive and teratogenic effects of fentanyl in Sprague-Dawley rats. Teratology. 1986;34:51–7.

23. Fujinaga M, Mazze RI, Jackson EC, Baden JM. Reproductive and teratogenic effects of sufentanil and alfentanil in Sprague-Dawley rats. Anesth Analg. 1988;67:166–9.
24. Fujinaga M, Baden JM, Mazze RI. Developmental toxicity of nondepolarizing muscle relaxants in cultured rat embryos. Anesthesiology. 1992;76:999–1003.
25. Fujinaga M, Mazze RI. Reproductive and teratogenic effects of lidocaine in Sprague-Dawley rats. Anesthesiology. 1986;65:626–32.
26. Fantel AG, MacPhail BJ. Teratogenicity of cocaine. Teratology. 1982;26:17–9.
27. Shepard TH, Lemire RJ. Catalog of teratogenic agents. 13th ed. Baltimore: Johns Hopkins University Press; 2010.
28. Milkovich L, Van den Berg BJ. Effects of prenatal meprobamate and chlordiazepoxide hydrochloride on human embryonic and g=fetal development. N Eng J Med. 1974;291:1268–71.
29. Saxen I, Saxen L. Association between maternal intake of diazepam and oral clefts. Lancet. 1975;2:498.
30. Safra MJ, Oakley GP. Association between cleft lip with or without cleft palate and prenatal exposure to diazepam. Lancet. 1975;2:478–80.
31. Shiono PH, Mills JL. Oral clefts and diazepam use during pregnancy. N Eng J Med. 1984;311:919–20.
32. Koren G, Pastuszak A, Ito S. Drugs in pregnancy. N Engl J Med. 1998;338:1128–37.
33. Mazze RI, Fujinaga M, Rice SA, et al. Reproductive and teratogenic effects of nitrous oxide, halothane, isoflurane, and enflurane in Sprague-Dawley rats. Anesthesiology. 1986;64:339–44.
34. Lane GA, Nahrwold ML, Tait AR, et al. Anesthetics as teratogens: nitrous oxide is fetotoxic, xenon is not. Science. 1980;210:899–901.
35. Baden JM, Fujinaga M. Effects of nitrous oxide in day 9 rat embryos grown in culture. Br J Anaesth. 1991;66:500–3.
36. Keeling PA, Rocke DA, Nunn JF, et al. Folinic acid protection against nitrous oxide teratogenicity in the rat. Br J Anaesth. 1986;58:528–34.
37. Fujinaga M, Baden JM, Yhap EO, Mazzel RI. Reproductive and teratogenic effects of nitrous oxide, isoflurane, and their combination in Sprague-Dawley rats. Anesthesiology. 1987;67:960–4.
38. Smith BE, Usubiage LE, Lehrer SB. Cleft palate induced by halothane anesthesia in C-57 black mice. Teratology. 1971;4:242.
39. Bussard DA, Stoelting RK, Peterson C, Ishaq M. Fetal changes in hamsters anesthetized with nitrous oxide and halothane. Anesthesiology. 1974;41:275–8.
40. Mazzel RI, Wilson AI, Rice SA, Baden JM. Fetal development in mice exposed to isoflurane. Teratology. 1985;32:339–45.
41. Harlap S, Shiono PH. Alcohol, smoking and incidence of spontaneous abortion in the first and second trimester. Lancet. 1980;2:173–6.
42. Kline J, Stein ZA, Susser M, Warburton D. Smoking: a risk factor for spontaneous abortion. N Engl J Med. 1977;297:793–6.
43. Spence AA. Environmental pollution by inhalation anesthetics. Br J Anaesth. 1987;59:96–103.
44. Shnider SM, Webster GM. Maternal and fetal hazards of surgery during pregnancy. Am J Obstet Gynecol. 1965;92:891–900.
45. Duncan PG, Pope WDB, Cohen MM, Greer N. The safety of anesthesia and surgery during pregnancy. Anesthesiology. 1986;64:790–4.
46. International Commission on Radiological Protection. Pregnancy and medical radiation. Ann ICRP. 2000;30:1–43.
47. Radiation and pregnancy: A fact sheet for clinicians. Center for Disease Control Prevention. http://www.bt.cdc.gov/radiation/prenatalphysician.asp.
48. Lowe SA. Diagnostic radiography in pregnancy: risks and reality. Aust N Z J Obstet Gynacol. 2004;44:191–6.
49. Vorhees CV, Acuff-Smith KD, Schilling MA, et al. Behavioral teratologic effects of prenatal exposure to continuous-wave ultrasound in unanesthetized rats. Teratology. 1994;50:238–49.
50. Hande MP, Devi PU. Teraogenic effects of repeated exposure to X-rays and/or ultrasound in mice. Neurotoxicol Teratol. 1995;17:179–88.
51. Brent R, Jensh RP, Beckman DA. Medical sonography: reproductive effects and risks. Teratology. 1991;44:123–46.
52. Werboff J, Gottlieb JS. Drugs in pregnancy: behavioral teratology. Obstet Gynecol Surv. 1963;18:4203.
53. Smith RE, Bowman RE, Katz J. Behavioral effects of exposure to halothane during early development in rat: sensitive period during pregnancy. Anesthesiology. 1978;49:319–23.
54. Armitage SG. The effects of barbiturates on the behavior of rat offspring as measured in learning and reasoning situations. J Comp Physiol Psychol. 1952;45:146–52.
55. Chalon J, Walpert I, Ramanathan S, et al. Meperidine-promethazine combination and learning function of mice and of their progeny. Can Anaesth Soc J 1982;29:612–6.
56. Jevtovic-Todorovic V, Hartman RE, Izumi Y, et al. Early exposure to common anesthetic agents causes widespread neurodegeneration in the developing rat brain and persistent learning deficits. J Neurosci. 2003;23:876–82.
57. Committee on drugs of the American Academy of. Pediatrics and the committee of obstetrics and maternal and fetal medicine of the American College of Obstetricians and Gynecologists: effect of medication during labor and delivery on infant outcome. Pediatrics. 1978;62:402–3.
58. Ingalls TH, Curley FJ, Prindle RA. Anoxia as a cause of fetal death and congenital defect in the mouse. Am J Dis Child. 1950;80:34–5.
59. Pitt DB. A study of congenital malformations. II Aust N Z J Obstet Gynaecol. 1962;2:82–90.
60. Warkany J, Kalter H. Congenital malformations. N Eng J Med. 1961;265:1046–52.
61. Khazin AF, Hon EH, Hahre FW. Effects of maternal hyperoxia on fetus. I. Oxygen tension. Am J Obstet Gynecol. 1971;109:628–37.
62. Walker A, Madderin L, Day E, Renow P, et al. Fetal scalp tissue oxygen measurements in relation to maternal dermal oxygen tension and fetal heart rate. J Obstet Gynaecol Br Commonw. 1971;78:1–12.
63. Levinson G, Shime J, Paul WM, Hoskins M. Oxygen administration during labor. Am J Obstet Gynecol. 1969;105:954–61.
64. Motoyama EK, Rivard G, Acheson F, Cook CD. The effect of changes in maternal pH and PCO2 on the PO2 of fetal lambs. Anesthesiology. 1967;28:891–903.
65. Lee A, Ngan Kee WD, Gin T. A quantitative, systemic review of randomized controlled trials of ephedrine versus phenylephrine for the management of hypotension during spinal anesthesia for cesarean delivery. Anesth Analg. 2002;94:920–6.
66. Ngan Kee WD, Khaw KS, Tan PE, et al. Placental transfer and fetal metabolic effects of phenylephrine and ephedrine during spinal anesthesia for cesarean delivery. Anesthesiology. 2009;11:506–12.
67. Shnider SM, Webster GM. Maternal and fetal hazards of surgery during pregnancy. Am J Obstet Gyncol. 1965;92:891–900.
68. Crawford JS, Lewis M. Nitrous oxide in early human pregnancy. Anesthesia. 1986;41:900–5.
69. Mazze RI, Kallen B. Appendectomy during pregnancy: a Swedish registry study of 778 cases. Obstet Gynecol. 1991;77:835–40.
70. Doyle LW. Antenatal magnesium sulfate and neuroprotection. Curr Opin Pediatr. 2012;24:154–9.
71. Shim JY, Park YW, Yoon BH, et al. Multicentre, parallel group, randomized, single-blind study of the safety and efficacy of atosiban versus ritodrine in the treatment of acute preterm labour in Korean women. BJOG. 2006;113:1228–34.

72. McKellar DP, Anderson CT, Boynton CJ, Peoples JB. Cholecystectomy during pregnancy without fetal loss. Surg Gynecol Obstet. 1992;174:465–8.
73. Coleman MT, Trianfo VA, Rund DA. Nonobstetric emergencies in pregnancy and surgical conditions. Am J Obstet Gynecol. 1997;177:497–502.
74. Fatum M, Rojansky N. Laparscopic surgery during pregnancy. Obstet Gynecol Surv. 2001;56:50–9.
75. Bhavani-Shankar K, Steinbrook RA, Brooks DC, Datta S. Arterial to end-tidal carbon dioxide pressure difference during laparoscopic surgery in pregnancy. Anesthesiology 2000;93:370–3.
76. Buser KB. Laparscopic surgery in the pregnant patient results and recommendations. JSLS. 2009;13:32–5.
77. Guidelines Committee of the society of American Gastrointestinal. Endoscopic surgeons. Guidelines for diagnosis, treatment, and the use of laparoscopy for surgical problems during pregnancy. Surg Endosc. 2008;22:849–61.
78. The task force on obstetrical anesthesia. Practice guidelines for obstetrical anesthesia. Anesthesiology. 1999;90:600–11.
79. Sanders RD, Weimann J, Maze M. Biologic effects of nitrous oxide: a mechanistic and toxicologic review. Anesthesiology. 2008;109:707–22.
80. Steinbrook RA, Brooks DC, Datta S. Laparoscopic cholecystectomy during pregnancy: review of anesthetic management, surgical consideration. Surg Endosc. 1996;10:511–5.
81. Biehl DR. Foetal monitoring during surgery unrelated to pregnancy. Can J Anaesth Soc J. 1985;12:455–9.
82. American College of Obstetricians and Gynecologists. Nonobstetric surgery under pregnancy. ACOG Committee opinion No 474. Obstet Gynecol. 2011;117:420–1.
83. Kilpatrick CC, Puig C, Chohan L, et al. Intraoperative fetal heart rate monitoring during nonobstetric surgery in pregnancy; a practice survey. South Med J. 2010;103:212–5.

Part XI
Pediatrics

Section Editors: Craig D. McClain and Kai Matthes

Craig D. McClain
Department of Anesthesiology, Perioperative and Pain Medicine,
Boston Children's Hospital, Boston, MA, USA

Craig D. McClain
Harvard Medical School, Boston, MA, USA

Kai Matthes
Division of Gastroenterology, Department of Anesthesiology,
Perioperative and Pain Medicine, Boston Children's Hospital,
Harvard Medical School, Boston, MA, USA

Neonatal Resuscitation

52

Jonathan R. Meserve and Monica E. Kleinman

CASE

A 28-year-old G1P0 female at 35 weeks gestation is brought to the OR for emergent C-section following a non-reassuring fetal heart tracing of late decelerations. She presented 12 h prior with spontaneous rupture of membranes and had previously had an uneventful labor. General anesthesia with a rapid sequence intubation is achieved and the infant is delivered shortly thereafter. No neonatology team is present at the time of delivery.

Maternal Medications:	Prenatal Vitamins
Allergies:	NKA
Maternal Past Medical History:	Gestational Diabetes

Please Note

1. **Which infants require newborn resuscitation?**

When asked to evaluate a newborn for possible resuscitative measures, three questions should be asked

(1) Is this a term gestation?
(2) Is the newborn crying or breathing?
(3) Is there good muscle tone? [1]

If the answer is yes to these three questions, the child should remain with the mother for skin-to-skin care to facilitate bonding, covered with a dry clean cloth for warmth.

If the answer is "no" to any of these questions, the child should immediately be evaluated for resuscitative measures, which could include: initial stabilization (provide warmth, clear airway, dry, stimulate), ventilation, chest compressions, or administration of epinephrine or volume expanders.

10% of newborns will need resuscitation to transition to extrauterine life with 1% requiring involved resuscitative measures. Worldwide, birth asphyxia accounts for approximately 23% of the 4 million neonatal deaths [2].

2. **How does neonatal circulatory system differ from adult circulation?**

Fetal intrauterine oxygen delivery is dependent upon maternal oxygenation and placental transfer to fetal red blood cells. Following transfer of oxygen to the Hgb F-rich fetal red blood cells, the oxygenated blood returns to the fetus via the umbilical vein (PaO_2 = 30 mmHg). 75–80% of blood from the umbilical vein bypasses the fetal liver via the ductus venosus. Blood then enters the right atrium, where two-third of the blood flows through the foramen ovale into the left atrium. From the left atrium, blood passes into the left ventricle out the aorta where it perfuses the brain and upper extremities.

Pulmonary vascular resistance is high in utero and only one-third of blood flow from the ductus venosus exits the right ventricle. Only a small portion of this flow will reach the lungs as the majority of blood flows through the Patent Ductus Arteriosis (PDA) to the descending aorta, mixing with blood from the left ventricle. Most of the circulation to the lower body is supplied by the PDA, whereas the brain and upper extremities are perfused by blood leaving the left ventricle. Blood then enters the two umbilical arteries (PaO_2 = 20) and flows to the placenta. At birth, the lungs begin to expand and the increase in PaO_2 begins the process by which the ductus arteriosis and the foramen ovale close.

J.R. Meserve (✉) · M.E. Kleinman
Department of Anesthesiology, Perioperative and Pain Medicine, Boston Children's Hospital, 300 Longwood Avenue, Boston, MA 02115, USA
e-mail: jonathan.meserve@childrens.harvard.edu

M.E. Kleinman
e-mail: monica.kleinman@childrens.harvard.edu

© Springer International Publishing AG 2017
L.S. Aglio and R.D. Urman (eds.), *Anesthesiology*,
DOI 10.1007/978-3-319-50141-3_52

3. **What are "normal" umbilical artery and umbilical vein blood gases?**

In the fetal system, umbilical venous blood returning from the placenta is more highly oxygenated than the arterial blood.

(1) Normal umbilical venous blood gas: pH: 7.35, PO_2: 30 (25-25), PCO_2: 40, and base excess: −3.3.
(2) Normal umbilical artery blood gas: pH of 7.26, PO_2: 20 PCO_2: 55, base excess: −3.4 [3].

A scalp pH < 7.2 indicates fetal distress and warrants immediate delivery. Severe cord blood acidemia (pH < 7.00) is suggestive of intra-partum asphyxia and may warrant postnatal interventions to limit neurologic sequelae including hypothermic cooling.

4. **What are the initial steps of neonatal resuscitation?**

After determining that an infant requires resuscitation (see question 1), three initial resuscitative steps should be performed, in the first 30 s of life. They include

(1) Provide warmth—the infant should be placed under a radiant warmer, uncovered by blankets to allow gross inspection of the infant.
(2) Position the infant—the neck should be slightly extended to facilitate unrestricted air entry. Both hyperextension and flexion may compromise the neonatal airway. The airway and nose (mouth first, nose second) may be cleared with a bulb suction if excessive secretions are impairing breathing, but routine use of bulb suctioning is no longer recommended.
(3) Dry, stimulate, reposition—using pre-warmed blankets, dry the infant to prevent evaporative heat loss. Discard wet linens. Reposition the head to ensure adequate breathing. Additional brief stimulation may be provided to help the infant transition. Approved stimulation includes: slapping or flicking soles of the feet, gently rubbing the back, trunk, or extremities.

5. **How does the presence of meconium affect your resuscitative efforts?**

Additional airway resuscitative measures may be required in the event of meconium depending on the newborn's level of activity. In all instances the infant should be brought to the warmer and the airway should be positioned as outlined in the initial resuscitative steps (see question 3). An infant born with meconium that exhibits vigorous behavior (strong respiratory effort, good muscle tone, and HR > 100), need no further airway manipulation than that outlined in the initial steps. Continue with drying, stimulation, and positioning as per routine resuscitation.

Should the infant emerge with depressed respirations, decreased tone, and/or HR < 100, an attempt should be made to suction the mouth and trachea. A laryngoscope should be inserted to facilitate intubation with an endotracheal tube (ETT). The ETT should be connected to a Meconium Aspirator connected to wall suction. The trachea should be suctioned for several seconds then slowly withdrawn. This step may be repeated for copious meconium but it must not delay other resuscitative efforts should the infant's HR remain depressed (<100) at 30 s. Of note, previous iterations of the NRP guidelines recommended airway intervention based on the quality of the meconium (thick vs. thin). This distinction no longer affects decision-making and airway intervention depends on solely neonatal qualities (vigorous vs. non-vigorous) [4].

6. **After the initial resuscitative efforts, the infant's heart rate is 45 beats per minute. What resuscitative effort should be employed?**

Following the three Initial Resuscitative Steps, the infant should be evaluated for respirations and HR. The initial Resuscitative Steps should take no longer than 30 s, and at this point the infant should demonstrate good chest movement and have a HR > 100. If the HR < 100, the infant is gasping or apneic despite stimulation you should proceed to Positive Pressure Ventilation (PPV). Assisting ventilation with effective PPV is the most critical intervention in resuscitating the compromised newborn.

PPV can be achieved with several devices including a self-inflating bag, flow-inflating bag, and T-piece Resuscitator. Most commonly a flow-inflating Jackson-Rees (modified Mapelson type F) bag is utilized. Initial inspiratory pressures should be 20 cm H_20. Rising HR is the best indicator of adequate ventilation. Breaths should be delivered at a rate of 40–60 breaths/minute.

7. **After 30 s of PPV the infant's HR remains below 60. What are the next resuscitative steps?**

If the HR remains below 100 bpm after 30 s of PPV, corrective ventilatory steps should be taken. These corrective steps include

(1) Mask adjustment—maintain a good airway seal
(2) Reposition the airway—place head in a sniffing position, avoiding hyperextension and flexion
(3) Suction the nose and mouth—ensure secretions are not obstructing ventilation efforts

(4) Open the mouth—utilize a jaw thrust maneuver with the fourth and fifth digits to slightly open the mouth.
(5) Increase PPV pressure—increase PPV with each breath until bilateral breath sounds or chest rise is observed
(6) Consider alternative airway—discuss ETT or laryngeal mask airway placement with team members.

If there is clinical concern for cyanosis or if you desire continuous HR monitoring, consider use of pulse oximeter to aid clinical decision-making. There are no definitive recommendations for if and when to use of pulse oximetry in NRP, though clinical practice typically dictates use expeditiously in the event of persistent bradycardia or concerns for cyanosis. Place the pulse oximeter probe on the right arm (pre-ductal saturation), typically over the hypothenar eminence. The use of oximetry must not delay other resuscitative actions including ventilation, compression, or medication administration.

8. **What fractional inspired oxygen concentration (FiO_2) should be routinely used for resuscitation of the newborn?**

Supplemental oxygen is no longer routinely used in the early stages of resuscitation for term newborns [5]. An air-oxygen "blender" should be routinely used, and the FiO_2 should be set to 21% at the beginning of resuscitative efforts. Increases in FiO_2 should be guided by pulse oximetry, targeting expected peripheral capillary oxygen saturations (SpO_2) values for age of the infant.

When resuscitating preterm infants, balancing the need to treat early hypoxemia with risks for oxygen toxicity is more complicated. Resuscitation should begin with a pulse oximeter and air-oxygen blender. In clinical practice, most practitioners utilize an FiO_2 of 40% to start resuscitation in neonates born before 32 weeks despite increased risk for oxygen toxicity in preterm infants.

9. **At 2 min of life the child's SpO_2 is 68% despite effective PPV with an FiO_2 of 21%. What should the FiO_2 be adjusted to?**

No changes to the FiO_2 should be made. FiO_2 should be adjusted to target expected SpO_2 values for newborn infant. As the infant transitions from neonatal circulation to breathing room air, the SpO_2 will gradually increase. At 1 min of life, the expected SpO_2 is 60–65%. This increases 5% for every minute of life thereafter until 5 min when the expected SpO2 is 80–85%. At 10 min the expected SpO_2 is 85–95%. Thus, at 2 min of life the expected SpO_2 is 65–70%.

10. **A newborn is quickly identified to require resuscitative measures, and receives 60 s effective PPV while a second team member applies a pulse oximeter. At 90 s of life, the pulse oximeter shows a heart rate (HR) of 40, confirmed by a third team member who palpates the umbilical cord for a pulse. What steps should be taken next?**

When an infant demonstrates a HR < 60 after 1 min of effective PPV, rescuers should perform chest compressions. Significant acidosis and low oxygen stores begin to compromise neonatal cardiac output in a short period of time. Chest compressions are necessary to maintain cardiac output and vessel rich organ perfusion.

11. **How should chest compressions be delivered to the neonate?**

Unlike adult chest compressions, neonatal chest compressions should be delivered with a second provider providing PPV at a ratio of 3 chest compressions to 1 breath (3:1).

Two techniques are approved for chest compressions:

(1) The "thumb-technique" involves encircling the chest and torso with both hands so that the fingers support the spine. Both thumbs are then used to compress the sternum.
(2) Alternatively, a "2-finger-technique" may be employed whereby the middle and index finger compress the sternum while the other hand is placed underneath in the infant to support the back.

The "thumb-technique" is the preferred method for delivering chest compressions as it is believed to better control the depth of compression. Goal chest compression depth is one-third of the anterior-posterior distance. Compressions should be delivered to the lower third of the sternum in plane with a line drawn between the infant's nipples.

Chest compressions should be delivered with PPV at a rate of 120 events per minute. At a ratio of 3:1, in one minute, 90 compressions should be delivered with 30 breaths. Note that the 30 breaths per minute rate of PPV is less than the 40–60 breaths/minute performed when no chest compressions are being administered.

12. **When can you stop chest compressions?**

Once the HR increases above 60, rescuers can stop chest compressions and continue PPV. PPV should be delivered at a rate of 40–60 breaths/minute until the child begins to breathe spontaneously and HR rises above 100.

13. **What steps should be taken if the HR remains below 60 after 30 s of chest compressions with effective PPV?**

After 30 s of chest compressions with adequate PPV, pharmacologic measures should be employed to increase the HR in an infant with a HR less than 60. Approved medications for use in neonatal resuscitation according to the 2010 American Heart Association®/American Academy of Pediatrics® Neonatal Resuscitation guidelines include epinephrine and volume expansion with crystalloid or blood products in the event of hypoperfusion from severe blood loss. Epinephrine can be delivered via intravenous or endotracheal administration. IV access is the most effective and predictable means of delivery, though often endotracheal access is faster than IV access in the newborn. Epinephrine used in neonatal resuscitation should be the 1:10,000 concentration.

IV dosing: 0.1–0.3 mL/kg of 1:10,000 epinephrine (0.01–0.03 mg/kg) [6].

ETT dosing (to be given only while IV access is being obtained): 0.5–1 mL/kg of 1:10,000 epinephrine (0.05–0.1 mg/kg) [7].

14. **How should IV access be obtained in the neonate?**

The umbilical vein provides the fastest and most reliable IV access in the neonate. If resuscitation is anticipated prior to delivery, a dedicated team member can prepare for umbilical vein access and begin the process immediately after the initially resuscitative steps. Umbilical vein access should be undertaken in a sterile manner, though complete sterility during emergent placement remains challenging. The umbilical stump is cleaned and a sterile cord is placed around the umbilical stalk to minimize blood loss. The cord is then transected with a scalpel and a 3.5 or 5F catheter (previously flushed with normal saline) is inserted into the single umbilical vein.

15. **How far should an umbilical catheter be inserted during neonatal resuscitation?**

The catheter should be inserted 2–4 cm until blood is easily aspirated. In premature infants the distance may be less. Note that this placement is not truly central IV access. For central insertion the catheter is advanced further, though the catheter may alternatively be inserted into the liver. Infusion of medications directly into the liver may cause hepatic injury, and therefore, the catheter should only be inserted a short distance during emergent neonatal resuscitation.

Should the infant require further umbilical access in the NICU following the initial resuscitation, the umbilical catheter should be replaced in a sterile fashion, as there is high risk for contamination of sterility during emergent placement. The new catheter can then be advanced centrally and confirmed by X-ray.

16. **What conditions are associated with neonatal hypovolemia?**

If the neonatal HR remains <60 after administration of epinephrine, one must consider acute blood loss and hemorrhage in the neonate. Conditions associated with acute blood loss include placenta previa, placenta abruption, vasa previa, twin pregnancies with twin-twin transfusion syndrome, hydrops fetalis, and umbilical cord blood loss. Signs of hypovolemia include bradycardia, delayed capillary fill, pale appearance, and weak pulses.

17. **What are acceptable volume expansion fluids in the newborn?**

Acceptable crystalloid solutions for the newborn include isotonic 0.9% NaCl (normal saline) and Ringer's Lactate solutions. Alternatively, packed red blood cells (PRBC's) may be considered in the event of known or suspected severe fetal anemia [8]. During initial resuscitation there is rarely time for blood typing or cross matching of unit specific blood products and instead non-crossmatched O^- emergency release blood must be used. Judicious use of volume expanders is recommended as even small volumes of intravenous fluids may precipitate heart failure in the transitioning neonatal circulation. Additionally, rapid administration of volume may result in intracranial hemorrhage, with preterm infants being the most susceptible [9]. The recommended initial volume expansion dose should be 10 mL/kg of either isotonic crystalloid fluids or pRBC's. This may be repeated if the clinical picture continues to demonstrate hypovolemia with cardiovascular compromise.

18. **When should the neonate be intubated?**

Unlike PPV or chest compressions, where defined recommendations for initiating therapy exist, the timing of intubation of the neonate is based on the clinical scenario. Some infants require intubation immediately, such as the depressed, meconium-stained infant or the severely preterm infant that has expected ventilatory needs.

Some indications for intubation include

(1) The depressed, meconium-stained infant.
(2) Failed PPV—PPV is indicated, yet the newborn is not demonstrating clinical improvement or there is no chest rise.
(3) Provide airway for mechanical ventilatory support—PPV is predicted to be necessary for more than several minutes.
(4) If chest compressions are necessary—intubation should be performed to help coordinate the 3:1 compression to ventilation ratio, as well as to ensure the breaths provided are maximally effective.
(5) The preterm infant—if the newborn is suspected to require ventilator support or surfactant administration.
(6) Severe neonatal blood loss—where significant resuscitative efforts are predicted
(7) Individual circumstances or congenital anomalies where PPV is not desirable—example: congenital diaphragmatic hernia, omphalocele, gastroschisis.
(8) Overcome critical airway obstruction—Congenital anomalies such as Pierre Robin sequence, or macroglossia with trisomy 21.

During resuscitation, intubation can be considered at any step during the NRP algorithm, including with initiation of PPV at 30 s, corrective ventilator steps at 60 s, or with initiation of chest compressions at 90 s for persistent bradycardia. In all instances, intubation should occur expeditiously so as not to delay other therapies. It should also not be undertaken until all necessary equipment and staff are available, as intubation is not urgent provided PPV can adequately ventilate the newborn. If intubation attempts take longer than 30 s, stop and ventilate the patient to prevent hypoxia and bradycardia.

19. **How is the neonatal airway different from the adult airway?**

Compared to the adult, the neonatal larynx and tracheal are funnel shaped with anterior slanting vocal cords. The narrowest part of the pediatric airway is subglottic as compared to the glottic opening in the adult. Additionally the glottis is at the level of the C3–C4 vertebra in term neonates and even higher at C3 in preterm infants as compared to C5 in the adults. Neonates have a comparatively larger tongue and occiput, which makes the head more prone to move from side to side during intubation attempts. The larger occiput additionally increases flexion, which combined with the more anterior airway, may make intubation more challenging. Many providers employ a rolled baby blanket under the shoulders to neutralize this flexion [10].

Straight Miller laryngoscope blades size 00, 0, or 1 are commonly used. Uncuffed, non-tapered, sterile endotracheal tubes (ETT) should be used. The choice of laryngoscope blade and ETT size are determined by infant birth weight

(1) Less than 28 weeks (below 1000 g): Miller 00, 2.5 mm tube size (inside diameter)
(2) Between 28 and 34 weeks (1000–2000 g): Miller 0, 3.0 mm tube size (inside diameter)
(3) Between 34 and 38 weeks (2000–3000 g): Miller 0 or 1, 3.5 mm tube size (inside diameter)
(4) Above 38 weeks (above 3000 g): Miller 1, 3.5–4.0 mm tube size (inside diameter)

20. **How do you confirm ETT placement after intubation?**

Confirmation of tracheal placement should be performed with a CO_2 detector. While watching the tube pass through the cords, auscultating breath sounds, and confirming chest rise are all signs of tube placement, true confirmation is best achieved with CO_2 detection. Sounds are easily transmitted in the neonate and esophageal or stomach ventilation may deceptively produce breath sounds when auscultating the chest wall. Either a capnograph with CO_2 waveform or calorimetric CO_2 device should be utilized. Note that if a colorimetric CO_2 detection device is used, you must ensure it has not already changed color in the package. Additionally, the addition of epinephrine though an ETT may falsely change the colorimetric device if epinephrine contaminates the sensor.

The ETT should be inserted to the mid carina. Typical insertion relies on a simple algorithm of the infant's weight in kilograms (kg) plus 6 to equal the number of centimeters from the tip of the tube to the vermillion border of the upper lip. For example: a 2 kg, 30-week infant should have a 3.0 uncuffed ETT inserted 8 cm (2 + 6) as measured from the vermillion border. Following resuscitation, tube placement should be confirmed with a chest X-ray.

21. **A term neonate requires PPV at 30 s of life for apnea, which quickly resolves. At 4 min the child is noted to have increasing respiratory distress, decreasing SpO_2, and asymmetric breath sounds. What steps should be taken?**

Pneumothorax is a common, and potentially life threatening complication of the newborn. The risk is increased for those infants that require PPV during initial resuscitation. A tension pneumothorax may quickly form, impeding lung expansion and compromising cardiac output as demonstrated by bradycardia, hypoxia, and respiratory distress. Congenital pleural effusions may additionally present with symptoms of respiratory distress, hypoxia, and asymmetric breath sounds. While definitive diagnosis is made with a chest X-ray, urgent intervention may preclude the use of this diagnostic modality. Transillumination of the chest cavity may assist providers in making the diagnosis of pneumothorax. This is done by placing a bright light on the infant's posterior chest wall. A pneumothorax will appear brighter than the contralateral expanded lung.

Percutaneous catheter placement is indicated if the newborn is demonstrating significant respiratory distress or bradycardia. A 20- or 18-Gauge needle may be inserted into either:

(1) The fourth intercostal space at the anterior axillary line or,
(2) The second intercostal space at the mid-clavicular line

As with an adult, the needle should be inserted above the lower rib to avoid trauma to the intercostal artery. A three-way stopcock should be affixed to a 20 mL syringe which connects to the catheter. This allows for air to be aspirated via the syringe, with subsequent closing of the stopcock to prevent the re-accumulation of air.

22. **What is a congenital diaphragmatic hernia and how should infants initially be resuscitated?**

A congenital diaphragmatic hernia (CDH) is a posterolateral defect of the diaphragm that results in failed closure of the diaphragm in the eighth week of gestation. The subsequent migration of abdominal viscera into the chest cavity results in mild to severe pulmonary hypoplasia, which may threaten oxygenation and ventilation of the infant. Presenting symptoms include severe respiratory distress and a scaphoid abdomen, with reduced breath sounds on the affected lung side (90% left, 5% right, 5% bilateral). PPV in these infants will result in intestinal dilation, which may further compromise lung ventilation as the viscera expands in the chest cavity. As such, these infants should be intubated quickly with the additional rapid placement of an orogastric tube to decompress the abdominal viscera. Note that many of these infants have pulmonary hypertension and associated congenital cardiac anomalies. Pneumothorax can be particularly deleterious, as any impediment to the sole functional lung may prevent adequate gas exchange.

23. **What considerations must be given to the preterm neonate?**

Both early preterm infants (before 34 weeks) and late preterm infants (34–36 weeks) are likely to require some degree of resuscitation. The appropriate resources and personnel should be available and mobilized. The initial resuscitation of the preterm infant follows that of the term newborn as outlined in the preceding questions. In addition, the ambient room temperature should be increased (25–26 °C) and a radiant warmer should be preheated. Infants born significantly preterm (before 29 weeks gestation) are placed in a food or medical-grade polyethylene bag to prevent heat and evaporative losses. An oxygen blender with a FiO_2 of 40% and pulse oximeter should be routinely utilized for infants born before 32 weeks. Consider intubation and the administration of surfactant via the ETT for neonates born before 30 weeks as they are the most likely to develop Respiratory Distress Syndrome (RDS). Be mindful that in addition to hypothermia, preterm infants are at risk for hypoglycemia, infection, retinopathy of prematurity, and intracranial hemorrhage secondary to a germinal matrix hemorrhage. Immediate transport to a NICU in a pre-warmed transport incubator after the initial resuscitation is necessary to prevent adverse sequelae from these common conditions.

24. **A term infant is born via a c-section for a non-reassuring fetal heart tracing. He is brought to the warmer and is dried and stimulated. At one minute of life the infant is grimacing but quiet, retracting while breathing, HR is 110 bpm, with flexed extremities and blue hands and feet. What is the child's APGAR score?**

The APGAR score is typically assigned at 1, 5, and 10 min of life. The purpose is to identify those newborns that require additional resuscitative efforts. It is not intended to determine long-term neurologic sequelae. The score is assigned using the mnemonic APGAR: **A**ppearance (skin color), **P**ulse (heart rate), **G**rimace (reflex irritability), **A**ctivity (muscle tone), and **R**espiration. A total of two points may be assigned for each criteria for a maximum score of 10. Scores 7–10 are normal, 4–6 low, and 0–3 regarded as critically low.

In the vignette above, the child has an APGAR score of 6 (1 respiratory effort, 2 for HR >100, 1 for flexed extremities, 1 for peripheral cyanosis and 1 for facial grimace). Infants with APGAR scores less than 7 at 1 min typically require additional resuscitation. In this case, PPV should be considered with a FiO_2 of 21% for the ongoing retractions.

The concept of a newborn resuscitation grading criteria was developed in 1952 by Anesthesiologist Dr. Virginia Apgar [11] (see Table 52.1) Arguably the most famous American anesthesiologist of the twentieth century, she contributed to the fields of anesthesiology, neonatology, and obstetrics. She was one of the first to recognize the

Table 52.1 APGAR score

Score	0	1	2
Heart rate	None	<100 bpm	>100 bpm
Respiratory effort	Apnea	Irregular, slow	Crying, good effort
Muscle tone	Limp	Flexed extremities	Actively moving
Irritability	No response	Facial grimace	Cough, cry
Color	Blue or pale	Peripheral cyanosis	All pink

importance of preterm birth and championed neonatal health though the March of Dimes Foundation.

25. **What post-resuscitative care should be provided for newborns?**

While every child should be returned to the mother as quickly as possible to facilitate bonding, infants who require resuscitative measures are prone to deterioration and may well require additional resuscitative care. Additionally, resuscitative efforts themselves may cause complications such as pneumothorax secondary to PPV. As such, newborns should be transported to a location where close monitoring can be provided with staff ready to assist in the event of clinical change. Every attempt to include the parents for bonding should be given provided it does not interfere with a provider's ability to care for the infant.

References

1. Kattwinkel J, Perlman JM, Aziz K, Colby C, Fairchild K, Gallagher J, et al. Neonatal resuscitation: 2010 American heart association guidelines for cardiopulmonary resuscitation and emergency cardiovascular care. Pediatrics. 2010;126(5):e1400–13.
2. Rajaratnam JK, Marcus JR, Flaxman AD, Wang H, Levin-Rector A, Dwyer L, et al. Neonatal, postneonatal, childhood, and under-5 mortality for 187 countries, 1970-2010: a systematic analysis of progress towards millennium development goal 4. Lancet. 2010;375(9730):1988–2008.
3. Goldaber KG, Gilstrap LC III, Leveno KJ, Dax JS, McIntire DD. Pathologic fetal acidemia. Obstet Gynecol. 1991;78(6):1103–7.
4. Halliday HL. Endotracheal intubation at birth for preventing morbidity and mortality in vigorous, meconium-stained infants born at term. Cochrane Database Syst Rev 2001;1(1):CD000500.
5. Saugstad OD, Ramji S, Vento M. Resuscitation of depressed newborn infants with ambient air or pure oxygen: a meta-analysis. Biol Neonate. 2005;87(1):27–34.
6. Perondi MB, Reis AG, Paiva EF, Nadkarni VM, Berg RA. A comparison of high-dose and standard-dose epinephrine in children with cardiac arrest. N Engl J Med. 2004;350(17):1722–30.
7. Barber CA, Wyckoff MH. Use and efficacy of endotracheal versus intravenous epinephrine during neonatal cardiopulmonary resuscitation in the delivery room. Pediatrics. 2006;118(3):1028–34.
8. Wyckoff MH, Perlman JM, Laptook AR. Use of volume expansion during delivery room resuscitation in near-term and term infants. Pediatrics. 2005;115(4):950–5.
9. Kattwinkel J, Perlman JM, Aziz K, Colby C, Fairchild K, Gallagher J, et al. Neonatal resuscitation: 2010 american heart association guidelines for cardiopulmonary resuscitation and emergency cardiovascular care. Pediatrics. 2010;126(5):e1400–13.
10. Thomas J. Reducing the risk in neonatal anesthesia. Paediatr Anaesth. 2014;24(1):106–13.
11. APGAR V. A proposal for a new method of evaluation of the newborn infant. Curr Res Anesth Analg 1953;32(4):260–267.

53 Gastroschisis and Omphalocele

Laura Downey

CASE:

A 34-week, 4 h-old neonate born via emergent C-section for non-reassuring fetal heart rate is diagnosed with gastroschisis. The patient was intubated in the delivery room for respiratory distress and a peripheral IV was placed. The baby is emergently brought to the operating room with a large abdominal wall defect and dusky bowel with concern for bowel ischemia and possible obstruction.

Medications:	None
Allergies:	NKA
PMH:	Maternal history significant for 18-year-old G1P1 with premature ruptured membranes, smoking, no prenatal care. Received two doses of betamethasone prior to delivery
Physical Exam:	Weight 2.6 kg HR 190 RR 40 BP: 45/20 (28) SpO_2: 94% on 21% FiO_2
Head:	Normocephalic, Fontanelle depressed
Respiratory:	3.0 uncuffed ETT, FiO_2 21%, RR 40
CV:	No murmur, Weak distal pulses
Abdominal:	Large abdominal defect, bowel covered with plastic silo
Access:	24 g PIV in the left hand

Medical Disease and Differential Diagnosis

(1) What is the difference between gastroschisis and omphalocele?
Gastroschisis is the herniation of bowel contents through an anterior abdominal wall defect usually to the right of the umbilical ring. The umbilical cord is normal. In most cases, only the small and large intestines are involved. Since there is no covering membrane, the bowel is exposed to the intrauterine environment and may develop an inflammatory peel. Associated anomalies are rare, comprising about 2–10% of patients. Only 1–3% of these anomalies are cardiac defects. However, additional gastrointestinal problems such as malrotation, atresia, stenosis are common.
Omphalocele is a midline abdominal wall defect of the umbilical ring. Abdominal viscera herniate through the umbilical ring into the umbilical sac. The sac may include intestines, spleen, liver, or other abdominal viscera. If the defect is less than 4 cm, it is considered an umbilical hernia. The umbilical cord is inserted into the sac.
While both abnormalities are associated with other congenital malformations, the frequency of other abnormalities associated with omphalocele is 35–75% and only 2–10% for gastroschisis. The site of the umbilical cord may help distinguish between gastroschisis and omphalocele. In omphalocele, the cord insertion site is into an umbilical sac, whereas in gastroschisis, the cord insertion site is paraumbilical into an otherwise intact abdominal wall. Prematurity is more common in gastroschisis (60%) than omphalocele (33%) [1, 2]. See Table 53.1.

(2) What other anomalies are associated with omphalocele?
While gastroschisis is less likely to be associated with other syndromes or anomalies, 35–75% of neonates with omphalocele will have associated anomalies, usually related to midline defects including neural tube defects, cardiac defects, genitourinary anomalies, orofacial clefts, and diaphragmatic defects. Up to 50% of these patients may have congenital cardiac disease, including VSD, Tetralogy of Fallot, and extropia corpis. Chromosomal abnormalities are common, including trisomy 13, 18, and 21, as well as Turner Syndrome and rare chromosomal deletions. In addition to chromosomal abnormalities, several syndromes are associated with

L. Downey (✉)
Pediatric Cardiac Anesthesiology, Emory University, 1405 Clifton Road, Atlanta, GA 30322, USA
e-mail: ladowney@gmail.com

© Springer International Publishing AG 2017
L.S. Aglio and R.D. Urman (eds.), *Anesthesiology*,
DOI 10.1007/978-3-319-50141-3_53

Table 53.1 The differences between gastroschisis and omphalocele

	Gastroschisis	Omphalocele
Incidence	4.5: 10,000	3: 10,000
Embryology	Anterior abdominal wall defect, umbilical cord intact and to the right of defect. No membranous sac. Usually small and large intestines	Midline abdominal wall defect. Abdominal viscera herniated through the umbilical ring into a membranous sac. Sac may include small and large intestines, liver, spleen, and other viscera
Maternal risk factors	Young maternal age, cigarette smoking	Extremes of maternal age 20< or >40 years
Associated Anomalies	2–10% GI problems: malrotation, atresia and stenosis 1–2% with cardiac defects	35–75% Chromosomal abnormalities (Trisomy 13, 18, 21); Associated syndromes Up to 50% with cardiac defects
Prematurity (%)	60	33

omphalocele: CHARGE syndrome, Pentalogy of Cantrell (omphalocele, diaphragmatic hernia, sternal abnormalities, ectopic cordis), amniotic band sequence, OEIS syndrome (omphalocele, exstrophy of the bladder, imperforate anus, spinal defects), Carpenter syndrome, Beckwich Wiedemann syndrome (macroglossia, giantism, hypoglycemia, omphalocele) [1, 2].

(3) What maternal risk factors are associated with gastroschisis?
The two most important risk factors for gastroschisis are young maternal age and smoking. Other potential risk factors include use of recreational drugs, low socioeconomic status, poor nutritional status, young age at the time of first pregnancy and previous terminations [1, 3].

(4) Describe the associated risk factors in neonates born with gastroschisis?
Neonates born with gastroschisis are usually premature and small for gestational age (SGA).
Risk factors associated with **prematurity** are associated with immature organ systems—including the respiratory, cardiovascular, and renal systems. Consequences include respiratory distress syndrome (RDS), retinopathy of prematurity (ROP), electrolyte abnormalities and sepsis.

- **Respiratory Distress Syndrome**: Type II pneumocytes are responsible for surfactant production, but surfactant synthesis for appropriate pulmonary function is not adequate until 34–36 weeks GA. Maternal preterm betemethasone therapy 48 h prior to delivery has been shown to improve lung maturation in premature infants.
- **Retinopathy of Prematurity**: ROP is a progressive vascular overgrowth of the retinal vessels that lead to intraocular hemorrhage associated with hyperoxia. Therefore, FiO_2 should be minimized to reach a target saturation of 90–95% depending on the clinical or procedural circumstances.

Risk factors associated with **SGA** include hypoglycemia, electrolyte abnormalities, polycythemia, hyperbilirubinemia, and temperature instability [1, 4, 5].

(5) Describe potential GI complications associated with gastroschisis?
Up to 25% of neonates may have associated gastrointestinal atresias, which may require emergent surgery for bowel obstruction.
Second, when the bowel is exposed to the intrauterine environment with no protective sac, it is at risk for injury. An inflammatory peel may develop and cause the bowel loops to become indistinguishable from each other. Pathology can include localized atresias to volvulus with loss of the entire midgut. Intestinal atresia or volvulus may result in intestinal obstruction, rupture, and eventually sepsis [1].

Preoperative Evaluation and Preparation

(6) What other studies would you request prior to proceeding with the procedure?
Important laboratory studies prior to starting the procedure would include hematocrit, type, and cross for blood products, blood glucose level and standard electrolytes as this patient is at risk for large insensible loses, electrolyte abnormalities, and blood loss during the procedure.
If time permits, a chest X-ray and an echocardiogram would be useful in ruling out cardiac defects. However, due to the unstable nature of the patient, including dusky bowel, tachycardia and hypotension, there may not be time for additional studies. Cardiac defects are rare in gastroschisis patients and physical exam may help determine the likelihood of other abnormalities.

(7) Are these vital signs normal for a 34-week-old premature infant?

The respiratory rate and oxygen saturation are normal for a newborn. However, the heart rate is elevated in this patient, with an upper limit of normal around 170. The blood pressure is low, even for a preterm neonate. Traditionally, the gestational age has been used as the lower acceptable mean arterial pressure (MAP) for a preterm infant. Target MAPs for this patient should be 34 mmHg. While the there is large variation in "normal" blood pressure for neonates, neonatal literature suggests that all premature infants should have a MAP >30 mmHg. Additionally, the clinical condition should be evaluated and this patient is tachycardiac and hypotensive [4, 6]. See Table 53.2.

(8) What is the differential diagnosis for tachycardia and hypotension in a neonate with gastroschisis?
The most common causes of hypotension in neonates are hypovolemia (insensible losses or blood loss during delivery), hypoglycemia, hypothermia, sepsis, or oversedation.
The most likely cause of hypotension and tachycardia in this patient is hypovolemia. On exam the patient has decreased distal pulses and a sunken fontanelle. Neonates with gastroschisis have fluid losses that are at least 3–4 times that of a healthy newborn from insensible losses, heat, and fluid losses from the exposed bowel, and third spacing of fluid from sequestration of intestinal fluid. Maintenance fluids may be as high as 150–300 ml/kg per day to maintain normovolemia [5].

(9) The leak with a 3.0 uncuffed ETT is at 10 cm H_2O. Would you change the ETT prior to starting the procedure? Why or why not?
The patient has a large leak with a 3.0 uncuffed ETT and the tube should be replaced with a larger ETT or a cuffed ETT. During gastroschisis repair, replacing the viscera into an underdeveloped abdominal cavity can restrict diaphragmatic excursion, compress the lungs and cause high intra-abdominal pressures. As a result, a cuffed ETT would allow the anesthesiologist to use higher peak inspiratory pressures to adequately ventilate the patient. While uncuffed ETTs were preferred historically, recent literature suggests that intubation with a low pressure, low profile cuffed ETT is preferable in cases with changing abdominal pressures.

10) What vascular access would you want in this patient prior to proceeding with the procedure? Would you place umbilical lines?
This patient will need an arterial line in order to monitor hemodynamics and serial ABGs. During gastroschisis repair, large fluid requirements and returning abdominal contents to an underdeveloped cavity may cause large shifts in hemodynamics, which necessitate monitoring of arterial blood pressure. Large fluid requirements and potential for electrolyte derangement necessitate the need for serial labs and glucose levels.
This case may be done without a central venous line if time is of the essence. However, a patient with dusky bowel concerning for bowel obstruction and potential sepsis, in addition to the large fluid shifts associated with a large gastroschisis defect, may warrant a central line to monitor central venous pressure, mixed venous saturation, and deliver inotropes.
While it is possible to place umbilical lines in a patient with gastroschisis, practically these lines may be in the surgical field or become kinked or inaccurate during replacement of abdominal viscera.

(11) What is a normal hemoglobin and hematocrit in a newborn?
A normal hematocrit for a full term infant is 16–17 g/dL or 45–47%. A premature infant or SGA infant may have a normal range of 15–18 g/dL and 45–53% [4].

(12) What is the circulating blood volume of this baby?
The equation for estimating the circulating blood volume is:

$$\text{Estimated Total Blood Volume} = \text{Weight (in kg)} \times \text{Average Blood Volume per kg}$$

The average blood volume for a preterm neonate is 95 ml/kg. The circulating blood volume is BV = 2.6 kg × 95 ml/kg = 247 ml.
See Table 53.3 for Estimated Blood Volume based on age [7].

(13) What other intraoperative concerns do you have regarding a small for gestational age neonate?
As mentioned above, neonates born with gastroschisis are usually premature and small for gestational age (SGA). Risk factors associated with **SGA** include hypoglycemia, electrolyte abnormalities, polycythemia, hyperbilirubinemia, and temperature instability [1, 4, 5].
- *Hypoglycemia*: SGA infants are prone to hypoglycemia and therefore should have a glucose containing solution and have frequent glucose checks to avoid hypoglycemia.

Table 53.2 Neonatal vital signs

	Heart rate	Blood pressure	Respiratory rate
Premature	120–170	55–70/35–45	40–70
Infant	100–150	65–75/40–45	35–55

Table 53.3 Estimated blood volume based on age

	Estimated blood volume (ml/kg)
Premature newborns	95
Full term newborns	85
Infants	80
Adult Women	75
Adult Woman	65

- *Impaired renal function*: Premature or SGA infants do not have normal renal function and cannot concentrate sodium. As a result, they have large sodium and water losses during the perioperative period and require careful monitoring of electrolyte abnormalities perioperatively. Attention should be paid to medication dosage and dosing interval as these infants have decreased GFR and may have impaired drug clearance.
- *Temperature instability*: Neonates are extremely susceptible to rapid heat loss through evaporation, convection, conduction, and radiation. Factors that contribute to this rapid heat loss are the high ratio of surface area to body, reduced subcutaneous fat, and decreased mechanisms to conserve heat, including an underdeveloped shivering mechanism. Methods for reducing heat loss include:
  - Warming the operating room
  - Using a radiant warmer
  - Covering the infant with warm blankets
  - Using humidified breathing circuits
  - Warming IV and irrigation fluids

Intraoperative Management

(14) What are your anesthetic concerns for gastroschisis closure?
Management for gastroschisis repair includes meticulous attention to volume replacement, covering the mucosal surfaces with sterile, saline-soaked dressings to minimize evaporative and heat losses, and a rapid sequence induction if there is a need for intubation.
As abdominal closure is attempted, it is important to monitor for (1) decreased perfusion to abdominal organs, (2) decreased ventilation/oxygenation, and (3) decreased venous return. Impaired organ function/damage may lead to decreased drug metabolism, lactic acidosis, and renal congestion. It is important to monitor for UOP, lactic acidosis, and ventilator changes as well as electrolyte abnormalities that may develop as the abdomen is closed. In patients who have a large defect, the replacement of abdominal contents may lead to mechanical obstruction of the IVC and subsequent decreased venous return, lower body edema, and lactic acidosis. In these cases, the reduction of abdominal contents may be done in a staged procedure to allow for the body to adapt.

(15) The first ABG on 21% FiO_2 is pH 7.18 $PaCO_2$ 43 PaO_2 80 Base Deficit -8 Lactate 4. What is the appropriate initial treatment?
This ABG demonstrates a metabolic acidosis, likely from a lactic acidosis. There are several potential sources for the metabolic acidosis in this patient: hypovolemia, bowel ischemia or sepsis.
The patient likely needs large volume resuscitation in the setting of a large amount of bowel exposed to the environment and large insensible loses. Patients with gastroschisis may have 3–4 times the daily fluid requirements as other neonates, requiring up to 300 ml/kg/day. Crystalloid or colloid can be used depending on the patient's hematocrit and other electrolytes. Those patients with ischemic bowel and possible sepsis also have large fluid requirements and may require inotropic support if fluid resuscitation is not enough to maintain systemic perfusion.

(16) Describe appropriate fluid management for this patient.
Newborns are at risk for hypoglycemia and will require a glucose-containing solution for maintenance. Maintenance fluid for 2.6 kg baby would be 4 ml/kg/hr or 2.6 × 4 ml/kg/hr = 10.4 ml/hr.
Maintenance fluid:
- For 10 kg or less: 4 ml/kg/hr
- For 10–20 kg: For the first 10 kg = 4 ml/kg/h; then 2 ml/kg/hr for each additional kilogram over 10 kg
- For >20 kg: For the first 10 kg = 4 ml/kg/h; then 2 ml/kg/hr for each additional kg, then 1 ml/kg/hr for each additional kilogram over 20 kg

As discussed above, this patient will likely require 3–4 times normal daily fluid requirements—up to 300 ml/kg/day. Therefore, it is important to monitor for signs of hypovolemia, including hypotension, tachycardia, UOP, central venous pressure (CVP), arterial waveforms, and evidence of metabolic acidosis or electrolyte abnormalities on serial ABGs. An increase in blood pressure or decrease in HR with a 10–20 ml/kg bolus, suggests a fluid deficit. Intraoperative fluid losses in this patient may be from blood loss, capillary leak, anesthetic vasodilation, and evaporative losses from viscera and mechanical ventilation.

Isotonic crystalloid or colloid may be used as fluid replacement, but the type of fluid lost should dictate the decision. Blood loss is replaced at a 1:1 ratio with colloid (5% albumin or blood) or 3:1 with isotonic crystalloid. While there is some debate about absolute minimum hematocrit levels, most studies agree that a critically ill premature neonate should have a hematocrit of $\geq 30\%$ or higher if clinical evidence suggests the need for improved systemic oxygen delivery [4, 5, 7].

(17) After volume resuscitation with 30 ml/kg lactated ringers, UOP increases to 1 ml/kg, the patient's vital signs stabilize at HR 160 and BP 55/34. The surgeon begins the procedure and you notice that the baby's temperature is 34.5 °C. What is the mechanism for the rapid cooling in a neonate?

There are likely several major causes for hypothermia in this patient: (1) radiant heat loss to the cold operating room; (2) conductive heat loss from large volume resuscitation and irrigation with cold fluids; (3) increased heat loss through environmental exposure due to large surface area-to-body ratio, exposed viscera, and decreased subcutaneous fat; (4) anesthetic-induced inhibition of thermoregulatory mechanisms.

Several factors make neonates and infants more susceptible to hypothermia: immature thermoregulatory mechanisms, limited glycogen and brown fat stores, and physiologic factors that accelerate heat loss. Under anesthesia, vasodilation and blunting of the primary mechanisms to maintain normothermia (vasocontriction, increased metabolic rate and non-shivering thermogenesis) increase environmental heat loss in the operating room [4, 8].

(18) What risks are associated with hypothermia?

During periods of cold stress, metabolic rates may rise by two to threefold, leading to further heat loss and other physiologic consequences that may increase morbidity and mortality during prolonged hypothermia. Perioperative hypothermia in neonates and infants have several adverse effects: (1) increased metabolic rate, oxygen consumption and exhaustion of brown fat and glycogen stores; (2) increased bleeding risk due to inhibition of normal coagulation pathways; (3) increased wound infections; (4) diminished metabolism of anesthetic agents leading to prolonged opioid effects and neuromuscular blockade [9–11].

(19) The surgeon has identified the obstruction and is planning to resect the dead bowel. During the dissection, the heart rate increases to 190 and the blood pressure increases to 65/42. What is your differential diagnosis and how might you manage the patient?

The differential for tachycardia includes pain and noxious stimuli, hypovolemia, SIRs response to bowel ischemia. However, in combination with hypertension, it is most likely that the patient has light anesthesia. Therefore, the anesthetic should be deepened. Intravenous fentanyl is a hemodynamically stable opioid that is metabolized by neonates and can be used if the patient is on an ICU ventilator with no ability to deliver volatile anesthetic. Using volatile anesthetics is an option in these patients. However, the resulting vasodilation and depression of myocardial function in a patient that already has large volume requirements, bowel ischemia, and SIRS may not be the best option.

(20) The surgeon has replaced the abdominal contents and is closing the fascia, when you notice that the blood pressure has slowly been drifting down and now is reading 40/27. You have given an additional 30 ml/kg of 5% albumin, but the patient has no urine output in the last hour and the peak inspiratory pressures (PIP) have increased. What is your differential diagnosis for decreased UOP? How will you manage the patient?

Decreased UOP can be broken down into three etiologies: (1) Pre-renal (2) Renal and (3) Post-renal.

Renal: This patient has no known renal abnormalities and the cause is unlikely to be renal.

Pre-renal: In a patient that has large insensible loses and third spacing, pre-renal oliguria is also on the differential. It is important to review the fluid balance, CVP if available, arterial waveform and blood gases. A fluid challenge is also warranted if there is concern for hypovolemia.

Post-renal: Possibilities include kinked or clotted foley or a mechanical obstruction, including compression of the IVC.

For patients undergoing gastroschisis repair, who present with low blood pressures, decreased UOP and increased PIPs, abdominal compartment syndrome (ACS) is high on the differential. ACS is due to mechanical obstruction of the IVC from abdominal contents. This may cause mechanical obstruction of the ureters, leading to obstruction. These patients may develop "relative hypovolemia" from mechanical obstruction that prevents adequate venous return to the heart. The decreased preload results in decreased cardiac output and eventually decreased systemic perfusion. Assuming that you have adequately kept up with the fluid requirements of the patient, the best course of action is to reopen the abdomen and plan for staged closure of a large defect.

When attempting closures of large abdominal defects, it is important that the anesthesiologist be in close communication with the surgeon to prevent problems with impaired ventilation/oxygenation, decreased perfusion to abdominal organs, and decreased preload/cardiac output.

(21) The decision is made to leave the abdomen open. On 30% FiO_2, the blood gas is pH 7.20 CO_2 60 PaO_2 60 Base Deficit -6 Lactate 6. Interpret the blood gas.
This is a mixed metabolic and respiratory acidosis. There is a respiratory acidosis since a normal PCO_2 is 40 mmHg and the PCO_2 is 60 mmHg. Therefore, ventilation should be increased blow off the carbon dioxide. The patient continues to have a metabolic acidosis, likely from increased lactate production. Lactate is produced during organ ischemia. In this case, bowel ischemia and decreased perfusion during IVC obstruction likely resulted in a lactic acidosis. Now that perfusion has been restored to the abdominal organs, the metabolic acidosis should resolve. However, if the metabolic acidosis persists or worsens, the anesthesiologist should consider fluid resuscitation, adding inotropes, or a blood transfusion to increase systemic oxygen delivery.

(22) What concerns do you have regarding acidosis a neonate?
Metabolic acidosis in neonates may cause increases in pulmonary vascular resistance (PVR). Elevated PVR in an infant that is only a few hours old may result in reversal to fetal circulation. Blood shunts from right to left and may result in severe hypoxemia that does not respond to oxygen or other normal ventilation strategies. If not quickly reversed, this may result in persistent pulmonary hypertension of the newborn (PPHN). In a preterm neonate, an increase in right-to-left shunting through a large patent ductus arteriosus (PDA) may lead to systemic hypoperfusion and hypoxia [4, 12, 13].

(23) What is your plan for postoperative pain management?
In a neonate undergoing a small gastroschisis repair with minimal fluid resuscitation, it is reasonable to consider extubation and a neuraxial block, such as a caudal or epidural for pain control. However, this patient is a SGA premature patient with large volume resuscitation and a large abdominal defect that remains open with a silo. Therefore, this patient should remain intubated and sedated for the immediate perioperative period to monitor for worsening acidosis, respiratory complications, and hypovolemia. Pain may be managed with IV opioids.

References

1. Holland A, Walker K, Badawi N. Gastroschisis: an update. Pediatr Surg Int. 2010;26:871–8.
2. Christison-Lagay E, Kelleher C, Langer J. Neonatal abdominal wall defects. Semin Fetal Neonatal Med. 2011;16:164–72.
3. D'Antonio F, Virgone C, Rizzo G, Khalil A, Baud D, Cohen-Overbeek TE, Kuleva M, Salomon L, Flacco ME, Manzoli L, Giuliani S. Prenatal risk factors and outcomes in gastroschisis: a meta-analysis. Pediatrics. 2015;136(1):159e–69e.
4. Gregory G, Brett C. Neonatalogy for anesthesiologists. In: Davis PJ, Cladis FP, Motoyama EK, editors. Smith's Anesthesia for Infants and Children. 8th ed. Elsevier. Philadelphia, PA; 2011. pp. 512–553.
5. Brusseau R, McCann ME. Anaesthesia for urgent and emergency surgery. Early Human Dev. 2010;86:703–14.
6. Fanaroff J, Avroy Fanaroff. Blood pressure disorders in the neonate: hypotension and hypertension. Semin Fetal Neonatal Med. 2006;11:174–81.
7. Brett C. Pediatrics. In: Stoelting RK, Miller RD, editors. Basics of anesthesia. 5th ed. Elsevier: Philadelphia, PA; 2007. p. 504–17.
8. Luginbuehl I, Bissonnette B, et al. Thermoregulation: physiology and perioperative disturbances. In: Davis PJ, Cladis FP, Motoyama EK, editors. Smith's anesthesia for infants and children. Philadelphia, Mosby; 2011. p. 157–78.
9. Jonsson K, Jensen JA, et al. Tissue oxygenation, anemia, and perfusion in relation to wound healing in surgical patients. Ann Surg. 1991;214(5):605–13.
10. Kurz A, Sessler DI, et al. Perioperative normothermia to reduce the incidence of surgical-wound infection and shorten hospitalization. Study of wound infection and temperature group. New Engl J Med. 1996;334(19):1209–15.
11. Polderman KH, Herold I. Therapeutic hypothermia and controlled normothermia in the intensive care unit: practical considerations, side effects, and cooling methods. Crit Care Med. 2009;37 (3):1101–20.
12. Walsh-Sukys MC, Tyson JE, et al. Persistent pulmonary hypertension of the newborn in the era before nitric oxide: practice variation and outcomes. Pediatrics. 2000;105(1 Pt 1):14–20.
13. Murphy JD, Rabinovitch M, et al. The structural basis of persistent pulmonary hypertension of the newborn infant. J Pediatr. 1981;98 (6):962–7.

Congenital Diaphragmatic Hernia

54

Bridget L. Muldowney and Elizabeth C. Eastburn

CASE

A 4 day-old male presents for left congenital diaphragmatic hernia repair. The defect was diagnosed prenatally on ultrasound and the pregnancy was otherwise uncomplicated. The patient was intubated shortly after birth in the delivery room and transferred to the tertiary care children's hospital.

Medications:	Fentanyl 1 mcg/kg/h
Allergies:	NKDA
Birth history:	Born via NSVD to a 34 yo G3P2 serology negative female at 38 2/7 weeks gestation
Physical exam:	
Vs:	Weight 2.9 kg BP 76/42 HR 135 RR 28 O2 sat 96%
HEENT:	Intubated, nasogastric tube in place
CV:	Diminished breath sounds on left
Abdomen:	Scaphoid concave appearance of the abdomen with diminished bowel sounds
Access:	24 g PIV, umbilical artery catheter
Ventilator settings:	SIMV-PCV 16/4 RR 28 measured Vt 15 ml
CXR:	Bowel loops present in left chest cavity with slight right mediastinal shift

1. **What is a congenital diaphragmatic hernia (CDH)?**

A congenital diaphragmatic hernia is a defect in the diaphragm that occurs in utero allowing the abdominal contents to herniate into the thorax. The abdominal contents in the thorax impinge on the space for pulmonary development leading to unilateral irreversible pulmonary hypoplasia. In severe cases the abdominal contents will cause a mediastinal shift resulting in deleterious effects on pulmonary development bilaterally. Bowel compression of the developing lung causes arterial remodeling that can lead to persistent pulmonary hypertension, a major cause of morbidity and mortality in patients with a CDH. CDH lesions occur more frequently on the left side, and often in a posterior lateral location through the foramen of Bochdalek. Defects in an anterior parasternal location through the foramen of Morgagni and at the esophageal hiatus are less common [1].

2. **What is the incidence of congenital diaphragmatic hernia?**

Congenital diaphragmatic hernia occurs in 1 in 2500–3000 live births [2]. CDH is associated with significant morbidity and mortality [3]. Survival rates for patients with CDH vary based on the size and severity of the lesion. Survival rates range from 60 to 90% and are often higher at medical centers that do a high volume of cases [4].

3. **What is the embryologic origin of the defect?**

Formation of the diaphragm occurs between weeks four to ten of gestation. Four structures form the diaphragm: the septum transversum, the dorsal esophageal mesentery, the pleuroperitoneal membrane, and muscular ingrowth from the body wall [5]. Failure of these structures to properly develop leads to a diaphragmatic defect that allows the abdominal contents to herniate into the thorax.

B.L. Muldowney (✉)
Department of Anesthesiology, University of Wisconsin School of Medicine and Public Health, 600 Highland Ave., B6/319, Madison, WI 53792, USA
e-mail: blmuldowney@wisc.edu

E.C. Eastburn
Department of Anesthesiology, Perioperative and Pain Medicine, Boston Children's Hospital, 300 Longwood Ave., Bader 3rd Floor, Boston, MA 02115, USA
e-mail: Elizabeth.eastburn@childrens.harvard.edu

© Springer International Publishing AG 2017
L.S. Aglio and R.D. Urman (eds.), *Anesthesiology*,
DOI 10.1007/978-3-319-50141-3_54

4. **What is the risk of coexisting congenital anomalies?**

Approximately 40% of patients with a CDH have coexisting congenital anomalies that can occur as part of a known syndrome or as an isolated finding. Cardiovascular malformations occur in approximately 10–15% of non-syndromic cases, while central nervous system anomalies including neural tube defects and hydrocephalus occur in 5–10% of non-syndromic cases. Limb anomalies occur in approximately 10% of non-syndromic cases of CDH [6].

5. **Why are CDH defects not corrected on the first day of life?**

Historically a congenital diaphragmatic hernia was considered an emergency and was repaired shortly after birth. Newer evidence suggests that medical stabilization and delayed repair may improve survival [7]. Surgery should be delayed until the patient is hemodynamically stable, has adequate oxygenation and ventilation, and pulmonary hypertension has resolved or been medically optimized. Typically a neonate with a CDH will be intubated in the delivery room and initiated on gentle ventilation with permissive hypercapnia.

6. **What is transitional circulation?**

In utero, the pulmonary arteries have high vascular resistance while there is low systemic vascular resistance. The majority of oxygenated blood from the placenta enters the right heart and is shunted across the Eustachian valve to the left atrium to supply the brain, heart and upper body with relatively highly oxygenated blood. Immediately after birth the inflation of the lungs with the first few breaths causes a drop in the resistance to pulmonary blood. The majority of blood flow is now circulated through the lungs which replaces the placenta as the as the organ of gas exchange. The subsequent increase in left atrial blood flow from the pulmonary veins increases left atrial pressure and functionally closes the foramen ovale [8]. With these anatomic and flow changes the right heart and pulmonary artery pressures fall. In a healthy neonate the mean pulmonary artery pressure approaches 50% of mean systemic pressure by the end of day one of life, and should drop to the normal adult level by two weeks of age [9]. In the case of a neonate with a congenital diaphragmatic hernia the normal fall in pulmonary artery pressure may not occur and the degree of persistent pulmonary hypertension as a result of the defect will become apparent in the first few days of life.

7. **What additional diagnostic work-up is necessary for a patient presenting for CDH repair?**

Prior to any major thoracic or abdominal surgery in a neonate one should obtain a CBC, type and screen, and possibly coagulation studies. In a patient with a congenital diaphragmatic hernia an echocardiogram is absolutely necessary.

8. **What might you expect to see on the echocardiogram?**

Echocardiography is used to rule out any coexisting congenital cardiac anomalies. Of even more importance, though, it is used to confirm the presence and degree of pulmonary hypertension. This often will be quantified by actual pressure estimates and measurements, but may only be suggested by the presence of right to left shunting or the presence of right heart strain and dysfunction.

9. **Why might the ICU team order a head ultrasound?**

Head ultrasounds are commonly done on patients with a CDH to assess for intracranial hemorrhage. Depending on the center they are preformed frequently, up to every two days, to monitor for bleeding. Intracranial hemorrhage is a contraindication to extracorporeal membrane oxygenation (ECMO) therapy. Therefore this monitoring should continue until there is confidence the patient will not need ECMO support.

10. **What is the role of extracorporeal membrane oxygenation therapy in patients with CDH?**

ECMO is often used as a rescue therapy in neonates with very low estimated lung volumes, those failing escalation of respiratory and hemodynamic support, and those who acutely decompensate. Respiratory indications for ECMO in the neonatal population include a high oxygen index (OI) ($OI = MAP \times FiO2 \times 100/PaO2$), high peek inspiratory pressures, and refractory hypercarbia [10]. Cardiac indications for ECMO in the pediatric population include a rising or persistently elevated lactate, long term need for high dose inotropic support, low mixed venous oxygen saturation, persistent arrhythmias, and severe cardiac dysfunction [11].

11. **What are contraindications to EMCO?**

Contraindications to ECMO include any situation in which systemic anticoagulation must be avoided, such as intracerebral hemorrhage, irreversible cardiac or respiratory failure where transplant or ventricular assist device (VAD) is not possible, gestational age <34 weeks, birth weight <2 kg, and other significant co-morbid conditions with a poor prognosis [12].

12. **What is the optimal ventilation strategy for a patient with CDH?**

Gentile ventilation with permissive hypercapnia is important. Improved outcomes are seen in patients with CDH when they are managed with very specific ventilation strategies, including low peak inspiratory pressures, adequate positive end expiratory pressure (PEEP), permissive hypercapnia, and high frequency oscillatory ventilation (HFOV) if necessary to prevent severe hypercapnia [13].

13. **What are options for ventilation in transport to the OR?**

The patient should remain on the ICU ventilator during transport when feasible. This will avoid delivering inadvertently high peak pressures and tidal volumes when the patient is switched to hand ventilation. The ventilator will also maintain lung recruitment that will be lost when disconnecting the patient from the circuit. If transport on the ICU ventilator is not possible hand ventilation should be done with a bag capable of delivering (PEEP) with a pressure valve to monitor the peak airway pressures delivered in transport.

14. **If the patient experiences sudden oxygen desaturation in transport what is the differential diagnosis and what treatments should be initiated?**

The differential diagnosis for oxygen desaturation in any patient should include lack of oxygen delivery, inadequate ventilation, and increased oxygen demand. First and foremost listen to the patient to ensure adequate breath sounds. In this case ensure that there is still an adequate source of oxygen to your ventilator or your inflation bag. Ensure patency of all connections. Check the endotracheal tube patency and look for kinks or plugs. Check the endotracheal tube depth and see if it is too low (mainstem intubation) or too high (inadvertent extubation).

In a patient with a congenital diaphragmatic hernia one must be suspicious of a pneumothorax on the side contralateral to the defect. If unilateral breath sounds are noted adjust endotracheal tube placement to ensure it is not in the right mainstem bronchus. In the case of suspected pneumothorax, a stat chest radiograph should be obtained to confirm the diagnosis. Should the patient continue to deteriorate, empiric treatment with needle decompression and chest tube placement is necessary.

15. **What intraoperative monitoring is necessary for this case?**

Standard ASA monitoring includes monitoring of the patient's oxygenation, ventilation, circulation, and temperature. In addition to standard monitoring an additional pulse oximeter to measure both pre-ductal and post-ductal oxygen saturation is warranted. A gradient that develops between the pre and post-ductal oxygen saturations may be the first indication of an exacerbation of pulmonary hypertension. Invasive arterial pressure monitoring is warranted as well. If the patient presents with an umbilical artery catheter it will need to be replaced at a site not interfering with the operative field. Finally, although continual CVP measurement is unlikely to guide management central access may be warranted to provide a safe route for inotropic support.

16. **What equipment modifications do you want to ensure adequate ventilation during the case?**

A circuit with the smallest volume and lowest compliance will allow the most accurate inspiratory pressure and tidal volume measurement. Many choose to have inhaled nitric oxide set up and ready to use in the event that the patient suffers a pulmonary hypertensive crisis during the procedure.

17. **What are the advantages and disadvantages of using an ICU ventilator for the case?**

Most anesthesia machines in use at major children's hospitals have the same technology, ventilation modes, and capabilities as the ventilators used in the ICU. The ICU may have circuits with lower compliance and a sampling port more proximal to the patient to more accurately measure end tidal CO_2. In many cases these circuits can be connected to the OR anesthesia machine.

The main disadvantage of using an ICU ventilator for the case is the inability to deliver potent inhaled anesthetics through the vaporizer of the anesthesia machine. This limits options for maintenance of anesthesia. Also most anesthesiologists are not familiar with the settings and functions of the ICU ventilator. Lack of familiarity with the ventilator is another major disadvantage of using the ICU ventilator. If the decision is made to use the ICU ventilator it is imperative to have a respiratory therapist or additional provider immediately available who is comfortable making adjustments and troubleshooting the ICU ventilator.

18. **What is a reasonable plan for maintenance of anesthesia for the case?**

Anesthesia is typically maintained with a balanced technique using potent inhalational agents, narcotics, and muscle relaxants. If the repair is done on ECMO anesthesia is often maintained with a narcotic relaxant technique. It is important to remember that the ECMO circuit increases the volume of distribution of drugs while the synthetic material of the circuit may absorb lipophilic medications such as midazolam and fentanyl, making their dosing unpredictable [14].

19. **What is the typical surgical approach to a CDH repair and how does that influence the anesthetic plan?**

Small defects can be treated with a primary repair in which the native diaphragm is sewn together. Some surgeons are attempting these smaller repairs via a minimally invasive thoracoscopic approach. Larger defects may require a synthetic patch to repair. The majority of large defects are repaired through an open subcostal abdominal approach. Lung isolation may be requested for a thoracoscopic approach.

20. **What are the options for lung isolation and one-lung ventilation in the neonatal and infant population?**

As the use of minimally invasive thoracoscopic procedures increases in the infant population there will be a greater number of requests for lung isolation. One-lung ventilation in the neonate and infant population is challenging. When right lung isolation is necessary the easiest method is often right mainstem intubation. If left lung isolation is needed it can be very challenging to mainstem an endotracheal tube in the left main bronchus even with fiberoptic bronchoscopy guidance. Fluoroscopic-assisted endobronchial intubation has been reported as a successful technique to achieve lung isolation [15]. Extraluminal use of the 5F endobronchial blocker has also been reported to achieve successful lung isolation in the infant population [16]. Such techniques are challenging and best preformed by experienced pediatric anesthesia providers. Intraoperative use of high frequency oscillatory ventilation (HFOV) has been reported in the surgical literature to provide good intraoperative exposure while facilitating excellent oxygenation and carbon dioxide elimination during thoracoscopic procedures in neonates [17].

21. **The procedure is underway via an open abdominal approach and the monitor shows a growing difference between the pre-ductal and post-ductal oxygen saturations. What could be going on?**

An exacerbation of pulmonary hypertension must be high on the differential diagnosis. Pulmonary hypertension can be exacerbated by the 5 H's: hypoxia, hypercarbia, H+ (acidosis), hypothermia, and hurts (pain). The status of all these factors should be evaluated and treated if necessary. The most likely cause in this case is small changes in ventilation worsening hypercarbia coupled with sympathetic stimulation in the form of pain.

22. **How do you treat an intraoperative pulmonary hypertensive episode?**

In this case ensure the patient and the room are as warm as possible. Modify ventilation strategies to treat any hypoxia or hypercarbia. Look for other causes of acidosis and treat if necessary. Finally increase the depth of anesthesia and administer additional narcotic to treat pain that might be a factor in the exacerbation.

If the above measures are not sufficient in treating pulmonary hypertension selective pulmonary vasodilators can be used including nitric oxide. Nitric oxide causes vasodilation in the pulmonary vascular bed without causing systemic vasodilation. Inhaled nitric oxide should only be used in cases of refractory pulmonary hypertension as it is very expensive and has not been shown to reduce the need for EMCO support nor improve mortality [18]. Initiation of phosphodiesterase inhibitors can also benefit children with pulmonary hypertension [19].

23. **What is the plan for emergence and extubation?**

Even after repair of a CDH patients are still at high risk of cardiac and respiratory decompensation after surgery. Extubation should only be considered in a stable patient who underwent a small repair. In the majority of cases the patient will remain intubated and transfer back to the ICU for continued medical management and stabilization.

24. **What are options for postoperative analgesia?**

As the majority of patients with CDH remain intubated a narcotic infusion such as fentanyl or morphine is often used. In the rare case of a small lesion where early extubation is planned one can consider placing an epidural catheter to facilitate pain control and early extubation. It is imperative to check coagulation studies before preforming regional anesthesia in neonates.

25. **What are the approaches to place an epidural in a neonate?**

Historically epidural analgesia was preformed through a caudal approach because it minimizes the risk of both spinal cord and dural puncture. Landmarks that surround the sacral hiatus include the 4th sacral spinous process cephalad, the sacral cornua lateral, and the coccyx caudad. In the case of epidural catheter placement an 18 gauge angiocatheter or a Tuohy needle is inserted in the sacral hiatus and passes through the sacrococcygeal ligament. Entry into the epidural space is felt via loss of resistance. An epidural catheter is then threaded cephalad to the desired location. It is important to verify the epidural tip location, often with fluoroscopic confirmation, when using a caudal approach to placement. One study found the catheter tip location to be inadequate in 32% of catheters threaded from a caudal location [20]. Caudal catheters are also at risk of bacterial contamination. Tunneling the caudal catheter will reduce the risk of bacterial colonization and may reduce the risk of infectious complications [21]. Many providers will remove a caudal catheter after an infant passes the first postoperative bowel movement for fear of fecal contamination at the entry site. With the risks just mentioned many experienced pediatric anesthesiologists may prefer to place the epidural directly at the desired site of action: a thoracic or lumbar approach.

References

1. Veenma DC, de Klein A, Tibboel D. Developmental and genetic aspects of congenital diaphragmatic hernia. Pediatr Pulmonol. 2012;47(6):534–45.
2. Langham MR Jr, Kays DW, Ledbetter DJ, Frentzen B, Sanford LL, Richards DS. Congenital diaphragmatic hernia. Epidemiology and outcome. Clin Perinatol. 1996;23(4):671–88.
3. Colvin J, Bower C, Dickinson JE, Sokol J. Outcomes of congenital diaphragmatic hernia: a population-based study in Western Australia. Pediatrics. 2005;116(3):e356–63.
4. Skari H, Bjornland K, Haugen G, Egeland T, Emblem R. Congenital diaphragmatic hernia: a meta-analysis of mortality factors. J Pediatr Surg. 2000;35(8):1187–97.
5. Clugston RD, Greer JJ. Diaphragm development and congenital diaphragmatic hernia. Semin Pediatr Surg. 2007;16(2):94–100.
6. Pober BR. Genetic aspects of human congenital diaphragmatic hernia. Clin Genet. 2008;74(1):1–15.
7. Logan JW, Rice HE, Goldberg RN, Cotten CM. Congenital diaphragmatic hernia: a systematic review and summary of best-evidence practice strategies. J Perinatol. 2007;27(9):535–49.
8. Finnemore A, Groves A. Physiology of the fetal and transitional circulation. Semin Fetal Neonatal Med. 2015.
9. Gao Y, Raj JU. Regulation of the pulmonary circulation in the fetus and newborn. Physiol Rev. 2010;90(4):1291–335.
10. ELSO Neonatal Respiratory Failure Supplement to the ELSO General Guidelines. 2013.
11. ELSO Pediatric Cardiac Failure Supplement to the ELSO General Guidelines. 2013.
12. Kim ES, Stolar CJ. ECMO in the newborn. Am J Perinatol. 2000;17(7):345–56.
13. Haroon J, Chamberlain RS. An evidence-based review of the current treatment of congenital diaphragmatic hernia. Clin Pediatr (Phila). 2013;52(2):115–24.
14. Wildschut ED, Ahsman MJ, Allegaert K, Mathot RA, Tibboel D. Determinants of drug absorption in different ECMO circuits. Intensive Care Med. 2010;36(12):2109–16.
15. Cohen DE, McCloskey JJ, Motas D, Archer J, Flake AW. Fluoroscopic-assisted endobronchial intubation for single-lung ventilation in infants. Paediatr Anaesth. 2011;21(6):681–4.
16. Stephenson LL, Seefelder C. Routine extraluminal use of the 5F arndt endobronchial blocker for one-lung ventilation in children up to 24 months of age. J Cardiothorac Vasc Anesth. 2011;25 (4):683–6.
17. Mortellaro VE, Fike FB, Adibe OO, Juang D, Aguayo P, Ostlie DJ, et al. The use of high-frequency oscillating ventilation to facilitate stability during neonatal thoracoscopic operations. J Laparoendosc Adv Surg Tech A. 2011;21(9):877–9.
18. Campbell BT, Herbst KW, Briden KE, Neff S, Ruscher KA, Hagadorn JI. Inhaled nitric oxide use in neonates with congenital diaphragmatic hernia. Pediatrics. 2014;134(2):e420–6.
19. Lowson SM. Alternatives to nitric oxide. Br Med Bull. 2004;70:119–31.
20. Valairucha S, Seefelder C, Houck CS. Thoracic epidural catheters placed by the caudal route in infants: the importance of radiographic confirmation. Paediatr Anaesth. 2002;12(5):424–8.
21. Bubeck J, Boos K, Krause H, Thies KC. Subcutaneous tunneling of caudal catheters reduces the rate of bacterial colonization to that of lumbar epidural catheters. Anesth Analg. 2004;99(3):689–93 (table of contents).

Pyloric Stenosis

55

Hyun Kee Chung

Introduction

Pyloromyotomy for PS is a common surgical procedure performed routinely at pediatric hospitals. It is the most common condition requiring surgery in the first few months of life [1]. Because of modern medical, surgical and anesthetic care, these patients do extremely well, with little morbidity and mortality [2]. A typical hospital course can consist of admission and diagnosis on hospital day one, medical treatment and stabilization overnight, surgery on hospital day two, and hospital discharged the next day. Pyloromyotomy is one of the most satisfying and rewarding cases for pediatric caregivers not only because the treatment is quickly successful, but also the patient swiftly recovers and is returned to a normal diet and activity within days [3]. The pediatric anesthesiologist plays a vital role in ensuring that these neonates safely undergo surgery with their perioperative risks minimized. This chapter will review the medical and surgical management of PS, and examine current anesthetic management techniques. Areas of controversy regarding induction and intubating methods and the use of regional anesthesia will also be discussed.

Incidence

PS is a relatively common condition. Rates of approximately 2–4 per 1000 live births in western countries have been reported [4–6]. The incidence is correlated with geographic location, season, and ethnic origin [7]. There is some evidence that in recent years the incidence in boys has increased in some parts of the United Kingdom [8–10]. The incidence has been reported to be four times lower in Southeast Asian and Chinese populations [4, 5, 7]. In fact, PS is considered relatively rare in patients of African, Chinese, and Indian extraction [11, 12].

Inheritance

Gender and genetics influence the incidence of PS. Males are affected four times more often than females [13]. Firstborn males are most commonly affected. Siblings of patients with PS are 15 times more likely to suffer the condition than those without a family history [14]. There is a higher incidence in the offspring of affected parents. Children of affected men are only affected 3 and 5% of the time, whereas children of affected women are affected between 7 and 20% of the time [15].

Pathogenesis

Though the etiology of PS is not fully understood, recent progress has been made in characterizing the condition. It is proposed that PS is inherited via a multifactorial threshold model. This model assumes that the ability to develop PS is affected by the additive effects of numerous genetic and environmental factors [16]. Although no specific gene has been linked to the pathogenesis of PS, genetic syndromes such as Smith–Lemli–Opitz, Cornelia de Lange, and other chromosomal abnormalities have been associated with it [17].

Recent studies suggest that, in pyloric stenosis, the smooth muscle cells of the pylorus are improperly innervated. Non-adrenergic, non-cholinergic nerves that mediate smooth-muscle relaxation are likely absent causing excessive contraction and hypertrophy of the pyloric muscle. The increased expression of certain growth factors and their receptors in the hypertrophied pyloric muscle suggests that the increased local synthesis of these factors play an important role in smooth-muscle hypertrophy. The circular

H.K. Chung (✉)
Division of Pediatric Anesthesia, Department of Anesthesiology and Perioperative Medicine, University of Massachusetts Medical School, University Campus, 55 Lake Avenue North, Worcester, MA 01655, USA
e-mail: hyun.chung@umassmemorial.org

© Springer International Publishing AG 2017
L.S. Aglio and R.D. Urman (eds.), *Anesthesiology*,
DOI 10.1007/978-3-319-50141-3_55

smooth muscle cells are actively synthesizing collagen, and this may be responsible for the characteristic "firm" nature of the pyloric tumor. Particular attention has been paid to the role of gastrin in the pathogenesis of PS. It has been suggested that repeated hyperacid stimulation of the duodenum induced by gastrin evokes repeated pyloric sphincter contractions causing hypertrophy of the pylorus [2].

Clinical Presentation and Evaluation

Feeding intolerance and gastroesophageal reflux are conditions considered in the early differential diagnosis of PS. When typical treatments for these conditions fail, and the patient's feeding intolerance worsens, PS should be considered. The typical PS patient is a full term, previously healthy infant 2–4 weeks old. The cardinal sign is a history of nonbloody, nonbilious emesis, often described as projectile in nature. 8% of patient may present with a temporary jaundice, but this reverses once feeding is resumed [11, 18]. The clinical presentation of patients with PS may vary widely, from a toxic infant who is severely dehydrated and malnourished, to a relatively healthy appearing infant. In recent years, due to earlier diagnosis, fewer patients present with severe symptoms [19]. A typical patient may be non-vigorous, mildly dehydrated, and have had a small amount of weight loss. Volume status is evaluated by assessing the fontanels, mucous membranes, skin turgor, and the absence of tears. Obtaining a history about the amount of wet diapers produced in a day (at least 5–6) is important in assessing the degree of dehydration. On the abdominal physical exam, one may palpate the classic "olive" between the midline and right upper quadrant, Gastric peristalsis may be observed. Blood chemistries are obtained when establishing intravenous (IV) access. Abnormally low chloride and high bicarbonate is characteristic of patients with PS. Arterial blood gas analysis is also obtained in the severely dehydrated patient to further assess the acid-base status. The finding of acidosis on arterial blood gas analysis is a sign of severe dehydration and organ hypoperfusion. The diagnosis of PS can be made with history and physical exam alone 90% of the time. However, in contemporary practice, patients almost always undergo radiolographic studies to confirm the diagnosis.

Radiolographic Studies

Ultrasound is the diagnostic modality of choice for evaluating suspected PS. A pyloric muscle thickness greater than 3 mm and a pyloric channel length of greater than 15 mm is considered diagnostic for PS [20, 21]. When ultrasound is inconclusive or unavailable, the upper gastrointestinal study is a reliable alternative. Poor gastric emptying in the presence of the classic string sign caused by the hypertrophied pyloric muscle is diagnostic for PS. If a contrast upper GI study has been performed, this must be taken into account during induction of general anesthesia.

Preoperative Medical Treatment

Careful preoperative management is likely the major factor in reducing the mortality related to PS to less than 0.5% [11, 19, 22–24]. PS is a medical emergency first. It is mandatory that the patient's volume status, acid-base balance, and electrolyte abnormalities are corrected prior to anesthesia and surgery to minimize the potential for intraoperative and postoperative complications. The hypochloremic, hypokalemic, metabolic alkalosis is a chloride-responsive alkalosis. The goals are to replenish the extracellular fluid volume, and to replace Na^+ and Cl^- to enable the kidney to excrete HCO_3^- and correct the alkalosis. The fluid deficit should initially be replaced with boluses of isotonic fluids. Maintenance fluids should be started using D5 0.45% NS or D5 0.2% NS. Once urine output is established, potassium is added to the maintenance fluid [25]. Once the fluid deficit is corrected, maintenance fluids of D5 0.45% NS or D5 0.2% NS with potassium may be given at a rate of 4 ml/kg/hr [26]. The plasma chloride concentration is used as a guide in the assessment and correction of the acid-base status of the patient. When the hypochloremia has been corrected, the correction of the alkalemia usually follows [27]. In infants, a chloride concentration of 95–105 mEq/L is considered normal [28]. Repeat laboratory studies prior to surgery must document the correction of the patient's metabolic status.

Pyloromyotomy

Fredet in 1908 was the first to suggest a full-thickness incision of the pylorus followed by a transverse closure. Ramstedt modified the technique and later described the sutureless, extramucosal longitudinal splitting of the pyloric muscle, which left the mucosa intact [29]. This technique is the guiding principal of the current surgical approaches for PS today [3]. There are three methods of operative treatment for PS: open (right upper quadrant incision), transumbilical, and laparoscopic. The laparoscopic technique is rapidly being acknowledged as the standard of care [30]. Advantages of the laparoscopic approach include a lower incidence of wound infection, shorter length of hospital stay, and decreased time to feeding. The complication rate for laparoscopic pyloromyotomy is similar to that of open procedures [31]. Surgical pyloromyotomy is considered the treatment of choice for PS [11].

Conservative Treatment

Atropine has been historically used as a non-surgical treatment for PS. The antispasmodic properties of atropine act to reduce pyloric muscle spasm. This modality has largely been abandoned over the past 40 years due to the excellent results with surgery. Recently, atropine's effectiveness as a nonsurgical alternative in the treatment of PS has been revisited. Studies of atropine treatment in PS have demonstrated success rates of 75–87% [32–34]. There may be a role for atropine treatment for PS but this must be further investigated [32]. Until then, surgical treatment remains the gold standard treatment.

Anesthesia

General Considerations

The relevant anesthetic issues for pyloromyotomy surgery for an infant are

1. General considerations of neonatal anesthesia including differences in physiology and pharmacology of infants.
2. Ensuring the restoration of intravascular volume preoperatively.
3. Correction of electrolyte abnormalities preoperatively.
4. Airway management of an infant while minimizing the risk of pulmonary aspiration in a patient with a full stomach.
5. Pain management, especially considerations of opioids in infants and the risk of postoperative respiratory depression.
6. Surgical approach—open versus laparoscopic.

It should be noted that only anesthesia providers experienced with pediatric care should perform anesthetics for neonates. This will often mean a pediatric anesthesiologist. If pyloromyotomy is not considered a routine case for the anesthesiologist, surgeon, or hospital, the patient should be transferred to an institution where appropriate personnel and resources are available. PS is not a surgical emergency, and therefore after medical stabilization is achieved, arrangements can be made for the safe transport of the patient to an appropriate facility.

Regional Anesthesia

Concerns regarding the possible adverse neurobehavioral effects of anesthetics on young children have prompted reevaluations and new investigations into regional anesthesia alternatives for surgery [35]. Currently general endotracheal anesthesia remains the standard technique.

Pyloromyotomy has been performed utilizing many regional anesthetic techniques. Historically, local anesthesia has been utilized, but with higher surgical complication rates [24]. Caudal block remains the standard anesthetic technique practice at the Hospital Infantil de México [36]. Willschke et al. [37] demonstrated the ability to provide anesthesia with an ultrasound guided single shot thoracic epidural injection for open pyloromyotomy. Spinal anesthetics for open and laparoscopic pyloromyotomy are possible [38, 39]. Spinal anesthetics have been considered in order to avoid (1) the issues of postoperative apnea and respiratory depression, (2) possible aspiration with induction, and (3) the stress of awake intubations. With the shift from open towards laparoscopic approaches, the only regional technique that may have potential application is the spinal. Currently the use of spinals for laparoscopic pyloromyotomy is not routinely recommended.

Regional blocks for postoperative pain control have also been investigated. Among them, the ultrasound guided rectus sheath block seems to be the simplest method for providing intra and postoperative analgesia for the open pyloromyotomy [40].

Preoperative Evaluation

Prematurity and postconceptional age (PCA, gestational age + chronological age) should be noted, as anesthetizing premature infants will require additional precautions. Premature infants less than 60 weeks PCA are at risk for apnea after general anesthesia and may require pediatric intensive care unit (PICU) admission postoperatively [41]. The fontanels, mucous membranes, skin turgor, and evidence of tearing should be examined to ensure that there has been adequate fluid resuscitation. The laboratory chemistries should be reviewed to ensure that metabolic disturbances have been corrected. Adequate IV access should be confirmed as well. Finally, informed consent for the anesthetic should be obtained from the parents. Parents should be reassured that their child will have adequate postoperative pain control, and that special precautions will be taken to avoid aspiration. As with any neonatal surgery, parents should be informed that their child may require postoperative intubation/ventilation and care in the ICU, but for an uncomplicated pyloromyotomy, this would be rare.

Preparation and Monitoring

The room, anesthesia machine, and all equipment should be appropriate for a neonate. An appropriately sized anesthesia circuit, reservoir bag, and mask should be utilized. Suction should be set up with an appropriately sized suction tip. Monitors should be of the appropriate size, and alarms should be set to a neonatal mode. Standard monitoring for neonates includes three lead EKG, noninvasive blood pressure cuff, pulse oximetry, end-tidal gas monitoring, and temperature probe. Airway set up includes appropriately sized masks, oral airways, endotracheal tubes, and laryngoscope blades. For the neonate, a 3.0 or 3.5 cuffed or uncuffed endotracheal tube are often appropriate. If a cuffed tube is used, meticulous management of cuff pressures is critical in this patient population. This can be done using a manometer or checking a tube/cuff leak using auscultation at the neck. A Miller 0 or 1 blade should be appropriate for laryngoscopy. A pediatric stylet should be loaded into the endotracheal tube in preparation for a rapid sequence induction. IV maintenance fluids of D5 0.45% NS with 20 mEq KCl should be administered at 4 ml/kg/hr via an infusion pump. 0.9% NS should be available for 10 mg/kg fluid boluses if needed. Angiocaths for intravenous access should be ready in case IV access is lost. All medications should be drawn up and ready for use. Many practitioners will have unit doses of medications available to decrease the chance of inappropriate dosing in infants. Atropine and succinylcholine should be ready with intramuscular needles in case IV access is lost. Propofol 2–3 mg/kg is a commonly used induction agent. Epinephrine should be immediately ready to administer in the event of cardiovascular collapse, which fortunately is an uncommon occurrence. Acetaminophen (IV or PR) is commonly administered intraoperatively for postoperative analgesia. The room should be warmed and a circulating air warming blanket should be turned on to warm the operating room table prior to the patient's arrival.

Preinduction

Once in the operating room, the patient's gown is removed and a warmed blanket is placed over the patient. All monitors are applied (except the temperature probe). IV Atropine is administered at a dose of 10–20 mcg/kg with a minimum dose of 100 mcg. Atropine premedication is used to prevent a vagal reflex when suctioning the stomach, and to prolong the time from oxygen desaturation to bradycardia if intubation is prolonged. A large-sized endotracheal suction catheter (12 french) is typically used to suction the stomach in an attempt to reduce the gastric volume and thereby reduce the aspiration risk. It must be clear that suctioning the stomach ***does not*** ensure an empty stomach, but it is recommended to reduce the gastric volume [42]. Orogastric suction is employed, and the patient is turned side to side with the catheter in place. Suction is intermittently applied. The catheter is removed, and the process is repeated once or twice until no fluid can be aspirated.

Orogastric tubes are replaced after intubation to decompress the stomach to ensure adequate surgical exposure. A decompressed stomach is required for safely accessing the abdominal cavity in laparoscopic surgery. Surgeons typically request the insufflation of air into the stomach after the pyloromyotomy is complete to ensure that the pyloric mucosa has not been perforated.

Induction and Intubation

Controversy still exists concerning induction techniques for pyloromyotomy. Mask inductions recommended by Stevens et al. [43] have gone out of favor, but the technique is still occasionally practiced. Recently Scrimgeour et al. [44] has suggested that inhalational induction it is no more risky than RSI and may confer some advantages. The proposed advantage was avoiding the RSI technique altogether. RSI may not decrease the risk of aspiration in PS patients while actually increasing the incidence of failed intubations. Controversy also exists concerning the method of intubation, awake versus asleep. Cook-Sather et al. [42] compared awake, RSI, and modified RSI intubating methods for PS. They concluded that intubations performed in unanesthetized and awake patients were not superior to intubations performed in anesthetized and paralyzed patients. Outcomes evaluated were maintenance of stable vital signs. Thus, they concluded that the practice of awake intubations should be abandoned in otherwise healthy infants. Of note, it was also determined that the modified RSI method, providing mask ventilation with cricoid pressure (CP), conferred no advantage over immediate tracheal intubations in preserving oxygen saturation [45].

Patients with PS are considered to have a full stomach and, although some practitioners perform them occasionally, mask inductions are generally not considered the safest induction technique is these patients. RSI is the preferred method of intubating patients with PS [46]. Awake intubations can be done safely, and may be an ideal alternative to RSI when a patient appears to have a difficult airway. Though Cook-Sather et al. [42] found that a modified RSI did not prevent oxygen desaturation, a simulation study by Eich et al. [47] found that a "controlled RSI" (non-depolarizing muscle relaxation and mask ventilation with CP) prevented hypoxemia and this in turn reduced operator stress and lead to fewer unsafe actions.

Muscle Relaxation

Though succinylcholine (SUX) is the ideal muscle relaxant for providing rapid intubating conditions, the use of Rocuronium (ROC) for RSI is an acceptable alternative. For patients with contraindications to SUX, ROC 0.7 mg/kg combined with Propofol 2–3 mg/kg should provide equally effective intubating conditions [48]. The standard RSI doses of ROC, 1–1.2 mg/kg, may produce prolonged muscle relaxation in the neonate and delay extubation. Practitioners must balance the risks of delayed onset of neuromuscular blockade with prolonged muscle relaxation. The dose of SUX in the neonate is 2 mg/kg.

There are a few considerations when using SUX in infants. Because neonates are resistant to SUX on a per-kilogram basis, a higher dose is required. Paralysis occurs within 20–30 s, and infants do not fasciculate. The duration of SUX in neonates is shorter. SUX is not recommended for routine use in pediatric patients, but the RSI is not considered a routine intubating method. SUX is a triggering agent for malignant hyperthermia. Pseudocholinesterase deficiency should be considered in the differential diagnosis in patients with delayed emergence after SUX administration [49].

Maintenance

Maintenance with volatile anesthetics is typical. Isoflurane and sevoflurane are currently the most commonly used agents. Use of nitrous oxide may be beneficial to reduce volatile anesthetic requirement, but may have unwanted side effects with laparoscopic procedures. Nitrous oxide can distend any gas filled bowel making laparoscopic exposure difficult. With open and laparoscopic procedures, additional muscle relaxation is typically not required especially if ROC was used for intubation. Positive pressure ventilation with appropriate levels of PEEP is recommended. Dextrose containing IV fluids are required to avoid hypoglycemia in the neonate due to reduced glycogen stores. Acetaminophen (IV at 10–12.5 mg/kg or PR at 30–45 mg/kg) may be administered for postoperative pain control [50, 51]. Body temperature is monitored either rectally or via esophageal temperature probe. Opioids are typically avoided due to the risk of respiratory depression and postoperative apnea related to the cerebrospinal fluid alkalosis associated with PS [25, 52]. Remifentanil may be a good alternative to volatile anesthetics in patients with a history of preoperative apnea. The study by Galinkin et al. [53] demonstrated that pre- and postoperative apnea occurs in term infants undergoing pyloromyotomy, and that a remifentanil-based anesthetic prevented new-onset postoperative apnea compared to halothane based anesthetics.

Emergence

Infants are extubated awake. Volatile agents should be eliminated; non-depolarizing neuromuscular blocking agents, if used, should be reversed. The patient should be breathing spontaneously with an appropriate end-tidal carbon dioxide level. The patient should be fully awake, vigorous, and demonstrating purposeful movement. Ideally the patient's eyes are open. When all these criteria are met, it is prudent to wait until one is absolutely certain that the patient will cry and cough immediately upon extubation. IV induction agents and airway equipment should be available for immediate use in the event that an emergent reintubation is required.

Pain Management

Pain control for pyloromyotomy is most commonly accomplished with local anesthetic wound infiltration by the surgeon and acetaminophen. Bupivacaine 0.25% with or without epinephrine 2.5 mg/kg (1 ml/kg of 0.25%) is the maximum recommended dose in neonates [54]. IV acetaminophen is commonly used although PR acetaminophen has a long history of use in this setting. A one time loading doses of 30–45 mg/kg of rectal acetaminophen is considered safe and effective [50, 51].

The routine use of opioids in PS patients is typically avoided. It is well known that the former premature infant that is less than 60 weeks PCA is at an increased risk of postoperative apnea after general anesthesia [41]. However, the incidence of apnea occurring in term neonates following general anesthesia is less clear, although it certainly exits [55]. Neonates respond to opioids differently than adults. They are more susceptible to the respiratory depressive effects of opioids. This is likely due to an incomplete blood-brain barrier allowing higher concentrations of opioids to reach the central nervous system [56]. Opioids are metabolized slower in neonates leading to higher plasma concentrations and longer elimination half-lives. [57]. The patient with PS has the additional risk of apnea related to cerebrospinal fluid alkalosis that may persist even though the acid-base balance of the blood has been corrected [23, 58]. A study by Habre et al. [59] on pain control after pyloromyotomy found that wound infiltration with bupivacaine delayed the need for other analgesics (acetaminophen) for up to 9 h. It was also noted that the use of intraoperative opioids was associated with naloxone administration in 10% of cases studied. If the practitioner feels that opioids must be administered, great care must be taken. Opioids should be given in the lowest effective doses after the patient is extubated, awake, and in an adequately monitored setting.

Breschan et al. [40] mentions the use of Ibuprofen and Tramadol for postoperative analgesia though these medications are typically not used in neonates.

Postoperative Management

Anesthetic considerations in the post anesthetic care unit (PACU) include

1. Ensuring adequate oxygenation and ventilation.
2. Ensuring effective analgesia.
3. Promotion of early feeding.
4. Ensuring appropriate IV fluid management and avoiding hypoglycemia.

All infants should receive supplemental oxygen while being transferred from the operating room to the post-anesthesia care unit (PACU). Supplemental oxygen should be routinely administered in the PACU until the patient's respiratory status returns to baseline [25]. All post pyloromyotomy patients should be on a cardiac and apnea monitor for 24 h once transferred to the pediatric floor [3]. Patients displaying any sign of altered respiratory status should remain in the PACU until stable. Patients that continue to display an altered respiratory status should be admitted to the PICU for observation.

If patients are inconsolable and exhibiting pain behavior, the judicious use of opioids may be required. A minimal dose of morphine at 0.02 mg/kg, (0.1 mg in a typical 4 kg patient) may be an effective rescue approach. It is recommended that a patient who recently underwent pyloromyotomy who is requiring opioids for effective analgesia should be admitted to the PICU for close monitoring. Acetaminophen 10–15 mg/kg, IV, orally, or rectally, every 6 h as needed, should be the only analgesic required on the floor [3].

Modern postoperative management advocates early feeding. Feeding within a few hours of surgery is safe and may hasten the tolerance of full feeds. Early feeding my also enable hospital discharge at 24–48 h postoperatively [60]. Allowing an infant to drink sugar water in the PACU can have a dramatic affect on calming the seemingly inconsolable patient. This may obviate the need for additional analgesics.

Dextrose containing maintenance fluids should be continued in the PACU. Postoperative hypoglycemia is a risk and dextrose containing IV fluids should not be discontinued abruptly [61]. IV fluids are discontinued when patients tolerate full enteral feeds.

Recommendations

1. PS is a relatively common condition. All anesthesiologists should be familiar with the pathophysiology of this disease, and be aware of the anesthetic implications. Practitioners with significant pediatric anesthesia experience should provide care for these neonatal patients.
2. The correction of volume status, acid-base disturbances, and electrolyte abnormalities is mandatory prior to surgery. Correction should be confirmed and documented with repeat laboratory studies.
3. General endotracheal anesthesia is considered the standard of care for open and laparoscopic pyloromyotomy.
4. All issues related to neonatal anesthesia apply. Intraoperative hypothermia and hypoglycemia must be prevented.
5. Patients with PS are considered to have a full stomach, and all precautions to prevent pulmonary aspiration should be taken. The RSI or awake intubation techniques are both effective in preventing aspiration with induction of anesthesia. Mask inductions are not recommended.
6. SUX and ROC are effective neuromuscular blocking agents for RSI in the neonate.
7. Gastric fluid volume should be reduced via orogastric suction prior to the induction of general anesthesia to reduce the risk of aspiration.
8. Infants have a higher vagal tone relative to sympathetic tone. Atropine (10–20 mcg/kg IV with a minimum dose of 100 mcg) should be administered prior to orogastric suction and RSI.
9. Opioids should be avoided intra- and postoperatively. Patients with PS are at particular risk for postoperative apnea and respiratory depression. Local anesthetic infiltration by the surgeon and acetaminophen provide adequate analgesia.

References

1. Puri P, Lakschmanadass G. Hypertrophic pyloric stenosis. In: Puri P editor. Newborn surgery. Oxford: Butterworth-Heinemann; 1996. p. 266–71.
2. Oshiro K, Puri P. Pathogenesis of infantile hypertrophic pyloric stenosis: recent progress. Pediatr Surg Int. 1998;13:243–52.
3. Pandya S, Heiss K. Pyloric stenosis in pediatric surgery, an evidence-based review. Surg Clin N Am. 2012;92:527–39. doi:10.1016/j.suc.2012.03.006.
4. Huang IF, Tiao MM, Chiou CC, et al. Infantile hypertrophic pyloric stenosis before 3 weeks of age in infants and preterm babies. Pediatr Int. 2011;53:18–23.
5. MacMahon B. The continuing enigma of pyloric stenosis of infancy: a review. Epidemiology. 2006;17(2):195–201.
6. Ramstedt WC, Clinic R, Sprincer D. Proffered review infantile hypertrophic pyloric stenosis: a review. Br J Surg. 1982;69:128–35.
7. Leck I. Descriptive epidemiology of common malformations. Br Med Bull. 1976;32:45–52.
8. Kerr AM. Unprecedented rise in incidence of infantile hypertrophic pyloric stenosis. Br Med J. 1980;281:714–5.
9. Knox EG, Armstrong E, Hayes R. Changing incidence of infant hypertrophic pyloric stenosis. Arch Dis Child. 1983;58:582–5.

10. Tam PKH, Chan J. Increasing incidence of hypertrophic pyloric stenosis. Arch Dis Child. 1991;66:530–1.
11. Spicer RD. Infantile pyloric stenosis: a review. Br J Surg. 1982;69:128–35.
12. Joseph TP, Nair RR. Congenital hypertrophic pyloric stenosis. Ind J Surg. 1974;36:221–3.
13. Stringer MA, Bereton RJ. Current management of infantile hypertrophic pyloric stenosis. Br J Hosp Med. 1990;43:266–72.
14. Finsen VR. Infantile pyloric stenosis-unusual family incidence. Arch Dis Child. 1979;54:720–1.
15. Carter CO, Evans KA. Inheritance of congenital pyloric stenosis. J Med Genet. 1969;6:233–54.
16. Carter CO. Inheritance of congenital pyloric stenosis. Br Med Bull. 1961;17:251–4.
17. Panteli C. New insights into the pathogenesis of infantile pyloric stenosis. Pediatr Surg Int. 2009;25(12):1043–52.
18. Woolley MM, Bertram FF, Asch MJ, et al. Jaundice, hypertrophic pyloric stenosis, and hepatic glucoronyl transferase. J Ped Surg. 1974;9:359–63.
19. Benson CD, Lloyd JR. Infantile pyloric stenosis: a review of 1,120 cases. Am J Surg. 1964;107:429–33.
20. Hernanz-Schulman M. Pyloric stenosis: role of imaging. Pediatr Radiol. 2009;39(Suppl 2):134–9.
21. Malcom GE 3rd, Rios CC, Del Rios M, et al. Feasibility of emergency physician diagnosis of hypertrophic pyloric stenosis using point-of-care ultrasound: a multi-center case series. J Emerg Med. 2009;37(3):283–6.
22. MacDonald NJ, Fitzpatric GJ, Moore KP, et al. Anaesthesia for congenital hypertrophic pyloric stenosis: a review of 350 patients. Br J Anaesth. 1987;59:672–7.
23. Daly AM, Conn AW. Anaesthesia for pyloromyotomy: a review. Can Anaesth Soc J. 1969;16:316–20.
24. Rasmussen L, Hansen LP, Pederson SA. Infantile hypertrophic pyloric stenosis: the changing trend in treatment in a Danish County. 1987;22:953–5.
25. Bissonnette B, Sullivan PJ. Pyloric stenosis. Can J Anaesth. 1991;38(5):668–76.
26. Steward DJ. Manual of pediatric anesthesia. 2nd ed. New York: Churchill-Livingstone Inc; 1985.
27. Goh DW, Hall SK, Gornall P, et al. Plasma chloride and alkalaemia in pyloric stenosis. Br J Surg. 1990;77:922–3.
28. Hatch DJ, Sumner E. Congenital pyloric stenosis. In: Hatch DJ, Sumner E, editors. Neonatal anaesthesia and perioperative care, 2nd ed. London: Edward Arnold Publishers; 1981. p. 145–7.
29. Garcia VF, Randolph JG. Pyloric stenosis: diagnosis and management. Pediatr Rev. 1990;11(10):292–6.
30. Oomen MWN, Hoeksra LT, Bakx R, et al. Open versus laparoscopic pyloromyotomy for hypertrophic pyloric stenosis: A systematic review and meta-analysis focusing on major complications. Surg Endosc. 2012;26:2104–10. doi:10.1007/s00464-012-217-y.
31. Sola JE, Neville HL. Laparoscopic versus open pyloromyotomy: a systemic review and meta-analysis. J Pediatr Surg. 2009;44 (8):1631–7.
32. Lukac M, Antunovic SS, Vujovic D, et al. Is abandonment of nonoperative management of hypertrophic pyloric stenosis warranted? Eur J of Pediatr Surg. 2013;23(1):80–4. doi:10.1055/s-0032-1333114.
33. Yamataka A, Tsukada K, Yokoyama-Laws Y, et al. Pyloromyotomy versus atropine sulfate for infantile hypertrophic pyloric stenosis. J Pediatr Surg. 2000;35(2):338–41, discussion 342.
34. Kawahara H, Takama Y, Yoshida H, et al. medical treatment of infantile hypertrophic pyloric stenosis: should we always slice the: olive? J Pediatr Surg. 2005;40(12):1848–51.
35. Consensus statement on the use of anesthetic and sedative drugs in infants, toddlers, and preschool children (Draft 2014 revision). International anesthesia research society. http://www.smarttots.org/resources/consensus.html. Accessed 31 Jul 2015.
36. Moyao-Garcia D, Garza-Leyva M, Velazquez-Armenta EY, et al. Caudal block with 4 mg/kg (1.6 ml/kg) of bupivacaine 0.25% in children undergoing surgical correction of congenital pyloric stenosis. Paediatr Anaesth. 2002;12:404–10.
37. Willschke H, Manchata A, Rebhandl W, et al. Management of hypertrophic pyloric stenosis with ultrasound guided single shot epidural anaesthesia-a retrospective analysis of 20 cases. Pediatr Anesth. 2011;21:110–5. doi:10.111/j.1460-9592.2010.03452.x.
38. Somri M, Gaitini LA, Vaida SJ, et al. The effectiveness and safety of spinal anaesthesia in the pyloromyotomy procedure. Paediatr Anaesth. 2003;13:32–7.
39. Islam S, Larson SD, Kays DW, et al. Feasibility of laparoscopic pyloromyotomy under spinal anesthesia. J Pediatr Surg. 2014;49: 1485–7. doi:10.1016/j.jpedsurg.2014.02.083.
40. Breschan C, Jost R, Stettner H, et al. Ultrasound-guided rectus sheath block for pyloromyotomy in infants: a retrospective analysis of a case series. Pediatr Anesth. 2013;23:1199–204. doi:10.111/pan.12267.
41. Kurth CD, LeBard SE. Association of postoperative apnea, airway obstruction, and hypoxemia in former premature infants. Anesthesiology. 1991;75:22–6.
42. Cook-Sather SD, Tulloch HV, Liacouras CA, et al. Gastric fluid volume in infants for pyloromyotomy. Can J Anaesth. 1997;44 (3):278–83.
43. Steven IM, Allen TH, Sweeney DB. Congenital hypertrophic pyloric stenosis: the anaesthetist's view. Anaesthesia Intensive Care. 1973;1(6):544.
44. Scrimgeour GE, Leather NWF, Perry RS, et al. Gas induction for pyloromyotomy. Pediatr Anesth. 2015;25:677–80. doi:10.111/pan.12633.
45. Cook-Sather SD, Tulloch HV, Cnaan A, et al. A comparison of awake versus paralyzed tracheal intubation for infants with pyloric stenosis. Anesth Analg. 1998;86:945–51.
46. Wang JT, Mancuso TJ. Ultrasound assessment of the gastric contents for the guidance of the anaesthetic strategy in infants with hypertrophic pyloric stenosis: a prospective cohort study. Pediatr Anesth. 2015;25:652–3. doi:10.111/pan.12690.
47. Eich C, Timmermann A, Russo SG, et al. A controlled rapid-sequence induction technique for infants may reduce unsafe actions and stress. Acta Anaesthesiol Scand. 2009;53:1167–72. doi:10.111/j.1399-6576.2009.02060.x.
48. Ghazal E, Amin A, Wu A, et al. Impact of Rocuronium versus succinylcholine neuromuscular blocking drug choice for laparoscopic pyloromyotomy: is there a difference in time to transport to recovery? Pediatr Anesth. 2013;23:316–21. doi:10.111/j.1460-9592.2012.03912.x.
49. Gregory GA. Pharmacology. In: Gregory GA, editor. Pediatric Anesthesia 4th ed. Australia: Churchill Livingstone; 2002. p. 5–33.
50. Montgomery CJ, McCormack JP, Reichert CC, et al. Plasma concentrations after high dose (45 mg/kg) rectal acetaminophen in children. Can J Anaesth. 1995;42:982.
51. Birmingham PK, Tobin MJ, Henthorn TK, et al. Twenty-four-hour pharmacokinetics of rectal acetaminophen in children: an old drug with new recommendations. Anesthesiology. 1997;87:244.
52. Holl JW. Anesthesia for abdominal surgery. In: Gregory GA, editor. Pediatric Anesthesia 4th ed. Australia: Churchill Livingstone; 2002. p. 569–80.
53. Galinkin JL, Davis PJ, McGowan FX, et al. A randomized multicenter study of Remifentanil compared with halothane in neonates and infants undergoing pyloromyotomy. II. Perioperative breathing patterns in neonates and infants with pyloric stenosis. Anesth Analg. 2001;93:1387–92.

54. Sethna NF, Berde CB. Pediatric regional Anesthesia. In: Gregory GA, editor. Pediatric Anesthesia 4th ed. Australia: Churchill Livingstone; 2002. p. 270–2.
55. Noseworthy J, Curan C, Khine HH. Postoperative apnea in a full term infant. Anesthesiology. 1989;70:879.
56. Kupfergerg HG, Way EL. Pharmacologic basis for the increased sensitivity of the newborn rat to morphine. Pharmacol Exp Ther. 1963;151:105.
57. Koren G, Butt W, Chinyanga H, et al. Postoperative morphine infusion in newborn infants: assessment of disposition characteristics and safety. J Pediatr. 1985;107:963.
58. Mendenhall MK, Ahlgren EW. Anesthetic considerations in surgery for gastrointestinal disease. Surg Clin North Am. 1979;59:905–17.
59. Habre W, Schwab C, Gollow I, et al. An audit of postoperative analgesia after pyloromyotomy. Paediatr Anaesth. 1999;9:253–6.
60. Puapong D, Kahng D, Ko A, et al. Ad libitum feeding: safely improving the cost-effectiveness of pyloromyotomy. J Pediatr Surg. 2002;37(12):1667–8.
61. Shumake LB. Postoperative hypoglycemia in congenital hypertrophic pyloric stenosis. South Med J. 1975;68:223–4.

Tracheoesophageal Fistula

56

Herodotos Ellinas

CASE

One-day-old 2000 g neonate, 34 week gestation presents to the operating room for a tracheoesophageal fistula (TEF) repair.

VS—temp 36.8C, RR 42, HR 135, BP 55/30 SpO_2 99% on RA, OG tube in place.

PIV 24G left saphenous vein, D10W infusing at 8 ml/h.

1. **How would you define a tracheoesophageal fistula (TEF)?**

TEF is a congenital anomaly that arises from an abnormal development of the tracheoesophageal septum. There are several theories regarding the embryological origin of the TEF but none have been definitively proven. Tracheoesophageal development from the foregut occurs around the 4–5th week of gestation. Foregut malformation with prevention of complete separation of the respiratory and gastrointestinal components creates a connection between the trachea and the esophagus. Its incidence ranges from 1:3000 to 1:4000 births with male preponderance (25:3) [1].

2. **What are the different types of a TEF?**

The most known classification systems are the Gross and Vogt (Table 56.1). As shown below they are defined as TEF with or without esophageal atresia (EA). The most common type is C/3b, esophageal atresia (blind end esophagus) with a fistula arising from the distal portion of the trachea [2, 3].

3. **What other anomalies are associated with TEF?**

About 25–50% of these neonates have other congenital anomalies such as congenital heart disease, genitourinary anomalies, gastrointestinal disorders, skeletal anomalies, and CNS disorders [4]. These anomalies have been incorporated into the acronym VACTERL (**V**ertebral anomalies, imperforate **A**nus, **C**ongenital heart disease, **TEF/EA**, **R**enal anomalies, **L**imb anomalies) (Table 56.2).

A less common association of TEF is with CHARGE syndrome (**C**oloboma of the eye, **H**eart defects, **A**tresia of the choanae, **R**etardation of growth/development, **G**enitourinary anomalies, **E**ar defects/deafness) [3, 5–9]. Chromosomal anomalies are also associated with TEF; specifically trisomy 18 (25%), 13 and 21 (1%). Therefore, karyotyping should be considered once in utero diagnosis has been confirmed [6, 10].

4. **How is the diagnosis made antenatally?**

Maternal polyhydramnios, due to inability to swallow the amniotic fluid, and consequent preterm labor due to the increased intrauterine volume has been associated with TEF. Further, an absent stomach bubble on ultrasonography can assist with diagnosis. Unfortunately the findings are nonspecific and prenatal detection rate is about 40–50% [11, 12].

5. **What is the clinical presentation of a TEF patient?**

TEF presents in the first week of life with symptoms such as excessive salivation, coughing, choking, and cyanosis with feeds and failure to pass an orogastric/nasopharyngeal tube to the stomach beyond 7–10 cm. Upon delivery, diagnosis can be confirmed by radiography of a radio-opaque oropharyngeal catheter unable to pass to the stomach [1, 5].

H. Ellinas (✉)
Department of Anesthesiology, Children's Hospital of Wisconsin, Medical College of Wisconsin, 9200 W. Wisconsin Ave., Milwaukee, WI 53226, USA
e-mail: hellinas@mcw.edu

© Springer International Publishing AG 2017
L.S. Aglio and R.D. Urman (eds.), *Anesthesiology*,
DOI 10.1007/978-3-319-50141-3_56

Table 56.1 Gross and Vogt TEF classifications [2, 3]

	EAgen	Isolated EA	pTEF/distal EA	dTEF/prox EA	prox/dist TEF	TEF/no EA, H-type	ES
Gross		A	B	C	D	E	F
Vogt	1	2	3A	3b	3c	4	
Frequency (%)		10	1	85	1	3	

EAgen Esophageal Agenesis, *ES* Esophageal Stenosis
pTEF proximal TEF, *dTEF* distal TEF

Table 56.2 VACTERL congenital anomalies

Anomalies	
Vertebral	Hemivertebrae, missing/extra vertebrae, scoliosis
Anorectal	Anal atresia and/or imperforate anus
Cardiac	VSD (most common), ASD, ToF, CoA, Right-sided aortic arch, Truncus, TGA
Tracheoesophageal Fistula	TEF
Esophageal Atresia	EA
Renal	Agenesis/dysplasia, hypospadias, polycystic kidneys, single umbilical artery
Limb	Radial agenesis/dysplasia, polydactyly/syndactyly

VSD Ventricular Septal Defect, *ASD* Atrial Septal Defect, *ToF* Tetralogy of Fallot
CoA Coarctation of the Aorta, *TGA* Transposition of the Great Vessels

6. **How would you manage this neonate preoperatively?**

Evaluation for other congenital anomalies prior to surgical procedure is mandatory due to the associations discussed above. A neonatologist should evaluate all neonates preoperatively unless the child is in extremis and truly emergent, life saving surgery is indicated. For children diagnosed with TEF, the minimum workup should include an echocardiogram to evaluate presence of congenital heart disease, a renal ultrasound to provide information about renal anomalies and a chest radiograph (CXR) should be obtained. Blood work to evaluate for electrolyte abnormalities is useful. Also, assessment of serum glucose (esp. if neonate is premature with increased secretions and frequent suctioning) and current hemoglobin and hematocrit (prematurity) are also recommended [13].

Since the most common tracheoesophageal defect is with an upper blind pouch (type C/3b TEF), an NG/OG with intermittent suction may prevent pulmonary aspiration with subsequent pneumonitis. Antibiotics should be considered to treat pneumonia/sepsis. Upright positioning and cessation of feeds should be initiated as soon as presumptive or definite diagnosis has been made [6].

7. **What is your plan for induction?**

- Standard ASA monitoring as recommended for all patients with temperature evaluation and active warming systems to avoid hypothermia and risk for bleeding
- Additional peripheral intravenous access (22G if possible) for volume resuscitation if needed
- Consider Near-Infrared Spectroscopy (NIRS) and/or arterial line for the neonate with congenital anomalies and
- Assure OG (or NG) is connected to suction and functioning well
- There are different approaches for induction. One possible method is rapid sequence induction (RSI) with or without cricoid pressure due to the high risk for pulmonary aspiration even with a gastric tube in place. The anesthesiologist must take into account the potential problems with positive pressure ventilation in a neonate with an uncontrolled TEF; namely, uncontrolled inflation of the stomach with consequent elevation of the diaphragm and severe respiratory compromise that can lead to arrest. If there is already a gastric vent placed, this technique may be considered.
- Medications for RSI: a sedative such as propofol (2 mg/kg) and either succinylcholine (2–3 mg/kg) or a non-depolarizer such as rocuronium (high dose 1.2 mg/kg); glycopyrrolate 10–15 mcg/kg will prevent bradycardia and decrease secretions.

8. **Would your plan change if the surgical colleague is planning a rigid bronchoscopy?**

Rigid bronchoscopy is performed to evaluate the anatomy of the airway prior to repair (missed secondary TEF, malacia, position of the fistula). Dependent on the size of the fistula, tracheal intubation or tracheobronchial intubation may be the choice with or without muscle relaxation. If the fistula is large, studies advocate for Fogarty catheter placement for occlusion to assure acceptable mechanical ventilation [12]. Thus, an alternative induction technique that many practitioners advocate would be slow IV or inhalational induction in order to maintain spontaneous ventilation and allow the surgeons to delineate the fistula (and control with a Fogarty catheter) during rigid bronchoscopy. A neonate who is spontaneously breathing is recommended by most to prevent the adverse effects of positive pressure ventilation (PPV) with increased abdominal distension and subsequent ineffective ventilation; medications recommended with this technique include volatile anesthetics and propofol or remifentanil infusion in addition to vocal cord local anesthesia (1–2% lidocaine max 4 mg/kg). Although ketamine administration may maintain spontaneous breathing, its association with neural apoptosis and its side effect of increased secretions render it a secondary agent [13].

9. **What are complications associated with either flexible or rigid bronchoscopy?**

If the airway is not adequately anesthetized, complications may include apnea and, coughing with laryngospasm, bronchospasm, and hypoxemia [14].

10. **What is the significance of a right-sided aortic arch?**

The usual positioning for the repair of a TEF is left lateral decubitus with a shoulder roll and a right thoracotomy approach. A left thoracotomy approach may be warranted in patients with a right-sided aortic arch in order to allow adequate visualization of the TEF and decrease the risk of injury to the aorta. However, it should be noted that successful repairs have been performed via a right thoracotomy even with a right-sided aortic arch [15].

11. **What are the advantages of a thoracoscopic approach?**

- Decreased stress response as reported in minimally invasive procedures in infants
- Avoidance of thoracotomy and thus concern for rib fusion/retraction and future high degree scoliosis
- Better visualization of the anatomy for fistula mobilization and ligation
- Less postoperative pain
- Cosmesis [16, 17].

12. **What are the disadvantages of a thoracoscopic approach?**

- Steep learning curve for the success of the operation
- Technically challenging anastomotic suture placement
- Higher incidence of post-repair anastomotic narrowing
- Hemodynamic collapse with insufflation (decreased venous return, compression of great vessels) [17].

13. **What would be your anesthetic maintenance plan intraoperatively?**

Volatile anesthetics are common for neonatal surgical procedures. However, neonates do not have the most robust myocardium and may experience significant hemodynamic compromise when exposed to volatile anesthetics, particularly at higher doses. In addition, opioids are used to decrease stress response esp. associated with initial airway manipulation (e.g., remifentanyl and fentanyl). Assuming intraoperative stability and successful fistula ligation, the plan for end of procedure extubation may be facilitated by low dose opioid (or complete avoidance of opioids) use intraoperatively. Extubation is preferred, if it can be done safely, to minimize ETT pressure over the anastomotic site. A worse problem would be the need for an emergent reintubation with possible damage to the fresh suture line. Thus, the benefits of immediate extubation must be balanced with the significant complications that can occur if the child needs to be reintubated in the OR or ICU.

14. **What would you do if you are having difficulty ventilating during repair?**

Ventilatory difficulty during TEF repair has been reported at approximately a 10% incidence [13, 18]. Ideal ETT placement (for a type C TEF) is distal to the TEF but above the carina. If the fistula is too close to the carina, the ETT may be forced down the right main stem bronchus. Single lung ventilation is not well tolerated in neonates especially those with cardiac anomalies and/or preexisting respiratory difficulties. A malpositioned ETT, the presence of excessive secretions or blood clots occluding the ETT, and surgical lung manipulation may all contribute to inadequate ventilation. Dependent on location of the fistula and the endotracheal tube (ETT) placement, adjustments can be made to improve ventilation. If the fistula is unintentionally intubated then the ETT can be withdrawn and the neonate can be hand ventilated until ligation is performed. If the fistula is large (>3 mm), a Fogarty balloon can be used to occlude the fistula prior to ligation. If there is persistent difficulty ventilating, emergent gastric decompression should be considered via a surgically placed gastric tube or vent. It has been suggested that in the premature infant with respiratory difficulties preoperatively, an emergent transpleural ligation of the TEF with reoperation in 8–10 days to complete the repair should be performed instead [13].

15. **What are your criteria for extubation at the end of the case?**

- Consideration of associated comorbidities (e.g. cardiac anomalies, respiratory distress)
- Ease of ventilation
- Intraoperative hemodynamic and respiratory stability
- Ease of surgical repair
- Procedure duration [13]
- Appropriate level of consciousness
- Adequate analgesia
- Complete reversal of muscle relaxation

16. **How would you manage perioperative pain?**

If thoracotomy is planned, most neonates remain intubated postoperatively and thus liberal use of opioids would be beneficial in reducing airway complications during bronchoscopy and reducing surgical stress response during repair. An opioid infusion should be used intra/postoperatively until extubation is considered. Alternatively, a thoracic epidural (or caudal to thoracic space catheter) with local anesthetic infusion with or without opioids can be combined with volatile agents to deliver a successful balanced intraoperative technique [19]. Epidural anesthesia has been associated with an improved response to surgical stimulation after major abdominal procedures in infants but local anesthetic infusion in neonates should be used with caution due to decreased clearance [13].

17. **What are complications post TEF repair?** [20, 21]

- Gastroesophageal reflux (GER) is the most common long-term complication
- Esophageal/laryngeal strictures secondary to GER
- Tracheomalacia, significant only in <10% of repairs but cause of reintubation
- Anastomotic leaks (up to 20%) resolve spontaneously or are recognized in the immediate postoperative period and get repaired
- TEF recurrence
- Scoliosis post thoracotomy
- TEF cough, present during childhood
- Dysphagia that improves with age
- Persistent pouch post repair. When these children return for other surgeries and tracheal intubation is required, the presence of a pouch must be considered when there is a lack of $ETCO_2$ and inadequate chest excursion after intubation. Veteran pediatric anesthesiologists know this to be a problem in these patients as they age and return for other procedures, but for some relatively inexperienced practitioners, this anatomic problem can come as a surprise.

18. **What are the prognostic indicators for long-term outcome?**

Three different classifications have provided information regarding survival rate: Waterson in 1962 modified by Spitz in 1994 and more recently by Okamoto in 2009. Initially three prognostic factors were included: birth weight, congenital anomalies and pneumonia. The two latter classifications removed pneumonia because of its rarity. The major risk factor contributing to all three classifications was cardiac anomalies (esp. with ductal dependent lesions [22]) reducing survival rate from 100 to 30% when present. Even with birth weights <2 kg and major heart defects, the survival rate was 27% [4, 12].

References

1. Lauder G, Hume-Smith H. Anaesthesia for specialist surgery in infancy. Anaesth Intensive Care Med. 2014;15(3):116–25.
2. Gross RE, DeBakey ME. The surgery of infancy and childhood; its principles and techniques. Philadelphia: Saunders; 1953. p. 1000.
3. Vogt E. Congenital esophageal atresia. Am J Roentgenol. 1929;22 (463–464):465.
4. Dave S, Bajpai M, Gupta DK, Agarwala S, Bhatnagar V, Mitra DK. Esophageal atresia and tracheo-esophageal fistula: a review. Indian J Pediatr. 1999;66(5):759–72.
5. Holzman RS, Mancuso TJ, Polaner DM. A practical approach to pediatric anesthesia. Seco ed. Philadelphia, PA: Wolters Kluwer; 2016. p. 384–90.
6. Brett C, Davis PJ. Anesthesia for general surgery in the neonate. Smith's Anesth Infants Child. 2011:554–588.
7. Roberts JD, Romanelli TM, Todres ID. Neonatal emergencies. Pract Anesth Infants Child. 2009:747–766.
8. Krosnar S, Baxter A. Thoracoscopic repair of esophageal atresia with tracheoesophageal fistula: anesthetic and intensive care management of a series of eight neonates. Paediatr Anaesth. 2005;15(7):541–6.
9. The charge syndrome foundation (1993–2015). www.chargesyndrome.org. Accessed Sep 2015.
10. Scott D. Esophageal atresia/tracheoesophageal fistula overview. In: Pagon RA, Adam MP, Ardinger HH, Wallace SE, Amemiya A, Bean LJH, Bird TD, Dolan CR, Fong CT, Smith RJH, Stephens K, editors. SourceGeneReviews® [Internet]. Seattle (WA): University of Washington, Seattle; 1993–2015. 12 Mar 2009 (updated 2014 Jun 12).

11. Houben CH, Curry JI. Current status of prenatal diagnosis, operative management and outcome of esophageal atresia/tracheo-esophageal fistula. Prenat Diagn. 2008;28(7):667–75.
12. Broemling N, Campbell F. Anesthetic management of congenital tracheoesophageal fistula. Paediatr Anaesth. 2011;21(11):1092–9.
13. Knottenbelt G, Costi D, Stephens P, Beringer R, Davidson A. An audit of anesthetic management and complications of tracheo-esophageal fistula and esophageal atresia repair. Paediatr Anaesth. 2012;22(3):268–74.
14. Parolini F, Boroni G, Stefini S, Agapiti C, Bazzana T, Alberti D. Role of preoperative tracheobronchoscopy in newborns with esophageal atresia: a review. World J Gastrointest Endosc. 2014;6(10):482–7.
15. Bicakci U, Tander B, Ariturk E, Rizalar R, Ayyildiz SH, Bernay F. The right-sided aortic arch in children with esophageal atresia and tracheo-esophageal fistula: a repair through the right thoracotomy. Pediatr Surg Int. 2009;25(5):423–5.
16. Rothenberg SS. Thoracoscopic repair of esophageal atresia and tracheoesophageal fistula in neonates, first decade's experience. Dis Esophagus. 2013;26(4):359–64.
17. Laberge JM, Blair GK. Thoracotomy for repair of esophageal atresia: not as bad as they want you to think! Dis Esophagus. 2013;26(4):365–71.
18. Davidson A. Anesthetic management of common pediatric emergencies. Curr Opin Anaesthesiol. 2013;26(3):304–9.
19. Lonnqvist PA. Regional anaesthesia and analgesia in the neonate. Best Pract Res Clin Anaesthesiol. 2010;24(3):309–21.
20. Gayle JA, Gomez SL, Baluch A, Fox C, Lock S, Kaye A. Anesthetic considerations for the neonate with tracheoesophageal fistula. Middle East J Anaesthesiol. 2008;19(6):1241–54.
21. Burge DM, Shah K, Spark P, et al. Contemporary management and outcomes for infants born with oesophageal atresia. Br J Surg. 2013;100(4):515–21.
22. Diaz LK, Akpek EA, Dinavahi R, Andropoulos DB. Tracheoesophageal fistula and associated congenital heart disease: Implications for anesthetic management and survival. Paediatr Anaesth. 2005;15(10):862–9.

Congenital Heart Disease: Atrioventricular Septal Defects

57

Viviane G. Nasr and Annette Y. Schure

Case

A 3-month-old, 3.5 kg male infant, born full term following a normal spontaneous vaginal delivery and diagnosed with Trisomy 21 and congenital heart disease at birth, is booked for an urgent inguinal hernia repair. He is scheduled for surgical repair of his atrioventricular septal defect the following week, but unfortunately presented to the ER with a poorly reducible right-sided inguinal hernia.

Medications:	Lasix
Allergies:	NKDA
Past Medical History:	Trisomy 21, Inguinal Hernia

PART A

1. **What is an atrioventricular septal defect?**

Congenital heart disease is the most common birth defect and affects approximately 1 in 100 newborns. There is a wide range: some defects resolve spontaneously over time (spontaneous closure of PDA, small ASDs or VSDs), others require multiple surgeries or even a heart transplant (single ventricle lesions) [1].

Atrioventricular canal defects (AVC) constitute 4–5% of congenital heart disease.

AV septal defects are a spectrum of malformations, which are characterized by a defect in the atrial septum, a defect in the ventricular septum and a defect in one or both atrioventricular (AV) valves (see below for the details) (Fig. 57.1).

AVC defects are often referred to as "mixing lesions." Depending on the size of the septal defects and the vascular resistances in the pulmonary and systemic circulations, deoxygenated blood from the right side of the heart and oxygenated blood from the left side of the heart will mix within the heart and determine the arterial oxygen saturation.

Left-to-right, right-to-left, or bidirectional shunting can be present.

2. **What is left-to-right shunting?**

In left-to-right shunting, oxygenated blood from the left side of the heart is shunted away from the systemic circulation and recirculates into the pulmonary circulation resulting in volume overload, poor cardiac output, congestive heart failure, and pulmonary edema.

Examples are large ventricular septal defects and complete AV canals with low pulmonary vascular resistance.

3. **What is right-to-left shunting?**

In right-to-left shunting, deoxygenated blood from the right side of the heart is shunted away from the pulmonary circulation and directly enters the systemic circulation, leading to cyanosis and poor tissue oxygenation. A classic example is Tetralogy of Fallot with pulmonary stenosis, one of the most common cyanotic heart defects.

4. **What is bidirectional shunting?**

In bidirectional shunting, the direction of the shunt usually changes with the cardiac cycle; it is different in systole versus diastole.

5. **Why is this child presenting for cardiac surgery now at the age of 3 months? Why not at the time of diagnosis?**

At birth the pulmonary vascular resistance is relatively high, but gradually decreases over time due to the ongoing maturation of the pulmonary arteries. Except for a murmur,

V.G. Nasr (✉) · A.Y. Schure
Department of Anesthesiology, Division of Cardiac Anesthesia, Perioperative and Pain Medicine, Harvard Medical School, Boston Children's Hospital, 300 Longwood Avenue, Bader 3, Boston, MA 02115, USA
e-mail: Viviane.Nasr@childrens.harvard.edu

A.Y. Schure
e-mail: Annette.schure@childrens.harvard.edu

© Springer International Publishing AG 2017
L.S. Aglio and R.D. Urman (eds.), *Anesthesiology*,
DOI 10.1007/978-3-319-50141-3_57

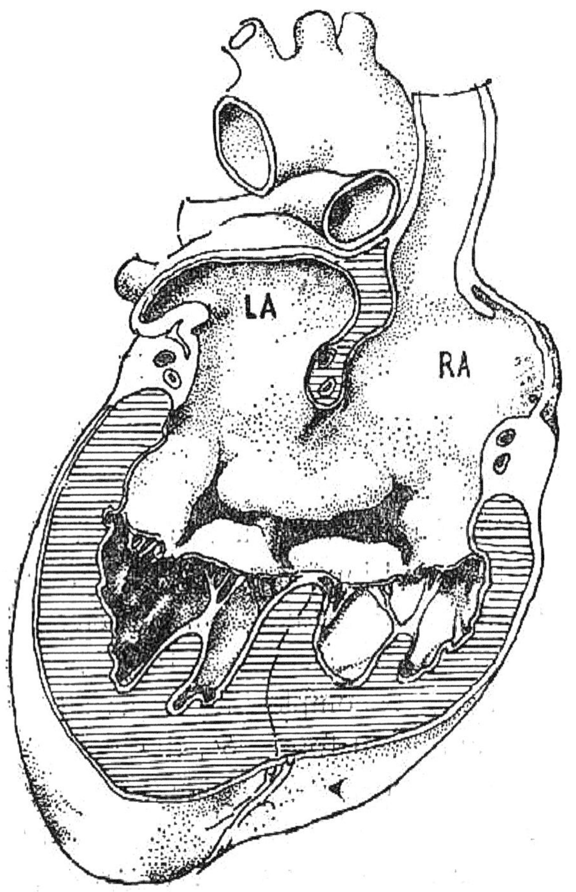

Fig. 57.1 Cross section of the heart showing mitral and tricuspid valve apparatus and common atrial and ventricular septal defects in a case of CAVC. Reproduced from Böök K, Björk V. O, Thorén C. (1986) "Complete atrioventricular canal." In: (Wu Y and Peters RM, eds.) International Practice in Cardiothoracic Surgery. Dordrecht: Springer Netherlands, pp. 779–785

many patients with AV defects are initially relatively asymptomatic and can be medically managed with diuretics and ACE inhibitors for afterload reduction. As the pulmonary vascular resistance drops further and reaches a nadir at about 2–3 months of age, the patients present with an increased left-to-right shunt and pulmonary overcirculation leading to congestive heart failure and poor growth. In addition, the complex surgical repair is easier to perform in an older and larger infant [2].

6. **How would you evaluate this infant? What are your specific concerns?**

Similarly to any patient presenting with an inguinal hernia, this patient needs to be evaluated for NPO status, presence of bowel sounds/obstruction or emesis. In terms of his cardiac status, it is important to review the history, existing imaging studies, current medications and assess the patient for signs and symptoms of congestive heart failure (Failure to thrive, poor feeding, cold sweating with feeding, tachypnea, history of recurrent respiratory infections, etc.) or pulmonary hypertension (hepatomegaly, tachypnea, cyanosis).

Furthermore, 25% of patients with CHD have other anomalies or associated syndromes, and this patient has already been diagnosed with Trisomy 21, so a thorough evaluation of potential airway problems, skeletal abnormalities, or endocrine issues is important. AV septal defects can also be associated with DiGeorge Syndrome, Tetralogy of Fallot, or double outlet right ventricle defects [3].

7. **What are you looking for on the physical exam?**

The findings on physical exam include signs and symptoms of congestive heart failure: tachypnea, increased work of breathing with retractions or nasal flaring, rales, cachexia, hepatomegaly, tachycardia, cool extremities, poor pulses, delayed capillary refill, and mottled appearance.

Focusing on the cardiac exam, findings may include a hyperactive precordium, normal or accentuated first heart sound, wide, fixed splitting of S2, pulmonary systolic ejection murmur with thrill, holosystolic murmur at apex with radiation to axilla, and mid-diastolic rumbling murmur at the left sternal border [3].

8. **Which preoperative tests would you like to see? Why? What do you expect to find?**

Preoperative testing should include: (1) a recent echocardiography for assessment of ventricular function, the severity of AV regurgitation, and the direction of shunting; (2) Electrocardiogram (EKG) looking at the rhythm and atrial or ventricular hypertrophy; (3) Chest X-ray (CXR) for the presence of pulmonary edema, infiltrates and cardiomegaly.

In addition to the imaging, laboratory testing is requested to check for polycythemia (secondary to cyanosis), anemia (physiologic nadir or secondary to malnutrition) and electrolyte disturbances, especially hypokalemia due to emesis and diuretic therapy.

9. **What are the anesthetic implications of Trisomy 21?**

Anesthetic implications of Trisomy 21 include (in addition to cardiac defects) cervical spine instability, large tongue, short and narrow trachea, muscular hypotonia, difficult vascular access, abnormal thyroid function, and early onset of pulmonary hypertension.

10. **The preoperative oxygen saturation is 95%. What if it is only 82%? Would this change your management?**

Decreasing arterial saturations are an ominous sign in patients with AV septal defects and can be caused by pulmonary hypertension or low cardiac output. In the presented case the differential diagnosis should include:

- Pulmonary hypertension secondary to increased pulmonary blood flow or vascular remodeling with increased vascular reactivity
- Coexisting pulmonary artery stenosis
- Pulmonary edema
- Low cardiac output, decreased tissue oxygenation, and mixed venous desaturation
- Aspiration or respiratory infection.

Obviously, the anesthetic management depends on the most likely cause, but should consider the increased risk for pulmonary hypertensive crisis, potential need for inotropic support, and invasive monitoring as well as appropriate postoperative monitoring (ICU).

11. **How would you induce this child for the inguinal hernia repair?**

An intravenous induction aiming for a well-balanced circulation (stable pulmonary vascular resistance/systemic vascular resistance (PVR/SVR) ratio) and normoventilation is safe while avoiding hyperventilation and high FiO_2. A high PaO_2 and low $PaCO_2$ decrease PVR, which will increase left-to-right shunting and decrease systemic cardiac output.

In addition, removing all possible bubbles in intravenous lines is a must to prevent a paradoxical air embolus.

12. **What are the factors that affect PVR?**

Factors that increase PVR include: Hypoxia, hypercarbia, acidosis, atelectasis, high hematocrit, and sympathetic stimulation.

Factors that decrease PVR include: oxygen, hypocarbia, alkalosis, normal FRC, low hematocrit, and attenuating sympathetic stimulation.

13. **How would you manage the airway?**

The management of the airway will involve a general anesthetic with endotracheal intubation allowing for control of ventilation and oxygen delivery. It is also necessary to avoid a potential pulmonary aspiration secondary to a non-reducible hernia. Shunt reversal (right-to-left) with severe hypotension or increase in PVR may occur following induction, bronchospasm, hypoxia, or acidosis, coughing, or breath-holding during emergence.

14. **Do you plan any invasive monitoring? Why?**

Two peripheral intravenous (PIV) lines should be inserted, using one PIV for bolusing medications and another PIV (e.g., external jugular venous line) for potential inotropic support. If insertion of a PIV is not possible, a central venous line (e.g., internal jugular) should be placed. Invasive blood pressure monitoring with an intra-arterial catheter is needed if the patient demonstrates signs of heart failure upon presentation for his inguinal hernia repair or instability at induction that requires constant resuscitation.

15. **After induction and institution of positive pressure ventilation with 100% FiO_2, the BP drops from 70/40 to 40/20 mmHg. What is your differential diagnosis? How do you treat it?**

Following induction and hyperventilation with a high $FiO_{2,}$ the PVR can fall significantly and lead to an increase in left-to-right shunting and a drop in systemic cardiac output. The decrease in sympathetic tone after induction of general anesthesia will often lead to significant hypovolemia, especially in volume depleted patients on chronic diuretic therapy. The use of cardiodepressant anesthetics, such as potent inhalation agents, can further decrease ventricular function and cardiac output. Treatment will include ventilatory changes to optimize PVR (lower FiO_2, low respiratory rate to allow elevation of CO_2, etc.), administration of volume and inotropic support if necessary. In patients with long standing diuretic therapy a slow bolus of calcium chloride or gluconate can also be helpful.

16. **Do you need Endocarditis Prophylaxis?**

Endocarditis prophylaxis is not recommended for this procedure. Although AVCs are considered an unrepaired cyanotic congenital heart disease, endocarditis prophylaxis is no longer recommended for routine gastrointestinal or genitourinary procedures.

According to the American Heart Association in 2007, the following conditions require endocarditis prophylaxis for dental procedures involving the gingival tissue or oral mucosa [4]:

- Prosthetic cardiac valve or prosthetic material used for cardiac valve repair
- Previous endocarditis

- Congenital Heart Disease (CHD)
  - Unrepaired cyanotic CHD, including palliative shunts and conduits
  - Completely repaired CHD with prosthetic material or device, whether placed by surgery or catheter intervention, during first 6 months after the repair
  - Repaired CHD with residual defects in the site or adjacent to the site of a prosthetic patch or prosthetic device (which inhibits endothelialization)
- Cardiac transplantation recipients who develop cardiac valvulopathy

17. **After an uneventful inguinal hernia repair, the surgeon would like to discharge the child home later in the day. Do you agree?**

The risk of a pulmonary hypertensive crisis remains postoperatively. Therefore, the patient needs to be admitted following surgery for a 24 h observation ensuring adequate pain control and monitoring of oxygen saturations in addition to routine vital signs.

PART B

One week later, after an uneventful recovery, the child is presenting for the surgical repair of the atrioventricular defect.

1. **What is the difference between an atrioventricular septal defect and an ASD or VSD?**

It is the presence of an abnormal AV valve that distinguishes this group of malformations from other types of endocardial cushion defects: atrial septal defects (ASDs) and ventricular septal defects (VSDs).

2. **How do AV defects develop? Embryology**.

All AV septal defects result from some degree of incomplete fusion of the endocardial cushions during the 5th week of fetal development. There are four endocardial cushions, which originate from the primitive mesoderm to form the atrioventricular (AV) valves, atrial and ventricular septum. The atrial portion of the AV septum develops from the growth of the endocardial cushion tissue toward the posterior wall of the common atrial chamber. The ventricular portion of the AV septum results from the growth of the endocardial cushion tissue toward the apex of the heart. As the endocardial cushion tissue continues to grow to the right and the left, it results in the formation of the tricuspid and mitral valves.

3. **How would you describe an atrial septal defect (ASD)?**

5–10% of CHD are isolated defects in the atrial septum, but ASDs are often part of other complex lesions. They are classified according to their location within the septum:

(1) ostium secundum defects, located in the fossa ovalis;
(2) ostium primum defects which can be associated with small clefts in the mitral valve;
(3) inferior and superior sinus venosus defects, often associated with partial anomalous return of pulmonary veins
(4) coronary sinus (CS) defects.

An ASD is a simple shunt, usually left-to-right, leading to progressive dilation of the right atrium and right ventricle. A small, restrictive defect will allow minimal shunt flow and often closes spontaneously within the first few years of life. A large defect is unrestrictive and might require interventions (device closure or surgical repair) [5].

4. **How would you describe a ventricular septal defect (VSD)?**

With 20–25% of all CHD, VSDs are the most common form of heart defects. A VSD is an opening in the ventricular septum allowing communication between the right and left ventricles. It may exist in one or more locations in the ventricular septum.

(1) Subpulmonary or supracristal defects located in the infundibular septum just below the pulmonary valve.
(2) Membranous or perimembranous defects. These defects comprise approximately 70–80% of all VSDs and are located in the subaortic region of the membranous septum.
(3) Conoventricular defects: Similar to perimembranous defects but extend anteriorly and superiorly in the septum.
(4) Inlet or canal-type defects: posterior septum near the atrioventricular (AV) valves.
(5) Muscular defects: located in the lower trabecular septum, there are often multiple defects, which may be apical, midmuscular, anterior, or posterior (Swiss cheese VSDs).

30–40% of VSDs, especially small ones, will close spontaneously, the rest usually present with increasing left-to-right shunting and congestive heart failure [1, 5].

5. **Describe the different types of AV defects?**

AV defects are described as complete and incomplete. Incomplete AV septal defects have a divided AV valve orifice. Although the AV valve is abnormal, it is characterized by a trileaflet tricuspid valve on the right and a bileaflet mitral valve on the left, in association with an atrial defect, a ventricular defect, or both. Usually, there exists a cleft in the anterior leaflet of the mitral valve, which creates some degree of mitral insufficiency. When associated with simply a primum ASD, these defects are often referred to as a partial AV septal defect. When associated with a primum ASD and a small VSD, these defects are often referred to as a transitional AV septal defect. Complete AV septal defects have a common AV valve, usually with five leaflets and one large orifice, and both an ASD and VSD.

6. **How many types of complete AV septal defects exist?**

There are three types that are classified depending on the location of the chordal attachments of the anterior bridging leaflet of the common AV valve as Rastelli type A, B, or C.

(1) Type A: Anterior bridging leaflet is attached to the ventricular septum by multiple chordal attachments. The left ventricular outflow tract is narrow and elongated with Type A.
(2) Type B: Anterior bridging leaflet is attached to the right ventricular side of the ventricular septum by an anomalous papillary muscle
(3) Type C: Anterior bridging leaflet lacks attachments to the ventricular septum—"free-floating." The Rastelli type C is the most common and is defined by an anterior leaflet that lacks ventricular septal attachments and thus "floats" above the ventricular septum.

7. **What is a balanced AV septal defect?**

Balanced defects are those in which the common AV valve lies equally over both ventricles. Unbalanced defects are those in which the AV valve does not lie equally over both ventricles thus one ventricle predominates and the other ventricle is usually hypoplastic.

8. **What other anomalies can be associated with AV defects?**

AV septal defects are commonly associated with other major cardiac or extracardiac abnormalities. They may be seen especially in association with Tetralogy of Fallot and DiGeorge syndrome. AV septal defects are present in 20–50% of patients with Trisomy 21, 15% of patients with Noonan's syndrome, and 5% of patients with Ellis-van Crefeld syndrome.

PART C

1. **How do you evaluate this child for the cardiac surgery? Any specific concerns?**

Evaluation of this child includes a detailed history and review of existing diagnostic tests and laboratory results as well as a thorough physical exam with specific focus on airway, cardiac status, and vascular access. (See question # 6–9).

2. **What preoperative tests would you like to review? Do you need a cardiac catheterization?**

The preoperative testing including an echocardiogram, EKG, CXR, lab testing will be reviewed (see above Part A). If a catheterization is done, important data would include pulmonary vascular resistance (PVR), Qp:Qs (Shunt Fraction or ratio of pulmonary blood flow to systemic blood flow), and saturations. In patients with a large AV septal defect who have systemic or near systemic RV and PA pressures, it is essential to determine suitability for operative intervention by establishing whether the elevation in PVR is reversible. This is done by checking the response to O_2 and/or NO.

3. **How does the Nitric Oxide work?**

Inhaled NO selectively reduces pulmonary hypertension and improves ventilation/perfusion matching in a variety of disease states. Pulmonary selectivity is based on its gaseous state, small size and lipophilicity, and its avid binding to and rapid inactivation by hemoglobin prevents systemic vasodilatation.

4. **What is the difference between adult and pediatric cardiopulmonary bypass?**

Considerations for cardiopulmonary bypass in infants and children include: (1) smaller circulating volume, higher rate of oxygen consumption, reactive pulmonary vascular bed, immature organ systems, altered thermoregulation, poor tolerance to microemboli, and the presence of intra and extracardiac shunts. Figure 57.2 summarizes the differences between adult and pediatric cardiopulmonary bypass [6].

5. **What kind of monitoring do you need? Any specific equipment?**

Monitoring for repair with complete AVC would include a 5 lead ECG, invasive arterial line to assess for continuous blood pressure and blood testing, as needed, a central line

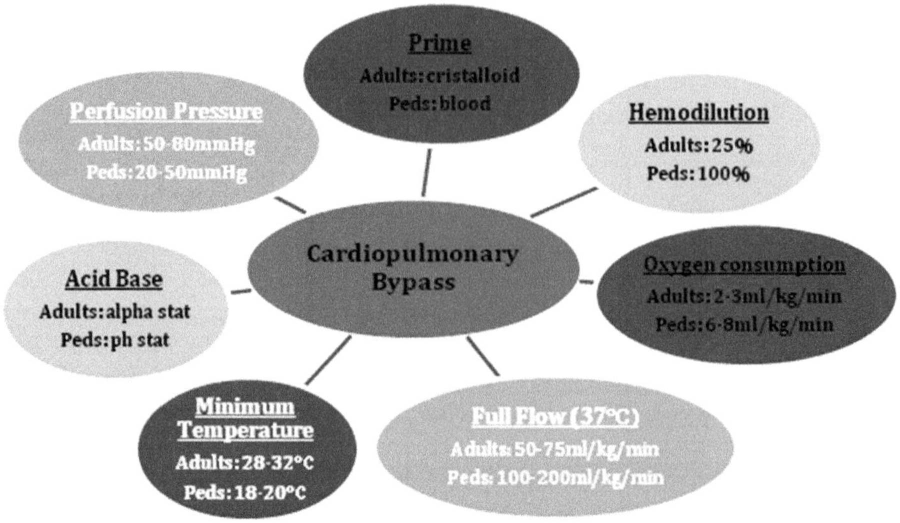

Fig. 57.2 Comparison between adult and pediatric cardiopulmonary bypass [1, 6]

placement for delivery of inotropic medications and mixed venous oxygen measurements, and near infrared spectroscopy for cerebral oxygenation.

6. **How would you induce this child?**

Because control of ventilation is the most reliable way to manipulate PVR, prompt and reliable control of the airway at induction is important. The goal should be to use a reduced FIO_2 and to maintain $PaCO_2$ at 35–40 mm Hg. Inhalational induction should be reserved for infants and children with small defects, no mitral regurgitation, and no Pulmonary arterial hypertension (PAH). Cardiac reserve often is limited or exhausted in patients with large shunts and high pulmonary blood flow. Moreover, the additional volume load imposed on the left ventricle by mitral regurgitation will further limit cardiac reserve. An intravenous induction and maintenance with fentanyl will provide better hemodynamic stability. In particular, for patients with reactive pulmonary vasculature, high doses of fentanyl will be useful in blunting increases in PVR associated with surgical stimulation. In addition, high doses of fentanyl will blunt stimulation-induced increases in systemic vascular resistance (SVR), which will increase the mitral regurgitant fraction.

7. **After induction, the oxygen saturation is 90% on an FIO_2 of 21%. How do you assess if the patient's cardiac output is adequate for systemic oxygen delivery?**

Assuming that only a L to R shunt exists, this saturation is representative of pulmonary vein desaturation (intrapulmonary shunt or V/Q mismatch). This in turn is the consequence of interstitial pulmonary edema. In the presence of bidirectional shunting the assessment is substantially more complicated. However, two facts are clear: (1) SaO_2 alone is a poor surrogate measure of Q_P:Q_S and (2) the best and easiest obtainable measure of the adequacy of systemic O_2 delivery is SaO_2—$SsvcO_2$. $SsvcO_2$ can be obtained from blood drawn from the proximal port of a CVP catheter. Alternatively, near infrared spectroscopy can be used as a surrogate trend marker for mixed venous saturations and cardiac output.

8. **Discuss the surgical repair**

Repair of these defects involves: (1) Septation of the common AV valve tissue into two separate competent, non-stenotic tricuspid and mitral valves. (2) Closure of the ostium primum ASD. (3) Closure of the inlet VSD.

There are two different surgical techniques. The patch technique whereby a single patch is used to close both the VSD and ASD and the reconstructed AV valves are resuspended by sutures to the patch. When the VSD is large and extends to other areas of the septum (as in TOF) two patches (atrial and ventricular) may be necessary. When the inlet VSD component is small, the AV valve tissue can be sutured down to the crest of the ventricular septum essentially closing the VSD. A patch is then sutured to the crest of the ventricular septum and is used to close the ASD [7].

9. **What are the risk factors for surgery?**

Risk factors for surgical repair include: young age and prematurity, preoperative severity of common AV valve incompetency, preoperative functional class and presence of associated cardiac and noncardiac malformations.

10. **What are the major postoperative complications?**

Major postoperative complications include residual VSD or ASD, residual mitral regurgitation, complete heart block, and right ventricular dysfunction [8].

11. **Describe the overall mortality and long-term outcome after primary repair of AV septal defects?**

The overall mortality for primary repair of a complete AV septal defect is <5%. Long-term survival is excellent and, in most cases, there is no need for further surgery. The overall prognosis is related to the repair of the left-sided AV valve [9].

12. **What are your concerns for subsequent noncardiac surgeries?**

Patients with repaired CAVC may present with residual mitral valve disease, pulmonary hypertension, right ventricle dysfunction and arrhythmias including heart block and sinus node dysfunction.

References

1. DiNardo JA, Zvara DA. Anesthesia for cardiac surgery. 3rd ed. Oxford: Blackwell Publishing; 2008 (Chapter 6).
2. Bent ST. Anesthesia for left-to-right shunt lesions. In: Andropoulos DB, Stayer SA, Russell IA, editors. Anesthesia for congenital heart disease. Massachusetts: Blackwell Publishing Inc; 2005.
3. Keene JF, Lock JE, Fyler DC. Nadas' pediatric cardiology. 2nd ed. Philadelphia: Saunders; 2006.
4. Prevention of infective endocarditis: guidelines from the American Heart Association: a guideline from the American Heart Association Rheumatic Fever, Endocarditis, and Kawasaki Disease Committee, Council on Cardiovascular Disease in the Young, and the Council on Clinical Cardiology, Council on Cardiovascular Surgery and Anesthesia, and the Quality of Care and Outcomes Research Interdisciplinary Working Group. Circulation. 2007 Oct 9; 116 (15):1736–54.
5. Odegard KC, DiNardo JA, Laussen PC. Anesthesia for congenital heart disease. In: Gregory GA, Andropoulos DB, editors. Gregory's pediatric anesthesia. 5th ed. Oxford: Wiley-Blackwell; 2012.
6. DiNardo JA. Chapter 12 in Lake L, Booker PD: Pediatric Cardiac Anesthesia, 4th ed. Lippincott: Williams & Wilkins.
7. Jonas RA. Comprehensive surgical management of congenital heart disease. 2nd ed. New York: Oxford University Press Inc; 2014.
8. Pilchard J, Dadlani G, Andropoulos D, Jacobs JP, Cooper DS. Intensive care and perioperative management of patients with complete atrioventricular septal defect. World J Pediatr Congenit Heart Surg. 2010;1(1):105–11.
9. Ginde S, Lam J, Hill GD, Cohen S, Woods RK, Mitchell ME, Tweddell JS, Earing MG. Long-term outcomes after surgical repair of complete atrioventricular septal defect. J Thorac Cardiovasc Surg. 2015;150(2):369–74.

Premature Infant

58

Lisa M. Hammond

Case

7-day-old ex 29-week premature infant, weighing 900 g, presents to the operating room for patent ductus arteriosus (PDA) closure.

Past Medical History:
Respiratory Distress Syndrome
Hypoglycemia
Hypotension
Intraventricular hemorrhage, grade III
Medications:
D10 infusion 110 ml/kg/day
Dopamine infusion 5 mcg/kg/min
Midazolam infusion 0.05 mg/kg/hr
PRN fentanyl boluses
Allergies: NKDA
Physical Exam:
VS: 166 bpm, 53/32, 93% on 30% FiO_2
Sedated
Intubated, with mechanical ventilation PVC 21/3 × 24, FiO_2 30%
3/6 machinery-like murmur throughout precordium
Rales bilaterally
Mildly distended abdomen, positive bowel sounds
24 g PIV in situ left saphenous
Labs: HCT 29%, PLTs 46 k, otherwise unremarkable

1. **How is prematurity defined? How does the degree of prematurity correlate to morbidity and mortality?**

Premature infants are defined as infants born prior to 37 weeks gestational age (GA). Specifically, these infants can be defined as low gestational age (LGA) newborns, born between 27 and 32 weeks GA, or extremely low gestational age newborns (ELGAN), born between 23 and 27 weeks GA. In addition, these neonates are often of low birth weight, given inadequate time for intrauterine growth, and therefore can be further classified based on the birth weight.

- Low birth weight (LBW): <2500 g
- Very low birth weight (VLBW): <1500 g
- Extremely low birth weight (ELBW): <1000 g.

Morbidity and mortality track much more closely with GA compared to BW. This is thought to be based on the organ prematurity associated with low GA, that may not be found to the same degree in term infants that may have isolated intrauterine growth restriction (IUGR) and resultant low birth weight [1].

In general, morbidity and mortality of premature infants has declined significantly with the advent of antenatal glucocorticoid use, specialization of NICUs, advancements in mechanical ventilator therapy, and development of multidisciplinary care team models. In ELBW newborns, the overall mortality in level 3 NICUs was estimated to be less than 30% in 2011, compared to greater than 80% in 1980 [2].

2. **What is the difference between gestational age, chronological age, postmenstrual age, and corrected age?**

These are all terms used to define a neonate's perinatal age, and therefore potential degree of prematurity.

L.M. Hammond (✉)
Department of Anesthesia, Harvard Medical School, Clinical Instructor, Boston Children's Hospital, 300 Longwood Avenue, Boston, MA 02115, USA
e-mail: lmhammond@gmail.com

© Springer International Publishing AG 2017
L.S. Aglio and R.D. Urman (eds.), *Anesthesiology*,
DOI 10.1007/978-3-319-50141-3_58

- Gestational Age: Time elapsed between the 1st day of the last menstrual period and the day of delivery
- Chronological Age: Time elapsed since birth
- Postmenstrual Age: Gestational age + chronological age
- Corrected Age: Chronological age reduced by the number of weeks born before 40 weeks of gestation.

3. **What are some of the cardiovascular physiologic differences to consider in premature infants?**

There are several structural and functional differences in the cardiovascular system of premature neonates. In general, there is more connective tissue in the myocardium, with less organized contractile elements, and an increased dependence on extracellular calcium concentrations. The myocardium is also less compliant, with a flatter Frank-Starling Curve, which renders these neonates to some degree preload-dependent, but also at increased risk of fluid overload with rapid volume increases. In addition, their small circulating blood volume compared to term neonates puts these patients at increased risk for fluid overload with IV medication administration followed by even small flush boluses. Because of a relatively fixed stroke volume, these patients are even more heart rate dependent compared to term neonates. The cardiovascular system of premature neonates functions at near-maximal baseline beta-adrenergic stimulation, and therefore these neonates are less responsive to augmentation with exogenous catecholamines.

4. **What is a patent ductus arteriosus (PDA)? What are the potential implications?**

PDAs result from persistent patency of the ductus arteriosus, a central shunt between the main pulmonary artery and the aorta that, in utero, preferentially shunts blood away from the pulmonary circulation into the systemic circulation in the setting of high intrauterine pulmonary vascular resistance (PVR) compared to lower systemic vascular resistance (SVR). Typically, the ductus arteriosus functionally closes soon after birth (by about 10–15 h after delivery). The exact mechanism of ductal closure is not clear. Several factors seem to play a part in closure including increased arterial oxygen tension, decreases in circulating prostaglandins after delivery and bradykinin release following lung expansion. In preterm infants, the ductus arteriosus has a thinner, poorly contractile muscular layer, and diminished responsiveness to the increasing arterial oxygen tension after birth resulting in failure of closure. Furthermore, preterm infants often suffer from respiratory distress syndrome (RDS), and resultant hypoxemia with reductions in arterial oxygen tension.

With resolution or optimization of underlying pulmonary pathology, such as RDS, lower PVR allows reversal of flow across the PDA, such that blood is shunted preferentially from the systemic circulation to the pulmonary circulation. This often results in pulmonary vascular congestion with worsening respiratory failure, hypotension, and ultimately left heart failure.

5. **How would you diagnose and treat a PDA?**

It is estimated that 50% of neonates weighing less that 1000 g and 20% of neonates weighing less than 1750 g will suffer from hemodynamically significant PDAs requiring intervention [3]. Therefore, high clinical suspicion in this patient population is appropriate.

Initial clinical presentation may be consistent with sudden increase in respiratory failure, tachycardia, tachypnea, widened pulse pressure, and hypotension. Physical exam may reveal a classic machinery murmur, but this is not always present.

The diagnosis is confirmed with echocardiography that demonstrates left atrial enlargement. Continuous-wave doppler or color doppler can be used to confirm abnormal flow in the pulmonary artery.

Management of a PDA can be either medical or surgical. Medical management involves fluid restriction, diuretic administration, minimizing exogenous oxygen exposure, and indomethacin, which, if effective, will usually close the PDA within 24 h. If there are contraindications to indomethacin administration, or medical therapy fails, surgical ligation is the definitive therapy.

6. **What is Respiratory Distress Syndrome (RDS)? How would you diagnosis and treat RDS?**

RDS is a life-threatening pulmonary complication of prematurity. The cause of RDS has been associated with a deficiency in alveolar phospholipid surfactant, produced by type II alveolar cells and necessary for the maintenance of alveolar stability. This pathology has been correlated with a high mortality in premature neonates, and its occurrence is inversely proportional to birth weight in premature neonates. The estimated occurrence is greater than 86% of ELBW neonates, and 27–48% of LBW neonates [3].

Clinical presentation of neonates with RDS would be consistent with hypoxia, cyanosis, and tachypnea. Physical examination would likely reveal intercostal and accessory muscle retractions, and bilateral rales on auscultation of lung fields. Chest X-ray often shows diffuse bilateral infiltrates.

Both a decrease in severity, and an increase in survival of neonates with RDS have been attributed to maternal steroid administration and exogenous neonatal surfactant administration. In addition, ventilator optimization and therapeutic inhaled nitric oxide (iNO) have also been described to improve oxygenation in these patients. There is, however, no good data that rescue or routine use of iNO improves survival in preterm neonates with RDS [4].

7. **How would you manage a ventilator for a patient with RDS?**

Mechanical ventilation is often necessary in patients with RDS secondary to (1) the greater inspiratory pressures required to initially expand surfactant deplete alveoli, (2) poor overall lung compliance with resultant increased work of breathing, and (3) hypoxemia resulting from poor V/Q matching in the setting of highly atelectatic lung tissue. Small tidal volumes (4–6 ml/kg), with greater inspiratory rates, minimal FiO_2 to maintain oxygen saturations within 90–94% range, and PEEP sufficient to avoid alveolar collapse reduce long-term lung injury in premature lungs [5]. In addition, randomized controlled trials have demonstrated that the use of permissive hypercapnia (PaCO2 45–55 mmHg) with shorter periods of assisted ventilation, may reduce the incidence of bronchopulmonary dysplasia (BPD) without adverse neurodevelopmental effects [6]. For patients that are refractory to conventional ventilator management, high frequency oscillatory ventilation (HFOV) has gained increasing popularity in the management of premature infants with RDS.

8. **What is Bronchopulmonary Dysplasia (BPD)? How is the severity graded? What are the implications of BPD?**

BPD is a chronic lung disease of prematurity as a result of remodeling that occurs after prolonged exposure (weeks) of supplemental oxygen therapy in the postnatal period. Like RDS, the occurrence of BPD is inversely proportional to birth weight in premature neonates. The mechanism of injury on lung parenchyma has been attributed to mechanical ventilation (atelectrauma and volutrauma to a greater extent than barotrauma), oxygen toxicity, infection, or a combination of any of these insults. The end result is various degrees of interstitial fibrosis, lobar emphysema, and increased reactivity of airways. This constellation of problems may require persistent exogenous oxygen, steroids, or prolonged mechanical ventilation. BPD is graded based on a severity index assessment at 36 weeks postmenstrual age, and has been shown to identify a spectrum of risk for adverse pulmonary and neurodevelopmental outcomes in preterm infants [2].

- Mild BPD: breathing RA
- Moderate BPD: need for <30% FiO_2
- Severe BPD: need for >30% FiO_2, and/or PPV or CPAP

9. **What are apnea spells? What are possible causes?**

Apnea of prematurity occurs in more than 85% of preterm infants, and its occurrence is inversely proportional to gestational age. Apnea spells are defined as cessation of breathing lasting more than 20 s, or more than 10 s if associated with desaturation and/or bradycardia. The mechanism can be attributed to both central and obstructive etiologies. Central etiologies are related to CNS immaturity and decreased chemoreceptor sensitivity to hypoxia and Hypercarbia. This may be exacerbated by abrupt changes in oxygen tension, pulmonary mechanics, brain hemorrhage, hypothermia, or even airway stimulation. Obstructive etiologies occur from pharyngeal muscle dyscoordination resulting in occlusion of the pharynx and/or larynx and may be exacerbated by residual anesthesia. Preterm infants with apnea do not increase ventilation in response to hypercapnia compared with those without apnea, thereby prolonging the apneic episode. Repeat episodes of apnea increase the potential for CNS damage because of repetitive exposure to hypoxemia [3]. The main treatment for apnea of prematurity is methylxanthine (e.g., caffeine).

Patients with apnea of prematurity are also at increased risk for postoperative apnea. Risk factors for postoperative apnea include postconceptional age <60 weeks, hematocrit <30, and major surgeries. The greatest risk factor is a postconceptional age <60 weeks. Postoperative apnea usually begins within 1 h after surgery, and in extreme premature infants can occur up to 48 h postoperatively. Because postoperative apnea is more common after major surgical procedures, there is some suggestion that the neurohormonal response to surgery and pain may play a role.

Management for neonatal apnea is centered on close observation, administration of IV methylxanthines (caffeine, theophylline), and prevention of anemia and hypovolemia.

10. **Are premature infants at risk for hypoglycemia or hyperglycemia? Why? How do you manage this?**

Premature infants are at risk for *both* hypoglycemia and hyperglycemia. Therefore, close glucose monitoring is imperative in this patient population.

Premature infants have decreased glycogen and body fat stores, predisposing them to hypoglycemia. Whipple's triad (low glucose, symptoms of hypoglycemia, and resolution of symptoms when glucose level is normalized) was classically used to diagnose neonatal hypoglycemia. Clinical signs of neonatal hypoglycemia include jitteriness, cyanosis, seizures, apnea, tachypnea, weak or high-pitched cry, floppiness, or lethargy, poor feeding, and eye rolling, many of which may not be appreciable under anesthesia, which may delay or obscure diagnosis. Further confounding the diagnosis, blood glucose concentrations as low as 30 mg/dL are common in healthy neonates at 1-2 h after birth. There is no strict consensus regarding when screening for hypoglycemia should occur or what serum glucose level would require intervention in asymptomatic patients [7]. A reasonable practice would be to administer exogenous glucose (D10 W infusion of 80–100 ml/kg/day, or 2 mL/kg of D10 W) for symptomatic patients with serum glucose levels of <40–45 mg/dL and asymptomatic patients with serum glucose levels <35–40 mg/dL.

Neonatal hyperglycemia is also common in premature infants, estimated to occur in more than 50% of ELBW infants. Deceased insulin production, exogenous dextrose infusions, perinatal steroid exposure, and the use of parenteral nutrition are thought to be contributing factors to the development of neonatal hyperglycemia. It is defined as a serum glucose levels >150 mg/dL, and has been associated with increased morbidity related to intraventricular hemorrhage (IVH), retinopathy of prematurity (ROP), potential neurodevelopmental delays, and death. When compared to liberal glycemic control (BGC 8–10 mmol/L), tight glycemic control patients (BGC 4–6 mmol/L) had no change in mortality but increased risk of hypoglycemic episodes [8]. Reasonable management would therefore include an insulin infusion at 0.01 units/kg/min and appropriate titration to achieve liberal glycemic control.

11. **How does prematurity impact renal function?**

The premature infant has underdeveloped kidneys and decreased renal function secondary to fewer overall nephrons and smaller glomerular size. During the first 40 days of life, premature infants are at significantly increased risk for renal injury secondary to low cardiac output, hypotension, and nephrotoxic drugs, as it is within this period of time that glomeruli continue to form postnatally. As a result of renal immaturity, plasma creatinine levels are often elevated initially and decline over the first 3 weeks of life. Hyponatremia may also occur in premature infants, with severity correlating to degree of prematurity. This is the result of reduced proximal tubular reabsorption of sodium and water, and reduced overall renal hormonal responsiveness [2].

12. **What is necrotizing enterocolitis (NEC)? How does it present? Is this patient at risk for NEC?**

NEC is a life-threatening condition that involves abdominal distension, ileus, and potential intestinal perforation. Its occurrence is inversely proportional to gestational age, with an estimated incidence of 5–10% in ELBW premature infants. As such, the patient presented above would be at risk for the development of NEC. The pathogenesis of NEC is incompletely understood, although etiologies implicated include intestinal immaturity, intestinal mucosal ischemia, abnormal microbial colonization secondary to antibiotic therapy, highly immunoreactive intestinal mucosa, gastric alkalinity, and low systemic cardiac output.

Clinical presentation includes feeding intolerance, abdominal distention with increased work of breathing from abdominal competition for diaphragmatic excursion, lethargy, temperature instability, with subsequent development of hypotension, sepsis, coagulopathy, and multisystem organ failure. The onset of NEC can be subdivided into early and late onset. Early onset is more common in premature infants with birth weights >1000 g, and typically occurs within the first 7 days of life. Late onset is more common in premature infants with birth weights <1000 g and typically occurs after 4 weeks of life [9].

13. **How do you diagnose and treat NEC?**

Diagnosis is largely clinical, and supported by the classic radiographic findings of gas in the intestinal wall (pneumatosis intestinalis) and biliary tract, as well as free air within the abdominal compartment. The degree of radiographic findings in the context of clinical suspicion are known as Bell's Classification, and can help determine the severity of NEC:

- Bell's Stage I: Ileus
- Bell's Stage II: Pneumatosis intestinalis
- Bell's Stage IIIa: Pneumatosis intestinalis + systemic illness
- Bell's Stage IIIb: Pneumatosis intestinalis + systemic illness + perforation

Treatment may be medical and/or surgical. Medical therapy is centered on appropriate antibiotic management, fluid resuscitation, and bowel rest. Extreme premature infants are more likely to fail conservative therapy, requiring surgical intervention, which carries mortality rates of up to 50%. Definitive surgical therapy involves laparotomy, peritoneal drain placement, and/or resection of necrotic bowel.

14. **Are premature infants at risk for any neurologic complications? What is intraventricular hemorrhage (IVH)?**

Premature infants are at risk for both immediate perinatal neurologic complications, as well as long-term neurodevelopmental abnormalities. Intraventricular hemorrhage (IVH) is hemorrhagic rupture of the endothelial lining of immature vessels within the germinal matrix secondary to venous stasis, which typically occurs within the first few weeks of life. IVH is often complicated by hydrocephalus secondary to post-hemorrhagic adhesive arachnoiditis. Risk factors for the development of IVH include prematurity, early sepsis, severe hypo/hypercapnia, need for mechanical ventilation, use of vasopressor infusions, and rapid fluctuations in cerebral blood flow, cerebral blood volume, or cerebral venous pressure.

IVH grade is based on the degree of hemorrhagic extension into the ventricular system on evaluation by head ultrasound:

- IVH Grade I: hemorrhage limited to the germinal matrix
- IVH Grade II: hemorrhage extending into the ventricular system
- IVH Grade III: hemorrhage extending into the ventricular system with associated ventricular dilation
- IVH Grade IV: hemorrhage extending beyond the ventricular system into brain parenchyma

Patients with severe IVH (grade III or IV) have more episodes of apnea crisis, hydrocephalus, periventricular leukomalacia, and longer hospital stays compared to premature infants without IVH. In addition, regardless of grade, premature infants with evidence of IVH display poorer neurodevelopmental outcomes long-term compared to those without IVH [10].

Only an estimated 25% of ELBW infants have normal neurologic development by 5 years of age, with developmental disabilities such as cerebral palsy, cognitive deficits, behavioral abnormities, hearing or visual impairment, and lower verbal and IQ performance scores being commonplace [11, 12].

15. **What is retinopathy of prematurity (ROP)? Is this patient at risk for developing this? Is there any way to reduce the risk of developing ROP?**

ROP results from damage of the spindle cells in the retina with the potential to cause permanent retinal scarring and visual impairment. It occurs in approximately 50% of ELBW premature infants, with the incidence being inversely proportional to both birth weight and gestational age. As such, this patient would be at significant risk for the development of ROP. The pathogenesis is not completely understood, but fluctuations in arterial oxygenation, and exposure to bright light have been implicated as contributing factors, resulting in a combination of hyperoxic vasoconstriction of retinal vessels, induction of vascular endothelial growth factor, and free radical injury to the retina. To decrease the risk of developing ROP, it is recommended to minimize FiO_2 concentrations to maintain oxygen saturations between 90 and 95%, which may limit the development of oxygen free radicals and diminish the effect of hyperoxic vasoconstriction of retinal vessels [2].

16. **Is the patient's hematocrit of 29% and platelet count of 46 k normal given this patient's age and size? Would you transfuse this patient preoperatively?**

The ideal hematocrit for premature infants remains controversial, however, a hematocrit of 29% is certainly low for any neonate at 7 days of life, regardless of prematurity. In addition, hematocrits <30% may increase risk for the development of postanesthetic apnea. It is reasonable to try to maintain a goal hematocrit of 44–48% in premature infants, to improve tissue oxygen delivery in the setting of reduced oxygen saturation and decreased cardiac output. In studies that look at liberal (HCT 46%) versus restrictive (HCT 34%) transfusion management in ELBW and LBW premature neonates, restrictive transfusion management was associated with increased incidence of intraparenchymal brain hemorrhage, periventricular leukomalacia, and apnea [13]. Therefore, it would be appropriate to transfuse this patient preoperatively.

The incidence of thrombocytopenia (PLT <150 k) is greater than 70% in ELBW premature neonates. The etiology is thought to be multifactorial including early onset infection, thrombi, DIC, and severe hemorrhage [14]. New onset thrombocytopenia is an indication for head ultrasound to evaluate for possible intracranial hemorrhage. It is considered reasonable practice to transfusion platelets preoperatively in the setting of clinical bleeding and PLT <100 k, or for prophylaxis against bleeding with PLT <50 k in patients with prematurity or other significant risk factors for intracranial hemorrhage [9].

17. **How does temperature regulation differ in premature infants?**

Premature infants lose heat by the usual four mechanisms of heat transfer: radiation, conduction, convection, and evaporation. They are however, at significantly increased risk of hypothermia, as insensible fluid loss and evaporative heat loss are markedly elevated secondary to a keratin-deficient epidermis layer, rending the skin "semi water-permeable" [2]. Conductive and convective heat loss are also increased because there is little soft tissue and fat for insulation and a large surface area to mass ratio.

The main mechanism of thermogenesis in premature infants, like term infants, is non-shivering thermogenesis by brown fat. Brown fat comprises 2–6% of a premature infant's body weight, and is located between the scapulae, mediastinum, nape, and surrounding the kidneys and adrenal glands. The mechanism of brown fat thermogenesis is by uncoupling protein resulting in oxidation of food to heat rather than energy-rich phosphate bonds [9].

Premature infants may have intact thermoregulatory systems, however may still demonstrate temperature instability secondary to a more narrow control range than term infants or adults. Thermoregulation in the face of hypothermia, in particular thermogenesis, occurs at the expense of oxygen consumption, and may impair growth and development of premature infants compared infants that remain thermoneutral [15].

To optimally maintain normal temperature ranges in premature neonates, transport to the operating room should occur in a double-walled transport incubator if available. Otherwise, the infant should be covered with Saran Wrap, a warm blanket, and importantly, a hat. There is evidence that the use of a 3-layer hat significantly decreases oxygen consumption and extends the thermal range in nude VLBW premature infants when placed in a cool environment [9]. The operating room should be preemptively warmed to 78–80 °F, with overhead heating lamps and hot air mattress established.

18. **How does the anesthetic requirement of premature infants differ from those of an adult?**

Premature infants have an underdeveloped CNS, increased circulating concentrations of progesterone and beta-endorphins, with resultant decreased requirement in volatile minimum alveolar concentration (MAC) compared to that of an adult. Cardiovascular depression is increased in response to volatile anesthetic exposure secondary to greater myocardial depression and reduced peripheral response to catecholamines. In addition, the baroreceptor reflex is often poorly developed in premature infants and further blunted by volatile agents [3]. These patients are, therefore, at increased risk for anesthetic overdose and cardiovascular collapse.

19. **Is it ideal to utilize an intentionally "light anesthetic" technique in premature infants in order to prevent hemodynamic instability?**

A "light anesthetic" may decrease the risk of cardiovascular collapse. However, such a technique may also result in undesirable, and deleterious intracranial complications. Premature neonates lack the capacity for cerebral autoregulation, and abrupt increases in systemic perfusion pressure from inadequate depth of anesthesia may be transmitted directly to the cerebral circulation. Fluctuations in cerebral circulation have been implicated in the development of intraventricular hemorrhage. Therefore, an intentionally "light anesthetic" would not be ideal for this patient population.

20. **Would a narcotic/paralytic anesthetic technique be useful in this premature patient?**

Fentanyl and other opioids possess excellent analgesic and moderate sedative properties. They do not however, produce reliable amnesia, and therefore are rarely if ever used as an anesthetic technique in children or adults. The use of fentanyl as an anesthetic has been justified in premature neonates because of the immaturity of the central nervous system. These patients are deemed inherently amnestic by properties of age and degree of CNS immaturity. It is therefore reasonable to use a narcotic/paralytic anesthetic technique for this patient. Premature neonates that receive fentanyl IV in doses of 30–50 mcg/kg do not have significant tachycardia or hypertension in response to thoracotomy when undergoing PDA ligation, and therefore are felt to have adequate levels of anesthesia to prevent blood pressure fluctuations associated with intracranial morbidity. In addition, in preterm VLBW neonates, systemic blood pressure reductions of less that 5% occur with this technique when used to preform a PDA ligation, and is therefore viewed as a hemodynamically stable anesthetic option in patients at risk for cardiovascular instability [2].

21. **What monitors and vascular access would be necessary for this patient during the proposed PDA ligation procedure? Why?**

Often these patients will come with indwelling umbilical vein (UVCs) and/or umbilical artery catheters (UACs). If these catheters are placed properly, they are appropriate for use during this procedure. Confirmation of appropriate line placement should always be completed by radiographic review prior to use intraoperatively, as these lines are notorious for migrating to undesirable locations with untoward complications if missed. The ideal location for a UVC is in the cephalad portion of the IVC, however, they are easily misplaced in the portal veins, and splenic veins. Known complications associated with indwelling and newly placed UVCs include hepatic hematoma, intravascular thrombi, intimal injury, atrial perforation, pericardial effusion, and intra-peritoneal migration [16]. Ideal location for UACs may be either above the diaphragm at between T6 and T9 or just above the aortic bifurcation between L3 and L5; above the diaphragm placement has been associated with fewer vascular complications, reduction in aortic thrombus, and longer catheter lifespan [16].

If central access is not available, this case can be preformed with peripheral access alone. The PDA lies in close proximity to the aorta and pulmonary artery and therefore potential brisk and abrupt bleeding may occur. Thus, intravenous access should be adequate to allow for rapid volume resuscitation if the need arises. Pack red blood cells should be immediately available for transfusion. If arterial access is not readily available, proceeding with noninvasive blood pressure monitoring would be reasonable. Mean gradient comparison between the right upper extremity (pre-ductal pressure), and systemic pressure on any other limb (post-ductal pressure) should be noted. Pulse oximeter placement should occur in both pre- and post-ductal locations as well. This will help confirm appropriate surgical clamp placement on the correct vascular structure prior to definitive ligation [2]. Upon successful PDA ligation, systemic diastolic and mean pressures should increase; loss of post-ductal pulse oximeter output could indicate unintentional aortic ligation and warrants immediate attention.

22. **During surgical dissection there is a precipitous decline in oxygen saturation from 94 to 80%, with associated bradycardia, what is the likely etiology? How would you manage this event?**

Premature neonates are prone to the development of hypoxemia secondary to poorly compliant lungs, diminished FRC, atelectasis, poor V/Q matching, and risk for endotracheal tube occlusion by secretions and/or blood. In addition, surgical compression on the lungs may be an important contributing factor to consider, particularly with sudden intraoperative changes in oxygen saturation. PDA ligation is completed by left thoracotomy approach with ipsilateral lung retraction. This results in an increase in pulmonary resistance and decrease in pulmonary compliance, often leading to a moderate degree of hypoventilation with secondary hypoxemia and bradycardia [3]. The patient should be managed with cessation of surgical manipulation, and manual re-recruitment on transient 100% inspired oxygen.

As a result of these complex cardiopulmonary dynamics, as well as what is often a high dose narcotic/paralytic anesthetic technique, these patients are left intubated and transported to the neonatal intensive care unit (NICU) to allow for stabilization of cardiopulmonary physiology and anesthetic clearance.

23. **How can you minimize the risk of insult to the premature infant at the conclusion of this surgical procedure and on transport to the neonatal intensive care unit?**

Removal of drapes at the conclusion of surgical procedures involving premature infants should occur with even greater caution than with term infants of children. These infants are often so small that their location on the operating room table can be challenging to identify under drapes. Inadvertent dislodgement of endotracheal tube, and/or venous or arterial catheters may occur with removal of drapes. Thus, an additional degree of vigilance is warranted at this time. Continuous monitoring should occur on transport to the NICU with monitors used intraoperatively, and transit time should be minimized. Proactive approaches to maintaining a thermoneutral state should be performed with utilization of a heated isolette, plastic wrap, warm blankets, and a hat. In order to avoid consequences of hyperoxia in premature infants, transport should occur by bag-mask ventilation or mechanical ventilator with minimal inspired oxygen concentrations to maintain adequate oxygen saturation. Conclusion of the anesthesiologist's responsibilities occurs when care has been appropriately transferred to the NICU care team [3].

References

1. Holzman R, Mancuso T, Polaner D. A practical approach to pediatric anesthesia. Lippincott Williams & Wilkins; 2006.
2. Cote C, Lerman J, Anderson B. Practice of anesthesia for infants and children. 5th ed. Elsevier Saunders; 2013.
3. Yao F. Anesthesiology, problem-oriented patient management. 6th ed. Lippincott Williams & Wilkins; 2008.
4. Kumar P. Use of inhaled nitric oxide in preterm infants. Pediatrics. 2014;133(1):164–70.
5. Thome UH, Ambalavanan N. Permissive hypercapnia to decrease lung injury in ventilated preterm neonates. Semin Fetal Neonatal Med. 2009;14:21–7.
6. Miller JD, Carlo WA. Safety and effectiveness of permissive hypercapnia in the preterm infant. Curr Opin Pediatr. 2007;19: 142–4.
7. Adamkin DH. Postnatal glucose homeostasis in late-preterm and term infants. Pediatrics. 2011;127(3):575–9.
8. Alsweiler JM, Harding JE, Bloomfield FH. Tight glycemic control with insulin in hyperglycemic preterm babies: a randomized controlled trial. Pediatrics. 2012;129(4):639–47.
9. Fanaroff AA, Fanaroff JM. Klaus and Fanaroff's care of the high risk neonate. 6th ed. Elsevier Health Sciences; 2013.
10. Mancini MC, Barbosa NE, Silveira S. Intraventricular hemorrhage in very low birth weight infants: associated risk factors and outcome in the neonatal period. Rev Hosp Clin. 1999;54(5):151–4.
11. Mikkola K, Ritari N, Tommiska V, et al. Neurodevelopmental outcome at 5 years of age of a national cohort of extremely low birth weight infants who were born in 1996–1997. Pediatrics. 2005;116:1391–400.
12. Peterson BS, Vohr B, Staib LH, et al. Regional brain volume abnormalities and long-term cognitive outcome in preterm infants. JAMA. 2000;284:1939–47.
13. Bell EF, Strauss RG, Widness JA, Mahoney LT, Mock DM, Seward VJ, Zimmerman MB. Randomized trial of liberal versus restrictive guidelines for red blood cell transfusion in preterm infants. Pediatrics. 2005;115(6):1685–91.
14. Christensen RD, Henry E, Wiedmeier SE, Stoddard RA, Sola-Visner MC, Lambert DK, Ainsworth S. Thrombocytopenia among extremely low birth weight neonates: data from a multihospital healthcare system. J Perinatol. 2006;26(6):348–53.
15. Glass L, Silverman W, Sinclair J. Effects of the thermal environment on cold resistance and growth of small infants after the first week of life. Pediatrics. 1968;41:1033.

16. Appearance N, Positions A, Schlesinger AE, Braverman RM, Dipietro MA. Neonates and umbilical venous catheters: normal appearance, anomalous positions, complications, and potential aid to diagnosis. Am J Roentgenol. 2003;180(4):1147–53.
17. Lou HC, Lessen PH, Fris-Hansen B. Impaired autoregulation of cerebral blood flow in the distressed newborn infant. Pediatrics. 1979;94:118.

Part XII

Critical Care

Section Editor: Suzanne Klainer

Suzanne Klainer
Department of Anesthesiology, Perioperative
and Pain Medicine, Brigham and Women's Hospital,
Boston, MA, USA

59 Trauma Anesthesia

Kevin Handy

Trauma is the number one cause of death for individuals less than 45 years old in the United States, and the fourth leading cause of death across all ages. This tremendous impact is felt in both the millions of years of lives lost nationally, as well as the greater than $100 billion in annual medical expenses [1]. Anesthesiologists are often called to help manage the difficult airway when a new trauma patient arrives, to manage the critically injured in the operating room and stabilize that patient in the intensive care unit. Familiarity with trauma evaluation and management gives the trauma patient the best chance of survival.

As experts in managing airways, obtaining vascular access, resuscitation and pain management, anesthesiologists are uniquely positioned to help care for trauma patients. From their arrival in the emergency department, through both the operative and post-operative phase in the ICU, anesthesiologists play a critical role in their management.

CASE

A 45-year-old male helmeted motorcycle driver, who presents to the ED after head-on collision with automobile. Reportedly traveling 35 mph, when suspected drunk driver of automobile collided with motorcyclist. He was found 25 feet from the scene, where the GCS was reportedly 13. Upon arrival to the emergency department, his mental status deteriorated and he was intubated for airway protection.

Medications:	oxycodone 5–10 mg prn
	Lisinopril
	Atorvastatin
Allergies:	none
Past Medical History:	Chronic low back pain
	Hypertension
	Hyperlipidemia
Physical Exam:	
Neuro—GCS 8; pupils with sluggish response to light	
Cardiovascular—Tachycardic with muffled heart sounds; no discernible murmurs	
Pulmonary—Diminished breath sounds in left hemithorax	
Gastrointestinal—bowel sounds present; abdomen soft, unable to determine if pain with palpation	
Genitourinary—small amount of blood after Foley catheter placement	
Skin—multiple abrasions on face, bruising apparent over sternum, multiple superficial abrasions on bilateral lower extremities	

(1) What are the key features of the "prehospital" phase of ATLS?

The prehospital phase involves the arrival of emergency services, the securing of the scene, and mobilization of affected parties. A critical portion of this phase is *identification* of the closest hospital facility with adequate resources, so in-house trauma teams can mobilize and be present as the patient(s) arrives. *Stabilization* of the patient is one of the main goals of this period. Airway control, identification, and slowing of external bleeding and immobilization are crucial first steps while minimizing "scene" time. If possible, a brief history of the patient and surrounding events should be obtained. The timing and mechanism of the injury can be critical in later identifying injuries that may not be immediately present [2].

K. Handy (✉)
Department of Anesthesia, Critical Care and Pain Medicine, Massachusetts General Hospital, 55 Fruit Street, Boston, MA 02114, USA
e-mail: khandy@partners.org

© Springer International Publishing AG 2017
L.S. Aglio and R.D. Urman (eds.), *Anesthesiology*,
DOI 10.1007/978-3-319-50141-3_59

(2) **What are the key features of the "hospital" phase of ATLS?**

Assuming proper notification of the appropriate parties, the trauma services should be available and waiting for the patient in a dedicated trauma bay. All necessary equipment should be available and tested for efficacy prior to arrival, including airway equipment, warmed fluids, and protective equipment for providers. Once the patient arrives, the team should immediately proceed to the *primary survey* [2].

(3) **What is involved in the primary survey of a trauma patient?**

The primary survey follows the "ABCDE" rules. **Airway** examination should begin by attempting to have the patient speak. If able to phonate without distress, their airway likely is not imminently life threatening. Suction and inspection for potential obstruction or foreign items should be done promptly. Stabilization of the cervical spine is often necessary during airway manipulation as trauma patients with multisystem injuries have a potential cervical spine injury. *Repeated assessment* is key, as the airway can be lost at any point, especially with waxing/waning mental status. If a patient has a GCS score of <8, then endotracheal intubation is likely needed.

Breathing effectively cannot be assumed just because an airway is patent. Proper gas exchange is impaired by rib fractures, pneumothoraces, hemothoraces, etc., which should be identified on primary survey. **Circulation** broadly covers hemodynamic assessment. *Hemorrhage* is the predominant cause of preventable death after traumatic injury [2]. Assessment of circulatory status first involves determining level of consciousness, skin color, and pulse strength. Bleeding can be obvious at visible external sites, or internally in harder-to-assess compartments, such as the retroperitoneum. Rapid external bleeding should be controlled with direct pressure and/or a tourniquet, keeping the risk of potential ischemia in mind. Most likely areas of rapid hemorrhage include chest, abdomen, retroperitoneum, and pelvis.

The primary survey continues to examination of potential neurologic **disability.** Establishing a level of consciousness with a GCS score, and frequent reassessment can help guide potential subsequent therapies (e.g., Need for intubation, head imaging, etc.). **Exposure and Environmental** control involves completely undressing the patient, and removing any hazardous materials from their presence. Cutting off garments is frequently necessary, and providers should be mindful of subsequent hypothermia during examination.

(4) **What is the most rapid way to assess a patient on arrival?**

Simply asking a patient their name and having them explain what happened can give the providers many clues as to their physical and mental stability. Phonation without distress gives some assurance that the airway and breathing status of the patient are not immediately compromised. Their ability to think and process recent events is a good sign that circulation and perfusion are at least adequate, and neurologic disability becomes less likely. It is essential to *frequently reassess* the patient, as any of these systems may fail rapidly and without obvious prodromes.

(5) **What is the Secondary Survey? When should it begin?**

The *secondary survey should begin once the primary exam is complete, and appropriate measures have been made to stabilize the patient's vital signs.* It involves a more detailed assessment of the patient from head to toe, with necessary imaging also being performed. Reassessing the GCS is an important first step, as it may change rapidly after initial examination. A **full physical exam** should then take place, and proper imaging should be ordered (plain films, CT, MRI, etc.). A FAST (Focused Assessment with Sonography for Trauma), a four-view (RUQ, LUQ, Suprapubic, Pericardial) focused ultrasound exam able to detect fluid in the abdomen or pericardium, may be performed at this time [3].

During the physical exam, a thorough **history** of the patient and surrounding events should be taken. This may not always be possible, and questions may need to be directed toward family members, friends, and witnesses at the scene. The mnemonic ***AMPLE*** is a useful tool for providers. *Allergies* should be identified, with emphasis on those that cause life-threatening side effects. Any *medications* used by the patient should be identified, and may be a clue to underlying chronic illness. *Past Illness/Medical history* is obviously critical information, as is potential *pregnancy* status for female patients. When the patient had his/her *last meal* is important especially during airway manipulation, as aspiration is always a grave concern with trauma patients. Finally, the *events* and *environment* surrounding the injury are of utmost importance. As stated above, the differential for underlying critical injuries changes with the type of impact or exposure the patient was subjected to. If he or she were exposed to potential toxins, providers should be made aware as soon as possible for their own protection, as well as anticipation for potential future patients [2].

It is critical to remember that patients should only be sent off the floor for radiological imaging once they are stable, as further resuscitative measures are hampered in environments not suited to them.

(6) **When should a cricothyroidotomy be considered/performed?**

A cricothyroidotomy should be considered and planned for whenever the trauma team anticipates a potentially difficult or impossible airway. Any damage to a patient's head/face/neck should clue in providers to a potentially difficult intubation. The actual procedure is performed when intubation is unsuccessful, and a definitive airway is needed. The ability to mask ventilate a patient provides the trauma team time to use other noninvasive or invasive airway equipment to secure the airway. The situation of "*cannot intubate and cannot ventilate*" is when an emergent cricothyroidotomy is must be performed as a surgical airway is the ultimate step in all failed pathways of the *difficult airway algorithm*.

(7) **What are some of the complications of a surgical cricothyroidotomy?**

Procedure failure is the most feared of the many potential complications. Passage of the airway device into a false lumen is indicated by inability to detect end tidal CO2, subcutaneous emphysema, and failure to see adequate chest rise. Other complications include aspiration of blood into the airway, laceration of trachea or esophagus, vocal cord injury, and hematoma or hemorrhage. Confirmation of successful airway placement is confirmed by: direct bronchoscopic visualization, consistent end tidal CO2 waveform, and vital signs indicative of adequate ventilation [2].

(8) **What is shock?**

It is often quoted as a systolic blood pressure less than 90 mmHg, or mean arterial pressure less than 60 mmHg. A more accurate description is a state of **global hypoperfusion**, resulting in multiple sites of end organ damage, while being resistant to initial means of resuscitation. The most common form of shock seen in trauma settings is **hypovolemic shock**, usually from hemorrhage. ATLS classifies shock as I-IV, based on heart rate, blood pressure, and mental status parameters [2]. The details of classification will be discussed later.

(9) **What are the major types of shock?**

Hypovolemic shock is most often due to hemorrhage in trauma patients. Low circulatory volumes lead to a compensatory increase in heart rate to maintain cardiac output, which is hampered by low preload. Hypovolemic shock is treated with replacement of fluid and/or blood, depending on the clinical scenario. This is the *most common* cause of preventable death in trauma patients.

Cardiogenic shock is due to heart or "pump" failure, where delivery of oxygen is compromised by poor cardiac output, leading to a low mixed venous saturation (<70%). Reactive increases in both heart rate and SVR can actually worsen cardiovascular function. This is treated with inotropic medications, such as epinephrine, dopamine, and dobutamine. If these therapies fail or are deemed inadequate, an intraortic balloon pump can help augment cardiac output and coronary vessel perfusion.

Both hypovolemic and cardiogenic shock, if left untreated, can progress to the third major class of shock: **Distributive.** This is characterized by higher than normal cardiac output, low SVR, and high mixed venous saturation (>70%). It is most commonly caused by *septic shock, anaphylaxis, and neurogenic shock*. It is a common endpoint if treatment for either hypovolemic or cardiogenic shock is delayed or inadequate [2].

(10) **What are the classes of hemorrhage and how are they identified?**

Estimated blood volume for adults: Male—70 mL/kg, Female 60 mL/kg, Children 80–90 mL/kg.

Class 1 → up to 15% volume loss. Values similar to blood donation. HR typically less than 100, and can easily be replaced with crystalloid.

Class 2 → 15–30% volume loss. Heart rate typically 100–120 bpm. Systolic pressure still usually maintained by increased blood vessel constriction.

Class 3 → 30–40% volume loss, often quoted as 1.5–2L lost. Heart rate typically greater than 120 bpm, with decreases in systolic blood pressure and mental status changes. This stage usually necessitates blood and/or crystalloid replacement.

Class 4 → Greater than 40% volume loss. Urine output becomes negligible. Mental status and vital signs severely impaired, with emergent need for blood repletion [2].

(11) **What are the signs and symptoms of a tension pneumothorax?**

A high degree of suspicion is needed with chest wall trauma (bruises, cuts and/or chest pain) along with hemodynamic instability. Identification and treatment should be done during the *primary survey*, and should not be delayed for imaging. Tension pneumothorax is a clinical diagnosis. If there are no clear external signs of chest wall injury, a thorough physical exam is key to identification. The patient may complain of breathlessness or air hunger, and will likely present with absent breath sounds over the affected hemithorax, deviated trachea, tachycardia, hypotension, and eventual desaturation [2]. Pneumothorax can also be diagnosed with sonographic examination of bilateral hemithoraces as part for the Extended FAST (Focused Assessment with Sonography in Trauma) exam or E-FAST.

(12) **How should a tension pneumothorax be treated?**

Rapid decompression is key to restoring hemodynamic stability. A large caliber (14 g) needle should be inserted at the mid-clavicular line between the *2nd and 3rd* rib spaces. Using an 8-cm needle has a >90% chance of reaching the pleura, while a standard 5-cm needle is less than 50% [2]. A chest tube placed on the affected side is the definitive therapy, and can be placed first if readily available.

(13) **What are the signs and symptoms of pericardial tamponade?**

It occurs most commonly with penetrating trauma, but also seen with significant blunt force. Hemodynamic instability is usually seen with *rapid* accumulation of fluid into the fixed fibrous pericardial space. Even a small amount of fluid, if accumulated quickly, can cause hypotension. Patients with chronic, slow accumulation of fluid, a chronic pericardial effusion, may not have drastic hemodynamic changes early on.

The classic Beck's Triad of symptoms: elevated venous pressure, muffled heart sounds and arterial hypotension can be unreliable. A **FAST** (Focused Assessment with Sonography in Trauma) exam, with subxiphoid pericardial window, is the best method to rapidly diagnose (90–95%), and should be done during the *primary survey* if clinically indicated. If the effusion is large enough, **electrical alternans** may be seen on ECG [2].

(14) **How is pericardial tamponade treated?**

If hemodynamically significant, pericardial tamponade should be treated *prior* to induction of general anesthesia, as induction could lead to cardiac arrest through myocardial depression by anesthetic agents and by the decrease in venus return from positive pressure ventilation. **Pericardiocentesis** is both diagnostic and therapeutic therapy. However, a failed aspiration may be seen if blood is already clotted in the pericardial sac. Once stable enough to proceed to the OR, a pericardial window or pericardiotomy may ultimately be necessary if fluid/blood continues to reaccumulate.

(15) **What is the classic "lethal triad" of trauma patients?**

The lethal triad is classically described as *hypothermia, acidosis,* and *coagulopathy.* It is the close interplay of these factors that lead to exsanguination, and eventually death in trauma patients [4]. The causes of hypothermia in a trauma patient are multifactorial. Prolonged exposure time in the field, rapid infusion of cold fluids, and the vasodilating/cooling effects of general anesthesia are all contributing factors. Damaging clinical effects of hypothermia are often seen in the resultant coagulopathy. Cold temperatures impede platelet adhesion and dysregulate the coagulation factors and enzymes. This may not be evident on common testing parameters, as the blood samples are often warmed to physiologic temperatures [5].

Acidosis in the trauma patient is often due to a state of global hypoperfusion—defined as shock. Without adequate delivery of oxygen, cells turn to anaerobic metabolism and production of lactate. The resultant decrease in pH can also further disrupt the coagulation cascade and other protein-based enzymes. Along with the aforementioned causes, coagulopathy can result from a number of complex factors. One of the most common is attributed to dilution of intrinsic factors by fluid resuscitation. Studies have shown a correlation between increasing amounts of crystalloid administered with higher incidence of coagulopathies [6].

(16) **What is Damage Control Resuscitation?**

Damage Control Resuscitation (DCR) is a systematic approach to the trauma patient with severe injuries, starting in the emergency room and continuing through both operative and post-op management in the intensive care unit. It encompases damage control surgery and its tenants of temporizing surgical hemorrhage and gastrointestinal spillage as well as principles of balanced resuscitation [7]. The major goal of balanced resuscitation is prevention and immediate correction of coagulopathy, and minimizing use of crystalloid fluids. It was developed to achieve the following goals [8]:

- Treat intravascular volume deficits
- Correct the acute coagulopathy of trauma
- Preserve oxygen-carrying capacity

- Repair the endothelium
- Prevent dilutional coagulopathy

DCR was codified by the US Department of Defense in 2004, and has been standard of care in battlefield scenarios ever since. It has also since been implemented in many civilian trauma centers, and has been associated with improved outcomes compared with more traditional transfusion practices [9].

(17) **What is the Monroe-Kellie Doctrine?**

It states that the total volume of the intracranial space must remain *constant*, due to the rigidity of the skull. *Three components* (blood, brain tissue, csf) make up the normal intracranial space. When a disruption occurs, such as a hemorrhage or mass, the brain attempts to compensate by decreasing the amount of CSF and/or lowering cerebral blood flow (CBF). If a traumatic injury results in a rapid change that exceeds the brains ability to compensate, then an exponential increase in intracranial pressure (ICP) is seen, with eventual herniation of brain tissue without intervention [2].

(18) **What are some medical therapies used to decrease intracranial pressure?**

In the past, prolonged *hyperventilation* was frequently used to help decrease ICP, by means of cerebral vasoconstriction, with PaCO2 levels between 20 and 25 often being the target. However, aggressive and prolonged hyperventilation may lead to secondary brain injury via cerebral ischemia [2]. As a result, hyperventilation should only be used in moderation for a limited period of time.

Mannitol and *hypertonic saline* (3 and 23.4%) are hyperosmolar solutions used to lower the interstitial volume of brain tissue, by increasing osmotic pressure of the blood vessels. There is no difference in their ability to lower ICP, but caution should be used when administering both medications. Mannitol may cause a transient increase in BP and ICP before the osmotic effect takes place, and rapid infusion of hypertonic saline can cause a vasodilatory response. *Barbiturates* may be effective at reducing ICP refractory to other measures. They are not indicated in the acute resuscitation phase, as they may also cause hypotension [2].

(19) **What are the classifications of traumatic brain injury?**
Mild—GCS 13–15
Moderate—GCS 9–12
Severe—GCS 3–8

(20) **When should the provider suspect inhalational injuries in a burn situation?**

Airway protection should be the first priority of providers in a patient with burn injuries. The mucosa of the oropharynx is friable and extremely susceptible to burns, and may get rapidly worse after initial presentation. Once an inhalational injury is suspected, preparations should be made to transfer the patient to a burn facility, with securing the airway prior to transportation given strong consideration. Potential signs and symptoms of an inhalation injury are as follows [2]:

- Face and/or neck burns
- Singeing of the eyebrows and nasal passages
- Carbon deposits in the mouth/nose, or carbonaceous sputum
- Acute inflammation of the oropharynx
- Hoarseness
- History of impaired mentation, or known confinement in a burning building
- Explosions with burns to head and torso
- Carboxyhemoglobin levels greater than 10% in a patient involved in a fire

(21) **How do you estimate the extent of burn injuries in terms of body surface area (BSA)?**

The *Rule of Nines* is a practical guide to determine the extent of burn injury. In adults, the body is divided into anatomic regions that represent 9% of the BSA, or multiples of 9. The palmar surface represents 1% of BSA, including the fingers:

Rule of 9's for Adults: 9% for each arm, 18% for each leg, 9% for head, 18% for front torso, 18% for back torso

Rule of 9's for Children: 9% for each arm, 14% for each leg, 18% for head, 18% for front torso, 18% for back torso [10].

(22) **How do you calculate the fluid requirements for a patient with burn injuries?**

The *Parkland Formula*, proposed in 1974 and validated in 2002, calculates the estimated fluid requirements for burn patients in a 24 h period.

Fluid Requirements = TBSA burned (%) × Wt (kg) × 4 mL

Half of the total requirements should be given in the first 8 h, with the second have given over the next 16 [10].

(23) **Do regional anesthesia techniques have a role in trauma patients?**

One of the major benefits of early utilization of regional anesthetic techniques is profound pain relief, and decreased need for intravenous opioids. As a result, patients are less likely to suffer from respiratory depression, oversedation, nausea/vomiting, and confusion. A properly performed nerve block can also reduce the overall stress response. Some literature even suggests that early use of regional techniques has the potential to reduce the incidence and severity of chronic pain, as well as PTSD [11].

References

1. Miller MD, Howard J. Trauma Anesthesia. University of Colorado-Denver School of Medicine. Lecture.
2. Advanced Trauma Life Support. 9th ed. Chicago, Illinois: American College of Surgeons; 2012.
3. Wolfson A, Hendey G, Hendrey P, et al. Harwood and Nuss' clinical practice of emergency medicine. Lippincott: Williams & Wilkins; 2005.
4. Kaafarani HM, Velmahos GC. Damage control resuscitation in trauma. Scand J Surg 2015;0:1–8 (Web).
5. Wolberg AS, Meng ZH, Monroe DM 3rd, et al. A systematic evaluation of the effect of temperature on coagulation enzyme activity and platelet function. J Trauma. 2004;56(6):1221–8.
6. Maegele M, Lefering R, Yucel N, et al. Early coagulopathy in multiple injury: an analysis from the German trauma registry on 8724 patients. Injury. 2007;38(3):298–304.
7. Ball CG. Damage control resuscitation: history theory and technique. Can J Surg. 2014;57(1):55–60.
8. Holcomb JB, Tilley BC, Baraniuk S et al. Transfusion of plasma, platelets, and red blood cells in a 1:1:1 vs a 1:1:2 ratio and mortality in patients with severe trauma: the PROPPR randomized clinical trial. JAMA 2015;313.5:471–82 (Web).
9. Borgman MA, Spinella PC, Perkins JG et al. The ratio of blood products transfused affects mortality in patients receiving massive transfusions at a combat support hospital. J Trauma 2007;63 (4):805–13.
10. Baxter CR. Fluid volume and electrolyte changes in the early post-burn period. Clin Plast Surg. 1974;1:693–703.
11. Wu JJ, Lollo L, Grabinsky A. Regional anesthesia in trauma medicine. Anesthesiol Res Pract. 2011;2011:1–7.

Burns

60

Sara E. Neves

CASE:

71 years old 51 kg female presents to the emergency room after being rescued from her burning apartment. She lives in a basement apartment and was trying to cook when a grease fire erupted. She has 35% second and third degree burns on her neck, torso, and the upper extremities. Her eyebrows are singed off and she is breathing noisily. She presents for emergency escharotomy of the right upper extremity.

Medications:	Donepezil 10 mg		
	Lisinopril 5 mg		
Allergies:	NKA		
Past Medical History:			
Alzheimer's dementia			
HTN			
Hearing impairment			
Tobacco: 1 ppd smoker			
Alcohol: none			
Physical Exam:			
VS: BP 101/45 (63)	HR 119	RR 32	Oxygen saturation: 99% on room air
General: moaning in pain, but able to respond to simple questions			
Neuro: grossly moves all 4 extremities; unable to cooperate with sensory exam			
HEENT: soot covering face, eyebrows, nosehairs singed			
CV: tachycardic, regular, and without murmur			
Pulm: stridorous breathing, coarse breath sounds bilaterally			
Extremities: circumferential burn on right upper extremity			
Otherwise insignificant			
Labs: Na 146 K 4.5 Cl 103 HCO_3 15 BUN 31 Cr 1.09, ABG pH 7.21 pCO_2 31 pO_2 67 Hg 15 mg/dL Otherwise insignificant			

S.E. Neves (✉)
Department of Anesthesia, Critical Care and Pain Medicine, Beth Israel Deaconess Medical Center, 330 Brookline Avenue Boston, Cambridge, MA 02115, USA
e-mail: saraeneves@gmail.com

© Springer International Publishing AG 2017
L.S. Aglio and R.D. Urman (eds.), *Anesthesiology*,
DOI 10.1007/978-3-319-50141-3_60

1. **How are burns classified?**

Burns are classically described according to the skin layer involvement; namely, as first, second, or third degree burns. First-degree burns only involve the epidermis, are erythematous without blistering, and are painful. Second-degree burns involve the dermis; they are painful and are characterized by blistering and edema in addition to erythema. Third-degree burns involve all three layers of skin—epidermis, dermis, and subcutaneous tissue—and appear white or charred and indurated. These burns are painless as the nociceptive nerve endings have also been burned away. A less commonly described fourth-degree burn is a burn that involves not only the three layers of skin but also the destruction of fascia, muscle, and bone. First- and second-degree burns are also referred to as partial-thickness burns while third- and fourth-degree burns are full-thickness [1].

2. **How is the extent of burns described? Are pediatric burns measured in the same way?**

The management and prognosis of the burn patient is largely dictated by the extent of the burn, termed the Total Burn Surface Area (TBSA). TBSA is approximated using one of the several tools. The palmar surface area technique uses the principle that the surface area of the patient's palm (including fingers) represents approximately 1% of the total body surface area. This technique is reasonably accurate for small burns, or in calculating the uninjured area in very large burns and subtracting to get the large TBSA. The most common technique, the Wallace Rule-of-Nines, describes body part surface areas as multiples of 9 to approximate TBSA (see Fig. 60.1). This technique is easy to use and remember and is a good estimate of medium and large burns in adults; however, it is not accurate in children, who have a proportionally larger head and trunk surface area compared

Rule of nines

Head	9%
Anterior Trunk	18%
Posterior Trunk	18%
Right Upper Extremity	9%
Left Upper Extremity	9%
Right Lower Extremity	18%
Left Lower Extremity	18%
Perineum	1%

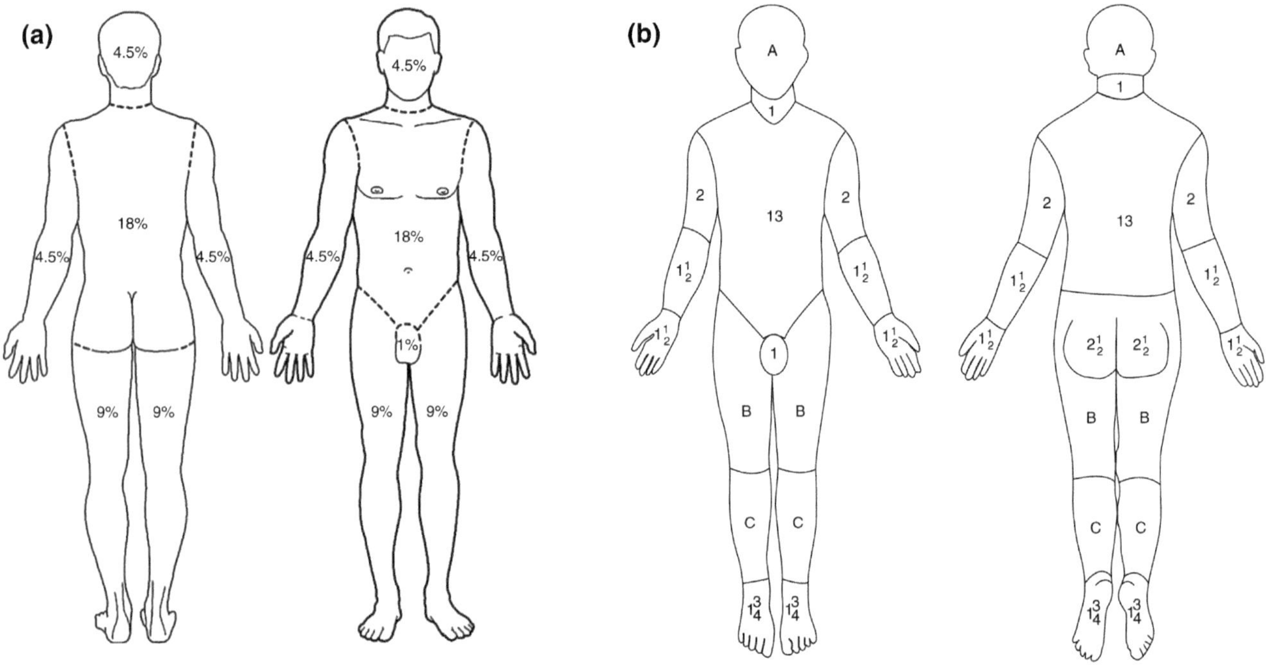

Fig. 60.1 **a** The rule of nines for estimating burn extent in adults. Reproduced from [21]. **b** Lund and Browder chart. Reproduced from [22]

to extremities. The most accurate technique is use of a Lund Browder chart, which takes into account the age of the patient and involves a more detailed calculation of burn surface area [2, 3].

3. **Does this patient have a major burn?**

The American Burn Association classifies a burn injury as a major burn requiring transfer to a burn unit if it includes any of the following criteria:

- Partial thickness (first or second degree) of more than 25% TBSA in adults (20% at extremes of age)
- Full thickness (third or fourth degree) of more than 10% TBSA
- Burns (any TBSA) of sensitive areas: face, hands, feet, perineum
- Inhalation burn injury
- Chemical burns
- Electrical burns
- Burns in patients with serious coexisting medical conditions.

Therefore, yes, this patient has a major burn as described by at least 2 criteria, >10% full-thickness burns and likely inhalational injury [4].

4. **What is the function of the skin?**

The skin is the body's first defense against the elements. It protects our vital organs from physical damage, maintains normothermia, preserves homeostasis of fluid and electrolytes, and is involved in vitamin D metabolism. It is the first barrier to infection; a physical wall between microorganisms outside and vulnerable tissues inside. The skin is also the medium through which we perceive the world using sensations such as touch, temperature, and pain.

5. **What are the major physiologic derangements after a thermal injury?**

The physiologic derangements seen after a thermal injury are the direct result of a disruption in the skin functions described above. Patients experience profound heat loss and the resulting hypothermia can result in cardiac arrhythmias, increased oxygen demand from shivering, and coagulopathy. Large insensible fluid losses due to evaporation result in fluid and electrolyte disturbances. Loss of skin surface area leaves these patients exquisitely vulnerable to infection. Damage to nerve endings in the skin makes burn pain severe and difficult to treat.

Most importantly, the injury triggers a large inflammatory response. It is not due to the tissue directly killed by thermal injury but by the surrounding tissue which is damaged but not dead. This damaged tissue produces local edema and inflammation, which then drives a systemic inflammatory response. It is this sublethally injured tissue that not only causes the problems but is also most at risk of further injury or death from poor perfusion or infection.

Local inflammatory mediators such as histamine, bradykinin, and prostaglandins, along with systemic mediators such as interleukins, TNF, nitric oxide, and endotoxin result in increased tissue permeability. Subsequently, a large amount of fluid moves from the intravascular space to the extravascular space in the wound, resulting in hemoconcentration and intravascular hypovolemia, even in the setting of extravascular volume overload. Intravascular volume depletion triggers a profound anti-diuretic hormone response resulting in low urine output or even anuria. This systemic inflammatory response syndrome (SIRS) leads to multiple organ failure, protein catabolism, and sepsis [5].

6. **Discuss the differences between a thermal burn, chemical burn, and electrical burn.**

A thermal burn is caused by extremes of temperature causing destruction of the skin layers. This can be due to extreme heat or extreme cold; cold burn injury (frostbite) has its own burn classification system yet can also be associated with SIRS.

A chemical burn is caused by exposure to a corrosive substance such as strong acid, strong base, or a vesicant. They do not require heat and are sometimes not evident until several hours to days after the exposure. They have a similar classification to thermal burns, but treatment is further specialized depending on the offending agent. An additional consideration is ensuring proper protection of the staff caring for the patient to limit further exposure.

An electrical current transmitted through the body causes an electrical burn. Often the only superficial sign of electrical injury is local burn at the contact point; for example, burns on the hands where they held high voltage wire. However, the majority injury lies below the surface where electrical energy is converted to thermal energy as the current encounters resistance of various tissues in its path. In addition, damage to the heart makes it vulnerable to malignant arrhythmias [3].

7. **What are the effects of burn injuries to the respiratory system?**

There are several different ways in which thermal injury can affect the respiratory system. Direct injury to the upper airway can quickly lead to complete airway obstruction. Even less severe injury can result in local swelling that can obstruct the airway. Inhalational injury—breathing in smoke, steam, or other noxious products of combustion—can cause both thermal and chemical damage to the smaller airways, causing significant shunting and hypoxemia. Furthermore, smoke inhalation can lead to carbon monoxide poisoning, cyanide poisoning, and other toxin exposures which vary depending on products of combustion. This can directly damage pulmonary tissues as well as decrease oxygen delivery.

Finally, the increased vascular permeability of SIRS predisposes these patients to Adult Respiratory Distress Syndrome (ARDS), which can be profound and difficult to treat due to these patients' high fluid requirements.

8. **What are the cardiovascular effects of a burn injury?**

The initial and rapid sequestration of fluid to the burned area results in a hypovolemic shock. The drop in intravascular volume is translated to a decrease in preload and cardiac output drops. As a result, catecholamine release triggers vasoconstriction to preserve central circulation, but this comes at a cost of ischemia to other organs such as brain, bowel, and kidneys. In addition, acidosis from carbon monoxide poisoning or hypoperfusion can directly depress cardiac function. Furthermore, hypothermia and electrolyte abnormalities from fluid shifts can predispose the heart to ectopy [5, 6].

9. **What are predictors of mortality in burn patients? Discuss the prognosis of this patient.**

Mortality in burn patients is directly related to the TBSA. In adults, age also directly correlates with mortality. In all patients, the presence of inhalational injury dramatically increases mortality, as do coexisting medical conditions.

Our patient is 71 years old with 35% TBSA and inhalational injury. Furthermore, she may have underlying COPD resulting from her heavy tobacco use. She also appears to have some degree of renal impairment as a Cr 1.09 is inappropriately high for someone of her age. Therefore, her mortality from this burn injury would be quite high. Burn centers have long used a Baux score, defined as age + TBSA to gauge mortality from an injury. Injuries with Baux scores greater than 140 were thought to be unsurvivable. However, treatment of these injuries has improved over the years and many advanced burn centers now associate a Baux score of 140 with about 50% mortality [7]. A modified Baux score has been developed which takes into account the presence of inhalational injury, which adds about 17 years (or 17% TBSA) to the Baux score. Therefore our patient's Baux score would be

$$\text{Age}\,(71) + \text{TBSA}(35) + \text{Inhalational injury}(17) = 123,$$

which is survivable by definition, but would be with a relatively high mortality [8].

10. **What is the most common cause of death for the burn patient?**

The most common early cause of death is asphyxiation from airway obstruction due to smoke inhalation. These patients usually do not survive to be admitted to the hospital. After this early period, the most common cause of death is sepsis; in developing countries hypovolemic shock remains an important cause of mortality [8, 9].

11. **How will you resuscitate this patient? What fluids should you use?**

The current standard of care for resuscitation uses the Parkland formula to guide fluid administration:

For the first 24 h, 4 ml/kg/% TBSA of lactated Ringer's solution should be administered; half of the total solution given in the first 8 h, the other half given over the next 16 h. Additional crystalloid given as needed to maintain urine output at 0.5–1.0 ml/kg/hr. For the next 24 h, 5% dextrose in water can be given to maintain serum sodium in normal range (135–145 mEq/L) and colloid may be given at a range of 0.3 ml/kg/% TBSA for patients with 30–50% burn. Urine output should still be maintained between 0.5 and 1 ml/kg/hr.

Vasopressors and inotropes to maintain blood pressure should be used very judiciously; it is usually more fluid that is required, not pharmacologic agents. Additionally, diuretics such as furosemide should not be used to maintain urine output during the initial fluid resuscitation phase at risk of further damage to renal function.

For our patient at 51 kg with 35% TBSA, she should receive approximately 7.2 L fluid in the first 24 h. 3.6 L should be given in the first 8 h, 1.8 L in the next 8 h, and 1.8 L in the last 8 h. Her urine output should be above 25 ml/hr at all times [10, 11].

12. **What are your endpoints to determine adequate resuscitation?**

In burn patients, one of the best markers of adequate resuscitation is urine output. In the absence of any drugs (diuretics, mannitol) or conditions (diabetes insipidus, uncontrolled hyperglycemia) that would falsely elevate urine output, amounts greater than 0.5 ml/kg/hr indicate a patient with adequate intravascular volume.

Other markers can offer clues to a patient's volume status but are less reliable. Tachycardia can be due to hypovolemia or pain; the absence of tachycardia may be due to chronic beta blocker therapy, not euvolemia. Blood pressure is highly variable in patients. While mean arterial pressures (MAP) less than 60 mmHg in an adult nearly always indicate under-resuscitation, MAP greater than 60 mmHg is no guarantee of adequate perfusion of vital organs. Intense peripheral vasoconstriction may produce MAPs greater than 60 mmHg, but organs distal to the vasoconstriction are at peril. Moreover, patients with longstanding hypertension may require a higher MAP to maintain adequate perfusion pressure. Measurements of CVP can be useful at the extremes of measurement, or in observing a trend, but are largely inaccurate, particularly in patients under positive pressure ventilation. Pulmonary artery catheters can measure cardiac output, stroke volume, and estimate left atrial pressure via pulmonary capillary wedge pressure to a reasonable level of accuracy, yet the risks involved in placement and management of PA catheters preclude their use in a majority of patients. Less invasive continuous cardiac output measurements, based on arterial pulse contour, can be used as well. These allow measurement of stroke volume variation, an indicator of fluid responsiveness and therefore under-resuscitation [6, 10, 11].

13. **What is the cause of the patient's acidosis?**

This patient has an anion gap metabolic acidosis with a low pH and low bicarbonate.

Anion gap = Na − (Cl + HCO_3); normal is 8–16.

$$146 - (103 + 15) = 28$$

Winter's formula show that this is a pure metabolic acidosis with appropriate respiratory compensation:

Winter's formula: pCO_2 (expected) = 1.5 (HCO_3) + 8 ± 2

$$1.5(15) + 8 = 30.5 \pm 2$$

In addition, the acidosis is pure high anion gap metabolic acidosis, not mixed gap and non-gap metabolic acidosis, through determination of the delta gap ratio:

(Patient's anion gap) − 12/24 − (patient's bicarbonate) = 1 − 2: pure high anion gap, less than 1: mixed gap and non-gap metabolic acidosis

$$(28 - 12)/(24 - 15) = 1.7$$

Causes of pure metabolic acidosis can be remembered according to the mnemonic MUDPILES: Methanol, Uremia, Diabetic ketoacidosis, Paraldehyde, Infection, Lactic acidosis, Ethylene glycol, Salicylic acid. In light of the patient's history, the cause of the anion gap acidosis is likely lactic acidosis due to poor oxygenation of tissues, caused by inadequate perfusion, or of inadequate oxygen extraction due to carbon monoxide poisoning [6].

14. **Discuss the diagnosis and treatment of carbon monoxide (CO) poisoning**

Patients with carbon monoxide (CO) poisoning presents with nonspecific symptoms such as headache, myalgias, dizziness, confusion, and loss of consciousness. The diagnosis requires a high index of suspicion and is supported by the patient's presenting history. Endogenous carbon monoxide exists as a neurotransmitter and modulates cell proliferation and inflammation. However, CO can quickly become poisonous at higher levels.

Carbon monoxide binds hemoglobin with over 200 times as much affinity as oxygen. This means that only a relatively small concentration is required to produce a pathologic effect. As it binds hemoglobin, it forms carboxyhemoglobin and induces a conformational change resulting in the oxygen already bound to the hemoglobin to be bound more tightly. This shifts the oxyhemoglobin dissociation curve to the left, favoring less oxygen delivery to the tissues. Furthermore, CO has other effects, such as binding to platelet heme proteins which then release nitric oxide. The nitric oxide impairs the mitochondrial cellular respiration, triggering anaerobic metabolism and the production of lactate. CO also induces neutrophil degranulation, releasing myeloperoxidase and producing reactive oxygen species. It is these reactive oxygen species that induce oxidative stress and an inflammatory response which causes the neurologic and cardiac injury.

Standard pulse oximetry cannot distinguish between oxyhemoglobin and carboxyhemoglobin species. Carboxyhemoglobin absorbs the same amount of red light as oxyhemoglobin and standard pulse oximeters may in fact overestimate the oxygen saturation. Co-oximetry, however, measures light absorption at multiple wavelengths and is therefore able to detect other hemoglobin species including carboxyhemoglobin, reduced hemoglobin, and methemoglobin. Many laboratory machines still use standard oximetry for ABG-reported oxygen saturations as well, though practice is shifting toward increased use of co-oximetry. Furthermore, as CO produces a functional hypoxia, there is no absolute reduction in O_2, so P_aO_2 detected on arterial blood gas (ABG) analysis will show normal partial pressures of O_2 dissolved in the plasma. The CO poisoning can be detected by a co-oximeter, but obtaining a venous CO saturation is the usual method of diagnosis. Levels greater than 3% in nonsmokers or greater than 10% in smokers make the diagnosis. Levels greater than 40% are associated with shock, coma, seizures, and death. In our patient with a heavy smoking history, her CO level would have to exceed 10%.

The treatment of CO poisoning is straightforward in most cases. While the first step in management of CO poisoning is to stop the exposure to CO, the half-life of carboxyhemoglobin in a patient breathing room air is roughly 300 min. This is reduced to 90 min in a patient breathing 100% oxygen. Standard supportive therapy applies; patients who have altered mental status may require intubation for airway protection [12].

15. **How can oxygen content and oxygen delivery be determined?**

The oxygen content of the blood includes the amount of oxygen bound to hemoglobin as well as the amount of oxygen dissolved in the plasma. It is dependent on the O_2 saturation (SpO_2), hemoglobin (Hb) concentration, and partial pressure of O_2 (p_aO_2).

$$\text{Oxygen content } (C_aO_2) = 1.31(\text{Hb})(SpO_2) + 0.003\,(p_aO_2)$$

As shown above, changes in hemoglobin or oxygen saturation have a more profound effect on oxygen content than does a change in p_aO_2. Oxygen content driven by a cardiac output provides oxygen delivery to the tissues.

$$\text{Oxygen delivery } (DO_2) = C_aO_2 \times \text{cardiac output}$$

If we use our patient's vital signs and laboratory results at face value, we will calculate a normal C_aO_2 and DO_2; however, the SpO_2 is falsely elevated as it does not distinguish normal oxyhemoglobin from abnormal carboxyhemoglobin. Carboxyhemoglobin traps the oxygen to the hemoglobin molecule and makes it unable to be released to the tissues. So to be more precise, the oxygen is still delivered to the tissues, but the tissues are unable to extract the oxygen from the hemoglobin. If we obtained the mixed venous oxygen content (C_vO_2), we could calculate the oxygen extraction fraction:

$$\text{Oxygen extraction fraction} = (C_aO_2 - C_vO2)/C_aO_2$$

In the setting of CO poisoning, the C_vO_2 would be pathologically elevated, and the oxygen extraction fraction will be decreased [13].

16. **What are the most common surgical procedures in burn patients?**

Burn eschar provides a robust medium for bacterial proliferation. Therefore, early excision and grafting provides the best chance of reducing infection risk and promoting healing. Split-thickness autologous skin-grafting appears to be the optimal technique, but allografting is sometimes necessary in patients without a good source of unburned skin to use.

Emergency escharotomies are indicated when circumferential burns create a compartment syndrome for the affected part of the body. This can be in an extremity or on the torso or abdomen, where it can restrict chest wall movement or cause renal failure and bowel ischemia in the abdominal compartment, respectively [3].

These patients also tend to have long hospitalizations, and in severe cases may require tracheostomy for prolonged mechanical ventilation or enteric feeding tube access due to increased nutrition requirements. Intravascular access can also be difficult depending on the location of burn wounds and may require surgical or radiological assistance in placement. Finally, burn patients frequently have other trauma associated with the inciting event (for example, long bone fractures in a patient who was in a motor vehicle collision) and management of these patients for non-burn-related surgeries can be challenging.

17. **What are the anesthetic goals for intraoperative management for this patient?**

The anesthetic goals for this patient would be to maintain hemodynamic and respiratory stability in the setting of SIRS and hypovolemic shock while still providing analgesia and anesthesia for the patient. Neuromuscular blockade will provide a quiescent field for the surgeon and assist in ventilation.

18. **The patient's family is concerned about the effects of general anesthesia on her cognitive function. What can you tell them?**

The patient is at risk for post-operative delirium and cognitive dysfunction. Delirium is a state of waxing and waning consciousness and confusion. Predisposing factors include organic causes such as infection, pain, and metabolic disturbances. Post-operative cognitive dysfunction is cognitive dysfunction that persists for months following surgery. Most mild cases resolve in the first three months following surgery; however in this patient, her likelihood of prolonged hospitalization and critical illness will confound the diagnosis and predictions of recovery. She has pre-existing cognitive impairment from Alzheimer's dementia, and her mental status is already further impaired from critical illness preoperatively; namely, metabolic acidosis and presumed carbon monoxide poisoning. Post-operatively, she will still be critically ill, likely requiring invasive treatments and several medications for some time. At this time she will be at her highest risk of delirium. Her history of hearing impairment will make attempts at reorientation difficult, but maintaining normal sleep-wake cycles and the presence of family members will increase her chances of recovery. It is difficult to predict the degree of long-term cognitive dysfunction that may occur, but the risk is increased given a prolonged hospitalization. Given these considerations, the patient's cognitive function will likely be affected even without a general anesthetic. Finally, the patient may require multiple surgeries to treat her burn wounds which compound the risk.

However, as anesthesiologists we can limit the number of additional factors that can predispose the patient to delirium and cognitive dysfunction. Removal of toxins can be started right away with administration of supplemental oxygen and correction of acidosis and electrolyte abnormalities. Certain medications, such as benzodiaezepines, have been shown to increase the risk of and worsen delirium; these can be avoided. While uncontrolled pain worsens delirium, limiting sedating medications such as narcotics to the minimum effective dose can help the patient return to an alert state as soon as possible [14].

19. **Would a regional technique be appropriate for this patient?**

Intuitively it would seem that regional anesthesia would be associated with less post-operative delirium; however evidence shows that there are similar amounts of post-operative delirium with either regional or general anesthesia.

Regional anesthesia would be inappropriate for this patient for several reasons. The patient has an unstable airway and requires intubation regardless of the need for surgery. She is critically ill and may demonstrate hemodynamic instability; general anesthesia will facilitate significant intraoperative resuscitation. Finally, peripheral nerve blockade may preclude an accurate neurologic exam post-operatively and may confound the etiology of nerve damage.

20. **What other concerns do you have given this patient's advanced age?**

We can expect this patient to exhibit physiologic changes appropriate for someone her age. Although her pre-injury exercise capacity has not been verified, advanced age results in a reduced ability to increase heart rate, stroke volume, and cardiac output to meet increased demands, which would increase her risk for ischemia. Her vasculature will have poor compliance and will not be able to adjust to acute changes in blood pressure, making her blood pressure labile. Her hypertension is likely chronic, which will have shifted her auto-regulatory curves; she may need a higher MAP to maintain adequate perfusion of her organs. The patient's age-related reduction of her protective cough and swallowing reflexes put her at a higher risk of aspiration. Work of breaking is increased as respiratory muscles weaken and chest wall elasticity is reduced. Closing capacity and residual volume increase with age and cause ventilation and perfusion mismatching. In addition to these age-related respiratory changes the patient likely has airway obstruction related to her heavy smoking history.

As people age, muscle mass decreases and a corresponding decrease in creatinine level is observed. This patient's creatinine level may be close to normal for a young adult, but represents a significant renal impairment at this patient's age. We can also expect her to have a reduced hepatic metabolism which will affect drug clearance. Age-related reductions of marrow function and cellular immunity will impair her ability to respond to blood loss and will put her at increased risk of infection [14].

21. **Would you like any other preoperative testing done? Which tests?**

The patient should have a preoperative electrolyte panel and complete blood count. A preoperative EKG is indicated based on her age being greater than 50 and state of critical illness; in this patient with significant smoking history and inhalation injury a preoperative CXR would help demonstrate underlying pulmonary disease. Pulmonary function tests are impractical in this setting and would not change management.

This patient has no Revised Cardiac Risk Index factors—presence of coronary artery disease, diabetes mellitus requiring insulin, creatinine >2.0, congestive heart failure, or history of cerebrovascular accident—and no acute coronary syndromes. Her functional capacity is unconfirmed, but she was at least ambulating at the time of her accident. This, combined with the intermediate risk and emergent nature of the surgery indicates that no further preoperative cardiac testing is indicated [15].

22. **What monitoring do you want for this patient?**

Standard ASA monitoring is of course indicated, EKG, pulse oximetry, blood pressure, temperature, and end-tidal carbon dioxide monitoring. Invasive blood pressure monitoring via arterial line is indicated because of predicted hemodynamic instability as well as need for frequent ABGs and blood draws both intra- and postoperatively. Large bore IV access is mandatory; central venous access would be prudent as this patient will require secure IV access for some time and peripheral access may be difficult to obtain due to her wounds. Furthermore, the patient may require pressor therapy and central venous pressure monitoring may assist fluid resuscitation. The patient should have a Foley catheter for strict urine output monitoring.

23. **Is a pulmonary artery (PA) catheter indicated?**

This patient does not have preexisting cardiac disease or signs of heart failure. If needed, cardiac output monitoring may be obtained using peripheral continuous cardiac output monitoring devices which are most efficacious in intubated, mechanically ventilated patients in normal sinus rhythm. The patient has no indication for PA catheter placement at this time; the risks of complications outweigh the benefits of measurements that may be obtained [16].

24. **Is intubation indicated? What if this patient were not going to the OR?**

Despite her indication for surgery, this patient requires emergent intubation due to the presence of inhalation injury exhibited by her noisy breathing and evidence of smoke and fire exposure on the patient's face. If her airway is not secured, swelling will increase, causing complete obstruction and making attempts at intubation extremely difficult if not impossible. She will likely require postoperative mechanical ventilation due to blossoming lung injury from her burns and fluid resuscitation, and metabolic acidosis. She will also need supplemental oxygen for carbon monoxide poisoning. Currently, she is maintaining her own airway and her respiratory status is adequate though tenuous.

25. **How would you intubate this patient?**

Spontaneous ventilation should be maintained. Airway swelling will make mask ventilation difficult, so an awake fiberoptic intubation would be the safest approach. Supplemental oxygen should be delivered through a nasal cannula as the airway is topicalized with local anesthetic. Sedatives should be avoided and narcotics limited. If the patient is unable to cooperate with awake intubation, a sedative that preserves spontaneous ventilation such as ketamine or dexmedetomidine should be considered. If assessment of the airway predicts difficult fiberoptic intubation, then a surgical airway kit and qualified personnel should be standing by. Finally, rescue equipment such as a laryngeal mask airway and a variety of endotracheal tube sizes and airway assist devices (e.g., bougie) should be immediately available.

26. **How would you induce anesthesia in this patient?**

After the airway is secured, anesthesia should be quickly but carefully induced to limit discomfort to the patient. Hemodynamic instability on induction should be expected due to interruption of endogenous catecholamine support. This effect can be limited through a careful induction using potent opioid in conjunction with small amounts of inhaled anesthetic, or a hemodynamically stable intravenous (IV) anesthetic such as ketamine. Even propofol could potentially be used, provided it was titrated carefully to use the minimum effective dose and was infused with prophylactic doses of a vasopressor such as phenylephrine to limit a decrease in blood pressure. Etomidate is best avoided; though controversial, some suggest that there is a higher risk of etomidate-induced corticosteroid deficiency in this patient population [17]. We suggest avoiding benzodiazepines if possible to reduce the risk of post-operative delirium, yet small doses may decrease the amount of vasodilation-producing agent required for anesthesia.

Once anesthesia is induced, a non-depolarizing neuromuscular blocking agent may be administered. In our scenario, we plan to intubate this patient while awake; therefore a rapid sequence induction is not required. However, if a patient is to be intubated after induction, a rapid sequence induction is suggested due to decreased gastric transit time resulting from trauma and the inflammatory state. Succinylcholine is used with caution in burn patients, and is discussed further below.

27. **What would you use for maintenance of anesthesia?**

The goal is to maintain a balanced anesthetic that addresses amnesia, analgesia, and immobility. A non-depolarizing neuromuscular blocking agent will keep the patient immobile. A multimodal approach to analgesia can provide the best pain control; IV narcotics are first line, but IV acetaminophen or an alpha-agonist such as dexmedetomidine can be valuable adjuncts if they are available. Non-steroidal anti-inflammatory drugs (NSAIDs), such as ketorolac, are best avoided in this initial phase as the patient is at risk for further renal injury. Inhalational agents, which can cause vasodilation and depress cardiac function, should be used with caution. Using them in conjunction with a opioid infusion may reduce the amount required to provide amnesia. Once again, a versatile agent like ketamine can cause amnesia and analgesia while limiting hemodynamic insult. Benzodiazepines infusions should be reserved for those patients too hemodynamically unstable to tolerate any amount of inhalational or IV anesthetic.

28. **Can succinylcholine be used in burn patients? What about non-depolarizing neuromuscular blockers?**

A burn injury triggers an upregulation of post-junctional acetycholine receptors (AChR). This occurs in the immediate area of injury, from local inflammation and muscle denervation, but later on at sites distal to the injury, presumably due to prolonged immobilization common in this patient population. Up-regulation of AChRs results in a significant increase in the amount of potassium released from the cells upon activation of the receptors by succinylcholine. Lethal and sub-lethal levels of hyperkalemia have been noted following succinylcholine administration in these patients. The up-regulation takes several hours to develop, so succinylcholine may be used up to 24 h after the burn injury. After this initial window, succinylcholine should be avoided until some time well after the patient has healed completely; some recommend a period up to two years after the burn wound has healed.

Non-depolarizing neuromuscular blocking agents are not associated with the same life-threatening hyperkalemia and can be used safely in burn patients. However, because of the up-regulation of AChRs, patients are usually quite resistant to non-depolarizing agents so higher doses than usual will be required to produce the desired relaxation. Avoidance of histamine-releasing agents, such as vecuronium, would be preferred to limit further exacerbating the inflammatory response [5, 18].

29. **Are you concerned about hypothermia in this patient?**

The skin plays a vital role in maintaining normothermia. Burn patients have lost this adaptive tool and are limited in their ability to retain body heat. Heat is lost through four different mechanisms:

Conduction	transfer of heat between two materials of differing temperatures (laying on cold OR table)
Convection	transfer of heat as a molecule repeatedly rises to a warmer temperature and falls to a cooler temperature (cool air from the air conditioning in the OR flowing over a patient's body)
Radiation	transfer of heat from an object into the surrounding space without physical contact with another object (parts of the body that are uncovered and exposed to the surrounding environment)
Evaporation	transfer of heat in the conversion of liquid to the gaseous state (evaporation of sweat or the exposed interstitial fluid of the body in injured areas)

Conduction plays a limited role in heat transfer in the OR; the OR table and IV fluids and blood products can be warmed to limit this effect. In the burned patient, the ability to reduce heat lost by radiation and evaporation is limited—the areas of the body most vulnerable are the injured areas which are usually in the sterile field. This is not always the case, however, so the patient should be covered as much as possible. This leaves convection as the most practical method by which we can control a patient's body temperature. In a typical case, we use a forced-air warmer on the nonoperative sites of the body. It has been suggested, that the airflow from these machines tosses bacteria into the ambient air, though this is controversial. More frequently the areas of the body on which to place the forced air warmer are limited due to injury. The ambient temperature of the OR, therefore, is increased close to the level of ideal body temperature in order to preserve body heat.

Because of the loss of the protective and insulating layer of skin, burn patients lose heat rapidly. Hypothermia is associated with increased cardiac ectopy, coagulopathy, cold-induced diuresis, altered mental status, and increased oxygen consumption caused by shivering [13].

30. **What is the plan for emergence? Will you extubate this patient?**

This patient should remain intubated as she has not recovered from the event prompting intubation; namely, inhalational injury. Sedation can be lightened so the patient can follow commands, and analgesia no longer has to be strong enough to allow the patient to withstand surgical stimulation. Only the minimum amount needed to keep the patient covered should be used. Neuromuscular blockade may be reversed once muscular twitches have returned; however this is not strictly necessary in a patient who will require mechanical ventilation over several days. Care should be taken, however, to lighten sedation only when the patient has return of muscle function.

31. **Can this patient go to the PACU? Should she be admitted to the ICU?**

This patient meets ICU admission criteria because she requires mechanical ventilation. Other criteria for ICU admission include need for vasopressor/inotropes to maintain blood pressure, invasive cardiac monitoring such as PA catheters, hemodynamic instability or large fluctuations in fluid shifts, severe blood loss or metabolic derangements requiring frequent laboratory testing, and high nursing demands, such as that for wound dressing changes, hourly neuromonitoring or vascular checks, or uncontrolled delirium.

32. **If this patient is to remain intubated, what will you choose for her ventilator settings?**

This patient should have a lung protective ventilation strategy as defined by the ARDSnet protocol. She should be on a controlled setting, as opposed to a spontaneous mode, to reduce the work of breathing. Tidal volumes should be 4–6 ml/kg based on ideal body weight, plateau pressures should be less than 30 cm H_2O, positive end expiratory pressure of at least 5 cm H_2O, and FiO_2 should be weaned to the lowest amount possible, aiming for p_aO_2 of 60. RR should be titrated to a normal pH, without exceeding a respiratory rate of 35. While she may not meet ARDS diagnostic criteria at this time, it is highly likely that she will develop ARDS during the course of her hospitalization as a result of her injuries and inflammatory state [19, 20].

33. **How will you manage post-operative pain in this patient? What will you choose for sedation?**

Burn pain is notoriously difficult to treat. There is not only the nociceptive pain of a large amount of damaged tissue and inflammation, but also neuropathic pain from destruction of nerve endings in the skin. The approach to postoperative pain should be multimodal. Opioids, acetaminophen, adjuncts such as dexmedetomidine or clonidine, ketamine, and gabapentin can help control burn pain during and in-between surgeries and should be administered at regular scheduled intervals or as an infusion. NSAIDs can be considered once acute renal injury has been ruled out.

Sedation should be limited to the amount necessary to maintain ventilator synchrony and patient comfort. Often if pain is controlled, the patient will not require much sedation. Patients who are sedated should have a daily sedation holiday to assess neurologic status and actively assess ventilator dependence. Due to her age, limiting benzodiazepines may reduce her risk or at least the severity of postoperative delirium.

References

1. Nitzschke SL. Wound healing trajectories in burn patients and their impact on mortality. J Burn Care Res. 2014;35(6):474–9.
2. Hettiaratchy S, Papini R. Initial management of a major burn: II—assessment and resuscitation. BMJ. 2004;329(7457):101–3.
3. Orgill DP. Excision and skin grafting of thermal burns. N Engl J Med. 2009;360(9):893–901.
4. American Burn Association. Practice guidelines for burn care: chapter 1. J Burn Care Rehab. 2001:1S–3S.
5. Yao FF. Anesthesiology: Problem-oriented patient managment, 7th ed. Philadelphia: Lippincott, Williams & Wilkins; 2012. p. 1200–21.
6. Marini JJ, Wheeler AP. Critical care medicine: the essentials, 4th ed. Philadelphia: Lippincott, Williams & Wilkins; 2010. 676–685.
7. Osler T, Glance LG, Hosmer DW. Simplified estimates of the probability of death after burn injuries: extending and updating the baux score. J Trauma. 2010;68(3):7–609.
8. Ryan CM, et al. Objective estimates of the probability of death from burn injuries. N Engl J Med. 1998;338(6):362–6.
9. Hussain A, Dunn KW. Predicting length of stay in thermal burns: a systematic review of prognostic factors. Burns. 2013;39(7):1331–40.
10. Kahn SA, Schoemann M, Lentz CW. Burn resuscitation index: a simple method for calculating fluid resuscitation in the burn patient. J Burn Care Res. 2010;31(4):616–23.
11. Mitchell KB, et al. New management strategy for fluid resuscitation: quantifying volume in the first 48 h after burn injury. J Burn Care Res. 2013;34(1):196–202.
12. Weaver LK. Carbon monoxide poisoning. N Engl J Med. 2009;360(12):1217–25.
13. Morgan GE, Mikhail MS, Murray MJ. Clinical anesthesiology, 4th ed. United States: McGraw-Hill; 2006. p. 148–50, 561–5, 870–2.
14. Hines RL, Marschall KE. Stoetling's anesthesia and co-existing disease. 6th ed. Philadelphia: Elsevier; 2012. p. 642–54.
15. Fleischer LA, et al. A report of the American College of Cardiology/American Heart Association Task Force nn Practice Guidelines. J Am Coll Cardiol. 2014;64(22):e77–137.
16. American Society of Anesthesiologists Task Force on Pulmonary. Artery catheterization. practice guidelines for pulmonary artery catheterization: an updated report by the American Society of Anesthesiologists Task Force on Pulmonary Artery Catheterization. Anesthesiology. 2003;99(4):988–1014.
17. Mosier MJ, Lasinski AM, Gamelli RL. Suspected adrenal insufficiency in critically ill burned patients: etomidate-induced or critical illness-related corticosteroid insufficiency? A review of the literature. J Burn Care Res. 2015;36(2):272–8.
18. Martyn JAJ, Richtsfeld M. Succinylcholine-induced hyperkalemia in acquired pathologic states etiologic factors and molecular mechanisms. Anesthesiology. 2006;104(1):158–69.
19. Network The Acute Respiratory Distress Syndrome. Ventilation with lower tidal volumes as compared with traditional tidal volumes for acute lung injury and the acute respiratory distress syndrome. N Engl J Med. 2000;342(18):1301–8.
20. NIH-NHLBI ARDS Network. About the NHLBI ARDS Network. Retreived from http://www.ardsnet.org/. Accessed 23 July 2015.
21. Dibildox M, Jeschke MG, Herndon DN. Burn injury, rule of nines. In: Vincent J-L, Hall JB, editors. Encyclopedia of intensive care medicine. Berlin: Springer; 2012. p. 417–9.
22. McKinnell T, Pape SA. Measurements in burns. In: Mani R, Romanelli M, Shukla V, editors. Measurements in wound healing: science and practice. London: Springer; 2013. p. 259–90.

Index

Note: Page number followed by *f* and *t* indicate figures and tables respectively

A

Abciximab, 75
Abdominal aortic aneurysm (AAA), 215
  abdominal compartment syndrome (ACS), 217–218
  anesthetic technique for open surgery, 221
  antibiotics for, 221
  blood loss, management of, 224
  BNP ("B-type" or brain natriuretic peptide), 219
  cardiac workup, 218, 219
  classification, 216
  coagulation, addressing, 220
  continuous cardiac output monitors, 221
  dangers of open surgical repair, 217
  diabetes and, 220
  endovascular aortic repair (EVAR), 217
  endovascular repair, 216
  evaluating respiratory status in patients undergoing major vascular surgery, 220
  fluid management, 221
  hemodynamic management, 221
  impact of aortic cross-clamping, 223
  incidence and prevalence of, 215
  intraoperative monitors, 220–221
  intravenous fluids, use of, 221
  measuring hematocrit and creatinine to predict outcome, 219
  mesenteric and hepatic protection strategies, 223
  noninvasive diagnostic testing, 218
  open repair of, 216
  percutaneous coronary intervention (PCI), 218
  postoperative pain management strategies, 224
  pre-existing cardiac disease and, 218
  preoperative interventions, 220
  preoperative myocardial revascularization, 218
  preparation for surgery, 216
  renal protection instituted during aortic cross-clamping, 223
  reperfusion, 223–224
  risk factors for developing, 215
  ruptured, 217
  rupture of, 216
  screening, recommendations for, 216
  short- and long-term outcome differences between approaches, 217
  significance of poorly controlled preoperative hypertension, 218–219
  spinal cord monitoring, 224
  surgical approach, 221
  systemic hemodynamic response to aortic cross-clamping, 222
  thermoregulation, 224
  unclamping, management of, 223–224
  venous access, 221
Abdominal aortic aneurysm (AAA) repair
  endovascular repair, 231*t*
  impact of obesity outcome in, 228
Abdominal compartment syndrome (ACS), 217–218, 249, 419
Abdominal obesity, 241
ACC/AHA guidelines, 47–48
  for non-cardiac surgery, 8–10
ACE inhibitors, 220
Acetylcholine metabolism, 150
Acetylcholine receptors (AChR), 472
Acidosis, 462, 468–469
Acquired hemophilia A (AHA), 327, 329
Activated clotting time (ACT), 109
Activated factor VII, 322
Activated partial thromboplastin time (aPTT), 328
  assessment, 320
  increase in, 321
  performance, 320–321
Activated partial thromboplastin time (aPTT) assay, 320
Activated prothrombin complex concentrate (aPCC), 331
Acute chest syndrome (ACS), 334
Acute compartment syndrome (ACS), 368, 370, 374
Acute coronary syndromes (ACS), 7
Acute fatty liver of pregnancy, 202
Acute hemolytic transfusion reaction, 316
  treatment of, 316
Acute intraoperative atrial fibrillation in mitral stenosis, 39
Acute liver failure, 201
Acutely decompensated heart failure, signs of, 20
Acute normovolemic hemodilution (ANH), 345
Acute-onset atrial fibrillation, treatment of, 39
Acute tubular necrosis (ATN), 267
A-delta fibers, 373
Adenoidectomy, 297
  common indications for, 297
Adenosine diphosphate (ADP), 323
Adrenal gland, function of, 184
Adrenergic receptor blocking agents, 185
Adrenocorticotrophic hormone (ACTH) excess, 136
Adult respiratory distress syndrome (ARDS), 467
Airway, 287
  anesthesia practice, 291
  awake intubation
    attempting, 290
    awake fiberoptic intubation, 292
  bag mask ventilation, 293
  cervical collar, managing, 290–291

© Springer International Publishing AG 2017
L.S. Aglio and R.D. Urman (eds.), *Anesthesiology*,
DOI 10.1007/978-3-319-50141-3

cricothyrotomy, contraindications to, 294
difficult intubation, 294
drying agent, administering, 291
end-tidal CO_2, 293
evaluating patient's airway, 288
extubation, 294
foreseeing potential problems, 289
formulating the plan, 289
invasive airway access, 294
management of, 287–288
mask ventilation, 293
encountering problems with, 293
medical history of patient, 288
nasal approach to tracheal intubation, 290
obtaining prior medical records, 289
oxygenation, maintaining, 291
for patient involved in MVA, 287
physical examination, 288
principal adverse outcomes, 295
reasons for airway complications and management failures, 295–296
respiratory rate, 292
sedation for intubation, 292
special precautions, 295
topicalization of, 291
trauma imaging studies, 289
Airway Approach Algorithm (AAA), 289
Airway evaluation/management, key considerations of, 306
Airway fire, 300, 307
managing, 308
preventing, 308
Airway history, 288
Airway in acromegaly, 135
Airway physical examination, 288
Airway protection, 180, 181
Akinesis, 5
Albumin, causes and consequences of low level, 204–205
Aldosterone antagonists, 22
Alemtuzumab (Campath), 266
Alfentanil, 397
Allen's test, 76
Allogeneic blood transfusion (ALBT), 129
Alpha-adrenergic receptors, 184
Alpha 1-acid glycoprotein (AAG), 354
Alpha-1 antitrypsin (AAT) deficiency, 202
Alpha-glucosidase inhibitors, 169
Amaurosis fugax. *See* Transient monocular blindness
Ambulatory surgery, 240
role of OSA in, 240
American Spinal Injury Association (ASIA) impairment scale, 123
Amide, 347, 350
Aminotransferases (AST/ALT), 209
Amylin analogues, 169
Analgesia, 242
Anaphylactic reaction, signs and symptoms of, 315
treatment of, 315–316
Anastomotic leaks, 438
Android obesity, 238
Anemia, 264
Anesthetic induction agent, 277
Aneurysms, 216
Angina/dyspnea on exertion (Angina/DOE), 241
Antepartum hemorrhage, causes of, 389
Anterior cord syndrome (ACS), 123
Antibiotic prophylaxis in patients with structural heart disease, 36
Antibiotic regimens, open globe procedures, 278
Anticholinesterase drugs, 156, 157
Anticoagulants, 231
for heart failure, 22
Anticoagulated patients, regional anesthesia for, 368
Antifibrinolytics, role of, 331
Antimetabolite, 70
Antiplatelet/anticoagulants, 74–75
Antiplatelet therapy, 275, 323
Antiserotonergic agents, 259
Antisialogogues, 291
Anxiolytics/opioids, 158
Aortic cross-clamping, 223
systemic hemodynamic response to, 222*f*
Aortic neck length scoring, 230*t*
Aortic stenosis
changing the physiology of heart, 34
etiologies of, 33
grades of, 34*t*
hemodynamic goals for patients, 35
monitoring patients, 35
natural progression of, 33–34
Aortic valve replacement surgery, 36
Aortic valve surgery, 35, 36
APGAR score, of child, 412–413
Apnea, 240
Apnea hypopnea index (AHI), 240, 297
Apnea of prematurity, 451
Apnea spells, 451
Apneic deoxygenation, 242
Aprotinin, 79–80
Arterial kinking, 267
ASA monitors, 92, 115
Ascites, 205
Asphyxia, intrauterine, 399
Aspirin, 63, 75, 275, 323
Asynchronous pacing, 58
Atherosclerotic disease
common perioperative adverse outcomes, 6–7
extracardiac manifestations of, 6
Atlantoaxial instability (AAI), 298, 299
Atracurium, 186, 397
Atrial fibrillation (AF), 25, 69
Atrial flutter, 69
Atrial to atrial cuff technique, 69
Atrioventricular septal defects, 444
Atropine dose, 276
Atropine/glycopyrrolate, 26
Autonomic denervation, 69
Autonomic nervous system
effect on transplanted heart, 68
influence on cardiac function, 67
Autonomic neuropathy, 170
AV node, 4, 5
Avoidance, 152
Awake extubation, 283, 290
Awake intubations, 430
Axillary block, 349
Azathioprine, 157

B

Bacillus cereus, 278
Bag mask ventilation, 293
Balloon angioplasty, 15
Balloon tamponade, 203
Barbiturates, 397

Bariatric surgery, 238
Beck's Triad of symptoms, 462
Benzocaine, 350
Benzodiazepines, 276, 397
Beta-adrenergic receptors, 184
Beta-blockers, 39, 51, 220
Beta-1 receptors, 25
Beta receptor blockers (BRB), for heart failure, 22
Biguanides, 169
Biliary obstruction, 209
Bispectral index (BIS) monitoring, 129
Bivalirudin, 75
Block room, 370
Blood given in emergency resuscitation, 391
BNP ("B-type" or brain natriuretic peptide), 219
Body mass index (BMI), 237
  calculation, 237
  limitations of, 237
Body surface area (BSA), in estimating extent of burn injuries, 463
Bone cement implantation syndrome, 344
Brachial plexus, anatomy of, 369*f*
Brachial plexus block, 367
  anatomy relevant to, 368–369
  anesthesia choices, 367–368
  communication with the surgical team, 370
  contraindications for, 368
    in severe pulmonary disease, 369–370
  with nerve stimulator, 370
  paresthesia, landmark with, 370
  performing peripheral nerve blocks outside OR, 370–371
  preoperative concerns and recommended work up, 367
  regional anesthesia for anticoagulated patients, 368
  with ultrasound guidance, 370
Brachial plexus block (BPB), 368
Bradycardia, 26, 35, 300
Brain relaxation, 108
  hyperventilation in, 108
Breathing, 460
Broca's index, 243
Bronchial blockers, 90
Bronchoalveolar lavage, 196
Bronchopulmonary dysplasia (BPD), 451
Budd–Chiari syndrome, 202
Bulbar muscles weakness, 156
Bupivacaine, 351, 373, 374
Burn injuries
  calculating fluid requirements, 463
  effects
    cardiovascular effects of, 467
    to respiratory system, 467
Burn pain, 467, 473
Burn patients
  advanced age of patient, 471
  anesthesia
    inducing, 472
    maintenance of, 472
  anesthetic goals for intraoperative management, 470
  common cause of death for, 468
  general anesthesia, effects of, 470
  hypothermia, 472–473
  intubation, 471, 472
  monitoring, 471
  PACU, patient going to, 473
  plan for emergence, 473
  post-operative pain, managing, 473–474
  predictors of mortality in, 467–468
  preoperative testing, 471
  pulmonary artery (PA) catheter, 471
  regional technique, 470–471
  succinylcholine, 472
  surgical procedures in, 470
  ventilator settings, 473
Burns, 465
  classification, 465
  extent of, 465–466
  major burn, 466

C

Cadaveric kidneys, 267
Calcineurin inhibitor, 70, 71
Calcium channel blockers (CCB), 163, 186
  for heart failure, 22
Carbon dioxide (CO_2), 249
  disadvantages, 248
  embolism, 252
Carbon dioxide laser, 305
Carbon monoxide poisoning, 469
Carbon tetrachloride, 202–203
Carboxyhemoglobin, 469–470
Carcinoid crisis, 257, 258
  development of, 257
    risk in, 257
  management of, 260
  steps to minimize, 258
Carcinoid heart disease (CHD), 256
  laboratory evaluation of, 257
  pathophysiology of, 256
  preoperative assessment to evaluate, 257
Carcinoid syndrome, 255
  neuraxial anesthesia for, 259
  postoperative considerations for, 260
Carcinoid tumors, 255
  laboratory evaluation, 256
  preoperative considerations, 256
Cardiac allograft vasculopathy, 69
  treatment, 69–70
Cardiac arrest, therapeutic hypothermia after, 30
Cardiac arrhythmias, 249
Cardiac autonomic signaling, 67
Cardiac conduction system, perfusion of, 5
Cardiac implantable electrical device (CIED), 55, 56–57, 59
Cardiac output (CO), 249
Cardiac resynchronization therapy (CRT), 22
Cardiac tamponade. *See* Pericardial tamponade
Cardiogenic shock, 461
Cardiopulmonary bypass (CPB), avoiding, 76–77
Cardiovascular disease, diabetes mellitus and, 169
Cardiovascular physiologic changes seen in pregnancy, 390
Cardiovascular system changes in pregnancy, 396
Carotid artery (CA) disease, 113
  treatment, 114
Carotid endarterectomy (CEA), 113
  anesthetic management, 115–116
  blood pressure management, 116
  cerebral hyperperfusion syndrome, 117
  comorbid conditions associated with, 113
  cranial nerves at risk during, 117
  ICU admission after, 117
  identifying perioperative stroke, 117
  improving CA perfusion, 114
  medical therapies, 114

monitors, 115
neuromonitoring, 115
non-stroke related death after, 117
postoperative management issues after, 117
premedication, 115
preoperative evaluation, 113–114
regional anesthetic, 116
reperfusion injury after, 116
respiratory management with general anesthesia, 116
surgical or endovascular therapy, 114
transient monocular blindness, 113
Carotid Revascularization Endarterectomy *versus* Stenting Trial (CREST), 117
Cataract surgery, 275
preoperative testing, 275
Catecholamine releasing drugs, 259
Catecholamines, 183, 184, 187
Caudal catheters, 425
Ceftazidime, 278
Central cord syndrome (CCS), 123
Central obesity, 238
Central venous access, 98, 257
Central venous catheter (CVL), 24
Central venous line (CVL), 63
Central venous pressure (CVP), 2, 24
measuring, 230
Cerebral autoregulation, 104
Cerebral edema, cause of, 387
Cerebral hyperperfusion syndrome, 117
Cerebral ischemia, 116
Cerebral oximetry, 115
Cerebral perfusion pressure (CPP), 104, 108
Cerebral salt wasting (CSW) syndrome, 105, 138
Cerebrospinal fluid (CSF), rhinorrhea, 137
Cerebrospinal fluid drainage, 108
Cervical spinal stenosis, 122
Cervical spondylotic myelopathy (CSM), 122–123
C-fibers, 373
Chemical burn, 467
Chemoreceptor, 240
Chest radiography, 21, 55
Childbirth, basis of the pain in, 381
Child-Pugh (CP) score, 207
Chloroprocaine, 350
Cholangiography, intraoperative, 398
Cholestasis, 209
Cholestatic cirrhosis, 201
Cholinesterase inhibitors, side-effects of, 153
Chromogranin A, 256
Chronic kidney disease (CKD), 228
Chronic obstructive pulmonary disease (COPD), 91, 220–221, 306
in patients with AAA, 228
Chronic renal disease, 264
Chronological age, 450
Circulation, 460
Cirrhosis, 200–201, 202
Cisatracurium, 211
Clevidipine, 186
Clonidine, 220, 352
Clonidine suppression test, 185
Clopidogrel, 15, 75, 275, 342
Coagulation, impact of aortic cross-clamp on, 223
Coagulopathies, intraoperative, 319
activated partial thromboplastin time, 320
assessing coagulopathy in patients, 320
coagulation cascade, major steps of, 320
co-morbidities causing coagulation abnormalities, 321
drugs causing, 323–324
effects of temperature and pH, 322
intraoperative coagulopathy, major causes of, 321
platelet activity, monitoring, 323
prothrombin time, 320
recombinant activated human factor VII, 322
routine coagulation testing in preoperative patients, 319
shortest half-life, coagulation factor having, 322
thromboelastograph (TEG), 323
Coagulopathy, 203, 210, 462
Cocaine, 350
Codeine, 302
CO_2 embolism, 252
Combined spinal epidural (CSE), 380–381
Conduction system of the heart, 5
Conduit, 295
Conduit spasm, 82
Congenital diaphragmatic hernia (CDH), 412, 421
additional diagnostic work-up, 422
advantages and disadvantages of using ICU ventilator, 423
approaches to place epidural in neonate, 425
contraindications to EMCO, 422–423
echocardiogram, 422
embryologic origin of the defect, 421
emergence and extubation, plan for, 424
equipment modifications, 423
extracorporeal membrane oxygenation therapy in patients with, 422
ICU team ordering head ultrasound, 422
incidence of, 421
intraoperative monitoring, 423
intraoperative pulmonary hypertensive episode, 424
lung isolation and one-lung ventilation, options for, 424
neonate with, 422
options for ventilation in transport to OR, 423
postoperative analgesia, 424–425
pre- and post-ductal oxygen saturations, 424
reasonable plan for maintenance of anesthesia, 424
risk of coexisting congenital anomalies, 422
sudden oxygen desaturation in transport, 423
transitional circulation, 422
typical surgical approach to CDH repair, 424
ventilation strategy for, 423
Congenital heart disease (CHD), 41, 441
anesthetic implications of trisomy 21, 442
atrioventricular septal defect, 441
bidirectional shunting, 441
cardiac surgery at age of 3 months, 441–442
differential diagnosis, 443
discharge after inguinal hernia repair, 444
endocarditis prophylaxis, 443–444
evaluation, 442
factors affecting PVR, 443
inguinal hernia repair, 443
left-to-right shunting, 441
management of airway, 443
peripheral intravenous, 443
physical exam, 442
preoperative oxygen saturation, 443
preoperative tests, 442
right-to-left shunting, 441
risk factors for surgery, 446
Congestive heart failure. *See* Heart failure (HF)
Continuous invasive blood pressure, 24
Continuous spinal analgesia, 380
Co-oximetry, 469

Cor pulmonale, 240
Coronary artery bypass graft (CABG), 15, 73
  Allen's test, 76
  antiplatelet/anticoagulants, 74–75
  avoiding CPB, 76–77
  conduit spasm, 82
  conduits used for, 76
  coronary angiogram, 74
  coronary steal, 80
  epiaortic scanning, 82
  epidural, 80
  "Fast Track" cardiac surgery, 78
  indications for, 73
  internal mammary artery, 81
  intra-aortic balloon pump for, 81
  investigation of carotid arteries, 75
  ischemic preconditioning, 80
  issues faced by anesthetist, 77
  monitors, 79
  myocardial viability test, 76
  off-pump CABG, 77
  on-pump CABG, 76–77, 83
  predicted risk of mortality, 74
  principle of, 81–82
  risk factors, 74
  surgical risk assessment, 74
  temporary pacing, 83
  transesophageal echo, 78–79
  uneventful induction of anesthesia, 81
Coronary artery bypass graft (CABG), 7
  pulmonary artery catheter, 78, 79
Coronary artery disease (CAD), 3, 13
  ACC/AHA guidelines, 8–10
  anatomy of coronary vasculature, 4–5
  associated extracardiac manifestations of atherosclerotic disease, 6
  chronic CAD
    clinical manifestations of, 6
    chronic stable CAD, 7
  clinical vignette, 3
  common perioperative adverse outcomes, 6–7
  conventional therapies for stable angina and its acute thrombotic complications, 7
  definition, 4
  expected patterns of injury due to ischemia or infarction in each coronary territory, 5–6
  major adverse cardiac events, 6–7
  mechanism of
    chronic stable CAD, 7
    demand ischemia by reviewing key determinants of myocardial oxygen consumption, 8
  modern approaches to treat CAD and acute thrombotic complications, 7
  overarching goals of perioperative cardiac risk stratification, 8
  perfusion of cardiac conduction system, 5
  perioperative coronary events, 7–8
  risk factors for, 6
Coronary artery revascularization prophylaxis (CARP), 218
Coronary dominance, 4, 5
Coronary perfusion, effects of hypothermia on, 30
Coronary steal, 80
Coronary vasculature, anatomy of, 4–5
Corrected age, 450
Corticosteroids, 157
Corticosteroids/serotonin blockers, 258
Coumadin, 75
Creatinine, 219
Cricoid pressure, 195
Cricothyroidotomy, 461
Cricothyrotomy, contraindications to, 294
Cryoprecipitate, 322
Cushing's disease, 136
Cyclosporine, 71, 157
Cyproheptadine, 258

D

Damage control resuscitation (DCR), 462–463
Dantrolene
  preparation, 163
  side effects, 163
DDAVP, utility of, 324
DDD(R) pacing, 58
D-dimers, 322
DDI(R) pacing, 58
Deemed Status 1, 208
Deep extubation, 283–284
Defibrillator, 59
Delayed cerebral ischemia (DCI), 106, 107
Delayed hemolytic transfusion reaction, 316
  treatment of, 316–317
Delayed ischemic neurological deficits (DIND), 104, 106
Delirium, 470
Demand ischemia, mechanism of, 8
Depolarizing muscle relaxants, 150
Depolarizing neuromuscular blocking agents (Depolarizing NMBA), 143–147
  abnormal plasma cholinesterase, 144
  characteristics of neuromuscular blockade with, 146
  dibucaine number, 144
  intracranial pressure (ICP), elevation in, 145
  patient at risk for severe hyperkalemia, 145
  phase II block, 146
  succinylcholine (*see* Succinylcholine)
Depth of neuromuscular blockade, 152
Desflurane, 282, 397
Dexamethasone, 284, 301
Dexmedetomidine, 276, 282, 292, 301–302, 381
Diabetes insipidus (DI), 138
Diabetes mellitus (DM), 167, 229
  and abdominal aortic aneurysm, 220
  anesthesia, 170, 172
  characterization, 167
  common forms, 167
  complications, 169
    autonomic neuropathy, 170
    cardiovascular disease, 169
    diabetic retinopathy, 170
    gastroparesis, 170
    stiff joint syndrome, 170
  diabetic ketoacidosis, 171
  diagnostic criteria for, 168
  glucose intolerance, 168
  glycemic control, 169
  hyperglycemia, 167
  hyperglycemic hyperosmolar state, 171
  intraoperative considerations in, 172
  management strategies for, 168–169
  metabolic syndrome X, 168
  postoperative considerations in, 172
  preoperative considerations, 171–172
  prevalence, 168
  Type 1 DM, 167

Type 2 DM, 167
Diabetic ketoacidosis (DKA), 171
Diabetic retinopathy, 170
Dibucaine, 352
Dibucaine number, 144
Difficult airway, 289, 459
Difficult Airway Algorithm, 289
Difficult intubation (DI), 289
Difficult mask ventilation (DMV), 289
Digoxin, for heart failure, 22, 25
Dilaudid, 268
Dipeptidyl peptidase-IV (DPP-4) inhibitors, 169
Diphenhydramine, 284
Disopyramide, 51
Distal bundle of His and proximal Purkinje network, 5
Distributive shock, 461
Diuretics, for heart failure, 22
Dobutamine, 25
Door-to-balloon time, 14
Dopamine, 25, 223
Doppler ultrasound, 267
Double-lumen tubes (DLT), 90, 92
Down syndrome, 298, 300
Doxazosin, 186
Droperidol, 186, 284
Drug-eluting stent (DES), 15, 275
Drug pharmacokinetics, in ESRD, 265*t*
D-tubocurarine, 397
Dual antiplatelet therapy (DAPT), 15
  current guideline for, after PCI, 16
  implication of, in perioperative setting, 16–17
Dual-chamber pacing, 58
Dural puncture epidural (DPE), 380
Dyskinesis, 5

E

Echocardiography, 38, 50
Eisenmenger syndrome, 41
  anesthetic induction, 44
  case, 41
  complications of, 42*t*
  definitive management of, 45
  hemodynamic considerations for anesthetic, 42–43
  hypotension, medication for, 45
  induction strategy, 44
  invasive monitoring, 44
  maintenance of anesthesia, 44
  perioperative concerns relating to hematologic abnormalities, 43
  post-op recovery, 45
  predicted perioperative mortality for patients with, 42
  predictors of poor post-operative function, 42
  preoperative testing, 42
  pulmonary hypertension, 45
  pulmonary vascular resistance, 42
  regional anesthesia, 45
  risks related to perioperative arrhythmia in, 43
  special considerations for parturient with, 45
  special medications and equipment, 44
  targeted therapies for pulmonary hypertension, 43*t*
  ventilator settings, 44
Elective nasogastric tube, 241
Electrical burn, 467
Electrocardiography (ECG/EKG), 21, 50, 62, 251
Electroencephalogram (EEG), 115
Electromyography (EMG), 126–127, 156
Encephalopathy, 201, 203, 204, 208
Endobronchial intubation, 252
Endocarditis, 47
Endocarditis prophylaxis, 39
Endoleaks, types of, 233*t*
Endomyocardial biopsy (EMB), 70
Endothelin receptor antagonists, 43*t*
Endotracheal intubation
  advantages of, 307
  disadvantages of, 307
Endotracheal tubes (ETT), 298, 308, 309, 408, 411, 437
Endovascular aortic aneurysm repair (EVAR), 227
  aortic neck length scoring, 230*t*
  blood pressure management of, 232
  concerns with regard to blood loss, 232
  COPD in patients with AAA, 228
  current use, 230, 231*t*
  CVP, measuring, 230
  factors limiting success of local anesthesia, 233
  fluid management, 232
  Foley catheter, use of, 232
  general *versus* regional or MAC anesthesia, 230–231
  hemodynamics management, 231
  heparin anticoagulation, management of, 232
  impact of obesity outcome in AAA repair, 228
  implications of fluoroscopy, 228
  intraoperative monitoring, 233
  LBBB block of significance, 227
  long-term results of, 234
  versus open surgery, 229–230
  pain management, 234
  patient recovery, 234
  postimplantation syndrome, 234
  preoperative evaluation, 229
  proximal aortic diameter scoring, 230*t*
  in ruptured AAA, 232–233
  suitability for EVAR, factors determining, 228–229
  surgical decision-making for, 229
  thrombus scoring, 230*t*
  volume management, 230
Endovascular aortic repair (EVAR), 217
End-stage renal disease (ESRD), 263
  cardiovascular comorbidities, 264
  hematologic issues, 264
  use of sevoflurane, 265
Enhanced recovery after surgery (ERAS) protocols, 221
Enzyme-linked immunosorbent assays (ELISA), 324
Ephedrine, 260
Epiaortic scanning, 82
Epidural, 92
Epidural analgesia, 212
  advantages/disadvantages of, 379–380
  complications of, 380
  indications/contraindications for, 379
  side effects of, 380
Epidural anesthesia, 343
Epinephrine, 25, 63, 260, 282, 352, 410
ESLD, 209, 211
Esophageal atresia, 435
Ester local anesthetics, 347
Etidocaine, 351–352
Etomidate, 277
ETT, 300
  placement after intubation, 411
EuroSCORE, 74
Euthyroid, 179

Euvolemia, 221
Extracorporeal membrane oxygenation therapy, 422
Extraocular muscle (EOM), 276
Extubation, 197
Eye surgery, 273, 275, 276
Eye trauma, 274
  mechanism of, 274
  pain after, 278

F

Facial muscles weakness, 156
Facial nerve electromyography monitoring (FNM), 283
Facial nerve monitoring, 283
Factor IX (FIX), 328, 329–330
  half-life of, 330
Factor VIII (FVIII), 328, 329–330
  half-life of, 330
Fasciculation, 146
FAST (Focused Assessment with Sonography in Trauma) exam, 462
"Fast Track" cardiac surgery, 78
Febrile non-hemolytic transfusion reaction, 316
  treatment of, 316
Fenfluramine, 243
Fen–Phen, 241, 243
Fentanyl, 397, 454
Fetal heart rate (FHR), 382
Fetal heart rate monitoring (FHM), 382
Fetor hepaticus, 203
Fetus
  concerns for surgery performed during pregnancy, 396
  maternal carbon dioxide affecting, 399
  maternal hypotension affecting, 399
  ultrasonography on, 398
Fiberoptic bronchoscopy, 196
Fiberoptic intubation, 196
Fibrinogen degradation products, 322
Fibrinolysis, 211, 212
Fibrinolytic therapy, 14
5-hydroxyindole-3-acetic acid (5-HIAA), 256
Flow volume loops, 158
Fluid management, 418
Flumazenil, 209, 292
Fluoroscopy, 228
Foley catheter, use of, 232
Frank–Starling mechanism, 68
Free hepatic venous pressure (FHVP), 203
Fresh frozen plasma (FFP), 329
  indications for transfusion of, 322
Full stomach, 193
  cricoid pressure, 195
  extubation, 197
  fiberoptic bronchoscopy, 196
  fiberoptic intubation, 196
  gastric aspiration
    increase the likelihood of, 193
    obesity or GERD affecting the risk for, 194
    pharmacologic measures to minimize the risk of, 194
  lower esophageal sphincter pressure, factors affecting, 194
  Mendelson's syndrome, 196
  neuromuscular blocking drugs, 195
  placing nasogastric tube prior to induction of general anesthesia, 194–195
  plan for postoperative care of, 197
  pros and cons to MAC anesthesia, 195–196
  protected airway, 195
  radiographic findings in period following aspiration of gastric contents, 196–197
  rapid sequence induction, 195
  sequelae of gastric aspiration, care for, 197
  ventilator settings, 197
  vomiting during induction, handling of, 196
Fulminant hepatic failure, 201
Functional residual capacity (FRC), 396
Functioning tumors, 135
Furosemide, 108

G

Gas (or air) embolism, 252
Gastric aspiration, 193, 194
Gastric motility, 194
Gastric varices, 203
Gastroesophageal reflux (GER), 438
Gastrointestinal system changes in pregnancy, 396
Gastroparesis, 170
Gastroschisis
  anesthetic concerns for, 418
  differential diagnosis for tachycardia and hypotension in a neonate with, 417
  maternal risk factors associated with, 416
  potential GI complications associated with, 416
  preoperative evaluation and preparation, 416
  risk factors in neonates born with, 416
Gastroschisis and omphalocele, 415
  difference between, 415
  medical disease and differential diagnosis, 415
General anesthesia, 251, 275
Gestational age, 450
Glasgow Coma Scale (GCS), 104, 105*t*
Glaucoma, 274
Global hypoperfusion, 461
Glomerular filtration rate (GFR), 219, 228, 263
Glycemic control, 169
Glycosylated hemoglobin, 172
Goal-directed therapy (GDT), 232
Goiter, 179, 181
Goldblatt kidney, 268
GOLD criteria, for COPD patients, 248
GP IIb/IIIa inhibitors, 323
Graft rejection, 266
Great auricular nerve (GAN), 284
Growth hormone secreting tumors, 135
Gynecoid/peripheral obesity, 238

H

HACEK organisms, 47
Halothane, 397
H1 and H2 blockers, 258
Heart failure (HF), 19
  anesthetic perioperative risk between acute/new onset *versus* chronic/compensated heart failure, 20
  case, 19
  clinical signs of, 19
  common arrhythmias seen with HF, 25–26
  determinants of cardiac output, 23
  grading classifications, 20
  hemodynamic management, 25
    inotropic agents, 25
    vasodilators/inodilators, 25
    vasopressors, 25

hip replacement, anesthetic techniques for, 23
hypotension, risk for, 23
implantable cardioverter-defibrillator, management of, 22–23
inducing general anesthesia, 24
maintenance of anesthesia, 24
central venous catheter, 24
continuous invasive blood pressure, 24
monitoring hemodynamic parameters, 24
pulmonary artery catheters, 24
transesophageal echocardiography, 25
management
assessment of LV function, 21–22
chest radiography, 21
EKG, 21
laboratory work, 21
medications
ACEI/ARB, 22
aldosterone antagonists, 22
anticoagulants, 22
BRB, 22
CCB, 22
digoxin, 22
diuretics, 22
neuraxial anesthesia, 24
New York Heart Association (NYHA) functional classification, 20*t*
right ventricular failure, treatment of, 26
risk assessment based on left ventricular ejection fraction, 21
signs of acutely decompensated heart failure, 20
therapeutic options, 26
urgent *versus* emergent procedures, 20–21
HELLP syndrome, 385, 387
Hemarthrosis, 328
Hematocrit (Hct), 219
Hematoma, epidural, 231
Hemochromatosis, 202
Hemodialysis, 263
Hemoglobin A1c (HgbA1c), 169
Hemoglobin S, pathophysiological implications of, 333
Hemophilia, 327
acquired hemophilia A, 327, 329
activated PCC, 331
antifibrinolytics, role of, 331
categorization of, 328
choosing a particular anesthetic drug in patients with, 331
clinical aspects of, 327
clinical manifestations of, 328–329
coagulation status, to be corrected before surgery, 330
diagnosis of, 328
discharge after open inguinal hernia repair, 331
emergency surgery, management of hemophilia patient for, 332
factor VIII, 328, 329–330
factor level required for operative procedures in patients with, 325
factor IX, 328, 329–330
intramuscular injection, administering, 331
intraoperative management, 331
neuroaxial block, conducting, 331
other diseases to be considered in patients with history of, 330
postoperative management, 331
precautions should be taken in intubating patient with, 331
preoperative management, 330
recombinant activated factor VII, 331
role of desmopressin in patients with, 330–331
types of, 324–325, 327
Von Willebrand disease, 327
Hemophilia A, 319
Hemorrhage, 460
Hemorrhagic shock, 390
Heparin, 265
Heparin anticoagulation, management of, 232
Heparin-induced platelet aggregation assay (HIPA), 324
Heparin induced thrombocytopenia (HIT), 324
Hepatic encephalopathy, 208–209
Hepatic metastases, 256
Hepatic portal venous system, 200
Hepatic sinusoids, 199–200
Hepatic venous pressure gradient (HVPG), 203
Hepatitis, viral, 201–202
Hep A, 201
Hep B, 201
Hep C, 201
Hep D, 201
Hep E, 202
Hepatopulmonary syndrome (HPS), 205
Hepatorenal syndrome (HRS), 205
High frequency oscillatory ventilation (HFOV), 424, 451
Hip replacement, anesthetic techniques for, 23
Histamine provoking drugs, 186
Histamine release, 152
Hoarseness in acromegaly, 135
Hofmann elimination, 151
Hormones secreted by pituitary, 133
Horner's/voice hoarseness, 369
H-2 antagonist, 241
Hydralazine, 188
Hydroxyurea, 334
Hydroxyzine, 284
Hypercarbia, 248, 249, 250, 276
affecting central nervous system, 250
Hyperchloremic metabolic acidosis, 267
Hyperglycemia, 167
Hyperglycemic hyperosmolar state (HHS), 171
Hyperkalemia, 145, 264
Hypermagnesemia, 264
Hypertension, 116, 187, 259
Hyperthyroidism, 176
appropriate maintenance anesthesia, 180
complications of thyroid surgery, 181
diagnosis, 177, 178*t*
extubation, 181
monitoring during anesthesia, 180
postoperative monitoring, 181
pre-anesthetic considerations, 179
preoperative sedation, 179–180
prepare to intubation, 180
signs and symptoms, 177
thyroid storm, 177–178
thyroidectomy, 180
treatment for, 178
Hypertrophic cardiomyopathy (HCM), 49
anesthetic management, 51, 52
case, 49
definition, 49
diagnosis, 50–51
genetic background, 50
induction agents of choice for, 52
maintenance techniques, 52
monitoring techniques, 51–52
non-pharmacological management options, 51
pathophysiology, 49
pharmacological treatment, 51
preoperative evaluation data, 52
symptoms, 50

things to consider during emergence, 52
Hypervolemia, hypertension, hemodilution (Triple H) therapy, 107
Hypervolemia and hyperdynamic circulation, 265
Hypokinesis, 5
Hypotension, 23, 116
controlled, 211
Hypothermia, 29, 322, 462, 472–473
compartment/site to measure the temperature when rewarming on cardiopulmonary bypass, 31
definition of, 29
effects on
cerebral metabolism, 29
coronary perfusion, 30
heart rhythm and rate changes expected with, 30
impact of intraoperative hypothermia on patient morbidity, 31
mechanism of hypothermia leading to hypovolemia during hypothermia, 30
metabolic changes associated with, 29
phases of hypothermia treatment, 29
protective mechanisms of, 29
rewarming the patient after being cooled for cardiac/vascular surgery, 31
risk
for shivering, 30
of infection, increasing, 31
severe bleeding due to, 30–31
side effects of, during induction (cooling) phase, 29–30
temperature goal for therapeutic hypothermia after cardiac arrest, 30
Hypothermia, risks associated with, 419
Hypothermia After Cardiac Arrest Study Group (HACA), 30
Hypovolemia, 30
Hypovolemic shock, 461
Hypoxemia, 91, 92
Hypoxia, 276
Hypoxic pulmonary vasoconstriction, 91

I
Ibuprofen, 63
Ideal body weight (IBW), 243
anesthetic medications, 244
versus total body weight (TBW), 244
Immune-mediated rejection of the organ, 266
Immunoglobulins, 157
Immunosuppression methods, 266
Immunosuppressive regimen, 266
Immunosuppressive treatment, 266
Implantable cardioverter defibrillators (ICD), 51, 55, 57, 59
central venous access, 59
magnet response, 59
management of, 22–23
single-chamber ICD, 56*f*
Increased intracranial pressure (ICP), 103
Incretin mimetics, 169
Indomethacin, 63
Induction, 259
Induction therapy, 266
Inhalational anesthesia, 310
Inhaled anesthetics, 277
Inhaled nitric oxide (iNO), 450
Inotropic agents, 25
In-stent restenosis (ISR), 15
Insulin resistance syndrome. *See* Metabolic syndrome X
Insulin therapy, 168, 172
Intermittent apnea technique, 309
Internal mammary artery, 81
International normalized ratio (INR) value, 321
International Subarachnoid Trial (ISAT), 106
Intra-abdominal pressure, 249
Intra-aortic balloon pump (IABP), 74, 81
Intracranial aneurysm, 103
delayed ischemic neurological deficits, 104, 106
Fisher Grade, 107
Hunt and Hess Grade III, 104
rebleeding, 104, 106
subarachnoid hemorrhage (*see* Subarachnoid hemorrhage (SAH))
treatment options for, 105–106
triple H therapy, 107
vasospasm, 106–107
Intracranial pressure (ICP), elevation in, 145
Intramuscular injection, administering, 331
Intraocular pressure (IOP), 274, 275
affected by glaucoma, 274
physiologic or pathophysiologic factors, 274
Intraoperative aneurysm rupture management, 109
Intraoperative neuromonitoring (IONM), 124
modalities, 127
Intraoperative opioids, 301
Intrapulmonary vascular dilation (IPVD), 205
Intrathecal opioids
side effects of, 361
underlying pathophysiology of respiratory depression with, 361
working of, 361
Intrauterine growth restriction (IUGR), 449
Intraventricular hemorrhage (IVH), 452–453
Intravitreal gentamicin, 278
Intubation, 471, 472
Investigation of carotid arteries, 75
Iodine therapy, 176, 178, 179
Irreversible pulmonary hypertension, 41
Ischemia-reperfusion injury, 212
Ischemic preconditioning, 80
Isoflurane, 210, 397

J
Jet ventilation, 309
advantages of, 309–310
potential complications of, 310

K
Ketamine, 35, 259, 277, 292, 397
Kidney transplantation
advantages of living donor, 265–266
arterial line, 264
changes in physiology, 265
choices for anesthesia, 265
postoperative pain relief, 268
potassium levels, 264
preoperative considerations, 263
screening undertaken prior to, 263
surgical complications, 266–267
timing of dialysis, 267
type
of rejections, 266
of venous access, 264–265
use
of diuretics, 267
of pressors, 268
of sevoflurane, 265

L
Labetalol, 188
Labor and delivery, 379
  fetal heart rate, 382
  fetal heart rate monitoring, 382
  labor epidural (*see* Epidural analgesia)
  labor pain, origin of, 381
  neuraxial analgesia (*see* Neuraxial analgesia)
  sedation, 382
  uterine relaxation, 383
Labor pain, 381
  origin of, 381
Lactulose, benefit of, 209
Laparoscopy, 247
  advantages of, 247–248
  causes
    of hypercarbia, 249
    physiological changes, 249
  definition, 247
  disadvantages of, 248
  endobronchial intubation, 252
  intraoperative complications, 251
  intraoperative concerns, 249–252
  laparoscopic surgery, 247
  nitrous oxide, use of, 250
  postoperative issues, 252–253
  preoperative concerns, 248–249
  procedures, 247
Laryngeal laser surgery, options for airway management in, 307
Laryngeal mask airway (LMA), 300, 309
Laryngoscopy, 386–387
Laser, 305
  advantages of using, 305
  commonly used, 305
Laser surgery of the airway, 305
  anesthesia maintenance, plan of, 310
  key components required for surgical fire, 307–308
  laryngeal laser surgery, options for airway management in, 307
  managing airway fire, 308
  monitoring patient, 307
  neuromuscular relaxant, indication of, 310
  plan to induce general anesthesia, 307
  potential hazards in, 308–309
  preoperative smoking cessation, recommendation for, 306
  preoperative testing, 306
  preventing airway fire, 308
  recovery room, complications observed in, 310–311
Lateral decubitus position (LDP), 91
LDH, 209
Lean body mass (LBM), 244
Left anterior descending artery (LAD), 4, 5
Left circumflex artery (LCx), 4, 5
Left internal mammary arteries (LIMA), 76, 81
Left main coronary artery, 4
Left ventricular ejection fraction (LVEF), risk assessment based on, 21
Left ventricular function, assessment of, 21–22
Left ventricular hypertrophy (LVH), 49
Left ventricular outflow tract (LVOT), 49, 50*f*, 51, 52
Lens capsule, 274
Lethal triad, 462
LeVeen shunt, 205
Levobupivacaine, 351
Lidocaine, 282, 350–351, 360
"Light anesthetic" technique in premature infants, 454
Limb weakness, 156
Lipophilic drugs, 244
Liver
  acetaminophen toxicity, 201
  acute fatty liver of pregnancy, 202
  acute variceal bleeds management, 203
  alpha-1 antitrypsin (AAT) deficiency, 202
  anatomy of, 199
  ascites, 205
  blood supply to, 199
  Budd–Chiari syndrome, 202
  carbon tetrachloride, 202–203
  causes of liver failure, 201
  cirrhosis, 200–201
  dialysis, 208
  fetor hepaticus, 203
  functions of, 200
  healthy liver and sudden hemorrhage, 204
  hemochromatosis, 202
  portal HTN diagnosis, 203
  portal hypertension, 203, 204
  varices, 203
  viral hepatitis, 201–202
    risks of surgery, 202
  Wilson disease, 202
Liver acinus, 200
Liver disease, affecting drug metabolism and pharmacokinetics, 211
Liver function tests (LFTs), 209, 212
Liver transplantation
  allocation of available organs in the United States, 207
  anesthesia for, 199
  anesthetic challenges, 211
  anesthetic depth, maintaining, 210
  anhepatic phase, 211
  cardiopulmonary evaluation, 210
  Child-Pugh score, 207
  contraindications to, 207
  deemed Status 1, 208
  donors matching with recipients, 207
  epidural for post-op pain control, 212
  extrahepatic hepatic features of hepatic failure in, 204
  health issues to be considered before, 207
  immunosuppression, types of, 212
  indications for, 206
  inducing hypotension in, 211
  initial signs of graft function, 212
  liver dialysis, 208
  MELD score, 208
  post-anhepatic phase, 211
  preanhepatic phase, 211
  preoperative evaluation, 208, 209
  reperfusion, 211–212
  sources for donor organs, 207
  survival rates post-transplantation, 208
Local anesthesia, 233, 251, 275
Local anesthetic infiltration, importance of, 282
Local anesthetics, 347
  regional anesthesia, possible benefits of, 347
Local anesthetic systemic toxicity (LAST), 348, 353, 355, 370, 371
Long-term immunosuppression, 266
Loop diuretics, 267
Low-dose dopamine, 268
Low molecular weight heparin (LMWH), 75, 323
Lower esophageal sphincter (LES) pressure, 194
Lung anatomy, 89
Lung cancer patients, anesthetic considerations for, 90
Lung isolation, 90–91
Lung resection, preoperative risk assessment for, 89–90

M

MAC anesthesia, pros and cons to, 195–196
Magnesium sulfate, 400
  for seizure prophylaxis, 387
Magnesium therapy, 107
Major Adverse Cardiac Events (MACE), 6–7
Malignant hyperthermia (MH), 147, 161
  calcium channel blockers for, 163
  dantrolene
    preparation, 163
    side effects, 163
  diagnosis, 162
  differential diagnosis, 161
  laboratory abnormalities, 162
  management, 162–163
  muscular rigidity developing neuromuscular blockade, 163
  myopathies/syndromes associated with, 162
  in operating room, 163
  signs of, 162
  treatment, 162
  triggers for, 162
Mannitol, 108, 267
Manual in-line stabilization (MILS), 290
Mask inductions, 430
Mask ventilation, 289, 293
  encountering problems with, 293
Maternal carbon dioxide affecting fetus, 399
Maternal hypotension affecting fetus, 399
Maternal oxygen tension, 399
Mean arterial blood pressure (MAP), 249
Mean arterial pressure (MAP), 104, 468
Mechanical ventilation, need for, 158
Meconium, 408
Meglitinides, 169
Mendelson's syndrome, 196
Meperidine, 397
Mepivacaine, 351, 360
Metabolic alkalosis, 428
Metabolic syndrome, 238
Metabolic syndrome X, 168
Methadone, 397
Methionine, 397
Methyl methacrylate, 344
Metoclopramide, 277
Microangiopathy, 167
Midazolam, 284, 292, 299
Middle ear surgery, 282, 284
"Mill-wheel" murmur, 252
Milrinone, 25
Minimum alveolar concentration (MAC), 396, 454
Mitral regurgitation (MR), 49
  changing physiology of heart, 35
  etiologies for, 33, 34*t*
  natural progression of, 34
Mitral stenosis, 37
  anesthetic management, 38
  antibiotic prophylaxis before dental procedure, 39
  classification of pulmonary hypertension, 38
  common cause of, 37
  definition, 37
  echo findings, 38
  factors contributing to worsening pulmonary hypertension during perioperative period, 38
  grading, 38
  inducing anesthesia, 38–39
  management, 37–38
  monitoring patients, 38
  physical exam findings, 38
  pulmonary hypertension, 38
  signs and symptoms, 37
  treating hypotension shortly after induction, 39
  treatment of new acute-onset atrial fibrillation, 39
Mitral valve disease and tachycardia, 38–39
Mivacurium, 151–152
Model-for-End-Stage-Liver-Disease (MELD) score, 208
Molecular adsorbents recirculation system (MARS), 208
Molecular genetic testing, 162
Monroe-Kellie Doctrine, 463
Morbid obesity (MO), 243, 248
  airway challenges, 242
  challenges, 243
  inhaled anesthetics for, 244
  patient positioning, 242
  prone procedure, 243
Morphine, 186, 268, 397
Motor evoked potentials (MEPs), 115, 125–126
  anesthetic effects on, 126
  complications and contraindications of, 126
Multimodal analgesia, 242
Multimodal approach, 342
Multiple endocrine neoplasia (MEN), 255
  MEN2, 185
Muscle contraction, 149–150
Muscle relaxants, 158–159, 195, 210–211, 283
  depolarizing, 150
  nondepolarizing, 151
Muscle weakness, 153, 157
Muscular rigidity, developing neuromuscular blockade, 163
Myasthenia gravis (MG), 155
  anatomical origins of, 156
  anesthetic considerations, 158
  classifications, 156
  diagnostic tests for, 156
  differential diagnosis, 157*t*
  differential for weakness in MG patients after surgery, 159–160
  effects
    of IV drugs, 159
    of volatiles anesthetics, 159
  epidemiology of, 155
  management based on preoperative medications, 157–158
  need for mechanical ventilation, 158
  neuraxial anesthesia, 158
  number of functional receptors, reducing, 155
  pathophysiology for, 155
  patients paralyzed with nondepolarizing muscle relaxants, 158–159
  response to succinylcholine for, 159
  signs and symptoms, 156
  treatments for, 156–157
Myocardial infarction (MI), 13
  current guideline for DAPT after PCI, 16
  definition, 13
  fibrinolytic therapy, 14
  high-risk PCIs, 15–16
  implication of DAPT in perioperative setting, 16–17
  in-stent restenosis, 15
  percutaneous coronary intervention, 14
  reperfusion strategy, 15
  types of, 13–14
Myocardial viability test, 76

N

Nasogastric tube (NGT), 194–195
National Surgical Quality Improvement Program (NSQIP), 201, 231
Necrotizing enterocolitis (NEC), 452
 diagnosis and treatment, 452
Neonatal airway and adult airway, 411
Neonatal anesthesia, 429
Neonatal resuscitation, 407
 chest compressions, 409
  stopping, 409–410
 fractional inspired oxygen concentration, 409
 infant's HR, 408–409, 410
 initial steps of, 408
 intubation of the neonate, 410–411
 IV access, 410
 meconium, 408
 neonatal circulatory system and adult circulation, 407
 neonatal hypovolemia, 410
 "normal" umbilical artery and umbilical vein blood gases, 408
 resuscitative effort, 408
 resuscitative measures, newborn requiring, 409
 umbilical catheter, 410
 volume expansion fluids in newborn, 410
Neonate
 acidosis, 420
 mechanism for rapid cooling in, 419
 intubation of, 410–411
Nephrogenic hypertension, 268
Nerve supply, cutaneous,, 369*f*
Neuraxial analgesia, 80
 alternatives to, 381
 other options for, 380–381
Neuraxial anesthesia, 24, 36, 158, 259
Neuroaxial block, conducting, 331
Neuroendocrine tumors. *See* Carcinoid tumors
Neurological deficit (NND) rate, 124
Neuromonitoring, 115
Neuromuscular blockade
 depth of, 152
 prolonged, 153
 reversing, 71
Neuromuscular blocker(s), 152
Neuromuscular blocking drugs, 149, 195
Neuromuscular junction (NMJ), 152, 155
Neurotransmitters and receptors, 67
Newborn
 post-resuscitative care for, 413
 volume expansion fluids in, 410
Nicardipine/clevidipine, 25
NICE guidelines *versus* ACC/AHA guidelines, 47
Nitric oxide, 424, 445
Nitric oxide pathway, 43*t*
Nitroglycerin, 25
Nitroprusside, 25
Nitrous oxide, 282–283, 381
Non-cardiac surgery, 20
 after heart transplantation, 67
  antibiotics, 71
  atrial arrhythmias, 69
  cardiac allograft vasculopathy, 69
  clinical signs/symptoms of rejection, 70
  cyclosporine, 71
  hemodynamic response to medications, 68
  immunosuppressive medications, 71
  intraoperative awareness, 68
  maintenance of preload, importance of, 68
  management of intraoperative arrhythmias, 68
  neuraxial/regional anesthesia, 71
  pacemakers and ICDs, 68–69
  significance of right bundle branch block, 69
Non-depolarizer, 152
Non-depolarizing neuromuscular blockade (NDNMBs), 310
Nondepolarizing neuromuscular blocking agents, 149–153, 158
 acetylcholine metabolism, 150
 avoidance, 152
 categories of, 150, 151
 cholinesterase inhibitors, side-effects of, 153
 depth of neuromuscular blockade, 152
 difference between
  mature acetylcholine receptor and immature/fetal receptor, 150
  phase I and phase II block, 153
 durations of action of, 151
 histamine release, 152
 Hofmann elimination, 151
 mechanism of action of, 151
  depolarizing muscle relaxants, 150
 mivacurium, 151–152
 muscle contraction, 149–150
 neuromuscular blockade monitoring, 152
 neuromuscular blocker(s), 152
 neuromuscular blocking drugs, 149
 nondepolarizing muscle relaxants, 151
 post-tetanic potentiation, 152
 prolonged neuromuscular blockade, 153
 reversal agents, 152–153
 side-effects of pancuronium, 151
 succinylcholine
  duration of action of, 150
  metabolism, 150
  risk for hyperkalemia, 151
  side-effects of, 150–151
Non-dihydropyridine calcium channel blockers, 51
Non-functioning pituitary tumors, clinical presentations of, 133–134
Non-ST elevation MI (NSTEMI), 6, 7, 13
Non-stenotic plaques, 7
Non-steroidal anti-inflammatory drugs (NSAIDs), 63, 70, 80, 146, 301
Norepinephrine, 25, 63
North American Society of Pacing and Electro physiology and the British Pacing and Electrophysiology Group (NASPE/BPEG), 56
Novel oral anticoagulants (NOACs), 75
N-terminal pro-brain natriuretic peptide (NT-proBNP), 257

O

Obesity, 237
 definition, 237
 diseases associated with, 238
 impact on open and endovascular abdominal aortic aneurysm, 228
 physiologic changes, 238
 preoxygenation, 242
Obesity-hypoventilation syndrome, 240
Obstructive sleep apnea (OSA), 239, 248, 297
 concerns in patients, 303
 diagnosis of, 239–240
 discharge after surgery, 302
 incidence of, 239
 induction of anesthesia without intravenous (IV) access, 299
 intraoperative considerations, 242
 intraoperative opioids, 301
 preoperative considerations, 241
 risk for cor pulmonale, 297

screening, 239
sleep study, 298
symptoms of, in children, 297
systemic effects of, 240
trisomy 21, children with, 298
Octreotide, 256, 258, 259, 260
adverse effects of, 259
Ocular trauma
common causes of, 274
patients requiring anesthesia, 274–275
pediatric patients, 278
Off-pump CABG (OPCAB), 77
Omphalocele, anomalies associated with, 415–416
Ondansetron, 284, 301
One-lung ventilation, 89–93
anesthetic considerations for, 90
choice of anesthetic, 93
epidural, 92
extubation in OR, 93
fluid management, 93
postoperative concerns, 93
On-pump CABG, 76–77, 83
Open AAA repair, 220, 224
Open eye injury
anesthetic management of, 273–274
antibiotic regimens, 278
anxiolytics used in, 276
hospitalization, 274
pain management, 278
type of anesthesia used for, 275
Open repair, 229–230
Operating room fires, prevention of, 300
Ophthalmic Anesthesia Society, 276
Ophthalmologic surgery
extubation, 278
maintain anesthesia during, 277
Opioid analgesics, 381
Orlistat, 243
Orthodeoxia, 204
Orthotopic transplantation, 206–207
Oxygen content, determination of, 469
Oxygen delivery, determination of, 469
Oxygen index (OI), 422

P

Pacemakers, 55
function of, 57
magnet response, 59
malfunction, types of, 58
non-capture, 58–59
oversensing causes under pacing, 58
undersensing causes over pacing, 58
perioperative, 55
sensing and capture, 58
subcutaneous, 56*f*
transvenous, 56*f*
Pancuronium, 397
Paradoxical air embolism, 100
Parkland formula, 463, 468
Patent ductus arteriosis (PDA), 407
Patient-controlled analgesia (PCA), 244
Patient positioning, 343
for middle ear surgery, 282
Percutaneous coronary intervention (PCI), 14, 218
current guideline for DAPT after, 16
high-risk PCIs, 15–16
Percutaneous transluminal coronary angioplasty (PTCA), 7
Pericardial effusion
medical treatments for, 63
Pericardial tamponade, 61
anesthetic agents for, 63
causes of, 61–62
complications, 64
definition, 61
diagnostic criteria for, 62
hemodynamic goals for tamponade, 63
indications for pericardiocentesis and pericardial window, 64
medical treatments for pericardial effusion, 63
noninvasive and invasive testing, 62–63
physical exam findings, 62
signs and symptoms of, 462
treatment, 462
vascular access, 63
Pericardiocentesis, 462
Perioperative antibiotics, 342
Perioperative arrhythmias, 43
Perioperative cardiac risk stratification, overarching goals of, 8
Perioperative MI, 7–8
Perioperative risk stratification, 8–10
Peripheral nerve block, 346
Peripheral nerve injury (PNI), 348
Persistent pulmonary hypertension of the newborn (PPHN), 420
Phase I and phase II block, difference between, 153
Phase II blockade, 146
Phenoxybenzamine, 185–186, 188
Phenylephrine, 39
Pheochromocytoma, 183
anesthesia, 186, 188
anesthetic considerations, 186–187
catecholamine withdrawal after venous ligation, 187
clinical presentation of, 184–185
diagnosis, 185
hypertensive crisis, 184, 185
incidence of, 184
intraoperative considerations for, 187
pathophysiology of, 184
postoperative considerations, 187–188
pregnancy and, 187–188
preoperative adrenergic blockade and volume preparation of patient, 185–186
preoperative considerations for, 185
signs and symptoms, 184
surgery, 185–186
surgical approach and hemodynamic considerations, 187
treatment for, 185
Pickwickian syndrome, 240
Pituitary adenoma, 133
Pituitary apoplexy, 136
Pituitary gland, anatomy of, 133
Pituitary tumors
management of, 136
non-functioning, 133–134
types of, 133
Placental abruption, 387, 389
Placenta previa, risk factors for, 389
Plasma cholinesterase, 144
Plasmapheresis, 157, 266
Platelet factor 4 (PF4), 324
Platypnea, 204
Pneumocephalus, 99
Pneumoperitoneum, 248, 249, 251

affecting renal system, 250
gas of choice, 248
Pneumothorax, 251, 252, 371, 423
Porta hepatis, 199
Portal hypertension, 203, 204
Portal hypertension diagnosis, 203
Portopulmonary hypertension (PPHTN), 206
Portosystemic shunting, 209
Positive airway pressure (PAP), 240
Positive end expiratory pressure (PEEP), 92, 423
Positive pressure ventilation (PPV), 408, 411–412, 437
Post anesthesia care unit (PACU), 337, 473
Post-dural puncture headache (PDPH)
after spinal anesthesia, 362–363
diagnosing, 362
treatment options for, 363
Posterior descending artery, 4
Posterior fossa craniotomy, 97
anesthetic management, 97–98
central access, 98
contraindications of surgery in sitting position, 99
extubation criteria, 100
induction, 99
maintenance technique, 99–100
management considerations for sitting position, 98–99
positioning a critical decision, 98
preoperative evaluation, 97
preoperative neurologic deficits, 98
prone/lateral position, management considerations for, 99
risks of, 97
special monitoring, 98
special positioning hazards, minimizing, 99
venous air embolism, 100–101
volume status, management of, 98
Postimplantation syndrome, 234
Postmenstrual age, 450
Postoperative apnea, 431
Postoperative cognitive dysfunction (POCD), 77
Postoperative nausea and vomiting (PONV), 282, 283
and tympanomastoidectomy, 281, 284
Postoperative vision loss (POVL), 130
Postpartum hemorrhage (PPH), 391–392
Potassium levels rise, 264
Potassium Titanyl Phosphate–Neodymium–Yttrium aluminum garnet laser (KTP-Nd-Yag), 306
Prasugrel, 17, 75
Prazosin, 186
Predicted risk of mortality (PROM), 74
Preeclampsia, 385
arterial catheter, placing, 386
cerebral edema, cause of, 387
combined spinal–epidural, placing, 386
cure for, 386
delivery of child, 386
diagnosis of, 385
HELLP syndrome, 385, 387
laryngoscopy, 386–387
magnesium sulfate infusion for seizure prophylaxis, 387
minimum platelet count for performing neuraxial technique, 386
placental abruption, risk of, 387
placing an epidural for labor analgesia, 386
prophylactic medication for, 386
risk factors for developing, 385
STAT Cesarean delivery, 386–387
uterotonics, 387
Preganglionic neurons, 67
Pregnancy, nonobstetric surgery during, 395
acute abdominal disease
diagnosis of, 400
incidence of, 400
anesthesia, responsiveness of pregnant women to, 396
anesthetic gases, effects of trace concentrations of, 397–398
anesthetic management, 400–401
behavioral teratology, 398–399
cardiovascular system changes in pregnancy, 396
concerns for fetus when surgery is performed during pregnancy, 396
effects of ultrasonography on fetus, 398
gastrointestinal system changes in pregnancy, 396
incidence of positive pregnancy tests in women of childbearing age for elective surgery, 395
incidence of surgery during pregnancy, 395
inhalation anesthetic agents effect
on animal fetus, 397
on human fetus, 397
intraoperative cholangiography, 398
intrauterine asphyxia, 399
laparoscopic surgery, 400
maternal carbon dioxide affecting fetus, 399
maternal hypotension affecting fetus, 399
maternal oxygen tension, 399
nonobstetric surgery, timing to perform, 400
nonobstetric surgical procedure performed during pregnancy, 395
pregnancy tests before surgery, 395
preterm labor
anesthesia increasing incidence of, 400
surgical procedure causing, 399
tocolytic agents to prevent, 400
respiratory system changes in pregnancy, 395–396
systemic anesthetic drugs effect
on animal fetus, 396–397
on human fetus, 397
teratogenicity of hypoxia and hypercarbia, 399
teratogens, 396
undergoing surgical procedure under anesthesia, 398
vasopressor, 399
Premature infant, 449
anesthetic requirement of, 454
cardiovascular physiologic differences to consider in, 450
diagnosis and treatment, 450
hematocrit for, 453
"light anesthetic" technique in, 454
minimizing the risk of insult, 455
narcotic/paralytic anesthetic technique, 454
oxygen saturation, decline in, 455
patent ductus arteriosus, 450
during PDA ligation procedure, 454–455
and renal function, 452
risk
for any neurologic complications, 452–453
for hypoglycemia/hyperglycemia, 451–452
temperature regulation difference in, 453–454
thrombocytopenia, incidence of, 453
Prematurity, 415, 416, 449
Preoperative anxiolysis, 258
Preoxygenation, 242, 291
Preterm neonate, 412
Prilocaine, 351
Procaine, 350
Prochlorperazine, 284
Proinflammatory cytokines, 238
Prolactin secreting tumor, 135

Promethazine, 284, 301
Propofol, 210, 265, 284
Prostanoids, 43*t*
Protected airway, 195
Proteinuria, 385
Prothrombin complex concentrate (PCC), 329
Prothrombin time (PT), 320
  assessment, 320
  increase in, 321
  performance, 320–321
Proximal aortic diameter scoring, 230*t*
Pruritus, 380
Pseudocholinesterase, 144
Pulmonary arterial hypertension (PAH), 446
Pulmonary artery catheter (PAC), 24, 36, 78, 230, 471
Pulmonary function tests (PFTs), 158
Pulmonary hypertension, 37, 38, 45, 424
  classification of, 38
  targeted therapies for, 43*t*
Pulmonary vascular resistance (PVR), 42, 45, 240, 441, 450
Pulsed dye laser (PDL), 306
Pulse oximetry, 302
Pulsus paradoxus, 62
Pyloric stenosis, 427
  anesthesia, 429
    emergence, 431
    general considerations, 429
    induction and intubation, 430
    maintenance, 431
    muscle relaxation, 430–431
    preinduction, 430
    preoperative evaluation, 429
    preparation and monitoring, 429–430
    regional anesthesia, 429
  clinical presentation and evaluation, 428
  conservative treatment, 429
  incidence, 427
  inheritance, 427
  pain management, 431
  pathogenesis, 427–428
  postoperative management, 432
  preoperative medical treatment, 428
  pyloromyotomy, 428
  radiolographic studies, 428
Pyloromyotomy, 428
Pyridostigmine, 156

Q
Qualitative test, 144

R
Radioimmunoassay, 156
Radiolabeled octreotide, 256
Ramping, 242
Rapid infusion system, 210
Rapid sequence, 430
Rapid sequence induction (RSI), 195, 210, 277
Recombinant activated factor VII (rFVIIa), 331
Recombinant activated human factor VII (rFVIIa), 322
Recombinant factor VIII (rFVIII) and IX (rFIX), 325
Recurrent laryngeal nerve, 176
Red cell alloimmunization, 336
Regional anesthesia, 23, 36, 115, 116, 163, 265, 343, 464
  advantages of, 343
  for anticoagulated patients, 368
  choosing, 349
  contraindications for, 347–348
  monitors and equipment required to perform, 349
  most commonly used local anesthetics, 349
  possible complications of, 348
  for ruptured eye surgery, 275
Regional neuraxial anesthesia, 251
Remifentanil, 282, 283
Remote preconditioning, 80
Renal artery stenosis (RAS), 218
Renal failure, 264
Reperfusion injury, 116
Reperfusion therapy, 15
Respiratory distress syndrome (RDS), 412
  diagnosis and treatment, 450–451
  managing ventilator for patient with, 451
Respiratory distress syndrome (RDS), 416, 450
Respiratory system
  changes in pregnancy, 395–396
  effects of burn injuries to, 467
Respiratory weakness, 156
Resting heart rate, in transplanted patients, 68
Resuscitation, 468
Retinopathy of prematurity (ROP), 416, 453
Rhabdomyolysis, 242
Rheumatic heart disease, 37
Rheumatoid arthritis (RA), 341
Right coronary artery (RCA), 4, 5
Right coronary dominance, 4
Right internal mammary arteries (RIMA), 76
Right to left shunt, 44
Right ventricular failure, treatment of, 26
Rigid bronchoscopy, 436–437
  complications associated with, 437
Rocuronium (ROC), 277, 430
Role of desmopressin (DDAVP) in patients with, 330–331
Ropivacaine, 351, 373
Roux-en-Y gastric bypass, 239
Rule of Nines, 463
Ryanodine receptor protein (RYR1), 161

S
Saline, 267
SA node, 4, 5
Scopolamine, 284
Secondary failure, 373
Seizure prophylaxis, magnesium sulfate infusion for, 387
Sellick's maneuver. *See* Cricoid pressure
Semi-Fowler's position, 244
Serotonin, 206
Serotonin receptors antagonists, 284
Serotonin release assay (SRA), 324
Serum potassium level, 264
Sevoflurane, 210, 282, 300, 397
Shortness of breath (SOB), 19
Sickle cell disease, 333
  anesthesia, inducing, 336
  anesthetic maintenance, plan for, 336
  anesthetic management goals for patients with, 335
  anesthetic modality, 335
  arterial line, necessity of, 336
  central venous pressure catheter, 336
  clinical manifestations of, 334
  commonly performed surgical procedures, 334

extubation criteria, 337
fluid management goals, 335–336
hemoglobin level, normal, 334
hydroxyurea used in, 334
incidence of, 334
increasing perioperative complications, 336
intravenous fluid used during surgery, 336
morbidity and mortality, causes of, 334
pain management during surgical procedure, 336–337
post anesthesia care unit, 337
postoperative management goals, 337
premedication, 335
preoperative arterial blood gas, 335
preoperative assessment, 334
preoperative electrocardiogram, necessity of, 335
preoperative hemoglobin level, 335
preoperative neuroimaging, necessity of, 335
pulmonary function tests, 334–335
secure the airway, 336
supplemental oxygen, 337
surgical procedure performed under regional anesthesia, 335
tourniquet, 335
transfusion of patient, 336
for transfusion therapy, 336
urinalysis, 335
Sickle cell pain crisis, 334
Side-effects of pancuronium, 151
Single-chamber ICD, 56*f*
Single-chamber pacing, 57
Sinusoids, 199
Skin, function of, 466
Sleep apnea, types of, 240
Sleep study, 298
Sleeve gastrectomy, 239
Small for gestational age (SGA), 417
Smoking cessation, 90, 220, 306
Sodium citrate, 277
Somatosensory-evoked potential (SSEP), 115, 124–125
alarm criteria, 125
anesthetic effects on, 124–125
disadvantages of, 125
systemic factors, 125
Somatostatin receptor scintigraphy, 256
Spinal anesthesia, 343, 357
absolute and relative contraindications to, 361
blood supply of spinal cord, 358
correct intervertebral space, identifying, 357–358
current recommendations for treatment of hypotension during, 364
factors influencing block level/distribution during, 360
implications
of antiplatelet agents, 364
of pregnancy on, 364
indications for, 357
intrathecal opioids
side effects of, 361
underlying pathophysiology of respiratory depression with, 361
working of, 361
level of, for different surgeries, 359
local anesthetics, 360–361
lumbosacral approach to the spinal space, 364
mechanism of action of local anesthetic injected into subarachnoid space, 358–359
physiologic alterations, 359
cardiovascular system, 359
central nervous system, 359
gastrointestinal system, 359
pulmonary system, 359
thermoregulation, 359–360
urinary system, 359
placement of, 358
possible complications of, 361–362
post-dural puncture headache (PDPH)
after spinal anesthesia, 362–363
diagnosing, 362
treatment options for, 363
saddle block, 363
side effects of, 361
using lidocaine/mepivacaine for, 360
Spinal column and spinal cord, anatomy of, 121–122
blood supply to, 122
spinal cord, anatomy of, 122
Spinal cord blood flow (SCBF), 122
Spinal cord injury, 123, 128
Spinal shock, 123
Spine surgery
airway management, 128
allogeneic blood transfusion, 129
anesthetic management, 129
bispectral index monitoring, 129
electromyography during, 126–127
fluid management during, 129–130
indications for, 122
and intraoperative monitoring, 121
intraoperative neuromonitoring (IONM), 124
IONM modalities, 127
monitors, choice of, 129
mortality rate of, 124
motor evoked potentials, 125–126
neurological deficit rate for, 124
physiological effects of prone position, 128–129
plan for extubation after 7 h of, 130
positions used during, 128
postoperative pain management, 130–131
postoperative vision loss, 130
preoperative concerns for, 128
preoperative laboratory tests, 128
SSEP
amplitude reduction, 130
monitoring, 124–125
Spontaneous bacterial peritonitis (SBP), 205
ST elevation MI (STEMI), 13, 15
ST segment elevation myocardial infarction (STEMI), 6, 7
Stable angina, conventional therapies for, 7
STAT cesarean delivery, 386–387
Statin therapy, 107, 220
Stent, 114, 117
Stent thrombosis, 15
Stiff joint syndrome, 170
STOP-BANG questionnaire, 239
STOP-BANG screening tool, 239
Streptococcus bovis, 47
String sign, 428
Stroke, 77, 117
Stroke volume variation (SVV), 221
Structural heart disease antibiotic prophylaxis, 36
STS score, 74
Stylet (intubating bougie), 295
Subacute bacterial endocarditis prophylaxis, 47
antibiotic prophylaxis, 47
case, 47
causative organisms of subacute bacterial endocarditis, 47
endocarditis prophylaxis, 47

NICE guidelines *versus* ACC/AHA guidelines, 47–48
Subarachnoid hemorrhage (SAH), 103
ability for cerebral autoregulation, 104
anesthetic management, 108–109
brain relaxation, 108
hyperventilation in, 108
cerebral perfusion pressure, 108
clinical grading, 104
intraoperative aneurysm rupture management, 109
physiologic abnormalities, 104–105
risk factors for, 103–104
signs and symptoms, 103
transmural pressure, 108
treatment, 105–106
Succinylcholine, 195, 276, 277, 472
appropriate dose of, 144
cardiac side effects of, 145–146
duration of action of, 150
fasciculation seen following administration of, 146
incidence of anaphylaxis related to, 144
mechanism of action of, 143–144
metabolism, 144, 150
onset and expected duration of action of, 144
rapid sequence induction and intubation, performing, 145
renal failure and, 145
response to, for patients with MG, 159
risk for hyperkalemia, 151
serum potassium and, 145
side-effects of, 150–151
Succinylcholine administration
negative side effects of, 144
in pediatric population, 147
significance of trismus following, 147
Succinylcholine (SUX), 430
Sufentanil, 397
Sugammadex, 277
Sulfonylureas, 169
Supplemental oxygen, 409
Supplemental oxygen, delivery of, 291
Supraclavicular block
shortness of breath after, 371–373
ventricular tachycardia and cardiovascular collapse after, 371
Supraclavicular catheter, 373
Supraglottic ventilation, 292
Surgical Care Improvement Project (SCIP), 31
Surgical drainage, 64
Surgical fire, key components for, 307–308
fuels, 308
ignition source/laser, 308
oxidizers, 308
Surgical microscope, 282
Surgical repair, 446
Surgical site infections (SSI), 31
Syndrome of inappropriate ADH secretion (SIADH), 105, 138
Syndrome X, 168
Synthetic epo- or darbepoetin, 264
Synthetic liver function, 209
Systemic inflammatory response syndrome (SIRS), 467
Systemic vascular resistance (SVR), 23, 43, 45, 63, 249, 446, 450
Systolic anterior motion of mitral valve (SAM), 49

T

Tachycardia, 35, 39
Temporary pacing, 83
Tensilon test, 156
Tension pneumocephalus, 99
Tension pneumothorax, signs and symptoms of, 462
Teratogenicity of hypoxia and hypercarbia, 399
Terazosin, 186
Tetracaine, 350
Tetrahydrofolate (THF), 397
Thermal burn, 467
Thermal injury, physiologic derangements after, 467
Thermoregulatory mechanisms, 419
Thiamylal, 396–397
Thiazolidinediones, 169
Thionamide, 178, 179
Third trimester, normal vital signs for pregnant patient in, 389–390
Thoracic epidural analgesia (TEA), 92
Thoracic ultrasound, 372
Thrombin, 391
Thrombin inhibitors, 323
Thrombocytopenia, 204, 386
Thromboelastograph (TEG), 323
Thrombus scoring, 230*t*
Thumb-technique, 409
Thymectomy, 157
Thyroidectomy, 180
Thyroid gland, 175–176
function of, 176
Thyroid storm, 177–178
Thyrotoxicosis. *See* Hyperthyroidism
Ticagrelor, 17, 75
Tonsil size evaluation, 298
Tonsillectomy, 297, 301, 302–303
common indications for, 297
Topicalization of airway, 291
Total blood volume, of baby, 417
Total burn surface area (TBSA), 465
Total hip replacement, 341
intraoperative considerations, 343–345
postoperative considerations, 345–346
preoperative considerations, 341–342
Total intravenous anesthesia (TIVA), 109, 277, 283, 310
Tourniquet pain, 373
Tracheoesophageal fistula (TEF), 435
anesthetic maintenance plan, 437
clinical presentation of, 435–436
complications post TEF repair, 438
definition, 435
different types of, 435
extubation, criteria for, 438
maternal polyhydramnios, 435
other anomalies associated with, 435
perioperative pain, managing, 438
plan for induction, 436
prognostic indicators for long-term outcome, 438
right-sided aortic arch, significance of, 437
rigid bronchoscopy, 436–437
complications associated with, 437
thoracoscopic approach
advantages of, 437
disadvantages of, 437
ventilatory difficulty during TEF repair, 437–438
Tracheomalacia, 179, 181, 438
Train-of-four (TOF) stimulation, 146*f*
Tranexamic acid (TXA), 344–345
Transcatheter aortic valve replacement (TAVR), 35
Transcranial Doppler (TCD), 106
Transcutaneous electrical nerve stimulation (TENS), 353
Transesophageal Doppler, 252

Transesophageal echocardiography (TEE), 25, 36, 38, 51, 78–79, 100, 218, 230
Transfusion-associated bacterial sepsis (TABS), 317
treatment, 317
Transfusion reactions, 315
acute hemolytic transfusion reaction, 316
anaphylactic reaction, signs and symptoms of, 315
delayed hemolytic transfusion reaction, 316
febrile non-hemolytic transfusion reaction, 316
transfusion-associated bacterial sepsis (TABS), 317
transfusion-related
acute lung injury, 317
circulatory overload, 317
urticarial transfusion reaction (UTR), 315
Transfusion-related acute lung injury (TRALI), 317
treatment, 317
Transfusion-related circulatory overload (TACO), 317
treatment, 317
Transient ischemic attack (TIA), 113, 114
Transient monocular blindness, 113
Transient neurologic symptoms (TNS), 353
Transitional circulation, 422
Transjugular intrahepatic portosystemic shunting (TIPSS) procedure, 206
Transmural pressure, 108
Transsphenoidal hypophysectomy, 133–139, 136
advantages of, 137
anesthetic plan, 137
complications of, 138
diabetes insipidus, 138
indications for, 136
patient positioning in operating room, 137
postoperative concerns, 137–138
preoperative work up, 136
surgical approach of, 137
syndrome of inappropriate ADH secretion, 138
venous air embolism, 138–139
Transthoracic echocardiography (TTE), 50, 62, 218
Transvenous pacemaker, 56*f*
Tranversus abdominal plane (TAP) block, 224
Trauma anesthesia, 459
body surface area, estimating extent of burn injuries, 463
complications of surgical cricothyroidotomy, 461
cricothyroidotomy, 461
damage control resuscitation, 462–463
hemorrhage, classes of, 461
intracranial pressure, medical therapies used to decrease, 463
key features
of "hospital" phase of ATLS, 460
of "prehospital" phase of ATLS, 459
lethal triad, 462
pericardial tamponade
signs and symptoms of, 462
treatment, 462
primary survey of trauma patient, 460
rapid way to assess patient on arrival, 460
secondary survey, 460–461
shock, 461
types of, 461
suspect of inhalational injuries in burn situation, 463
tension pneumothorax, 462
traumatic brain injury, classifications of, 463
Trendelenburg position, 242, 249
affecting cardiovascular system, 250
affecting respiratory system, 250
Trismus, 147
Trisomy 21, children with, 298
2-finger-technique, 409
Tylenol metabolism, 268
Tympanomastoidectomy, 281
ETT, 283
facial nerve monitoring and anesthesia plan, 283
intraoperative considerations for, 282
LMA, 283
local anesthetic infiltration, importance of, 282
nitrous oxide, use of, 282–283
plan for emergence of anesthesia, 283–284
precautions regarding patient positioning, 282
preoperative assessment, 281
risks of general anesthesia, 281–282
role of PONV, 284
surgical microscope, use of, 282

U

Ultrasonography, effects on fetus, 398
Unfractionated heparin (UFH), 75, 323
U.S. Eye Injury Register, 278
Upper respiratory infections (URIs), 298
Urticarial transfusion reaction (UTR), 315
treatment of, 315
Uterine atony, 392
risk factors for, 392
Uterine rupture, risk factors for, 389
Uterotonics, 387

V

VACTERL (Vertebral anomalies, imperforate Anus, Congenital heart disease, TEF/EA, Renal anomalies, Limb anomalies), 435
Valsalva maneuver, 274
Valvular heart disease, 47, 257
anesthetic considerations in, 33
case, 33–36
grades for mitral regurgitation, 34*t*
grades of aortic stenosis, 34*t*
induction of anesthesia in patients with multiple pathologies, 35
Vancomycin, 278
Vanillylmandellic acid (VMA), 185
Varices, 203
Vasoactive hormone, 264
Vasodilators/inodilators, 25
Vasodilatory agents, 249
Vaso-occlusive crisis (VOC), 334
Vasopressin, 25
Vasopressor, 25, 259–260, 399
preterm labor
anesthesia increasing incidence of, 400
surgical procedure causing, 399
tocolytic agents to prevent, 400
Vasospasm, 106–107
predictors of, 107
treatment, 107–108
Vecuronium, 210, 397
Venous air embolism (VAE), 100–101, 138–139
Venous thromboembolism (VTE), 344
Venovenous bypass (VVB), 211
Ventricular arrhythmias, 69
Ventricular fibrillation (VF), 25
Ventricular septal defect (VSD), 444
Ventricular tachycardia (VT), 25
Verapamil, 107–108/

Veress needle, 251
Video assisted thoracoscopic surgery (VATS), 90
Viral hepatitis, 201–202
  risks of surgery, 202
Viridans streptococci, 47
Volatiles anesthetics, 159
Volume expansion fluids in newborn, 410
Volume resuscitation, 418, 419
Von Willebrand disease (vWD), 319, 324, 327
V/Q matching, 91
V/Q ratio, 91
VVI® pacing, 57

W
Warfarin, 275
Wedged hepatic venous pressure (WHVP), 203
Weight loss
  preoperative concerns, 241
  surgical procedures, 239
Whipple's triad, 451
Wilson disease, 202
World Federation of Neurological Surgeon's Grading System (WFNS), 104

X
X-linked recessive pattern of inheritance, 325, 327